The Jing Luo

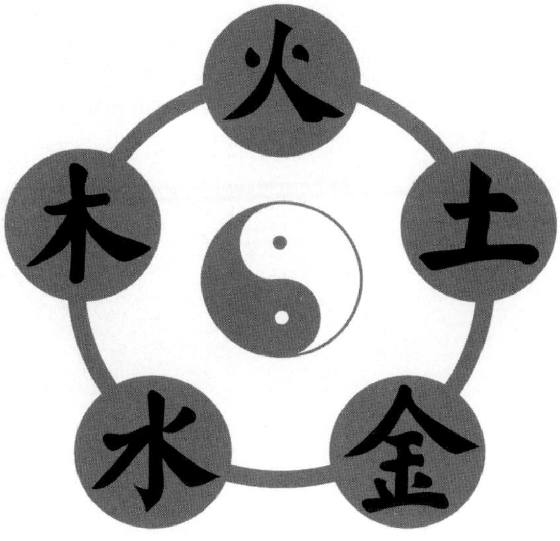

The Jing Luo

The Definitive Guide to Point Location

Edited by

Dean Lander Ac. M.; M.B.Ac.C.

The College of Traditional Acupuncture
Haseley Manor
Hatton
Warwick

Published by **The College of Traditional Acupuncture**

First Published April 2006

General Editor. Julian Morris,

ISBN Nos. 978-1-873272-01-5

Printed in Great Britain by Warwick Printing Company Ltd.

FOREWORD

It gives me great pleasure to introduce *The Jing Luo*. This textbook marks the culmination of over 10 years of investigation and research, carried out by College staff, into the entire area of point location in modern acupuncture practice. The College is greatly indebted to Dean Lander, senior faculty member and editor of the *Jing Luo*, for his dedication and perseverance in seeing this project through to publication.

Traditional acupuncture is, today, a richly diverse field of study and practice. Accurate point location is essential for effective practice, and the variety of descriptions, locations, and maps available to us can appear bewildering for practitioners and students alike. Many of these have been handed down to us as fixed, inflexible "traditions", with little apparent attempt made to research the evidence for what is taught or to place the tradition in the wider context of practice around the world.

The College has a longstanding commitment to critical enquiry and reflective practice as tools for personal and professional development. This led us, years ago, to initiate a search for the roots of our own tradition, with a willingness to critically examine any evidence that would support, or contradict, the point location model we had inherited. This exploration yielded an enormous amount of information about the diverse streams of knowledge and experience that informed our own, and also many other, approaches to the art of point location. The results of this wide-ranging enquiry can be found here.

We view this process as an ongoing initiative aimed at supporting continuous refinement of point location skills. In addition, it may further a deepening appreciation of the variety of approaches that co-exist under the banner of traditional acupuncture. I hope that this textbook will provide not just a valuable resource for study and practice, but will also inspire others to take a similar journey in relation to their own particular approach to acupuncture theory and practice.

"Let One Hundred Schools of Thought Contend".

Ken Shifrin, M.Ac., FBAcC

College Dean

March 2006

ACKNOWLEDGEMENTS

This project would not have been possible without the vision and commitment of the Acupuncture Master and teacher, J.R. Worsley, who developed the tradition of Five Element Acupuncture and inspired so many of us to learn this wonderful approach to practice.

The roots of the College's point location tradition are based on J.R. Worsley's publication in 1982 of "Traditional Chinese Acupuncture – Volume 1 – Meridians and Points". In the early 1990s, Allegra Wint carried out original research into the traditions of point location and inspired the College faculty to investigate further.

The faculty undertook a comprehensive critical review, coordinated by Niki Bilton, of the sources of this point location tradition, and also the anatomical descriptions and guidelines. In this latter respect, particular thanks go to Lezli Lawrence and Paula Dunleavy. Thanks also to Sue Kingston for her preparatory work on the deep pathways.

The outcome of this review, in which a number of alterations were made to the tradition we inherited, was published in 1996 as The Jing Luo, a point location handbook for College students. This has been updated several times since. Lois Francis-Metford and Tim Metford produced a very helpful series of illustrations to accompany the Jing Luo.

Thanks are also due to numerous individuals for their extensive clinical knowledge in the development of this book. Particular acknowledgement is given to Celia Tudor-Evans for her diligent research of needle depths and moxa use; to Zita West for her advice on forbidden points in pregnancy; to Gill Kelsey and Linda Winstanley for their comprehensive proofreading skills; to Julian Morris, the College's Chief Executive Officer, who made the completion of this book possible, and was also the photographer for the book; and to Jo Radley for her time and patience in assisting with the selection, cutting, cropping and labelling of the photographs.

Finally I would like to thank College staff, friends and family for their support and patience over the years whilst I researched and edited this textbook.

Dean Lander Ac. M., M.B.Ac.C.

March 2006

College of Traditional Acupuncture

INTRODUCTION

The purpose of this textbook is primarily to assist both students and experienced practitioners of acupuncture to locate acupuncture points. As practitioners, we tend to have a repertoire of favoured points, often developed through familiarity because we know how to locate them. There may also be points we avoid using simply because we are unsure of their location. A patient's condition may fail to improve, or progress may be unnecessarily slow, simply because we decided to use familiar points rather than those that might have suited the patient better.

Throughout the history of acupuncture medical texts, some point locations have been agreed unaminously, while others have differed widely. This has arisen from the divergent styles of acupuncture practised in different regions, the ability of individual masters of acupuncture to access the qi in their own particular ways, and occasional mistranslations of original texts.

There are many traditions of acupuncture around the world, and these often include particular models of point location. The fact that certain locations differ between various traditions does not imply that they are mutually exclusive. Each point has particular uses, depending upon context, practice style, and the intention of the practitioner when treating. Differences in point location may therefore be seen as adding to the rich diversity of practice.

This textbook is designed to promote research into the different locations for the same point. There are notes after many of the "tips" sections indicating alternative descriptions to that described in the main "location" section. It should also be borne in mind that "new" locations are being discovered regularly across the globe. The locations described in this textbook do not imply any denigration of other traditions, or other point locations, many of which may be valid doorways to the qi.

After gaining an acupuncture qualification, practitioners are advised to continue to practice point location, particularly of infrequently used points, thus expanding their repertoire. This textbook is designed to provide a guide, using clear step by step tips, to accurately locate all the main channel points on the body.

Accurate point location requires sound knowledge of surface anatomy, finger tip sensitivity and good palpation techniques. The locations and tips (including the cun measurements) are designed as guides to assist in locating the point. Note that cun measurements are a proportional measurement, but it is palpation that provides the highest degree of accuracy.

CONTENTS

Notes on using the Jing Luo		**xii**
Point Location Terminology (including needle depth and Moxa use)		**xvi**
Source Books / References		**xxv**
Acupuncture Texts		**xxv**
Anatomy Texts		**xxvi**
Chapter 1	**Lung Channel**	**1**
Chapter 2	**Large Intestine Channel**	**23**
Chapter 3	**Stomach Channel**	**57**
Chapter 4	**Spleen Channel**	**140**
Chapter 5	**Heart Channel**	**183**
Chapter 6	**Small Intestine Channel**	**195**
Chapter 7	**Bladder Channel**	**224**
Chapter 8	**Kidney Channel**	**337**
Chapter 9	**Pericardium Channel**	**395**
Chapter 10	**Triple Heater Channel**	**409**
Chapter 11	**Gall Bladder Channel**	**437**
Chapter 12	**Liver Channel**	**524**
Chapter 13	**Ren Mai** *(an Extraordinary vessel)*	**558**
Chapter 14	**Du Mai** *(an Extraordinary vessel)*	**600**
Chapter 15	**Extraordinary Vessels:**	**655**
	Chong Mai	655
	Dai Mai	663
	Yin Qiao Mai	664
	Yang Qiao Mai	666
	Yin Wei Mai	673
	Yang Wei Mai	677
	Du Mai	680
	Ren Mai	687
Chapter 16	**Extra Points**	**689**

NOTES ON USING THE JING LUO:

The introduction gives details of the terminology adopted by the College of Traditional Acupuncture, how the channels are described, and cites the textual sources used.

The channels are presented in sequence from Lung to Liver. Each section begins with a detailed description of the energetic channels. The points are listed in numerical order with their precise anatomical location.

This is followed by the channels and points of the Ren Mai and Du Mai and a brief description of other Extraordinary Vessels and a selection of commonly used Extra points.

Throughout the book the nomeneclature of the channels is consistent with that given in the introduction (Lu, LI, St etc). For ease of reading through the point sections, however, all nomenclature has been capitalised when introducing a point and when put in to bold type.

Within the profession acupuncture groups of points are known to have a particular use but may have different names. This has been reflected throughout the book by giving a comprehensive list associated with a given group of points, for example, Alarm Points are also known as Front Mu, Front Collecting or Herald Points.

The Acupuncture Channels (or meridians) form a net over the whole body, linking the individual components (both Anatomical structures and Energetic aspects), and creating a unified whole.

The main channels (*jing)* are generally vertical channels, which run through deep tissue, and connect the peripheral limbs with the internal organs (the *zangfu).*

The collateral channels (*luo)* are generally horizontal channels, which run over superficial surfaces of the body, and connect the primary channels, connective tissues, and cutaneous regions.

The main channels include:	the 12 primary channels the 12 divergent channels the 8 extraordinary vessels
The collateral channels include:	the 15 great connecting channels the minute connecting channels the superficial connecting channels the blood connecting channels

The 12 primary channels

- are the most important channels, housing the Acupuncture points
- nourish the body with Qi and blood in health
- show pathological signs and symptoms in distress

◇ 3 yin channels of the hand:	lesser yin	Heart (Ht)
	greater yin	Lung (Lu)
	absolute yin	Pericardium (Pc)
◇ 3 yang channels of the hand:	lesser yang	Triple Heater (TH)
	yang brightness	Large Intestine (LI)
	greater yang	Small Intestine (SI)
◇ 3 yin channels of the foot:	lesser yin	Kidney (Ki)
	greater yin	Spleen (Sp)
	absolute yin	Liver (Liv)
◇ 3 yang channels of the foot:	lesser yang	Gall Bladder (GB)
	yang brightness	Stomach (St)
	greater yang	Bladder (Bl)

The 12 divergent channels

- are vertical branches of the primary channels

- link the yin channels/organs internally with their paired yang channels and organs :

- Lu/LI
  Sp/St
  Ht/SI
  Ki/Bl
  Pc/TH
  Liv/GB

  link physiologically-related channels/organs (e.g. Ki to Ht, Ht to St)

NOTES ON USING THE JING LUO

The 8 Extraordinary vessels

- have their own channels (which can be vertical or horizontal)
- utilise points from the primary channels rather than having their own, apart from the Ren Mai and Du Mai
- branch out from the primary channels
- connect different primary channels
- regulate the primary channels (draining and storing Qi and blood when the primary channels are in excess, supplying Qi and blood when the primary channels are deficient)

    - ◇ Du Mai (Governing Vessel)
    - ◇ Ren Mai (Conception/Directing Vessel)
    - ◇ Chong Mai (Penetrating Vessel)
    - ◇ Dai Mai (Girdle Vessel)
    - ◇ Yin Qiao Mai (Yin Heel Vessel/Yin Motility Vessel)
    - ◇ Yang Qiao Mai (Yang Heel Vessel/Yang Motility Vessel)
    - ◇ Yin Wei Mai (Yin Linking Vessel)
    - ◇ Yang Wei Mai (Yang Linking Vessel)

The 15 great connecting channels

- connect the paired yin and yang primary channels, but on the extremities
- supervise all the lesser connecting channels

    - ◇ 12 branch out from the primary channels
    - ◇ 2 branch out from two of the extraordinary vessels (Ren/Du)
    - ◇ the last is the Great Connecting Channel of the Spleen

The minute connecting/superficial connecting/blood connecting channels

- are tiny vessels on or near the surface of the body
- distribute Qi and blood to areas not directly crossed by other channels
- branch out from the great connecting channels

The 12 muscle channels

- connect the 12 primary channels with connective tissues (muscles, tendons, ligaments) and cutaneous regions
- connect with other muscle channels
- extend and flex the muscles and joints, and move the limbs

The 12 cutaneous regions

- are 12 areas of the surface of the body/skin
- lie superficial to the related connecting channels/primary channels
- rely on Protective Qi throughout the superficial tissues to ward off External Pathogenic factors of disease

Note: Acupuncture points mainly lie on the 12 primary channels and the Ren and Du Mai (of the 8 Extraordinary Vessels). There are, however, two other groups of points:

- Extra or Master points (which lie off the primary channels)
- Ahshi points (points of tenderness/pain on palpation, off the channels)

Point Location Terminology:

Cun A unit of Acupuncture Measurement (also referred to as an Anatomical Chinese Inch/ACI)

The 12 Primary channels:

The Lung Channel of the Hand (Tai Yin)	Lu	IX
The Large Intestine Channel of the Hand (Yang Ming)	LI	X
The Stomach Channel of the Foot (Yang Ming)	St	XI
The Spleen Channel of the Foot (Tai Yin)	Sp	XII
The Heart Channel of the Hand (Shao Yin)	Ht	I
The Small Intestine Channel of the Hand (Tai Yang)	SI	II
The Bladder Channel of the Foot (Tai Yang)	Bl	III
The Kidney Channel of the Foot (Shao Yin)	Ki	IV
The Pericardium Channel of the Hand (Jue Yin)	Pc	V
(The Heart Protector or Circulation/Sex or Heart Constrictor)		
The Triple Heater Channel of the Hand (Shao Yang)	TH	VI
The Gallbladder Channel of the Foot (Shao Yang)	GB	VII
The Liver Channel of the Foot (Jue Yin)	Liv	VIII

Note: There is no standard nomenclature for the channels and points! The WHO nomenclature has not been universally accepted, and readers of Acupuncture texts will come across a range of historical, regional and individual variations. The use of Roman numerals for the channels, however, can only be found in very few Western books, such as *Meridians and Points* by J.R.Worsley, and *Acupuncture Handbook* by D.and J.Lawson-Wood, where in fact this nomenclature is attributed to Dr.Roger de la Fuye.

The 8 Extraordinary Vessels:

The Conception Vessel	Ren Mai
The Governor Vessel	Du Mai
The Penetrating Vessel	Chong Mai
The Girdle Vessel	Dai Mai
The Yin Heel Vessel/Yin Motility Vessel	Yin Qiao Mai
The Yang Heel Vessel/Yang Motility Vessel	Yang Qiao Mai
The Yin Linking Vessel	Yin Wei Mai
The Yang Linking Vessel	Yang Wei Mai

Specific Points:

- Source Points (Yuan/Regulator/Primary)
- Tonification (Reinforcing)
- Sedation (Dispersing/Reducing)
- Junction Points (Luo/Connecting/Passage/Lo/Lê)
- Accumulation Points (Xi Cleft/Gueki)
- Entry Points
- Exit Points
- Wood Points
- Fire Points
- Earth Points
- Metal Points
- Water Points
- Horary Points
- Seasonal Horary Points
- Back Shu Points (Associated Effect Points/AEP's/Shu Transporting /Approval/Vesical Reinforcement)
- A.E. (Aggressive Energy Points)
- 7 Internal Dragon Points (I.D's)
- 7 External Dragon Points (E.D's)
- Window of the Sky Points (Window of Heaven)
- Mother Points
- Child Points
- Alarm Points (Front Collecting/Front Mu/Herald)
- The 5 Shu Points/Shu – Transporting/Antique
  - Jing-Well Points
  - Ying-Spring Points
  - Shu-Stream Points
  - Jing-River Points
  - He-Sea Points
- The 8 Extraordinary Channels Confluent Points (8 Extraordinary Meridians Confluent/8 Extraordinary Vessels Opening/Master)
- 8 Extraordinary Vessel Coalescent Points
- 8 Extraordinary Vessel Coupled Points
- The Reunion Points (Crossing/Meeting)
- The 8 Influential Points (Hui-Meeting/Gathering/Assembling)
- Greater Influential Points (Greater Gathering/Greater Assembling)
- Cousin Points
- Original Points
- Host/Guest Points
- Sea of Qi Points
- Sea of Nourishment Points (Sea of Waters and Grains)
- Sea of Blood Points

- Sea of Marrow Points
- Hua Tuo Points (M-BW-35) (Hua Tuo Jia Ji/Hua Tuo Back-Filling Points)
- Ahshi Points
- Ma Dan-Yang's Twelve Heavenly Star Points
- Sun Si-Miao Ghost (Gui) Points (13 Points)

Details of Specific Points:

12 Source (Yuan/Regulator/Primary) Points:

Lu 9, LI 4, St 42, Sp 3, Ht 7, SI 4,
Bl 64, Ki 3, Pc 7, TH 4, GB 40, Liv 3.

12 Tonification (Reinforcing) Points:

Lu 9, LI 11, St 41, Sp 2, Ht 9, SI 3, Bl 67, Ki 7,
Pc 9, TH 3, GB 43, Liv 8

12 Sedation (Dispersing/Reducing) Points:

Lu 5, LI 2, St 45, Sp 5, Ht 7, SI 8, Bl 65, Ki 1,
Pc 7, TH 10, GB 38, Liv 2

15 Junction (Luo/Connecting/Passage/Lo/Lê) Points:

Lu 7, LI 6, St 40, Sp 4, Ht 5, SI 7, Bl 58, Ki 4,
Pc 6, TH 5, GB 37, Liv 5, Ren 15, Du 1, Sp 21.

16 Accumulation (Xi Cleft/Gueki) Points:

Lu 6, LI 7, St 34, Sp 8, Ht 6, SI 6, Bl 63, Ki 5
Pc 4, TH 7, GB 36, Liv 6
Bl 59 (Yang Motility Vessel/Yang Heel
Vessel/Yang Qiao Mai),
Ki 8 (Yin Motility Vessel/Yin Heel Vessel/Yin Qiao Mai) .
Ki 9 (Yin Linking Vessel/Yin Wei Mai),
GB 35 (Yang Linking Vessel/Yang Wei Mai)

6 A. E. (Aggressive Energy) Points – Yin Officials Only (Needle Depth is 0.1 Cun):

Bl 13 (Lu), Bl 14 (Pc), Bl 15 (Ht), Bl 18 (Liv),
Bl 20 (Sp), Bl 23 (Ki)

Back Shu (Associated Effect Points/A.E.P's/Shu Transporting/Approval /Vesical Reinforcement) Points of the 12 Officials:

(Lu) Bl 13, (LI) Bl 25, (St) Bl 21, (Sp) Bl 20,
(Ht) Bl 15, (SI) Bl 27, (Bl) Bl 28, (Ki) Bl 23,
(Pc) Bl 14, (TH) Bl 22, (GB) Bl 19, (Liv) Bl 18.

12 Horary Points:

Lu 8 (3 am – 5 am); LI 1 (5 am – 7 am)
St 36 (7 am – 9 am); Sp 3 (9 am – 11 am)
Ht 8 (11 am – 1 pm); SI 5 (1 pm – 3 pm)
Bl 66 (3 pm – 5 pm); Ki 10 (5 pm – 7 pm)
Pc 8 (7 pm – 9 pm); TH 6 (9 pm – 11 pm)
GB 41 (11 pm – 1 am); Liv 1 (1 am – 3 am)

12 Seasonal Horary Points:

GB 41 & Liv 1: SPRING
SI 5 & Ht 8: SUMMER
TH 6 & Pc 8: SUMMER
St 36 & Sp 3: LATE SUMMER
LI 1 & Lu 8: AUTUMN/FALL
Bl 66 & Ki 10: WINTER

14 Entry Points:

Lu 1, LI 4, St 1, Sp 1, Ht 1, SI 1, Bl 1, Ki 1,
Pc 1, TH 1, GB 1, Liv 1, Ren 1, Du 1

14 Exit Points:

Lu 7, LI 20, St 42, Sp 21, Ht 9, SI 19, Bl 67,
Ki 22, Pc 8, TH 22, GB 41, Liv 14, Ren 24, Du 28

Fire Points:

Lu 10, LI 5, St 41, Sp 2, Ht 8, SI 5, Bl 60, Ki 2,
Pc 8, TH 6, GB 38, Liv 2

Earth Points:

Lu 9, LI 11, St 36, Sp 3, Ht 7, SI 8, Bl 40, Ki 3,
Pc 7, TH 10, GB 34, Liv 3

NOTES ON USING THE JING LUO

Metal Points:

Lu 8, LI 1, St 45, Sp 5, Ht 4, SI 1, Bl 67, Ki 7,
Pc 5, TH 1, GB 44, Liv 4

Water Points:

Lu 5, LI 2, St 44, Sp 9, Ht 3, SI 2, Bl 66, Ki 10,
Pc 3, TH 2, GB 43, Liv 8

Wood Points:

Lu 11, LI 3, St 43, Sp 1, Ht 9, SI 3, Bl 65, Ki 1,
Pc 9, TH 3, GB 41, Liv 1

Alarm (Front Collecting/Front Mu/Herald) Points:

(Lu) Lu 1; (LI) St 25; (St) Ren 12; (Sp) Liv 13; (Ht) Ren 14; (SI) Ren 4; (Bl) Ren 3; (Ki) GB 25; (Pc) Ren 17; (TH Main Alarm Pt) Ren 5; (TH Upper Jiao Alarm Pt) Ren 17; (TH Middle Jiao Pt) Ren 12; (TH Lower Jiao t) Ren 7; (GB) GB 24; (Liv) Liv 14.

Internal Dragon's (I.D's) Points – Without Depression – Commonly Used:

Ren 15 (Master Point), St 25, St 32, St 41

Internal Dragon's (I.D's) Points – With Depression: Rarely Used:

Ren 15 (Master Point), St 32, St 36.5 (M-LE-13), St 41

External Dragon's (E.D's) Points:

Du 20, Bl 11, Bl 23, Bl 61

Window of the Sky (Window of Heaven) Points:

Lu 3, LI 18, St 9, SI 16, SI 17, Bl 10,
Pc 1 (Male Only), Pc 2, TH 16, Ren 22, Du 16

The 5 Shu Points/Shu – Transporting/Antique:

12 Jing Well Points:

(6 Wood points on the Yin Channels)	Lu 11, Sp 1, Ht 9, Ki 1, Pc 9, Liv 1.
(6 Metal points on the Yang Channels)	LI 1, St 45, SI 1, Bl 67, TH 1, GB 44.

12 Yin Spring Points:

(6 Fire points on the Yin Channels)	Lu 10, Sp 2, Ht 8, Ki 2, Pc 8, Liv 2.
(6 Water points on the Yang Channels)	LI 2, St 44, SI 2, Bl 66, TH 2, GB 43.

12 Shu Stream Points:

(6 Earth points on the Yin Channels)	Lu 9, Sp 3, Ht 7, Ki 1, Pc 7, Liv 3.
(6 Wood points on the Yang Channels)	LI 3, St 43, SI 3, Bl 65, TH 3, GB 41.

12 Jing River Points:

(6 Metal points on the Yin Channels)	Lu 8, Sp 5, Ht 4, Ki 7, Pc 5, Liv 4.
(6 Fire points on the Yang Channels)	LI 5, St 41, SI 5, Bl 60, TH 6, GB 38.

12 He Sea Points:

(6 Water points on the Yin Channels)	Lu 5, Sp 9, Ht 3, Ki 10, Pc 3, Liv 8.
(6 Earth points on the Yang Channels)	LI 11, St 36, SI 8, Bl 54, TH 10, GB 34.

Mother Points:

Lu 9 (Earth), LI 11 (Earth), St 41 (Fire),
Sp 2 (Fire), Ht 9 (Wood), SI 3 (Wood),
Bl 67 (Metal), Ki 7 (Metal), Pc 9 (Wood),
TH 3 (Wood), GB 43 (Water), Liv 8 (Water)

Child Points:

Lu 5 (Water), LI 2 (Water), St 45 (Metal),
Sp 5 (Metal), Ht 7 (Earth), SI 8 (Earth),
Bl 65 (Wood), Ki 1 (Wood), Pc 7 (Earth),
TH 10 (Earth), GB 38 (Fire), Liv 2 (Fire)

He-Sea of Qi Points:

St 9, Bl 10 (or Du 14 & Du 15), Ren 17

He-Sea of Marrow Points:

Du 15, Du 16, Du 19, Du 20

He-Sea of Nourishment Points (Sea of Waters & Grains):

St 30, St 36

He-Sea of Blood Points:

Upper Body: Bl 11
Lower Body: St 37, St 39

Lower He-Sea Points:

St 37: (LI), St 36: (St), St 39: (SI), Bl 40: (Bl),
Bl 39 (TH), GB 34 (GB).

Re-Union (Crossing/Meeting) Points (Main Channels Only):

Pc 5: Three Yin (Arm) Channels: Pc, Ht & Lu (Hand Jue Yin, Hand Shao Yin and Hand Tai Yin Channels)
TH 8: Three Yang (Arm) Channels: TH, SI & LI (Hand Shao Yang, Hand Tai Yang and Hand Yang Ming Channels)
GB 39: Three Yang (Leg) Channels: GB, Bl & St (Foot Shao Yang, Foot Tai Yang and Foot Yang Ming Channels)
Sp 6: Three Yin (Leg) Channels: Sp, Ki & Liv (Foot Tai Yin, Foot Shao Yin and Foot Jue Yin Channels)
Liv 13: Yin Channels: Liv, Ht, Pc, Sp, Ki & Lu (Foot Jue Yin, Hand Shao Yin, Hand Jue Yin, Foot Tai Yin, Foot Shao Yin and Hand Tai Yin Channels)
Ren 12: Yang Channels: LI, St, SI, Bl, TH & GB (Conception/Directing Vessel with the Hand Yang Ming, Foot Yang Ming, Hand Tai Yang, Foot Tai Yang, Hand Shao Yang and Foot Shao Yang Channels
Du 14: Yang Channels: LI, St, SI, Bl, TH & GB (Conception/Directing Vessel with theHand Yang Ming, Foot Yang Ming, Hand Tai Yang, Foot Tai Yang, Hand Shao Yang and Foot Shao Yang Channels

8 Influential (Hui-Meeting/Gathering/Assembling) Points:

Lu 9: Blood Vessels/Channels (Meridians)
Bl 11: Bones
Bl 17: Blood
GB 34: Muscles and Tendons (Sinews)
GB 39: Marrow:
Liv 13: Zang Organs (Lu, Sp, Ht, Ki, Pc, Liv)
Ren 12: Fu Organs (LI, St, SI, Bl, TH, GB)
Ren 17: Qi

Greater Influential Points (Greater Gathering/Greater Assembling) Points:

LI 4: Face & Mouth
St 36: Stomach & Abdomen
SI 7: Head & Neck

8 Confluent Points:

Lu 7: (Ren Mai), SI 3: (Du Mai),
Sp 4: (Chong Mai), GB 41: (Dai Mai),
Ki 6: (Yin Qiao Mai), Bl 62: (Yang Qiao Mai),

Cousin Points:

LI 4 in association with St 36
St 34 in association with Bl 10
St 36 in association with LI 4
Sp 9 in association with GB 34
Bl 10 in association with St 34
GB 34 in association with Sp 9

Host/Guest Combination Points – Source Point Used with the Junction Point of It's Paired Official/Organ:

Lu 7 & LI 4; Lu 9 & LI 6; LI 4 & Lu 7;
LI 6 & Lu 9; St 40 & Sp 3; St 42 & Sp 4;
Sp 3 & St 40; Sp 4 & St 42; Ht 5 & SI 4;
Ht 7 & SI 7; SI 4 & Ht 5; SI 7 & Ht 7;
Bl 58 & Ki 3; Bl 64 & Ki 4; Ki 3 & Bl 58;
Ki 4 & Bl 64; Pc 6 & TH 4; Pc 7 & TH 5;
TH 4 & Pc 6; TH 5 & Pc 7; GB 37 & Liv 3;
GB 40 & Liv 5; Liv 3 & GB 37; Liv 5 & GB 40

5 Original Points (each of the 5 points are used for specific symptoms)

LI 4; St 42, SI 4, Bl 64, GB 40

13 Sun Si-Miao Ghost (Gui) Points:

Lu 11: Gui Xin – Ghost Faith
LI 11: Gui Tui – Ghost Leg, Ghost Minister
St 6: Gui Chuang – Ghost's Bed, Ghost Forest
Sp 1: Gui Lei – Ghost Fortress, Ghost Pile, Ghost Eye
Bl 62: Gui Lu – Ghost Path
Pc 5: Gui Cu – Ghost in the Cave, Ghost Road (Pc 8 is an alternative to Pc 5)
Pc 7: Gui Xin – Ghost Heart (Less Common is Lu 9 – Same Name)
Pc 8: Gui Cu – Ghost in the Cave (Pc 5 is an alternative to Pc 8)
Ren 1: Gui Cang – Ghost Store or Ghost's in the Hidden Place
Ren 24: Gui Shi – Ghost Market
Du 16: Gui Zhen – Ghost Pillow, Ghost Hole, Ghost Forest
Du 23: Gui Tang – Ghost Hall
Du 26: Gui Gong – Ghost Palace, Ghost Reception Room
M-HN-37: Gui Feng – Ghost Seal or Ghost's in the Enclosed Territory

12 Heavenly Star Points of Ma Dan-Yang:

Lu 7, LI 4, LI 11, St 36, St 44, Bl 40, Bl 57,
Bl 60, Ht 5, GB 34, GB 39, Liv 3

Needle Depth:

The needle insertion depths have been refererred as units of cun. In some texts the unit of "fen" or "pouce" have been used. 1 cun = 10 fen / 10 pouce, but remember that although a 1 inch needle = 1 cun or 10 fen or 10 pouce, most points have a maximum needle insertion depth of 0.1 to 0.3 cun which is 1 fen or 1 pouce to 3 fen or 3 pouce.

You need to be extremely cautious when inserting to a point of maximum insertion depth. Consideration of the person's size and shape is needed. eg. a point with a maximum needle depth of 0.5 cun or 5 fen may be less than half the length of the 1 inch needle on a slim person or may be slightly more if the person is overweight.

Needle depth figures are proportional measurements. Remember that the needle depths listed in this book and the accompanying chart are maximum depths. You may insert the needle and reach the depth of the point which is less than the maximum depth description in this book. The depths of the points are based on perpendicular insertion in to the body.

SOURCE BOOKS

ACUPUNCTURE TEXTS:

The Acupuncture texts listed below provided valuable insight into the history of the locations of points, and the differing contributions of individual Masters of Acupuncture.

Bertschinger, Richard. (1991). *The Golden Needle.* Edinburgh: Churchill Livingstone. ISBN: 0-443-04390-6.

Chaitow Leon (1976). *The Acupuncture Treatment of Pain.* Wellingborough: Thorsons Publishers. ISBN: 0-7225-0334-2.

Cheng Xinnong (Editor). *Chinese Acupuncture and Moxibustion.* (1987). Beijing: Foreign Language Press. ISBN: 0-8351-2109-7/7-119-00378-X.

Dale, Ralph Alan (1999), *Macro-Acupuncture Manual, The.* Florida: Dialectic Publishing Inc. ISBN: 1-877589-19-5

Deadman, Peter, Al-Khafaji, Mazin and Baker, Kevin. (1998). *A Manual of Acupuncture.* Hove: Journal of Chinese Medicine Publications. ISBN: 0-9510546-7-8.

Drs. Lo Chi Kwong and Tsui Sui King. (1979). *Acupuncture in Clinical Practice.* Hong Kong: The Commercial Press. ISBN: 962-07-3050-X.

Dr. Roger De la Fuye. (1956). *Traiteé d'Acupuncture* Publisher Unknown. No ISBN Number.

Dr. Wu Wei-P'ing. (1973). *Chinese Acupuncture.* Trans: Dr. J. Lavier (French), Philip Chancellor (English). Northampton: Health Science Press. ISBN: unknown.

Eachou Chen. (1995). *Cross-sectional Anatomy of Acupoints.* Edinburgh: Churchill Livingstone. ISBN: 0-443-04974-2.

Ellis, Wiseman and Boss. (1989). *Grasping the Wind.* Brookline, MA: Paradigm Publications. ISBN: 0-912111-19-4.

Henry C. Lu. (1973). *The Chinese Versions of Modern Acupuncture.* Vancouver: The Academy of Oriental Heritage. ISBN: unknown.

Hicks, Sara. (1985). *Catalogue of Acupuncture Point Translations.* Oxford: Sara Hicks. ISBN: unknown.

Huang-fu Mi. Trans: Yang Shou-zhong and Charles Chace (1993). *The Systematic Classic of Acupuncture & Moxibustion – A Translation of the Jia Yi Jing.* Boulder, CO: Blue Poppy Press. ISBN: 0-936185-29-5.

James Tin Yau So (Dr). (1985). *The Book of Acupuncture Points.* Brookline, MA: Paradigm Publications. ISBN: 0-912111-02-X.

Jayasuriya Anton. (1982). *Clinical Acupuncture.* Sri Lanka: Asia printers. ISBN: unknown.

Katsusuke Serizawa. (1983). *Tsubo – Vital Points for Oriental Therapy.* Japan Publications, Inc.. ISBN: 0-87040-350-8

Lavier, J (Dr). (1974). *Points of Chinese Acupuncture.* Trans: P. M. Chancellor. Northampton: Health Science Press. ISBN: unknown.

Lawson-Wood, Denis. (1973). *Acupuncture Handbook.* Whitstable: Straker Brothers Ltd. ISBN: 0-85032-105-0.

Legge, David. (1997). *Close to the Bone.* Woy Woy, New South Wales. Sydney College Press. ISBN: 0-7316-9117-2.

Legge, David. (1999). *Acupuncture Points and Meridians.* Sydney College Press. ISBN: 0-9577392-0-6

Li Ding (Prof.). (1991). *Acupuncture, Meridian Theory and Acupuncture Points.* Beijing: Foreign Languages Press. ISBN:0-8351-2221-2

Lotan, Alon. (2000). *Acupoint Location Guide.* Israel: Etsem Publications. ISBN:965-222-735-8.

Low, Royston. (1988) *The Non-Meridial Points of Acupuncture.* Wellingborough: Thorsons Publishers Ltd. ISBN: 0-7225-1483-2.

Maciocia, Giovanni. (1995). *The Foundations of Chinese Medicine.* Edinburgh: Churchill Livingston. ISBN: 0-443-03980-1.

Mann, Felix (1962). *Acupuncture*. Birkenhead: Willmer Brothers and Haram Ltd. ISBN: unknown.

Masayoshi Hyodo, MD. (1975). *Ryodoraku Treatment.* Osaka, Japan: Japan Ryodoraku, Autonomic Nerve Society. ISBN: unknown.

Matsumoto, Kiiko and Birch, Stephen. (1986). *Extraordinary Vessels.* Massachusetts: Paradigm Publications. ISBN: 0-912111-35-6.

Professor Yang Jiasan (Editor) (1982) *The Way to Locate Acu-Points..* Beijing: Foreign Language Press. ISBN: unknown.

Qiu Mao-liang. (1993/1996). *Chinese Acupuncture and Moxibustion.* Edinburgh: Churchill Livingstone. ISBN: 0-443-04223-3.

Shandong Medical College and Shandong College of Traditional Chinese Medicine (1982) *Anatomical Atlas of Chinese Acupuncture Points..* Jinan: Shandong Science and Technology Press. ISBN: unknown.

Shanghai College of Traditional Medicine. (1981). *Acupuncture (A Comprehensive Text).* Trans: John O'Connor and Dan Bensky. Washington: Eastland Press. ISBN: 0-939616-00-9.

Shanghai College of Traditional Chinese Medicine. (1993). *Applied Anatomical Charts of Acupuncture and Moxibustion.* Shanghai: Publishing House of Shanghai College of Traditional Chinese Medicine. ISBN:7-81010-209-5

Soulie De Morant, George. *Chinese Acupuncture.* Trans: (1994). Brookline: Paradigm Publications. ISBN: 0-9121111-31-3.

The Academy of Traditional Chinese Medicine. (1975). *An Outline of Chinese Acupuncture*. Peking: Foreign Languages Press. ISBN: unknown.

The Location of Acupoints. (1990). Beijing: Foreign Languages Press. ISBN: 0-8351-2749-4 /7-119-01368-8.

Therapy). Trans: Stephen Brown. Washington: Eastland Press. ISBN: 0-939616-11-4.

Voisin, H (Dr) (1974). *Essentials of Acupuncture.* Quebec: Edisem Inc. ISBN: unknown.

West, Zita. (2001). *Acupuncture in Pregnancy and Childbirth.* Edinburgh: Churchill Livingston. ISBN: 0-443-06138-6

Worsley, J.R.. (1975). *Acupuncturists' Therapeutic Pocket Book. "The Little Black Book".* Columbia, Maryland: The Centre for Traditional Acupuncture, Inc. ISBN: unknown.

Worsley, J.R. (1982). *Traditional Chinese Acupuncture (Volume I Meridians and Points).* Wiltshire: Element Books. ISBN: 0-906540-03-8.

Woollerton, Henry and McLean, Colleen J. (1979). *Acupuncture Energy in Health and Disease.* Wellingborough: Thorsons Publishers Ltd. ISBN: 0-7225-0482-9.

Y. Nakatari and K. Yamashita. (1977). *Ryodoraku Acupuncture.* Tokyo: Ryodoraku Research Institute. ISBN: unknown.

Yoshiaki Omura. (1982). *Acupuncture Medicine*. Tokyo: Japan Publications Inc. ISBN: 0-87040-491-1.

ANATOMY TEXTS:

The following texts provided useful references in revising the anatomical descriptions:

Barbara Bates. (1974). *A Guide to Physical Examination*. London: Blackwell Scientific Publications. ISBN: 0-397-54151-1.

Dorland's Illustrated Medical Dictionary. (1974). Philadelphia: W. B. Saunders. ISBN: 0-7216-3148-7.

Elaine N. Marieb. (1992). *Human Anatomy and Physiology.* California: Benjamin/ Cummings Publishing Co. Inc. ISBN: 0-8053-4120-X.

Gary A. Thibodeau/Kevin T. Patton. (1992). *The Human Body in Health and Disease*. Missouri: Mosby Year Book. ISBN: 0-8016-6412-8.

Gray's Anatomy. (1973). Norwich: Longmans. ISBN: 0-443-01011-0.

Hogin McMurtrie, James Krall Rikel. (1991). *The Coloring Review Guide to Human Anatomy.* Dubuque, USA: W.C. Brown Publishers. ISBN: 0-697-03150-0.

John S. P. Lumley. (1990). *Surface Anatomy*. Edinburgh: Churchill Livingstone. ISBN: 0-443-04084-2.

Manchester University Department of Anatomy. (1985). *Atlas of Human Anatomy*. London: Gower Medical Publishing. ISBN: 0-906923-27-1.

McMinn and Hutchings. (1977). *A Colour Atlas of Human Anatomy*. London: Wolfe Medical Publications. ISBN: 0-7234-0709-6.

Pamela MacKinnon and John Morris. (1986). *Oxford Textbook of Functional Anatomy*. Oxford:Oxford University Press. ISBN: 0-19-2615173.

Stanley Hoppenfeld. (1976). *Physical Examination of the Spine and Extremities*. Connecticut: Appleton-Century-Crofts. ISBN: 0-8385-7853-5.

Wynn Kapit/Lawrence M. Elson. (1977). *The Anatomy Coloring Book*. New York: Harper and Row. ISBN: 0-06-453914-8.

THE LUNG CHANNEL OF THE HAND (TAI YIN)

Primary Channel

The Lung channel originates in the middle jiao, (around Ren 12). The channel descends behind the transverse colon, then in the region of Ren 9 loops back round the colon and travels through the upper (cardiac) orifice of the stomach. It joins the anterior median line (at Ren 13) to pass through the diaphragm. Continuing upwards it branches into the lungs, rejoining the median line at the trachea. It passes through the trachea and larynx, finally going transversely to the inferior border of the clavicle and from there to Lu 1, where the channel becomes superficial.

The channel arches up over the clavicle and axilla, descends the anterior aspect of the upper arm (lateral to the biceps brachii muscle) to the cubital fossa, then runs down the forearm to the wrist. Passing the thenar eminence it ends on the radial aspect of the thumb at Lu 11. A branch emerges from Lu 7 and runs directly to the radial side of the tip of the second digit, where it meets LI 1.

Divergent Channel

This leaves the primary channel at the axilla, travels anterior to the Pericardium channel into the chest where it connects with the lung, and then disperses in the large intestine. A branch rises from the lung to emerge at the clavicle (St 12), then ascends the throat to join with the Large Intestine channel.

Connecting Channel

Leaving the primary channel at Lu 7, this travels to the Large Intestine channel. Another branch follows the Lung channel to the palm of the hand, then spreads through the thenar eminence.

Muscle Channel

This begins on the thumb, binds with the thenar eminence, and crosses the wrist at the radial artery. It passes up the forearm to bind with the elbow, then continues up the medial aspect of the arm and enters the chest below the axilla. It reemerges at St 12, binding at the lateral aspect of the shoulder (LI 15). It binds at the clavicle and descends the chest to bind with the lungs, spreading over the diaphragm and converging again at the 12th rib.

THE LUNG CHANNEL OF THE HAND

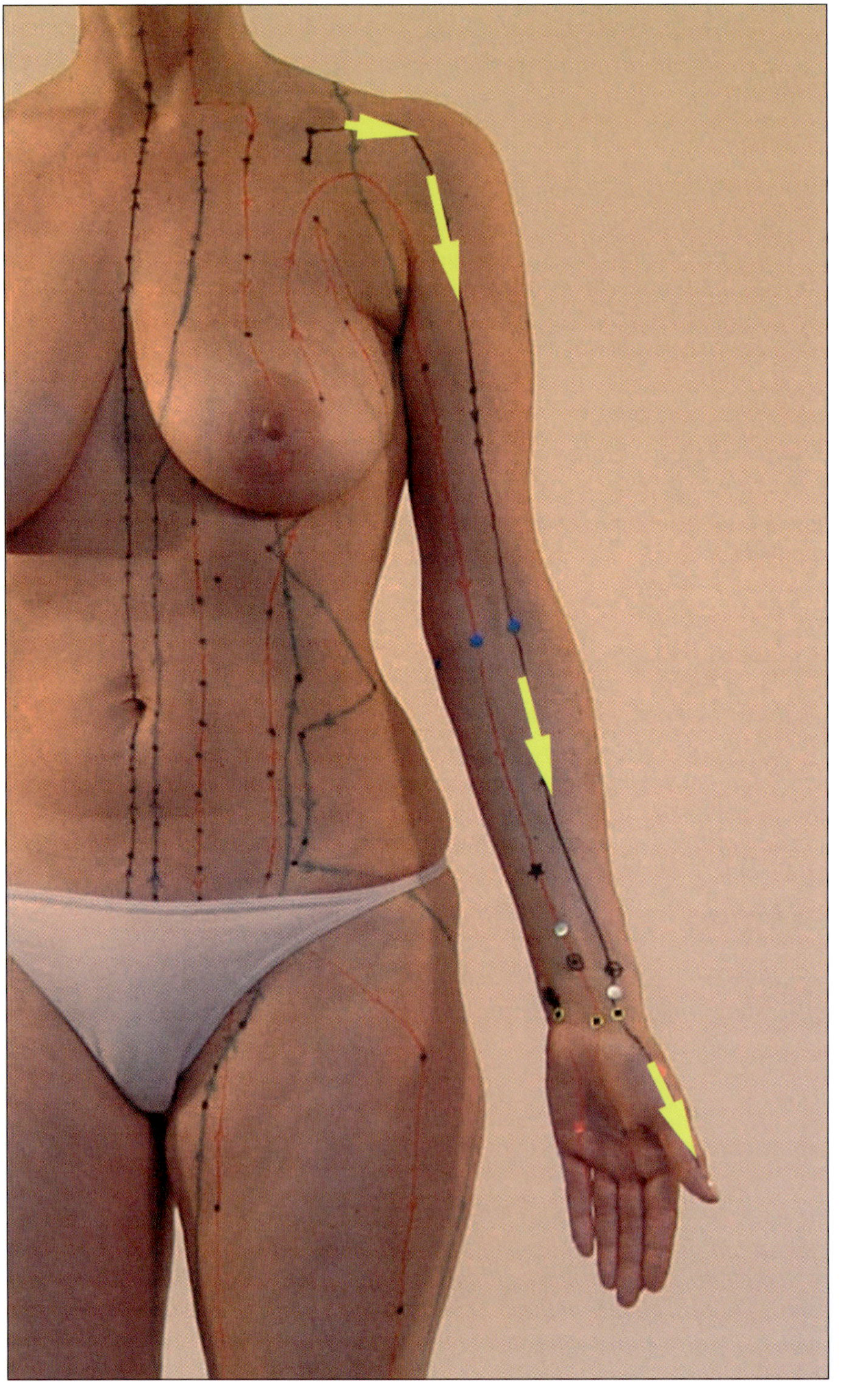

Points of the Lung Channel – Hand Tai Yin (Lu/LU/L/IX)

Lu 1 and Lu 2 are on the chest.

Lu 1 ZHONG FU – MIDDLE PALACE

⊥ ***0.3 TO 0.5 CUN (SEATED) 0.5 CUN (SUPINE)*** △ ***5 TO 10***

- ENTRY
- ALARM/Front Collecting/Front Mu/Herald Point of Lung
- RE-UNION/Crossing/Meeting Point of the Lung Channel with the Liver and Spleen Channels – Hand Tai Yin Channel with the Foot Jue Yin, and Foot Tai Yin Channels.

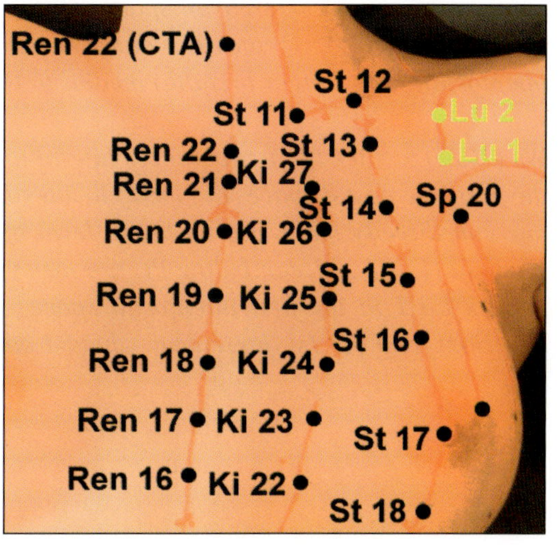

Pos: Position of patient: supine or seated.

Loc:
a) On the anterior torso.
b) On the chest (in the upper jiao).
c) On a level with the 1st intercostal space.
d) 6 cun lateral to the anterior median line.
e) 1 to 1.6 cun inferior to Lu 2.
f) In the pectoralis major muscle.

Tip:
a) To measure 6 cun lateral to the anterior median line (Ren channel) locate Lu 2.
b) Draw a vertical line inferior from Lu 2. Lu 1 is usually directly inferior to Lu 2. If there is a lot of breast tissue the arm will not necessarily be against the body. Therefore Lu 1 will be inferior and slightly lateral to Lu 2.
c) If there is a lot of breast tissue, it may be easier to have the patient in a seated position.
d) Using the flat part of the finger run along the 1st intercostal space from the sternal end to the drawn vertical line.
e) The distance between Lu 1 and Lu 2 is approximately the width of one intercostal space.
f) Ensure that the arm is against the body in the anatomical position when needling Lu 1.
g) Gently palpating the *men* (depression) prior to needling helps engage the Qi.

Note: Traditionally the distance between Lu 1 and Lu 2 has been given as 1 or 1.6 cun, indicating the width of the intercostal space. 1 cun is the current description for the upper intercostal spaces. Worsley (1982) locates IX 1 on the chest, on a level with the space between the first and second ribs, 1.6 ACI (Anatomical Chinese Inch) inferior to IX 2. Deadman (1998) locates LU 1 at 1 cun inferior to LU 2. Shanghai (1981) locates L1 at 1 unit below the lateral end of the clavicle in the lateral part of the first intercostal space.

Soulié (1994) locates LU 1 on the anterior upper shoulder at the level of the medial crease; at the inferior point of the projection of the coracoid process; in the angle of the superior edge of the second rib (the first under the clavicle) and of the medial superior edge of the tendon of the pectoralis minor, inserted on the coracoid process; in a hollow; three finger-widths below and medial to LU 2; three FW (Finger Width) medial and inferior to LI 15; three FW lateral to ST 14. Huang (1993) locates Lu 1 at 1 cun below Cloud Gate (Lu 2), in a depression in the breast above the third rib where a pulsating vessel is palpable. Masayoshi (1975) locates the point in the second intercostal space; So (1985) locates LU 1 between the second and third ribs. Voisin (1974), locates L 1 at the second rib, lower border (in the illustration – second intercostal), 2 fb (finger breadth) medial to the anterior axillary line.

Wu (1973) locates LU 1 two pouces lateral to the nipple and four pouces eight fen above it, in the first intercostal space. Li (1991) locates LU 1 at the level of the 3rd rib above the nipple, one cun directly below LU 2, at the level of the intercostal space. Shandong (1982) locate Zhongfu (Lu 1) at 1 cun below Pt. Yun men (Lu 2), in the 1st intercostal space. Legge (1999) locates Lu 1 in the first intercostal space, 1 cun inferior to Lu 2 and the tip of the (and superior) from the 1st intercostal; about 1 cun inferior (and lateral) to Lu 2.

Lu 2 YUN MEN – CLOUD GATE

⊥ ***0.3 TO 0.5 CUN (SEATED) 0.5 CUN (SUPINE)*** Δ ***5 TO 10***

Pos: Position of patient: supine or seated.

Loc: a) On the anterior torso.
b) On the chest (in the upper jiao).
c) Inferior to the acromial extremity of the clavicle in the infraclavicular fossa.
d) Between the upper border of the pectoralis major muscle and the anterior border of the deltoid muscle.
e) 6 cun lateral to the anterior median line.

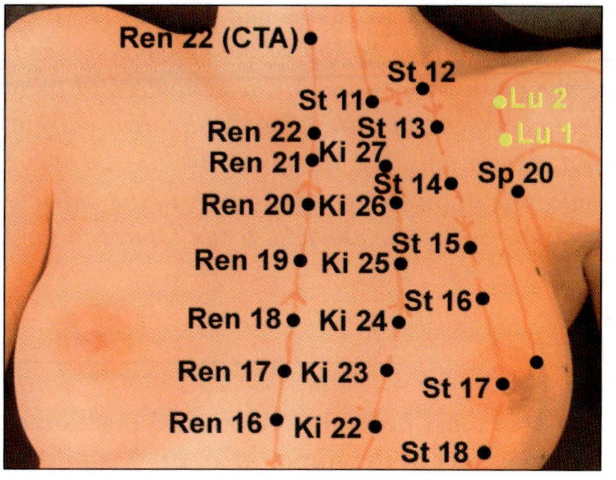

Tip: a) Lu 2 is located laterally at the obstruction formed by the humerus, clavicle and coracoid process.
b) The transverse measurement for the chest (upper jiao) is calculated as 8 cun from the anterior median line to the tip of the acromion process. Lu 2 is located at 6 cun lateral to the anterior median line (Ren channel).
c) Note that the point located relative to the anatomy is not always at 6 cun. 6 cun is only a guide as palpation of the anatomy gives a more accurate location.

Note: Wu (1973) locates LU 2 at two pouces lateral to the nipple and six pouces four fen above it, in the hollow of the subclavian artery below the clavicle. Voisin (1974) locates L 2 at the clavicle, lower border: 2 fb (finger breadth) medial to the anterior axillary line. Worsley (1982) locates IX 2 on the chest, in the depression which is found inferior to the clavicle and medial to the apex of the coracoid process. Huang (1993) locates Lu 2 under the clavicle, 2 cun lateral to St 13 with the patient's arm raised. So (1985) locates LU 2 at 1 and 3/8th divisions above LU 1 and 6 divisions lateral to the Conception (Ren) Vessel, between the first and second ribs. Academy (1975) locate Lu 2 below the acromial extremity of the clavicle in the depression lateral to the triangle of the m. pectoralis, 6 cun lateral to the midline of the chest.

Yang (1982) locates Lu 2 level with the lower border of the sternal extremity of the clavicle, and 2 finger breadths lateral to the mid-point of the clavicle. Soulié (1994) locates LU 2 on the superior anterior arm: three FW (Finger Width) under and exterior (lateral) to the projection between the humerus and thorax (coracoid process); in the angle of the superior edge of the three "major" muscles (pectoralis, latissimus dorsi, teres) and the lateral edge of the vertical tendon of the short head of the biceps (inserted on the coracoid process); in the hollow. On the medial edge of the tendon of the long head of the biceps; on the inferior edge of transverse insertion of the subscapularis muscle; three FW above LU 1; two FW lateral to

HT 1; four FW medial to LI 14. Deadman (1998) locates LU 2 below the lateral extremity of the clavicle, in the centre of the hollow of the delto-pectoral triangle. Shanghai (1993) locate LU 2 in the lateral inferior part of the clavicle, 6 cun lateral to the anterior midline, in the depression of the interior part of the coracoid process of the scapula.

Li (1991) locates LU 2 one cun directly above LU 1 and two fingers' width lateral to the mid-point of the lower border of the clavicle. Legge (1999) locates Lu 2 in the depression medial to the corocoid process of the scapula and below the clavicle, 6 cun lateral to the midline. Shanghai (1981) locate L 2 at the inferior margin of the clavicle, between the pectoralis major and deltoid muscles. Katsusuke (1983) locates LU 2 in the middle of the depression at the underside of the external extremity of the clavicle. One sun above LU 1. Lotan (2000) locates Lu 2 inferior to the clavicle, 6 cun lateral to the front midline; medial to the deltoid.

The arm must be in the anatomical position to locate Lu 3-5 . Lu 3-4 are on the antero-lateral aspect of the upper arm. Lu 5 is in the elbow crease.

The distance between the anterior end of the axillary fold (where the upper arm joins the torso) to the flexure of the elbow (the transverse cubital crease/elbow crease) is measured as 9 cun. To expose the biceps brachii muscle flex the elbow against resistance. To expose the flexure of the elbow, flex and extend the forearm.

Lu 3 TIAN FU – HEAVENLY PALACE

⊥ ***0.4 TO 0.8 CUN*** △ ***FORBIDDEN TO MOXA***

- WINDOW OF THE SKY/Window of Heaven

Pos: Position of patient: supine, in the anatomical position (arms at the side and flat on the couch with the palms facing upwards).

Loc:
a) On the antero-lateral aspect of the upper arm.
b) 6 cun proximal to the transverse cubital crease (at the anterior flexure of the elbow).
c) 3 cun distal to the anterior axillary crease.
d) In the groove formed by the lateral border of the biceps brachii muscle and the humerus.
e) 6 cun proximal to Lu 5.

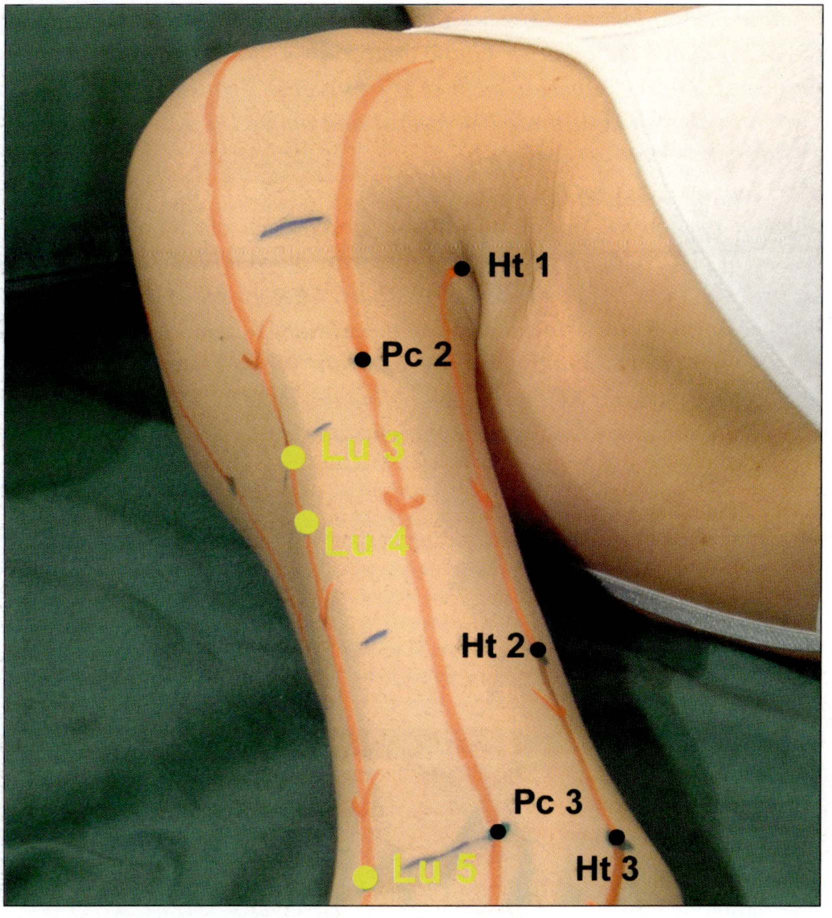

Tip: a) Flex the elbow against resistance to expose the lateral border of the biceps brachii muscle.

b) The distance between the anterior end of the axillary fold (where the upper arm joins the torso) to the flexure of the elbow (the transverse cubital crease/elbow crease) is measured as 9 cun.

c) Divide 9 cun into 3 equal measurements.

d) Lu 3 is approximately at 6 cun proximal to the flexure of the elbow.

e) Having earlier established the biceps brachii, ask the patient to relax their arm and run your finger down the Lung channel from the shoulder towards the elbow in the direction of the flow of the qi. When you arrive at 3 cun distal to the anterior axillary crease, palpate for the point.

f) Palpation gives you overall accuracy for the location of the point.

Note: Lavier (1974) measures 7 pouce from the elbow fold to the deltoid 'V'. He illustrates LU 3 as being located in between the two bellies of the biceps brachii muscle, on the anterior medianline of the upper arm. Wu (1973) locates LU 3 upon the anterior surface of the arm, upon the median line of the biceps, 6 pouces above the elbow, at the level of the "V" of the deltoideus. Soulié (1994) locates LU 3 on the biceps brachialis, mid-height, mid-width; four FW (Finger Width) above the anterior elbow crease, in a hollow between the short and long heads of the biceps. On the superior edge of a transverse ligament; two FW approximately medial and slightly above LU 4; three FW lateral and above HT 2,

Eachou (1995) locates LU 3 on the medial side of the arm 3 inches below the skin crease of the axilla, and at the lateral side of the biceps brachii muscle, at the same height as the nipples. Masayoshi (1975) locates LU 3 at the inferior margin of the deltoid muscle & sulcus of the biceps brachii, 3 sun below the axillary sulcus. Cheng (1987) locates L 3 on the medial aspect of the upper arm, 3 cun below the end of the axillary fold,on the radial side of m. biceps brachii. So (1985) locates LU 3 at 6 divisions above the elbow crease slanting up between the two muscles. Li (1991) locates LU 3 at 3 cun below the anterior end of the axillary fold. One simple way to locate the point is to ask the patient to extend his arm. The place where the tip of the nose touches is the point.

Lu 4 XIA BAI – VALIANT WHITE

⊥ ***0.3 TO 0.8 CUN*** △ **5**

Pos: Position of patient: supine, in the anatomical position (arms at the side and flat on the couch with the palms facing upwards).

Loc:
a) On the antero-lateral surface of the upper arm.
b) 5 cun proximal to the transverse cubital crease (at the anterior flexure of the elbow).
c) 4 cun distal to the anterior axillary crease.
d) In the groove formed by the lateral border of the biceps brachii muscle and the humerus.
e) 5 cun proximal to Lu 5.
f) 1 cun distal to Lu 3.

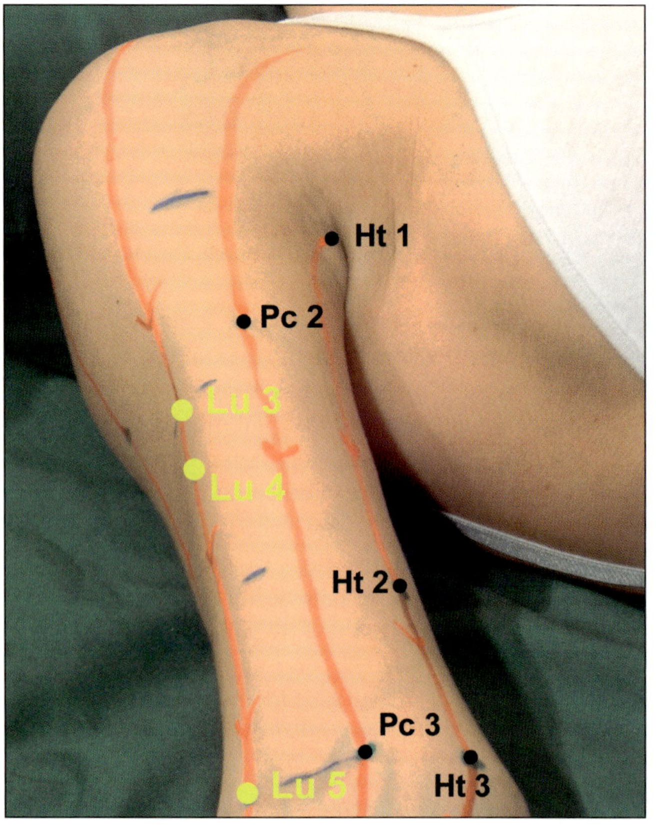

Tip: a) Flex the elbow against resistance to expose the lateral border of the biceps brachii muscle.
b) The distance between the anterior end of the axillary fold (where the upper arm joins the torso) to the flexure of the elbow (the transverse cubital crease/elbow crease) is measured as 9 cun.
c) Divide 9 cun into 3 equal measurements.
d) Lu 4 is approximately at 5 cun proximal to the flexure of the elbow.
e) Having earlier established the biceps brachii, ask the patient to relax their arm and run your finger down the Lung channel from the shoulder towards the elbow in the direction of the flow of the qi. When you arrive at 4 cun distal to the anterior axillary crease, palpate for the point.
f) Palpation gives you overall accuracy for the location of the point.

Lu 5 CHI ZE – OUTSIDE MARSH

⊥ ***0.3 TO 1.0 CUN*** △ ***3 TO 5***

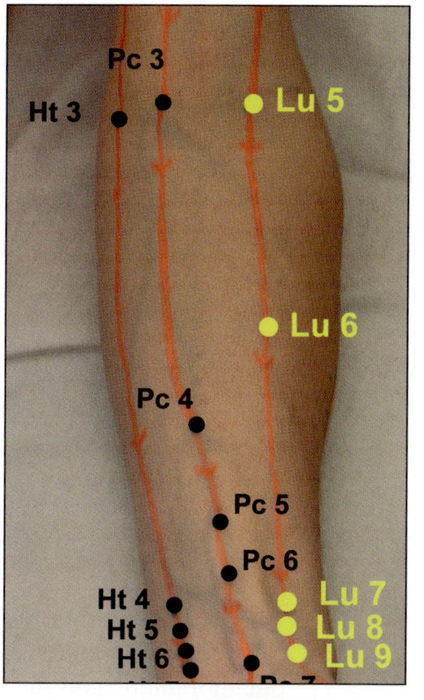

- WATER
- SEDATION/Reducing/Dispersing
- CHILD
- HE – SEA/Shu – Transporting/Antique

Pos: Position of patient: supine, in the anatomical position (arms slightly flexed with the palms facing upwards).

Loc: a) On the anterior surface of the forearm.
b) On the transverse cubital crease (at the anterior flexure of the elbow).
c) Just lateral to the tendon of the biceps brachii muscle, with the arm slightly flexed.

Tip: a) Flex the arm to expose the elbow crease and mark.
b) Use the most prominent crease if more than one is visible.
c) Slightly flex the elbow against resistance to expose the tendon of the biceps brachii muscle.
d) Run your finger in the direction of the flow of the qi along the lateral border of the biceps brachii muscle. Your finger should naturally fall into a *men* (depression) just lateral to the biceps brachii tendon in the elbow crease. This will determine how close the point is to the tendon.
e) Needling Lu 5 may cause discomfort if the arm is not supported and slightly flexed.

Note: The Chinese traditionally locate this point just lateral to the tendon, some Japanese texts locate it 1 cun lateral to the tendon. Voisin (1974) locates L 5 at the biceps, tendon, lateral border: elbow flexion fold. Worsley (1982) locates IX 5 on the elbow crease, at approximately 1 ACI (Anatomical Chinese Inch) lateral to the tendon of the biceps; Eachou (1995) locates LU 5 with an open hand and slightly flexing the elbow, on the skin crease of the elbow, in the fossa at the radial side of the tendon of the biceps brachialis muscle. So (1985) locates LU 5 at the crease of the elbow, on the lateral border of the tendon, between the tendon and the muscle. Bend the elbow and the point will be in a large hollow.

Li (1991) locates LU 5 at the midpoint of the transverse cubital crease, on the radial sde of m. biceps brachii. Soulié (1994) locates LU 5 on the front of the elbow, lateral third; in the angle of the superior edge of the large transverse bulge of the joint, of the medial edge of the large muscle (supinator longus) and of the inferior edge of the transverse tendon of the biceps; in a hollow; lateral to the deep radial artery; four FW (Finger Width) under LU 4; five FW above LU 6, three FW medial LI 11; three FW lateral to PC 3.

The arm must be in the anatomical position when locating Lu 6-11 . Lu 6-8 are on the anterior aspect of the forearm. The distance from Lu 9 (wrist flexure) and the flexure of the elbow is 12 cun.

Flex and extend the hand to locate the wrist flexure by palpating for the articulation between the radius and the scaphoid bones. The visible crease does not always relate to the wrist flexure.

Lu 6 KONG ZUI – GREATEST HOLE

⊥ ***0.5 TO 0.8 CUN*** △ ***5***

- ACCUMULATION/Xi Cleft/Gueki

Pos: Position of patient: supine, in the anatomical position (arms at the side and flat on the couch with the palms facing upwards).

Loc:
a) On the anterior surface of the forearm.
b) On the ulnar side of the radius.
c) Between the medial border of the brachioradialis and the lateral border of the flexor carpi radialis muscles.
d) On the line connecting Lu 5 to Lu 9.
e) 7 cun proximal to Lu 9 (wrist flexure).
f) 5 cun distal to Lu 5 (transverse cubital crease).

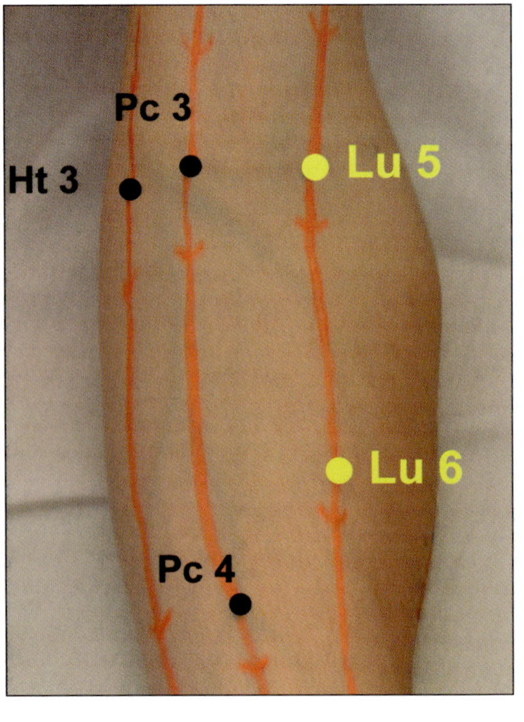

Tip:
- a) The most lateral muscle on the anterior surface of the forearm is the brachioradialis. The tendon inserts at its distal end into the tip of the styloid process of the radius bone. The tendon of the flexor carpi radialis muscle is medial to the brachioradialis muscle.
- b) If you run your finger with the flow of the channel from the flexure of the elbow you will be in between these two muscles. When you arrive at 5 cun distal to Lu 5 (or 7 cun proximal to Lu 9) palpate for the point.
- c) As the name of this point suggests, you are palpating for a relatively large men.
- d) The distance between Lu 5 (transverse cubital crease/elbow crease) and Lu 9 (wrist flexure) is 12 cun.
- e) The pronator teres muscle lies between the medial border of the brachioradialis and the lateral border of the flexor carpi radialis muscles. The pronator teres muscle cannot always be palpated at this level as it is positioned at a greater depth within the forearm.

Note: Wu (1973) locates LU 6 as above but also includes the point at 5 pouce below the elbow and outside of the palmaris longus. Voisin (1974) locates L 6 on the forearm, anterior aspect: 3 fb (finger breadth) below the elbow flexion fold, on the medial border of the radius. Soulié (1994) locates LU 6 on the anterior, external face of the forearm; six FW (finger width) above the wrist; in the angle of the medial edge (towards the ulnar bone), with the supinator longus of the radius and the edge of the insertions of the angular muscles coming from the inner elbow (pronator muscles); between the bone and the radial artery, very close to the bone; in a hollow. On the flexor longus of the thumb and deep to the common superficial flexors 9ungual phalangeal); five FW under LU 5; five FW above LU 7.

Katsusuke (1983) locates LU 6 on the thumb side of the inner surface of the forearm at a point about one third of the distance from the elbow to the wrist. Eachou (1995) locates LU 6 on a line between LU 5 and LU 9. The point is located 7 inches above LU 9 on the medial side of the forearm. So (1985) locates LU 6 at 5 divisions below LU 5, slanting down toward the radial bone on a muscle cleft.

Lu 7 LIE QUE – NARROW DEFILE

⊥ ***0.2 TO 0.5 CUN*** △ ***3 TO 5***

- JUNCTION/Luo/Connecting/Passage/Lo/Lê)
- EXIT
- 8 EXTRAORDINARY CHANNELS CONFLUENT/8 Extraordinary Meridians Confluent/8 Extraordinary Vessels Opening/Master Point of Ren Mai (Conception/ Directing Vessel)
- 8 EXTRAORDINARY VESSEL/Coupled Point of the Yin Heel/Yin Motility Vessel (Yin Qiao Mai)
- RE-UNION/Crossing/Meeting Point of the Lung Channel with the Large Intestine Channel – Hand Tai Yin Channel with the Hand Yang Ming Channel
- HOST/GUEST COMBINATION – Source Point with the Junction Point of its Paired Official/Organ Therefore Lu 7 is combined with LI 4
- ONE OF THE HEAVENLY STAR POINTS OF MA DAN-YANG (the others are: LI 4, LI 11, St 36, St 44, Bl 40, Bl 57, Bl 60, Ht 5, GB 34, GB 39 and Liv 3)

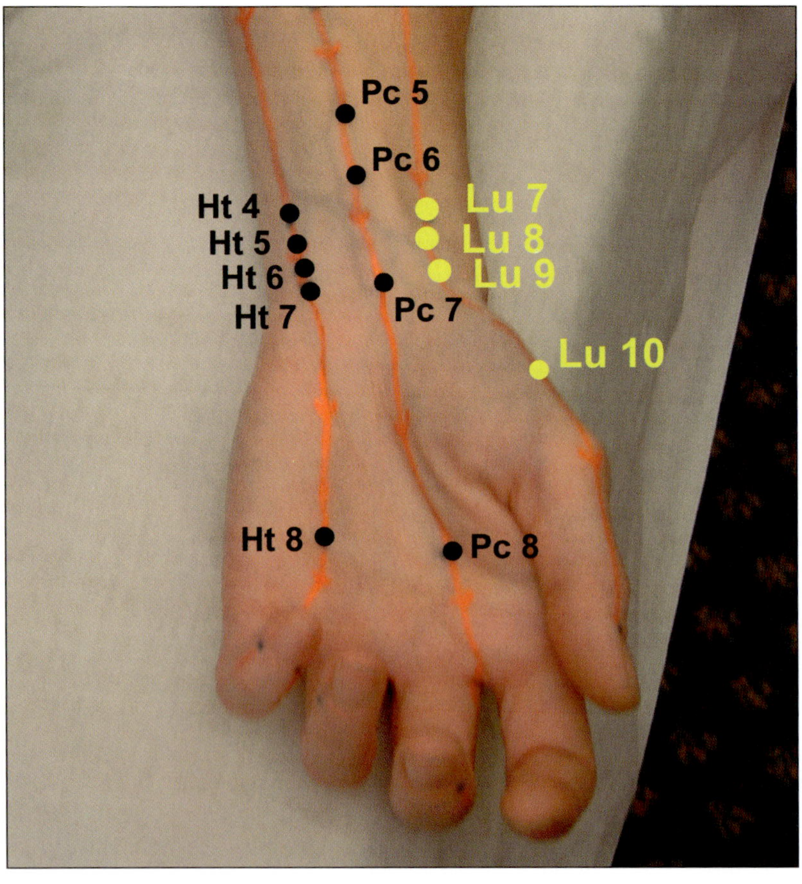

Pos: Position of patient: supine, in the anatomical position (arms at the side and flat on the couch with the palms facing upwards).

Loc:
a) On the anterior surface of the forearm.
b) On the ulnar side of the radius.
c) Proximal to the root of the styloid process of the radius.
d) Approximately 1.5 cun proximal to Lu 9 (wrist flexure).
e) In the hollow between the tendons of the brachioradialis and abductor pollicis longus muscles.

Tip:
a) The root of the styloid process of the radius is an important landmark. This determines the exact location of the point which may or may not be 1.5 cun proximal to the flexure of the wrist at Lu 9. The anatomy takes precedence over the cun measurement.
b) Extend the thumb to expose the tendon of the abductor pollicis longus muscle, which is lateral (radial) to the tendon of the brachioradialis muscle. Lu 7 lies in a *men* (depression) lateral to tendon of the brachioradialis muscle.
c) The tendon of the brachioradialis lies between the tendons of the abductor pollicis longus and the flexor carpi radialis muscles. The tendon of the brachioradialis lies at a deeper level than tendons of the abductor pollicis longus and the flexor carpi radialis muscles. To make this tendon more obvious semi-pronate the forearm against resistance.
d) To help locate this point run your finger with the flow of the channel from the elbow flexure towards the wrist flexure.
e) When Lu 7 is used to clear an entry/exit block between the Lung and Large Intestine, the channel between Lu 7 and LI 4 becomes more direct when the arm is semi-pronated. The lateral border of the radius is uppermost in this position, and Lu 7 can be palpated along the upper border.
f) The distance between Lu 5 (transverse cubital crease/elbow crease) and Lu 9 (wrist flexure) is 12 cun.
g) Lu 7 is 1.5 cun proximal to Lu 9 (wrist flexure).

Note: In Japan this point is located on the line connecting Lu 9 and Lu 5, at the root of the styloid process of the radius (1.5 cun proximal to the wrist flexure), just lateral to the radial artery. Matsumoto (1986) gives an interesting discussion on the Japanese versus Chinese approach to Lu 7. Wu (1973) locates Lu 7 upon the anterior surface of the forearm on the radial artery, at two pouce from the flexure of the wrist. Lavier (1974) in an illustration locates Lu 7 at 2 pouce from the flexure on the forearm. De la Fuye (1956) and Lawson-Wood (1973) locate Lu 7 at 2 cm above the lower extremity of the radius. Academy (1975) locates this point above the styloid process of the radius, 1.5 cun above the transverse crease of the wrist. By crossing the index fingers and thumbs of both hands, the point is in the depression that is under the tip of the index finger. Worsley (1982) locates IX 7 on the anterior surface of the forearm, 2 ACI (Anatomical Chinese Inch) proximal to IX 9 and just lateral to the radial artery. Voisin (1974) locates L 7 on the forearm, anterior aspect: 2-3 fb (finger breadth) above the wrist flexion fold, on the medial border of the radius. Masayoshi (1975) locates LU 7 at 2.5 cm proximal to the styloid process.

Soulié (1994) locates LU 7 on the anterior forearm, three FW (finger width) above the wrist (one above the head of the radius); on the line of the index finger; in the angle of the lateral (radial) edge of the large tendon (large palmar) and the inferior edge of a transverse bulge; in a hollow; on the medial (ulnar) edge of the radial artery; on pulse V (right, endocrines; left, organs of sense.); five FW under LU 6, alittle above LU 8; separated by the large palmar tendon from PC 6. Li (1991) locates LU 7 by making the index finger and thumb of one hand cross the index finger and thumb of the other with one index finger pointing at the styloid process of the other.

The point is located in the depression where the tip of the index finger touches, that is to say, at the distal point of the styloid process. Eachou (1995) locates LU 7 on the lateral and inferior part of the forearm above the styloid process of the radius, 1.5 inches above the skin crease of the wrist. Alternative method: ask the patient to cross both thumbs and index fingers with one hand's index finger pressing just above the styloid process of the radius of the other hand. The point is then located in the fossa under the index fingertip., Qiu (1995) locates Lu 7 superior to the styloid process of the radius, 1.5 cun above the transverse crease of the wrist. A simple way of locating this point is when the index fingers and thumbs of both hands are crossed with the index finger of one hand placed on the styloid process of the radius of the other, the point lies in the depression just under the tip of the index finger. Ellis (1991) locate Lu 7 in the crevice on the most lateral aspect of the radius, just proximal to the styloid process, 1.5" above the wrist crease.

When the thumb and index finger of each hand are interlocked, with the index finger of one hand resting on the styloid process of the other, the point is in the depression just under the tip of the index finger. Shanghai (1993) locates LU 7 in the superior lateral part of the styloid process of the radius, 1.5 cun above the carpal crease, between the tendons of the brachioradial muscle and of the long abductor muscle of the thumb. Shandong (1982) locate Lieque at 1.5 cun above the transverse wrist crease, above the processus styloideus of the radius. Jayasuriya (1982) – Lu 7; When the index finger and the thumbs of both hands of the patient are crossed, this point is at the tip of the upper index finger. This point is located by measuring 1.5 cun from the wrist-joint crease proximally on the outer (radial or lateral) border of the forearm. Cheng (1987) locates L 7 superior to the styloid process of the radius; 1.5 cun above the transverse crease of the wrist. When the index fingers and thumbs of both hands are crossed with the index finger of one hand placed on the styloid process of the radius of the other, the point is in the depression right under the tip of the finger. Lotan (2000) locates Lu 7 as one and the same, he also describes an alternate location for Lu 7, proximal to the radius styloid process, between the abductor pollicis longus and the extensor pollicis brevis; 1.5 cun proximal to the cubital (wrist) fold.

Lu 8 JING QU – MERIDIAN GUTTER

⊥ ***0.1 TO 0.3 CUN*** △ ***3***

- METAL
- HORARY from 3 a.m. to 5 a.m.
- SEASONAL HORARY – Autumn
- JING – RIVER/Shu – Transporting/Antique

Pos: Position of patient: supine, in the anatomical position (arms at the side and flat on the couch with the palms facing upwards).

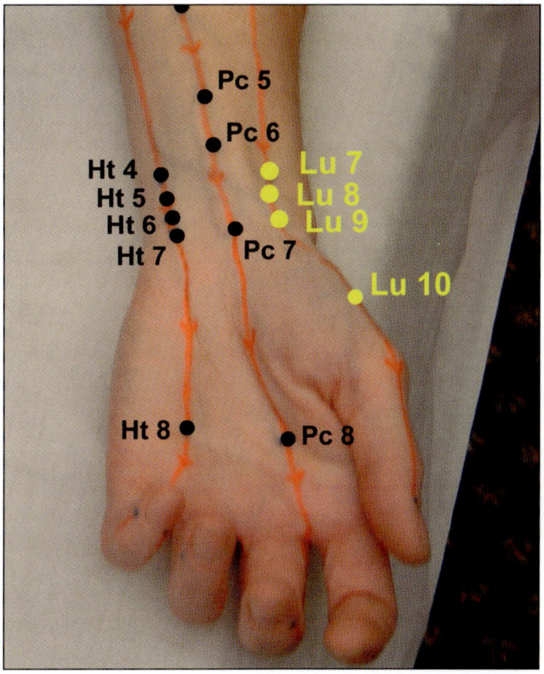

Loc:
a) On the anterior surface of the forearm.
b) On the ulnar (medial) side of the radius.
c) On the line connecting Lu 5 to Lu 9.
d) Approximately 1 cun proximal to Lu 9 (wrist flexure).
e) Level with and medial to the prominence of the styloid process of the radius.
f) On the lateral (radial) aspect of the radial artery.
g) Lateral to the tendon of the flexor carpi radialis.

Tip:
a) The prominence of the styloid process of the radius is the key landmark used in locating this point. The styloid process determines the exact location of the point which may or may not be 1 cun proximal to the flexure of the wrist at Lu 9.
b) To assist in locating this point run your finger along the flow of the channel from the elbow flexure towards the wrist flexure.
c) The distance between Lu 5 (transverse cubital crease/elbow crease) and Lu 9 (wrist flexure) is 12 cun.
d) Lu 8 is 1 cun proximal to Lu 9 (wrist flexure).

Note: Worsley (1982) locates IX 8 on the anterior surface of the forearm, 1 ACI (Anatomical Chinese Inch) proximal to IX 9, upon the radial artery. Wu (1973) locates LU 8 upon the radial artery at the styloid area, one pouce from the flexure of the wrist. So (1985) locates LU 8 in front of LU 7, one division below the radial eminence, 0.5 division proximal to the wrist crease. Eachou (1995) locates LU 8 at 1 inch above the skin crease of the wrist, on the medial side of the styloid process of the radius and the lateral side of the radial artery, in the fossa between the tendons of the carpi radialis and abductor pollicis longus muscles, or 1 inch above LU 9.

Soulié (1994) locates LU 8 on the anterior wrist (palm up, supination); external third (towards the thumb); on the superior edge of the internal extremity of the head of the radius; on the lateral edge of the large tendon of the palmaris longus; exactly at the angle of the bone and the medial edge of the artery; in a hollow; one FW (Finger Width) under LU 7; one FW above LU 9; separated from PC 7 by the tendon of the palmaris longus and at its level. Huang (1993) locates Lu 8 in a depression at the cun kou.

Li (1991) locates LU 8 on the medial aspect of the top of the styloid process of the radius, that is to say the "guan" position ("Cun, Guan and Chi" are the three divisions of the region for pulse palpation). Shanghai (1993) locate LU 8 on the radial side of the palmar surface of the forearm, 1 cun above the carpal crease, on the lateral side of the radial artery and exactly on the lateral side of the tendon of the radial flexor muscle of the wrist.

Lu 9 TAI YUAN – VERY GREAT ABYSS

⊥ ***0.2 TO 0.3 CUN*** **Δ *3***

- SOURCE/Yuan/Regulator/Primary
- EARTH
- TONIFICATION/Reinforcing
- MOTHER
- SHU – STREAM/Shu – Transporting/Antique
- INFLUENTIAL/Hui – Meeting/Gathering/Assembling Point of the Channels (Meridians)/Arteries/Blood Vessels
- RE-UNION/Crossing/Meeting Point of Arteries and Veins
- HOST/GUEST COMBINATION – Source Point with the Junction Point of its Paired Official/Organ Therefore Lu 9 is combined with LI 6
- SUN SI-MIAO GHOST (Gui) – Ghost Point Name: Gui Xin – Ghost Heart (Pc 7 is more common)

Pos: Position of patient: supine, in the anatomical position (arms at the side and flat on the couch with the palms facing upwards).

Loc: a) On the anterior flexure of the wrist.
b) In the articulation between the proximal edge of the scaphoid bone and the tip of the styloid process of the radius.
c) Between the tendons of the flexor carpi radialis and the abductor pollicis longus muscles.
d) On the lateral (radial) aspect of the radial artery.

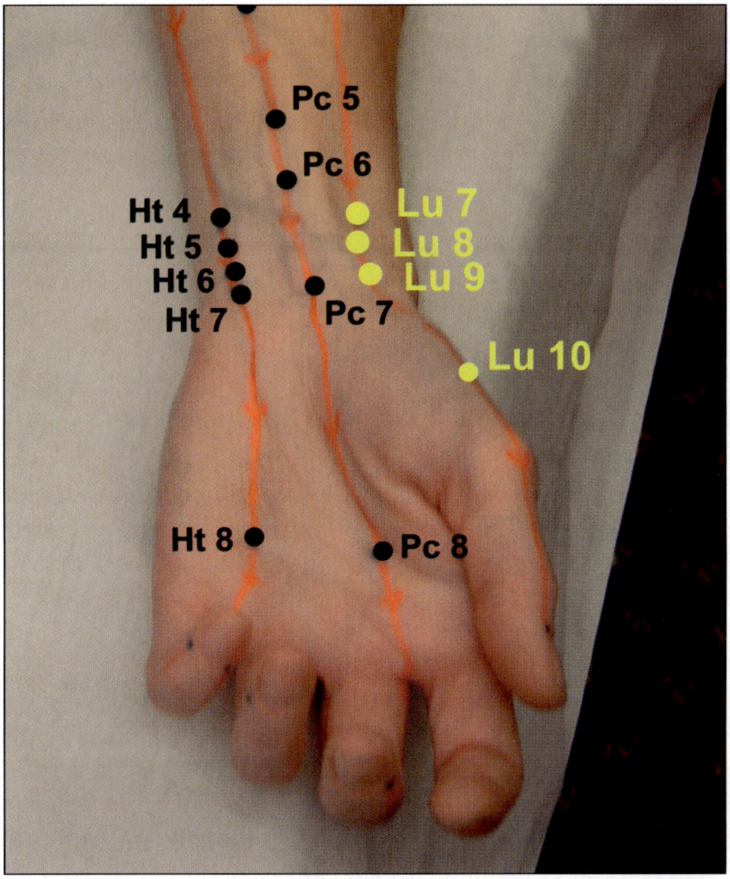

Tip:
a) Flex and extend the hand and palpate for the articulation at the wrist.
b) To expose two tendons in the middle of the wrist flex the wrist against resistance. The more lateral of the two tendons is the flexor carpi radialis and the more medial tendon is the palmaris longus.
c) To help locate this point run your finger with the flow of the channel from the elbow flexure towards the wrist flexure.
d) To minimise possible discomfort when needling this point it is important that the wrist is slightly flexed.
e) This point may be located on the wrist crease.

Note: Wu (1973) locates LU 9 upon the palmar flexure of the wrist, upon the radial artery between the radius and scaphoid. Worsley (1982) locate IX 9 on the crease of the flexure of the wrist, between the radius and the scaphoid bone, upon the radial artery. Lawson-Wood (1973) locates IX 9 on the anterior of the wrist on the radial groove at the wrist fold (antero-inferior of the tendon of the supinator longus. Shanghai (1981) locate L 9 with the palm facing up, this point can be found in a slight depression at the radial end of the transverse crease of the wrist. Qiu (1996) locates LU 9 at the radial end of the transverse crease of the wrist, in the depression at the lateral aspect of the radial artery.

Deadman (1998) locate LU 9 at the wrist joint, in the depression between the radial artery and the tendon of abductor pollicis longus, level with HE 7 (Ht 7) (the proximal border of the pisiform bone). Soulié (1994) locates LU 9 on the front of the wrist (palm up, supination); lateral third (lateral towards the thumb). In the large hollow between the carpal bone (bottom of thumb) and the radial bone; in the angle of the inferior edge of the carpal bone and the medial (ulnar) edge of the tendon of the palmaris longus and the radiopalmar artery, which detaches itself from the radial artery medial towards the palm; in a hollow; in the scaphoid-trapezoid joint; one large FW (Finger Width) below LU 8; one FW above LU 10; one large FW lateral to PC 7 and one FW above its level. Katsusuke (1983) LU 9 – When the fingers of the hand are outstretched to the maximum, a thick tendon becomes apparent at the base of the thumb.

This Tsubo is located on the thumb side of the tendon. Academy (1975) locate Lu 9 on the palmar surface, at the tip of the transverse crease of the wrist, in the depression on the radial side of the radial artery. Jayasuriya (1982) locates Lu 9 at the outer (lateral) end of the wrist crease, on the lateral side of the radial artery. So (1985) locates LU 9 in the hollow at the flexure of the wrist, between the radial bone and metacarpals, 0.5 division in front of LU 8. Huang (1993) locates Lu 9 in a depression proximal to the wrist.

Shanghai (1993) locate LU 9 on the radial side of the transverse crease of the wrist, in the depression between the tendons of the radial flexor muscle of the wrist and of the long abductor muscle of the thumb. Masayoshi (1975) locates LU 9 on the volar side of the wrist joint, recessed portion. Li (1991) locates LU 9 on the radial side of the large multiangular bone, in the depression on the radial side of the radial artery, above the 1st transverse crease of the wrist. Legge (1999) locates Lu 9 at the radial end of the transverse crease of the wrist, in the depression between the radial artery and the tendons (extensor pollicis brevis and abductor pollicis longus). Lotan (2000) locates Lu 9 in the carpal (wrist) joint, radial to the radial artery; search for the sensation of pulse; in the wrist transverse crease; ulnar to the abductor pollicis longus; between the radius and scaphoid (carpal bone); level with H 7.

Lu 10 YU JI – FISH REGION

⊥ ***0.5 TO 0.7 CUN*** △ ***FORBIDDEN TO MOXA***

- FIRE
- YING – SPRING/Shu – Transporting/Antique

Pos: Position of patient: supine, in the anatomical position (arms at the side and flat on the couch with the palms facing upwards) or seated.

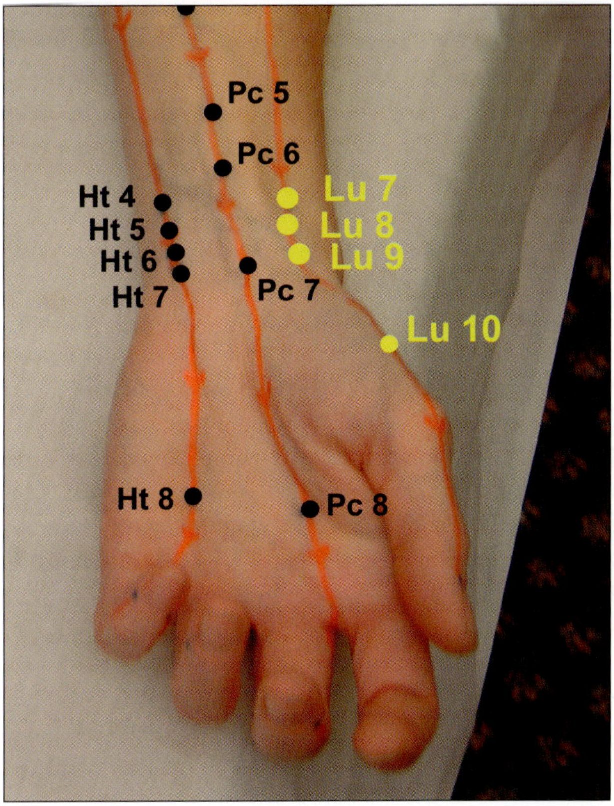

Loc:
a) At the radial extremity of the palmar surface of the hand.
b) At a point midway between the base and the head of the first metacarpal bone.
c) On the ulnar aspect of the first metacarpal bone.
d) In a channel on the radial (lateral) edge of the opponens pollicis muscle between the muscle and the 1st metacarpal bone.
e) At the junction of change in skin colour (red to white skin).

Tip:
a) Oppose the first and fifth digits to demonstrate the opponens pollicis muscle.
b) The opponens pollicis muscle is the most lateral of the group of muscles that form the thenar eminence at the root of the thumb.
c) The heads of the metacarpal bones are the "knuckles" of the hand.
d) Palpate for the point midway between the head and base of the first metacarpal bone, in a seam between the radial (lateral) edge of the opponens pollicis muscle and the first metacarpal bone.
e) If you are having difficulties locating the midway point of the first metacarpal bone, draw two marks, one on the prominence of the head and one on the prominence of the base of the first metacarpal bone, and divide the distance between the two marks in to two, and then palpate for the point.
f) Another guide is to see where the skin colour changes from red to white, ie. from the palmar aspect to the dorsal aspect of the hand.

Note: Lavier (1974), illustrates Lu 10, at a point midway between the proximal and distal ends of the first metacarpal bone at the mid-point of the thenar eminence, this is possibly a Japanese location. Worsley (1982) locates IX 10 on the palmar surface of the hand, mid-way along the ulnar side of the first metacarpal bone. The illustration locates IX 10 on the highest part of the thenar eminence where you can look down into a valley (to the middle of the palmar aspect of the hand). Wu (1973) locates LU 10 on the palmar surface of the hand, at the extremity of the thenar eminence behind the head of the first metacarpal.

Deadman (1998) locate LU 10 on the thenar eminence of the hand, in a depression between the midpoint of the shaft of the first metacarpal bone and the thenar muscles. Voisin (1974) locates L 10 on the thenar eminence: in a hollow above the head of metacarpal 1. So (1985) locates LU 10 on the palmar surface, at the anterior edge of the first metacarpal, behind the joint – bend the thumb to locate the joint. Masayoshi (1975) locates LU 10 on the radial metacarpophalangeal joint. Soulié (1994) locates LU 10 on the pal; base of the thumb (thenar eminence), one FW (finger width) above the wrist, about half width. Between the two muscles (lateral side of the thumb,of the short flexor of the thumb; medial to the short abductor of the thumb), at the angle of the inferior edge of the bony prominence (tubercle of the scaphoid bone) and of the insertion on it of the short abductor; deep: on the opposing muscle; in a hollow; one FW below LU 9; two fingers lateral to HT 7.

Eachou (1995) locates LU 10 on the thenar eminence 1 inch distal to LU 9, medial to the midpoint of the first metacarpal on the palmar side of the hand. Ellis (1991) locate LU 10 on the thenar eminence, midway along the first metacarpal bone, on the border of the red and white skin. Huang (1993) locates Lu 10 at the radial border of the thumb proximal to the base joint.

Lu 11 SHAO SHANG – LITTLE MERCHANT

⊥ ***0.1 CUN*** △ ***FORBIDDEN TO MOXA***

- WOOD
- JING – WELL/Shu – Transporting/Antique
- SUN SI-MIAO GHOST (Gui) – Ghost Point Name: Gui Xin – Ghost Faith

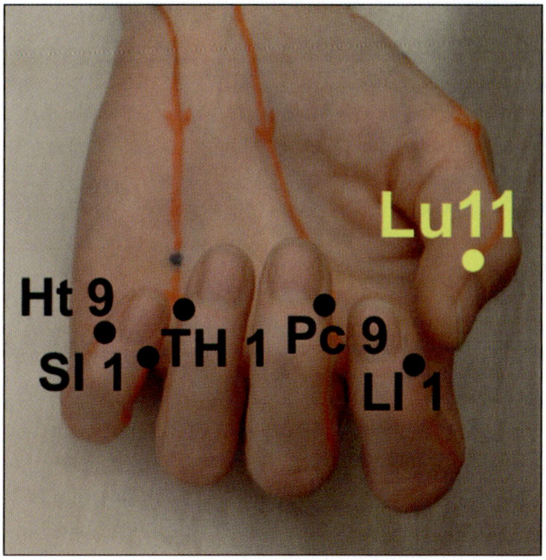

Pos: Position of patient: supine or seated.

Loc:
a) On the hand.
b) On the posterior aspect of the first digit (thumb).
c) The radial nail point of the first digit.
d) Approximately 0.1 cun proximal to the corner of the nail, just distal to the flare of the distal phalanx.

Tip:
a) The point is level with the nail bed (where the nail attaches to the skin) rather than the cuticle.
b) Draw a horizontal line across the nail bed.
c) Draw a vertical line from the radial border of the nail towards the nail bed.
d) The lines drawn from b) and c) (vertical and horizontal) form an intersection. This is approximately where the point is located.

Note: Ellis (1991) – the classical description from the Great Compendium locates this point on the inside (radial) of the thumb, about the width of a Chinese leek leaf from the corner of the nail. Huang (1993) locates Lu 11 at the tip of the inner (radial) aspect of the thumb, the distance of a leek leaf from the corner of the nail. Soulié (1994) locates LU 11 on the thumb, angular phalanx, index finger side (medial interior edge) about mid-width: at the angle of the inferior edge of the prominence of the bone near the joint and the dorsal edge of the palmar tendon (flexors), in a hollow.

Masayoshi (1975) locates LU 11 at 3-4mm radial from the ungual bed. So (1985) locate LU 11 on the inner side of the thumb. With the palms down, the side of the hand closer to the body is the "inner" side. The side moving away from the body is the "outer" side. With the palms up, the side closer to the body is also called the "inner" side. This is the Chinese habit, most books and charts in the West mislocate this point by mistranslating the Chinese idea of "inner." LU 11 is behind the edge of the cuticle 1/10th of an inch and directly behind the inner edge of the nail.

REFERENCES FOR THE LUNG CHANNEL

Worsley, J R 1982 Traditional Chinese Acupuncture Volume 1 – Meridians and Points. IX 1: 183; IX 2: 183; IX 5: 185; IX 7: 185; IX 8: 185; IX 9: 187; IX 10: 187

Deadman, Peter; Al-Khafaji, Mazin; Baker, Kevin 1998 Manual of Acupuncture, An – LU 1: 76; LU 2: 77; LU 9: 86; LU 10: 88

Shanghai College of Traditional Medicine 1981 Acupuncture – A Comprehensive Text – L 1: 176; L 2: 306; L 9: 243

Huang-fu Mi. Trans: Yang Shou-zhong and Charles Chace 1993 The Systematic Classic of Acupuncture & Moxibustion – Lu 1: 158; Lu 2: 158; Lu 8: 172; Lu 9: 172; Lu 10: 172; Lu 11: 171

Soulié De Morant, George. 1994 Chinese Acupuncture – LU 1: 341: LU 2: 342; LU 3: 340/342; LU 4: 340/343; LU 5: 343; LU 6: 344; LU 7: 344; LU 8: 345; LU 9: 346; LU 10: 346; LU 11: 347

Lawson-Wood, D&J 1973 Acupuncture Handbook – IX 7: 8; IX 9: 8

Masayoshi Hyodo 1975 Ryodoraku Acupuncture – LU 1: 30; LU 3: 30; LU 7: 30; LU 9: 30; LU 11: 30

So, James Tin Yau (Dr) 1985 The Book of Acupuncture Points: LU 1: 47; LU 2: 174; LU 3: 174; LU 4: 175; LU 5: 99; LU 6: 175; LU 8: 101; LU 9: 101; LU 10: 176; LU 11: 102

Voisin, Dr. H 1974 Essentials of Acupuncture – Herald: 30/31; L 1: 78/79; L 2: 78; L 4: 78/79; L 5: 78; L 6: 78; L 7: 78; L 10: 78

Wu, Wei-P'ing 1973 Chinese Acupuncture – LU 1: 59; LU 2: 59; LU 3: 59; LU 4: 59; LU 6: 60; LU 7: 60; LU 8: 60; LU 9: 60; LU 10: 61

Li Ding (Prof.). 1991. Acupuncture, Meridian Theory and Acupuncture Points – LU 1: 83/84; LU 2: 85; LU 3: 85; LU 5: 87; LU 7: 89; LU 8: 90; LU 9: 91

Legge, David 1999 Acupuncture Points and Meridians – Lu 1: 19; Lu 2: 19; Lu 9: 20

Lotan Alon (2000) – Lu 1: 17; Lu 2: 17; Lu 7: 19; Lu 9: 21

Academy of Traditional Chinese Medicine, The. 1975 – Outline of Chinese Acupuncture, An. Lu 2: 95; Lu 4: 97; Lu 7: 98; Lu 9: 98

Yang Jiasan (Prof) 1982 The Way to Locate Acu-Points – Lu 2: 4

Katsusuke Serizawa 1983 Tsubo – Vital Points for Oriental Therapy – LU 2: 230; LU 4: 91; LU 6: 91; LU 9: 91

Lavier, Dr. J 1974 Points of Chinese Acupuncture – Upper Arm Pouce Measurement: 8/9; LU 3: 8; LU 4: 8; LU 7: 14; LU 10: 21

Shandong Medical College and Shandong College of Traditional Chinese Medicine 1982 Anatomical Atlas of Chinese Acupuncture Points – Zhongfu (Lu 1): 8; Lieque (Lu 7): 8

Eachou Chen 1995 Cross-sectional Anatomy of Acupoints – LU 3: 13; LU 5: 18; LU 6: 22; LU 7: 30; LU 8: 32; LU 10: 39

Qiu Mao-Liang 1996 Chinese Acupuncture and Moxibustion – LU 7: 64/65; LU 9: 65

Ellis, Wiseman, Boss 1991 Fundamentals of Chinese Acupuncture – LU 7: 84; LU 10: 86; LU 11 (Classical Location): 87

Shanghai College of Traditional Chinese Medicine 1993 Applied Anatomical Charts of Acupuncture and Moxibustion – LU 2: 12; LU 7: 4; LU 8: 6; LU 9: 6

Cheng Xinnong (Editor) 1987 Chinese Acupuncture and Moxibustion – L 3: 128; L 4: 128; L 7: 129

Jayasuriya, Anton 1982 Clinical Acupuncture – Lu 7: 387; Lu 9: 387

Matsumoto, Kiiko and Birch, Stephen 1986— Extraordinary Vessels – Lu 7: ?

De la Fuye, Dr. Roger 1956 Traitée d'Acupuncture (le Francois) – Lu 7: no page number

THE LARGE INTESTINE CHANNEL OF THE HAND (YANG MING)

Primary Channel

The Large Intestine channel starts at LI 1 on the radial side of the second digit, and runs up the radial border of the forearm and the lateral aspect of the upper arm, remaining superficial as far as LI 14, (where a deep branch runs to TH 13 at the posterior border of the deltoid muscle). The channel continues over the shoulder joint to LI 16, then travels across the trapezius muscle to the posterior median line at the base of the 7th cervical vertebra, (Du 14). It crosses back over the shoulder to the supraclavicular fossa (St 12), where it divides.

One branch goes up from the lateral aspect of the neck, passing over the sternocleidomastoid muscle, into the lower part of the face. From the mandible it travels along the side of the mouth, crossing the median line below the nose and above the upper lip, and ends at the opposite side of the nose at LI 20 (where the LI channel links with the St channel).

Some Japanese texts include a channel encircling the mouth (LI 18/Ren 24/St 4/ Du 26/LI 19), and a branch from LI 20 to TH 20.

Another branch from the supraclavicular fossa passes through the chest and lung, goes down through the diaphragm and abdomen, and travels through the large intestine itself down as far as St 25. (Some historical texts include a deep channel running down from St 12 through the lung and large intestine to enter the lower limb, emerging at St 37.)

Divergent Channel

Leaving the primary channel on the hand, this passes up across the arm and shoulder to the breast. A branch separates at the top of the shoulder (LI 15), enters the spine at the nape of the neck (Du 14), and passes down to join with the large intestine and lung. A second branch ascends from the shoulder along the throat, emerging at the supraclavicular fossa (St 12) to rejoin the primary channel.

Connecting Channel

This leaves the primary channel at LI 6 to join the Lung channel. Another branch travels up the arm to the shoulder (LI 15), crosses the jaw and passes to the teeth. A third branch separates at the jaw and enters the ear to join the Chong Mai.

Muscle Channel

This originates at the tip of the first digit and binds at the dorsum of the wrist. It then travels across the forearm binding at the lateral aspect of the elbow, and continues up the arm to bind at the shoulder (LI 15). A branch encircles the scapula and attaches to the upper thoracic vertebrae at the spine. The main muscle channel travels from LI 15 at the top of the shoulder to the neck, where a branch separates to bind at the side of the nose, then continues upwards, anterior to the Small Intestine muscle channel. It crosses over the head, connecting at the mandible on the opposite side of the face.

THE LARGE INTESTINE CHANNEL OF THE HAND

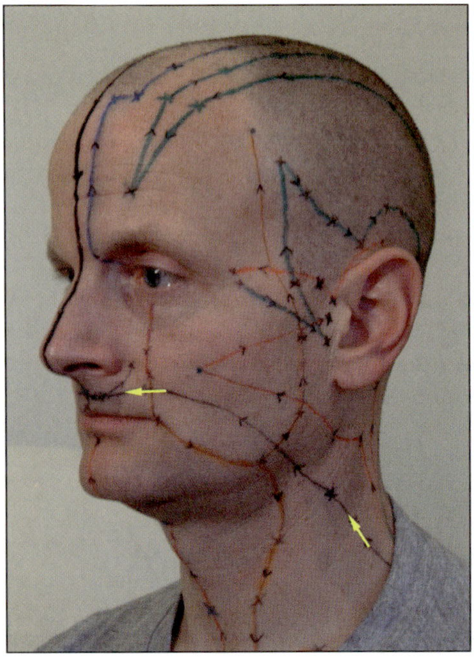

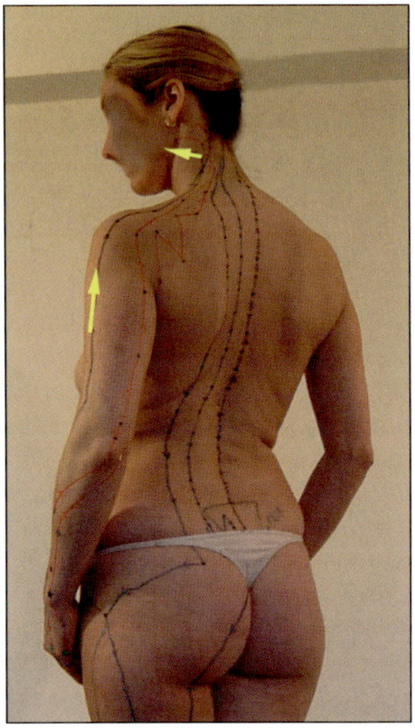

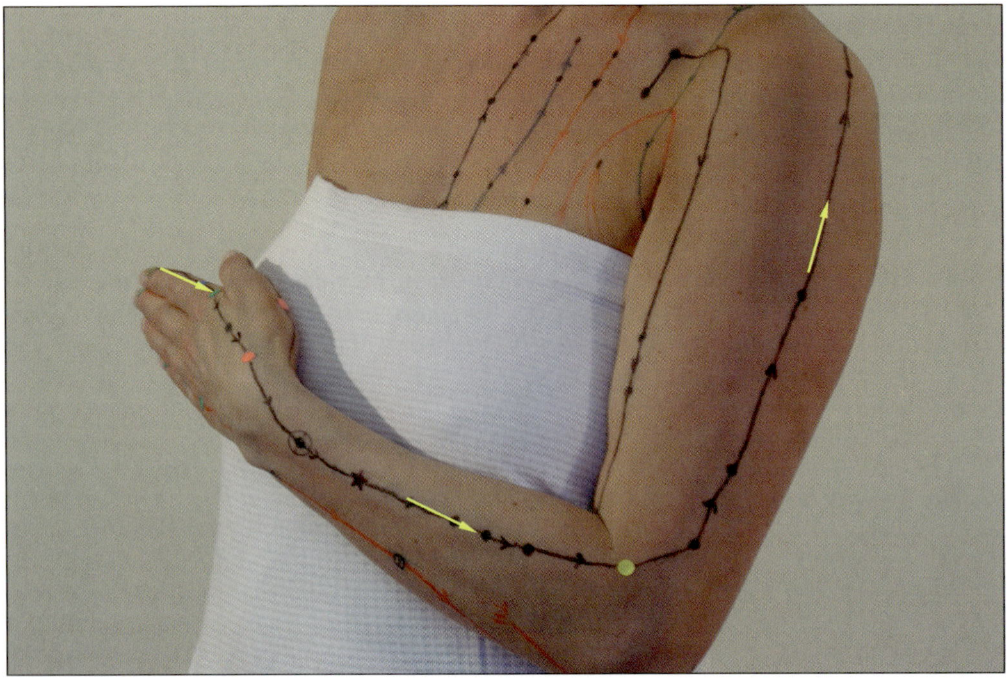

Points of the Large Intestine Channel – Hand Yang Ming (LI/Li/CO/X)

LI 1-4 are on the posterior aspect of the hand, LI 5 at the wrist.
To locate LI 1 to LI 5, place the forearm in the anatomical position and partially pronate the forearm so the radial border is uppermost.

LI 1 SHANG YANG – MERCHANT YANG

⊥ ***0.1 CUN*** ∆ ***3***

- METAL
- HORARY from 5 a.m. to 7 a.m.
- SEASONAL HORARY – Autumn
- JING – WELL/Shu – Transporting/Antique

Pos: Position of patient: supine or seated

Loc:
a) On the hand.
b) On the posterior aspect of the second digit (index finger).
c) The radial nail point of the second digit.
d) Approximately 0.1 cun proximal to the corner of the nail.
e) Just distal to the flare of the distal phalanx.

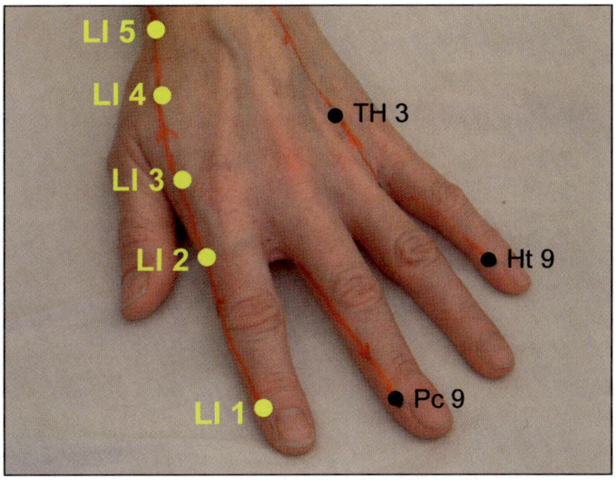

Tip:
a) The point is level with the nail bed (where the nail attaches to the skin) rather than the cuticle.
b) Draw a horizontal line across the nail bed.
c) Draw a vertical line from the radial border of the nail towards the nail bed.
d) The lines drawn from b) and c) (vertical and horizontal) form an intersection. This is approximately where the point is located.

Note: Ellis (1991) – the classical description from the Great Compendium locates LI 1 on the inside (radial side) of the index finger, the width of a Chinese leek leaf from the corner of the nail. Huang (1993) locates LI 1 on the radial aspect of the finger next to the thumb, the distance of a leek leaf from the corner of the nail. Masayoshi (1975) locates LI 1 at 2mm on the radial side of the ungual bed of the dorsal side of the index finger. So (1985) locates LI 1 on the pointing finger at the inner corner of the fingernail (see LU 11 for "inner" explanation).

LI 2 ER JIAN – SECOND INTERVAL

⊥ ***0.2 TO 0.3 CUN*** △ ***3***

- WATER
- SEDATION/Reducing/Dispersing
- CHILD
- YING – SPRING /Shu – Transporting/Antique

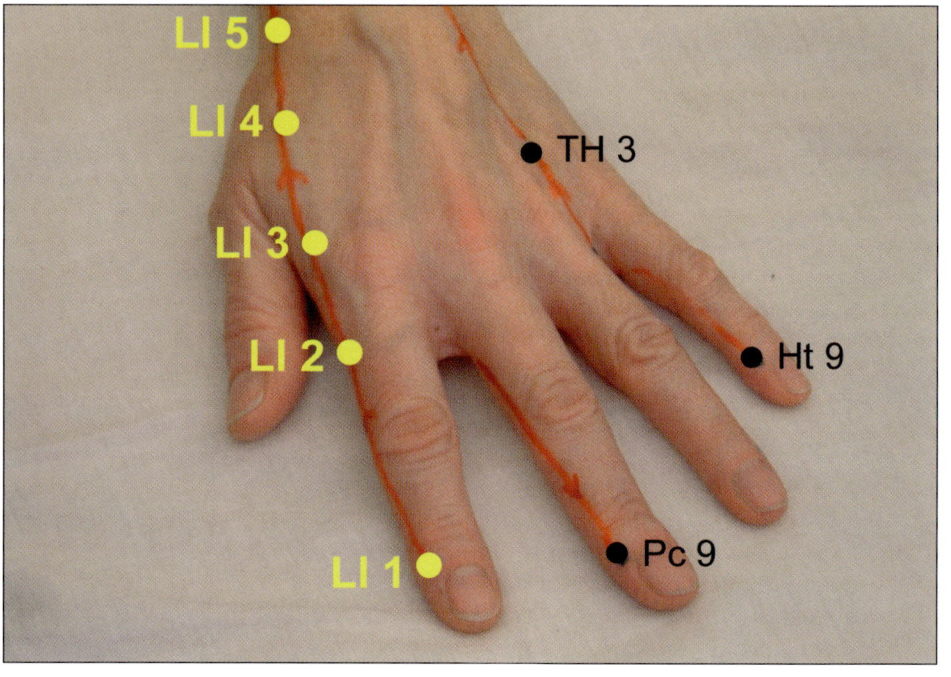

Pos: Position of patient: supine in the anatomical position, partially pronate the forearm so that the radial border is uppermost. The hand should be in a relaxed position so the fingers are curving slightly.

Loc:
a) On the hand.
b) On the midline of the radial surface of the second digit (index finger).
c) Distal to the metacarpo-phalangeal joint of the second digit.
d) Just distal to the flare of the base of the proximal phalanx of the second digit.

Tip:
a) This point is located with the finger slightly flexed.
b) Traditionally at the junction of the change in skin colour, where the palmar skin surface meets the posterior skin surface of the hand.
c) Run your finger with the flow of the channel from LI 1 towards the second metacarpo-phalangeal joint. The base of the proximal phalanx of the second digit begins to flare distal to the joint.
d) The point is located just distal to the flare at the base of the proximal phalanx.

Note: Lawson-Wood (1973) locates X 2 just below the metacarpo-phalangeal articulation on the index finger (thumb side). Worsley (1982) locates X 2 on the posterolateral surface of the index finger, just distal to the base of the proximal phalanx. Academy (1975) clenches the fist to locate the point.

LI 3 SAN JIAN – THIRD INTERVAL

⊥ ***0.3 CUN*** Δ ***3***

- WOOD
- SHU – STREAM/Shu – Transporting/Antique

Pos: Position of patient: supine with the posterior surface of the hand partially pronated (the first and second digits only visible). The hand should be in a relaxed position so the fingers are curving slightly.

Loc:
a) On the posterior surface of the hand.
b) On the radial side of the second metacarpal.
c) Proximal to the second metacarpo-phalangeal joint.
d) Proximal to the flare of the head of the second metacarpal bone.
e) Between the head of the second metacarpal and the first dorsal interosseous muscle.

Tip:
a) The heads of the metacarpal bones are the "knuckles" of the hand.
b) When a loose fist is made the point lies in a hollow between the head of the second metacarpal and the first dorsal interosseous muscle.
c) To expose the first interosseous muscle on the hand, firmly oppose the second digit against the first digit (index finger and thumb).

LI 4 HE GU – JOINING OF THE VALLEYS

⊥ ***0.3 TO 0.7 CUN*** Δ ***3 TO 7***

ALWAYS FORBIDDEN TO NEEDLE AND MOXA THIS POINT DURING PREGNANCY

- SOURCE/Yuan/Regulator/Primary
- ENTRY
- PATIENT BLACKOUT DURING ACUPUNCTURE TREATMENT
- RE-UNION/Crossing/Meeting Point of the Large Intestine Channel with the Lung Channel – Hand Yang Ming Channel with the Hand Tai Yin Channel
- CENTRE RE-UNION/Crossing/Meeting/General Point of Yang
- GREATER INFLUENTIAL /Greater Assembling Point of the Face and Mouth
- COUSIN in association with St 36
- ORIGINAL (one of 5 points for specific symptoms, the others are: St 42, SI 4, Bl 64 and GB 40)
- HOST/GUEST COMBINATION – Source Point with the Junction Point of its Paired Official/Organ
  Therefore LI 4 is combined with Lu 7
- ONE OF THE HEAVENLY STAR POINTS OF MA DAN-YANG (the others are: Lu 7, LI 11, St 36, St 44, Bl 40, Bl 57, Bl 60, Ht 5, GB 34, GB 39 and Liv 3)

Pos: Position of patient: supine with the posterior surface of the hand partially pronated so that the first and second digits are only visible. The hand should be in a relaxed position.

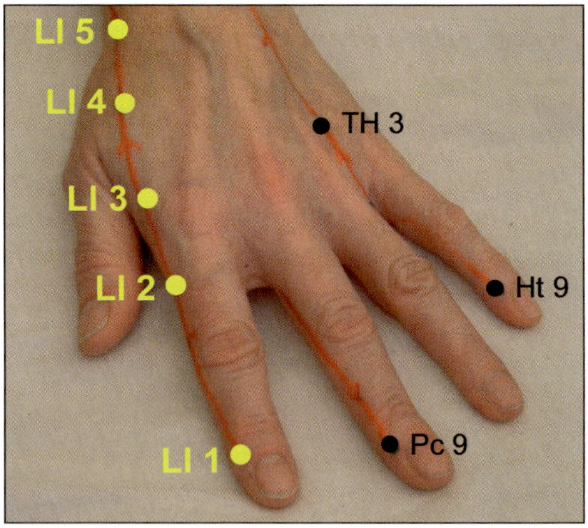

Loc: a) On the posterior surface of the hand.
b) Between the proximal ends of the first and second metacarpal bones.
c) Just distal to the flare of the base of the second metacarpal bone, on its radial surface.

Tip: a) To locate this point run your finger with the flow of the channel from LI 1 along the radial surface of the second metacarpal bone towards the junction of the bases of the first and second metacarpal bones.
b) Feel where the base of the second metacarpal begins to flare, this is just before where the bones meet.
c) The point lies just distal to the flare in the space between the bases of the first and second metacarpal bones.
d) The point lies slightly nearer to the radial border of the second metacarpal bone than the ulnar border of the first metacarpal bone.

Note: The Chinese currently locate LI 4 at the mid-point of the radial border of the second metacarpal bone, but there have been numerous historical and regional locations. Academy (1975) locates LI 4 in this position. Worsley (1982) locates X 4 on the dorsal surface of the hand, in the angle between the proximal ends of the first and second metacarpal bones. Jayasuriya (1982) locates LI 4 in the web between the forefinger and the thumb on the dorsal (posterior) aspect of the hand. Soulié (1994) locates LI 4 on the dorsal hand; between the superior (posterior) heads of the first and second metacarpals, just between the head of the metacarpal of the thumb and the dorsoradial artery; in a hollow; on the superior edge of a small ligament; two FW (Finger Width) above LI 3; two FW below LI 5. Cheng (1987) locates LI 4 on the dorsum of the hand, between the 1st and 2nd metacarpal bones, approximately in the middle of the 2nd metacarpal bone on the radial side.

Shandong (1982) locate Hegu (LI 4) on the middle point of the os metacarpale II, on the prominence of the 1st m. interossel dorsales slightly towards the side of the index. Lawson-Wood (1973) locates X 4 on the dorsum of the hand, in the angle formed by the first and second metacarpals. Legge (1999) locates LI 4 in the dorsal web space, between the 1st and 2nd metacarpal bones, approximately level with the midpoint of the 2nd metacarpal bone. Also – on the highest point of the bulge formed when the thumb is adducted. Lotan (2000) locates LI 4 on the dorsal side of the hand, in the depression, between the two heads of the first dorsal interosseous muscle, level with the midpoint (between head and base) of the second metacarpal.

Qiu (1996) locates LI 4 on the dorsum of the hand between the 1st and 2nd metacarpal bones, approximately in the middle of the 2nd metacarpal bone on the radial side. So (1985) locates LI 4 at the highest point on the muscle of the hand between the thumb and the first finger when the thumb and first finger are pressed together.

Shanghai (1993) locate LI 4 on the dorsum of the hand, between the 1st and 2nd metacarpal bones, approximatley in the centre of the 2nd metacarpal bone. Eachou (1995) locates LI 4 on the dorsum of the hand, between the first and second metacarpals at the midpoint of the radial margin of the second metacarpal bone. Alternative method: ask the patient to adduct the thumb and the index finger; the point is located at the highest spot of the first and second metacarpal muscles.

Ellis (1991) locate LI 4 in the centre of the flesh between the 1st and 2nd metacarpal bones, slightly closer to the 2nd metacarpal bone. If the transvers crease of the interphalangeal joint of the thumb of one hand is lined up with the margin of the web between the thumb and the index finger of the other hand, the point is where the tip of the thumb touches. Li (1991) locates LI 4 between the 1st and 2nd metacarpal bones. It can be located by following three methods: 1) Open the thumb and index finger, then put the transverse crease of the thumb of one hand on the midpoint of the extended margin between the thumb and index finger of the other. The place to which the tip of the thumb extends is LI 4; 2) a perpendicular crease will appear if the thumb and index finger are tightened, alongside of which there is a muscular process. The point is on the top of the muscle level with the end of the perpendicular crease; and 3) with the thumb and index finger separated, the point will be half way along the line linking the conjunction of the 1st and 2nd metacarpal bones and the midpoint of the margin of the web between the thumb and the index finger.

LI 5 YANG XI – YANG STREAM

⊥ ***0.3 TO 0.5 CUN*** Δ ***3 TO 5***

- FIRE
- JING – RIVER/Shu – Transporting/Antique

Pos: Position of patient: supine with the posterior surface of the hand partially pronated so that the first and second digits are only visible.

Loc:
a) On the radial surface at the flexure of the wrist.
b) Between the tip of the styloid process of the radius and the scaphoid bone.
c) Between the tendons of the extensor pollicis longus and extensor pollicis brevis muscles, (in the anatomical snuff box).

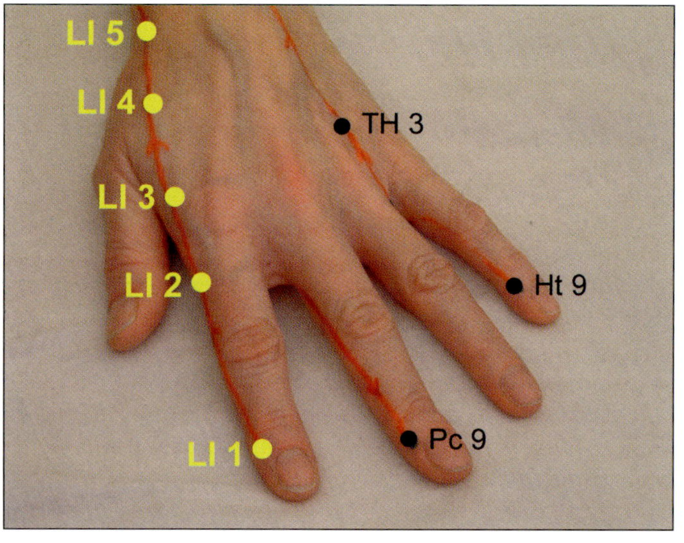

Tip:
a) Run your finger with the flow of the channel from LI 1, along the radial surface of the second digit and second metacarpal bone. Go proximal to the base of the second metacarpal bone into the anatomical snuff box at the wrist flexure.
b) To expose the anatomical snuff box, extend the thumb so the tendons of the extensor pollicis longus and extensor pollicis brevis muscles are exposed.
c) With your finger in the snuff box feel for the flexure of the wrist by abducting and adducting the wrist. You will be able to feel the gap between the styloid process of the radius and the scaphoid bones.
d) The point is located in the deepest part of the anatomical snuff box, between the tip of the styloid process of the radius and the scaphoid bone.

Note: Shandong (1982) locate Yangxi on the radial end of the dorsal crease of the wrist, when the thumb is tilted upward, it is in the depression between tendons of the m. extensor pollicis longus and brevis m.

LI 6 to LI 11 points are marked with the patient supine or seated with the forearm positioned so that the palmar surface of the hand and the anterior surface of the forearm are against the torso with the elbow flexed at 90 degrees. The distance between LI 5 and LI 11 is measured as 12 cun.

To mark out the cun measurements, keeping the elbow flexed at 90 degrees, draw a line from LI 5 across the posterior surface of the wrist to LI 11 on the lateral side of the flexure of the elbow, then measure 12 cun.

LI 6 to LI 11 lie on the posterior aspect of the forearm, on the posterior aspect of the radius.

LI 6 PIAN LI – SIDE PASSAGE

⊥ ***0.3 TO 0.5 CUN*** Δ ***3 TO 7***

- JUNCTION/Luo/Connecting/Passage/Lo/Lê
- RE-UNION/Crossing/Meeting Point of the Large IntestineChannel with the Lung Channel – Hand Yang Ming Channel with the Hand Tai Yin Channels
- HOST/GUEST COMBINATION – Source Point with the Junction Point of its Paired Official/Organ
  Therefore LI 6 is combined with Lu 9

Pos: Position of patient: supine or seated with the forearm positioned so that the palmar surface of the hand and the anterior surface of the forearm are against the torso with the elbow flexed at 90 degrees

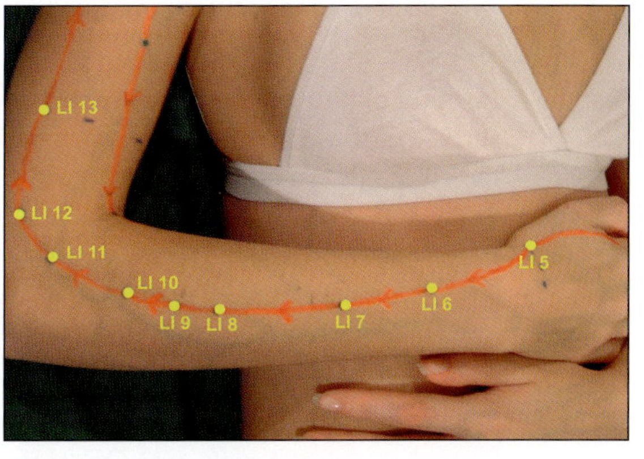

Loc: a) On the posterior aspect of the forearm.
b) On the ulnar aspect of the radius.
c) On the line connecting LI 5 with LI 11.
d) 3 cun proximal to LI 5 (wrist flexure).
e) On the intersection formed by the ulnar side of the radius and the seam between the extensor pollicis brevis and the abductor pollicis longus muscles.

Tip: a) The distance between LI 5 and LI 11 is 12 cun, this point is 3 cun proximal to LI 5.
b) Run your finger from LI 5 along the ulnar side of the radius into the seam formed by the extensor pollicis brevis and the abductor pollicis longus muscles.
c) When you follow this line with your finger to the 3 cun measurement a large men can be palpated.
d) The seam formed by these two muscles will be felt more easily by extending and flexing the thumb.

Note: Traditionally, to locate this point the elbow is in a flexed position with the radial side of the arm uppermost. The traditional description for this point is at 3 cun proximal to LI 5, but does not mention any anatomical features, only that this point lies on the line connecting LI 5 to LI 11, Academy (1975) describes the point 3 cun above LI 5. Voisin (1974) locates LI 6 on the forearm, posteriior aspect, close to the radius: 4 fb (finger breadth) proximal to the dorsiflexion fold of the wrist.

Deadman (1998) also locates the point using the 3 cun measurement and the line between LI 5 and LI 11. Soulié (1994) locates LI 6 on the dorsal side of the forearm (palm up, supination; three FW (Finger Width) above the wrist; at the angle of the medial (ulnar) edge of the radius and the inferior edge of the transverse prominence (inferior insertion of the flexor longus?) of the thumb; between the bone and the supinator longus; separated from LI 5 by the head of the radius; three FW under LI 7. Masayoshi (1975) locates LI 6 at the lower 1/3rd of the dorsal side of the foreearm.

LI 7 WEN LIU – WARM CURRENT

⊥ ***0.3 TO 0.8 CUN*** Δ ***3 TO 30***

- ACCUMULATION/Xi Cleft/Gueki

Pos: Position of patient: supine or seated with the forearm positioned so that the palmar surface of the hand and the anterior surface of the forearm are against the torso with the elbow flexed at 90 degrees.

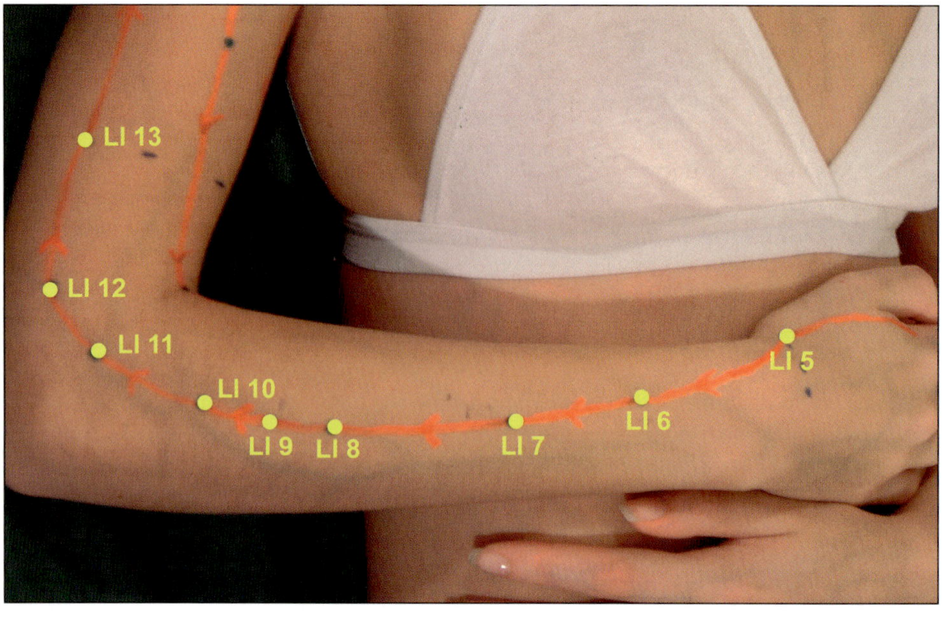

Loc: a) On the posterior aspect of the forearm.
b) On the ulnar aspect of the radius.
c) On the line connecting LI 5 with LI 11.
d) In the seam between the extensor digitorum and the extensor carpi radialis muscles.
e) 5 cun proximal to LI 5 (wrist flexure).
f) 7 cun distal to LI 11 (transverse cubital crease).

Tip: a) The distance between LI 5 and LI 11 is 12 cun, this point is 5 cun proximal to LI 5.
b) To expose the seam between the extensor digitorum and the extensor carpi radialis muscles flex and extend the digits (wiggle the fingers). You should feel the extensor digitorum muscle move. The seam is located on the radial side of this muscle.
c) To locate this point lightly place your finger along this seam with the direction of the flow of the channel towards the elbow until you are at 5 cun proximal to the wrist flexure.
d) Palpating the point is more accurate than the cun measurement which only provides an area for palpation.

Note: This point has traditionally been placed at either 5 or 6 cun above the flexure of the wrist. Traditionally, to locate this point the elbow is in a flexed position with the radial side of the arm uppermost. The traditional description gives this point at 5 cun proximal to LI 5, but does not mention any anatomical features, only that this point lies on the line connecting LI 5 to LI 11. Voisin (1974), locates LI 7 at on the forearm, posterior aspect, 6-7 fb (finger breadth) proximal to the wrist, (about midway along the radius).

Worsley (1982) locates X 7 on the posterior radial surface of the forearm, 7 ACI (Anatomical Chinese Inch) proximal to the flexure of the wrist.. With the anterior surface of the forearm across the chest, the point lies on the radial border of the extensor digitorum. Lavier (1974) on an illustration locates this point at 7 pouce proximal to LI 5. Wu (1962) locates CO 7 upon the posterior-external surface of the forearm, seven pounce below the flexure of the wrist. With the hand pronate, the point lies at the cubital side of the radius.

Katsusuke (1983) locates LI 7 on the thumb side of the arm at a point half way between the wrist and the elbow. Soulié (1994) locates LI 7 on the forearm, palm up, supination; six FW (Finger Width) above the wrist (mid-length of the forearm); at the angle of the anterior edge of the bone and of the inferior edge of a transverse eminence; between the supinator and flexor longus of the thumb; in a hollow; on the posterior edge of the supinator longus; on the anterior edge of the posterior radial artery coming from the posterior side; palm down (pronation), on the ulnar edge of the radius; 3 FW proximal to LI 6; one FW under LI 8, at the level of TW 9.

So (1985) locates LI 7 at 3 divisions above LI 6, along the outer edge of the radial bone, following the Large Intestine line up to the elbow. Ellis (1991) locates LI 7 with the ulna facing down and the elbow flexed, this point is 5" above LI 5. Locate the point while making a fist. Li (1991) locates LI 7 at two cun above LI 6 on the lateral side of the radius. Masayoshi (1975) locates LI 7 onthe centre of the radius of the extending side of the forearm.

LI 8 XIA LIAN – LOWER SIDE

⊥ *0.4 TO 0.8 CUN* Δ *3 TO 7*

Pos: Position of patient: supine or seated with the forearm positioned so that the palmar surface of the hand and the anterior surface of the forearm are against the torso with the elbow flexed at 90 degrees.

Loc:
a) On the posterior aspect of the forearm.
b) On the ulnar aspect of the radius.
c) On the line connecting LI 5 with LI 11.
d) In the seam between the extensor digitorum and the extensor carpi radialis muscles.
e) 8 cun proximal to LI 5 (wrist flexure).
f) 4 cun distal to LI 11 (transverse cubital crease).

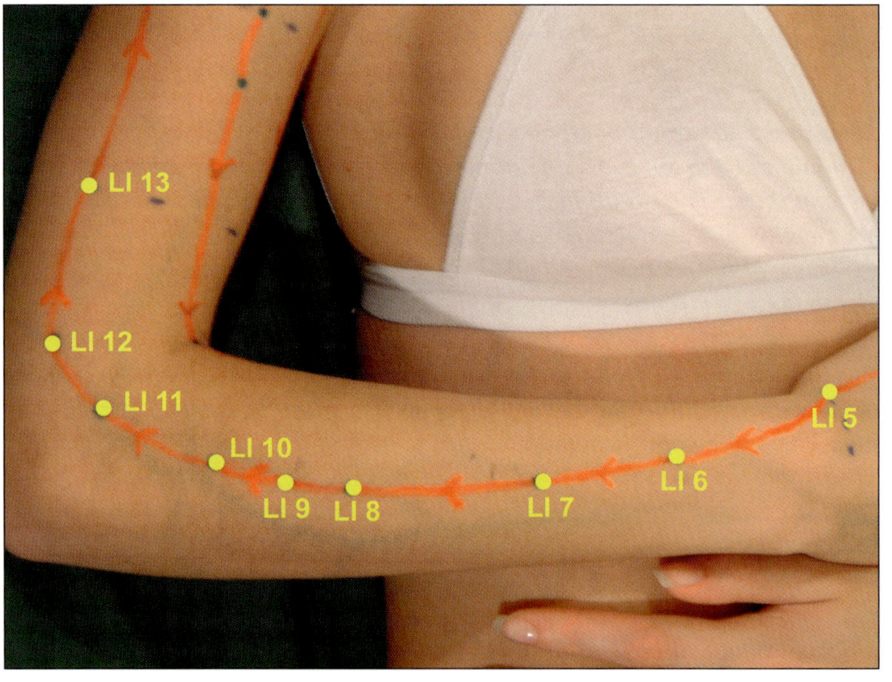

Tip
a) The distance between LI 5 and LI 11 is 12 cun, this point is 8 cun proximal to LI 5.
b) To expose the seam between the extensor digitorum and the extensor carpi radialis muscles flex and extend the digits (wiggle the fingers). You should feel the extensor digitorum muscle move. The seam is located on the radial side of this muscle.
c) To locate this point lightly place your finger along this seam with the direction of the flow of the channel towards the elbow until you are at 8 cunproximal to the wrist flexure.
d) Palpating the point is more accurate than the cun measurement which only provides an area for palpation.

Note: Traditionally, to locate this point the elbow should be in a flexed position with the radial side of the arm uppermost. The traditional description gives this point at 8 cun proximal to LI 5, but does not mention any anatomical features, only that this point lies on the line connecting LI 5 to LI 11. Wu (1973) locates CO 8 upon the posterior-external surface of the forearm, on the extensor digitorum communis, four pouce below the radial extremity of the flexure of the elbow. Voisin (1974) locates LI 8 on the forearm, posterior aspect, 1.5 fb (finger breadth) proximal to Large Intestine 7.

Soulié (1994) locates LI 8 on the forearm, palm up, in supination: seven FW (Finger Width) above the wrist (five large FW below the head of the radius). Just at the anterior edge of the radius with the supinator longus; at the angle of the inferior edge of a transverse eminence (the inferior insertion of the shorter supinator); in a hollow; on the inferior edge of the insertion of the pronator; one FW above LI 7; 1 FW under LI 9. So (1985) locates LI 8 at 2 divisions above LI 7 on top of the muscle.

Li (1991) locates LI 8 at three cun above LI 7 and 4 cun below LI 11. Huang (1993) locates LI 8 at the radius one cun distal to Upper Ridge (LI 9). in a fissure within the external irregular (external oblique) and muscles. Masayoshi (1975) locates LI 8 at the mid portion of LI 7 and LI 9.

LI 9 SANG LIAN - UPPER ANGLE

⊥ 0.3 TO 0.8 CUN ∆ 3 TO 10

Pos: Position of patient: supine or seated with the forearm positioned so that the palmar surface of the hand and the anterior surface of the forearm are against the torso with the elbow flexed at an angle of 90 degrees.

Loc:
a) On the posterior aspect of the forearm.
b) On the ulnar aspect of the radius.
c) On the line connecting LI 5 with LI 11.
c) In the seam between the extensor digitorum and the extensor carpi radialis muscles.
d) 9 cun proximal to LI 5 (wrist flexure).
e) 3 cun distal to LI 11 (transverse cubital crease).

Tip
a) The distance between LI 5 and LI 11 is 12 cun, this point is 9 cun proximal to LI 5.
b) To expose the seam between the extensor digitorum and the extensor carpi radialis muscles flex and extend the digits (wiggle the fingers). You should feel the extensor digitorum muscle move. The seam is located on the radial side of this muscle.
c) To locate this point easily lightly place your finger along this seam with the direction of the flow of the channel towards the elbow until you are at 9 cun proximal to the wrist flexure.
d) Palpating the point is more accurate than the cun measurement which only provides an area for palpation.

Note: Traditionally, to locate this point the elbow is in a flexed position with the radial side of the arm uppermost. The traditional description gives this point at 9 cun proximal to LI 5, but does not mention any anatomical features, only that this point lies on the line connecting LI 5 to LI 11. Wu (1973) locates CO 9 upon the dorsal surface of the forearm upon the extensor digitorum communis at three pouce below the radial extremity of the flexure of the elbow. Voisin (1974) locates LI 9 on the forearm, posterior aspect, 3 fb (finger breadth) proximal to Large Intestine 7. Li (1991) locates LI 9 at one cun above LI 8 and 3 cun below LI 11 lateral to the radius.

Huang (1993) locates LI 9 at the radius one cun distal to Three Li (LI 10) at the place where the external oblique (muscle) meets the yang (ming vessel). Masayoshi (1975) locates LI 9 on the upper 1/3rd of the radial extending side of the forearm. Soulié (1994) locates LI 9 on the forearm, thumb up: four FW (Finger Width) from the head of the radius (under the epicondyle). Just at the edge of the anterior angle of the radius; on the radial edge of the internal radial muscle; deep to the superior edge of the insertion of the flexor longus of the thumb; in a hollow; one FW above LI 8; two FW below LI 10.

LI 10 SHOU SAN LI – ARM THREE MILES

⊥ ***0.3 TO 1.0 CUN*** △ ***3 TO 10***

Pos: Position of patient: supine or seated with the forearm positioned so that the palmar surface of the hand and the anterior surface of the forearm are against the torso with the elbow flexed at an angle of 90 degrees.

Loc:
a) On the posterior aspect of the forearm.
b) On the ulnar aspect of the radius.
c) In the seam between the extensor digitorum and the extensor carpi radialis muscles.
d) 10 cun proximal to LI 5, on the line connecting LI 5 with LI 11.
e) 2 cun distal to LI 11.

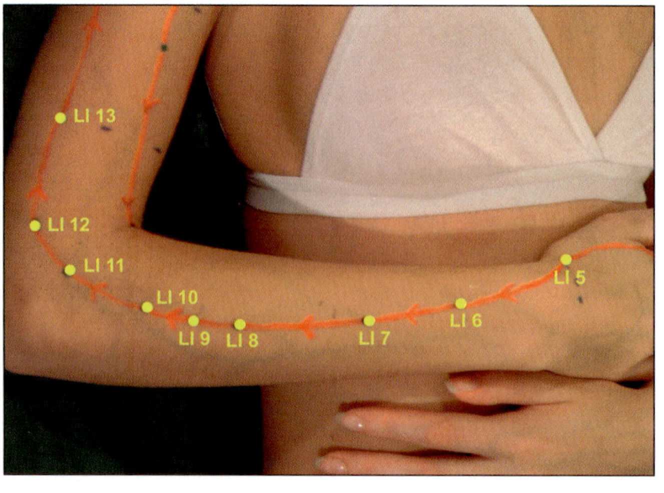

Tip
a) The distance between LI 5 and LI 11 is 12 cun, this point is 10 cun proximal to LI 5.
b) To expose the seam between the extensor digitorum and the extensor carpi radialis muscles flex and extend the digits (wiggle the fingers). You should feel the extensor digitorum muscle move. The seam is located on the radial side of this muscle.
c) To locate this point easily lightly place your finger along this seam with the direction of the flow of the channel towards the elbow until you are at 10 cun proximal to the wrist flexure.
d) Palpating the point is more accurate than the cun measurement which only provides an area for palpation.

Note: Traditionally, to locate this point the elbow is in a flexed position with the radial side of the arm uppermost. The traditional description gives this point at 10 cun proximal to LI 5, but does not mention any anatomical features, only that this point lies on the line connecting LI 5 to LI 11. Wu (1973) locates CO 10 upon the dorsal surface of the forearm upon the extensor digitorum communis at two pouce below the radial extremity of the flexure of the elbow. Voisin (1974) locates LI 10 on the forearm, posterior aspect, 3 fb (finger breadth) distal to the lateral extremity of the elbow flexion fold.

Katsusuke (1983) locates LI 10 on the thumb side of the forearm in line with the index finger and two sun from the bend of the elbow. Legge (1999) locates LI 10 at 2 cun LI 11 on a line connecting LI 11 and LI 5, over the often tender tendon of extensor carpi radialis brevis. Eachou (1995) locates LI 10 with the elbow flexed, the point is located on the radial side of the elbow on the line between LI 11 and LI 5, and 2 inches below LI 11; or clenching the hand firmly and flexing the elbow, the point is located in the fossa of the brachioradialis muscle. Huang (1993) locates LI 10 one cun distal to Pool at the Bend (LI 11) at a place where pressure causes the end of a tapering muscle to be raised up.

Soulié (1994) locates LI 10 on the forearm, thumb up; two large FW (Finger Width) under the round head of the radius (which is above the epicondyle). On the posterior edge of the sharp edge of the radius; just in the angle of a curve of the radius; between the two radial muscles, above a transverse bulge; deep to the short supinator. Palm down (pornation); ulnar edge of the radius; two FW above LI 9; one large FW under LI 11. Separated by the supinator longus from LU 5.

LI 11 QU CHI – CROOKED POND

⊥ ***0.5 TO 1.0 CUN*** △ ***3 TO 10***

- EARTH
- TONIFICATION/Reinforcing
- MOTHER
- HE – SEA/Shu – Transporting/Antique
- ONE OF THE HEAVENLY STAR POINTS OF MA DAN-YANG (the others are: Lu 7, LI 4, St 36, St 44, Bl 40, Bl 57, Bl 60, Ht 5, GB 34, GB 39 and Liv 3)
- SUN SI-MIAO GHOST (Gui) – Ghost Point Name: Gui Tui – Ghost Leg or Ghost Minister

Pos: Position of patient: supine or seated with the forearm positioned so that the palmar surface of the hand and the anterior surface of the forearm are against the torso with the elbow flexed at an angle of 90 degrees.

Loc: a) On the posterior aspect of the forearm.
b) On the ulnar aspect of the radius.
c) Approximately half way between the lateral edge of the tendon of the biceps brachii muscle and the lateral epicondyle of the humerus.
d) Towards the lateral end of the transverse cubital crease.

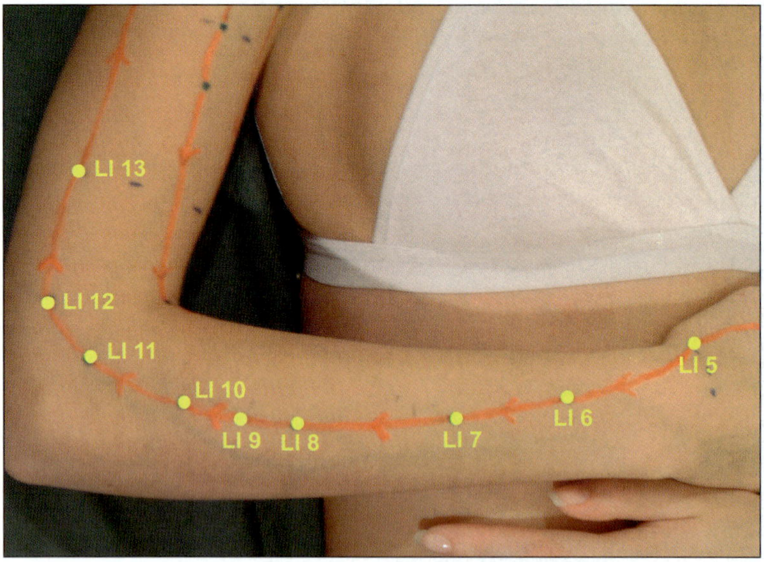

Tip: a) There is a lot of confusion on where to locate this point. In clinical practice the point does not always lie halfway between the tendon of the biceps brachii and the lateral epicondyle of the humerus because of the variable width of the tendon of the biceps brachii.

b) The transverse cubital crease varies so much in terms of its visibility and length, therefore using the lateral end of this crease as a landmark is only an approximation.
c) The best way to locate this point is to run your finger along the valley formed by the seam between the extensor digitorum and the extensor carpi radialis muscles. If you follow this valley it automatically takes you to the correct place on the transverse cubital crease. When you have done this you will need to palpate for the point.
d) Another way of locating this point is to place your finger on the olecranon, moving ove the lateral epicondyle of the humerus towards the transverse cubital crease. It is in the first available soft area when you have passed over the lateral epicondyle of the humerus.

Note: Jayasuirya (1982) locates LI 11 as above. He also locates this point midway between Lu 5 and the lateral epicondyle of the humerus. Cheng (1987) locates LI 11 with the elbow flexed, the point is in the depression at the lateral end of the transverse cubital crease, midway between L 5 (Lu 5) and the lateral epicondyle of the humerus. Worsley (1982) locates X 11 on the posterior radial surface of the forearm. With the anterior surface of the forearm across the chest, the point lies between the lateral end of the elbow crease and the lateral epicondyle of the humerus. Katsusuke (1983) locates LI 11 on the thumb side of the bend of the elbow. Legge (1999) locates LI 11 with the elbow flexed, the point is found midway between Lu 5 and the lateral epicondyle of the humerus. Also – at the lateral end of the elbow crease. Lotan (2000) locates LI 11 with the elbow in the flexed position, midway between Lu 5 and the humerus lateral epicondyle tip.

Soulié (1994) locates LI 11 with the elbow flexed, on the lateral side (extensors): in the radiohumeral articulation; in the angle of the superior edge of the round head of the radius, below the epicondyle and of the deep condyle of the humerus. When the elbow is extended, the point is covered by the supinator longus, which is on the anterior edge; one FW (Finger Width) above and in front of LI 10, four FW below LI 12; three FW anterior to Lu 5. Qiu (1996) locates LI 11 with the elbow flexed at a right angle, the point is in the depression at the lateral end of the transverse cubital crease, midway between Lu 5 and the lateral epicondyle of the humerus. Shanghai (1981) locate LI 11 with the arm flexed at the elbow, this point can be found midway between the end of the transverse crease of the elbow and the lateral epicondyle of the humerus.

Lawson-Wood (1973) locates X 11 on the antero-extern of the elbow, exactly at the extremity of the elbow-fold in hyperflexion. So (9185) locates LI 11 at the outer crease between the humerus and radius. Bend the arm resting the hand flat on the centre of the chest; at the highest part of the muscle is the point. If the patient is very thin, you cannot see this muscle; then the point will be found one division up toward the elbow crease from the meeting of the two bones. Shanghai (1993) locate LI 11 at the midpoint of the line between the radial end of the cubital crease and the external humeral epicondyle.

Eachou (1995) locates LI 11 with the elbow flexed at 90 degrees, the point is located at the anterior lateral elbow joint, in the midpoint between the radial side of the skin crease of the elbow and the lateral epicondyle of the humerus. Ellis (1991) locate LI 11 with the elbow flexed, in the depression at the lateral end of the transverse cubital crease, midway between LU 5 and the lateral epicondyle of the humerus. Li (1991) locates LI 11 on the lateral side of the transverse crease of the elbow approximately midway between Lu 5 and the lateral epicondyle of the humerus. Huang (1993) locates LI 11 between the elbow bones at the outer side of the elbow. Masayoshi (1975) locates LI 11 at one cun, exterior to the lateral epicondyle of the humerus, starting point of the brachial muscle; in a depression when the elbow is flexed.

LI 12-15 are on the lateral aspect of the upper arm, LI 16 on the superior aspect of the shoulder. There are 9 cun between the axillary fold and the transverse cubital crease.

To locate LI 12 to LI 15, with the patient supine or seated, with the forearm positioned so that the palmar surface of the hand and the anterior surface of the forearm are against the torso with the elbow flexed at an angle of 90 degrees. LI 16 can be located with the patient seated and the arms at the side.

Alternatively, with the patient supine, the forearm can be extended and partially pronated so that the radial border of the radius is uppermost.

LI 12 ZHOU LIAO – ELBOW BONE

⊥ ***0.3 TO 0.8 CUN*** △ ***3***

Pos: Position of patient: supine or seated with the forearm positioned so that the palmar surface of the hand and the anterior surface of the forearm are against the torso with the elbow flexed at an angle of 90 degrees. Alternatively, with the patient supine, the forearm can be extended and partially pronated so that the radial border of the radius is uppermost.

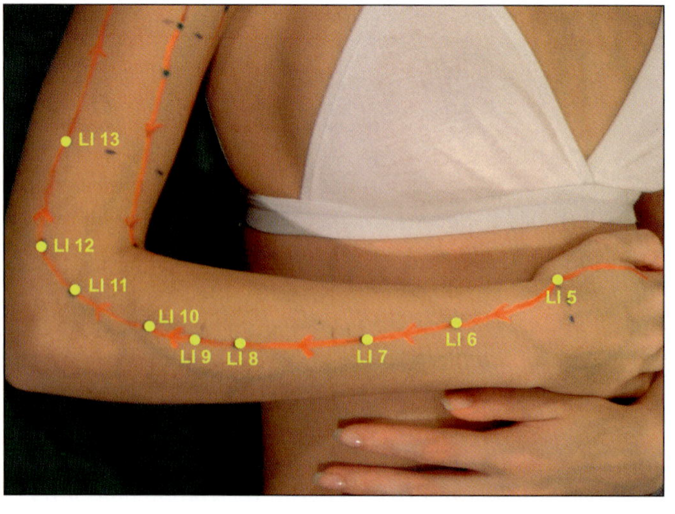

Loc: a) On the lateral aspect of the upper arm.
b) Superior to the lateral epicondyle of the humerus.
c) 1 cun proximal to LI 11, on the lateral border of the humerus.
d) On the anterior border of the triceps brachii muscle, when the arm is positioned as outlined above.

Tip: a) The distance between the transverse cubital crease and the axillary fold is 9 cun (where the upper arm joins the torso).
b) Run your finger from LI 11 proximally along the border of the humerus on the lateral surface of the upper arm towards the shoulder.
c) The point lies between the lateral surface of the humerus and the anterior border of the triceps brachii muscle, approximately 1 cun proximal to the flexure of the elbow at LI 11.
d) To expose the anterior border of the triceps brachii muscle ask the patient to press the hand and forearm down against resistance. This can be done with the elbow either in the flexed or extended position.

Note: This point has historically been located at both 1 and 2 cun above LI 11. Traditionally described as being 1 cun proximal to and 1 cun lateral to LI 11. It is also described as being superior to the lateral epicondyle of the humerus and anterior to the supracondylar ridge, or in a depression on the outer aspect of the large bone. Lavier (1974) measures 7 pouce from the elbow fold to the deltoid 'V'. Wu (1973) locates CO 12 upon the lateral surface of the arm, at two pouces above the flexure of the elbow. Worsley (1982) locates X 12 on the lateral surface of the arm, 2 ACI (Anatomical Chinese Inch) proximal to the lateral epicondyle of the humerus. Voisin (1974) locates LI 12 on the arm, posterolateral aspect: 2 fb (finger breadth) proximal to Large Intestine 11. Jayasuriya (1982) locates LI 12 with the arm extended, 2 cun proximal to LI 11; with the elbow semiflexed, about 1 cun superolateral to LI 11 and superior to the lateral epicondyle of the humerus on the medial border of the humerus. Cheng (1987) locates LI 12 with the elbow flexed, superior to the lateral epicondyle of the humerus, about 1 cun superolateral to LI 11, on the medial border of the humerus.

Soulié (1994) locates LI 12 on the lateral side of the arm: two FW (Finger Width) above the lateral epicondyle of the elbow, at the angle of the anterior edge of the humerus and the posterior, inferior edge of the muscle at an angle (brachialis anterior); four FW above LI 11; two FW below LI 13; two FW in front of TW 11; three FW posterior to LU 4. Qiu (1996) locates LI 12 when the elbow is flexed, the point is superior to the lateral epicondyle of the humerus, about 1 cun supero-lateral to LI 11, on the medial border of the humerus. So (1985) locates LI 12 one division slanting outwards from LI 11 in the corner of the humerus and radial bone; to locate this point, put the hand on the chest and bend the arm. Masayoshi (1975) locates LI 12 in a portion just above the lateral epicondyle of the humerus.

LI 13 SHOU WU LI – ARM FIVE MILES

⊥ ***0.5 CUN*** Δ ***3 TO 7***

Pos: Position of patient: supine or seated with the forearm positioned so that the palmar surface of the hand and the anterior surface of the forearm are against the torso with the elbow flexed at an angle of 90 degrees. Alternatively, with the patient supine, the forearm can be extended and partially pronated so that the radial border of the radius is uppermost.

Loc: a) On the lateral aspect of the upper arm.
b) Superior to the lateral epicondyle of the humerus.
c) On the line joining LI 11 and LI 15.
d) 3 cun proximal to the flexure of the elbow at LI 11.
e) Between the anterior border of the triceps brachii muscle and the lateral border of the humerus.

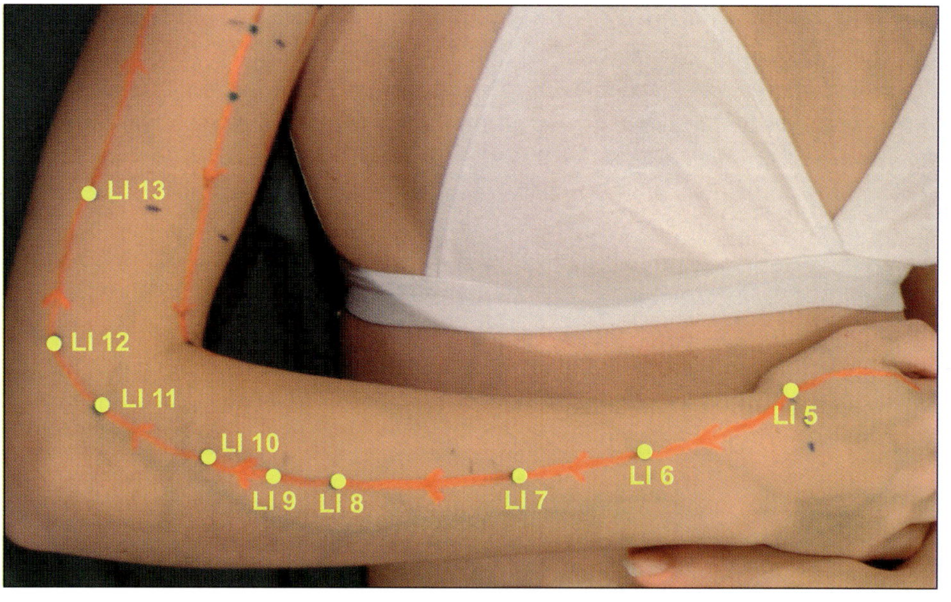

Tip: a) The distance between the transverse cubital crease and the axillary fold is 9 cun (where the upper arm joins the torso).
b) Run your finger from LI 11 proximally along the border of the humerus on the lateral surface of the upper arm towards the shoulder.
c) The point lies between the lateral surface of the humerus and the anterior border of the triceps brachii muscle, approximately 3 cun proximal to the flexure of the elbow at LI 11.
d) To expose the anterior border of the triceps brachii muscle ask the patient to press the hand and forearm down against resistance. This can be done with the elbow either in the flexed or extended position.

Note: Wu (1973) locates LI 13 on the lateral surface of the arm, at three and one half pouce from the flexure of the elbow. Lavier (1974) also demonstrates this on a diagram. He measures 7 pouce from the elbow fold to the deltoid 'V'. Worsley (1982) locates X 13 on the lateral surface of the arm, 3.5 ACI (Anatomical Chinese Inch) proximal to the lateral epicondyle of the humerus. Academy (1975) locates LI 13 on the antero-medial border of the humerus, also using the 3 cun measurement proximal to the elbow crease.

Deadman (1998) locate the point with the upper arm level with the shoulder (transverse) and the lower arm at right angles (vertically downwards). The point is then between the lateral border of the biceps brachii muscle and the humerus bone, 1 hand breadth superior to LI 11. or one third distance between LI 11 and the axillary fold. Vosin (1974) locates LI 13 on the arm, posterolateral aspect: 3fb (finger breadth) proximal to Large Intestine 11. Soulié (1994) locates LI 13 on the lateral side of the arm; five FW (Finger Width) above the lateral apicondyle of the elbow; on the humerus; on the anterior edge of the external posterior bony prominence of the humerus; on the inferior edge of the large opposite tendinous insertion of the brachialis and deltoid; two FW above LI 12; three FW under LI 14; three FW posterior to LU 4.

LI 14 BI NAO – OUTER BONE OF THE ARM

⊥ ***0.3 TO 0.7 CUN*** △ ***3 TO 7***

- RE-UNION/Crossing/Meeting Point of the Large Intestine Channel with the Small Intestine and Bladder Channels and the Yang Linking Vessel – Hand Yang Ming Channel with the Hand Tai Yang, and Foot Tai Yang Channels and the Yang Wei Mai

Pos: Position of patient: supine or seated with the forearm positioned so that the palmar surface of the hand and the anterior surface of the forearm are against the torso with the elbow flexed at an angle of 90 degrees. Alternatively, with the patient supine, the forearm can be extended and partially pronated so that the radial border of the radius is uppermost.

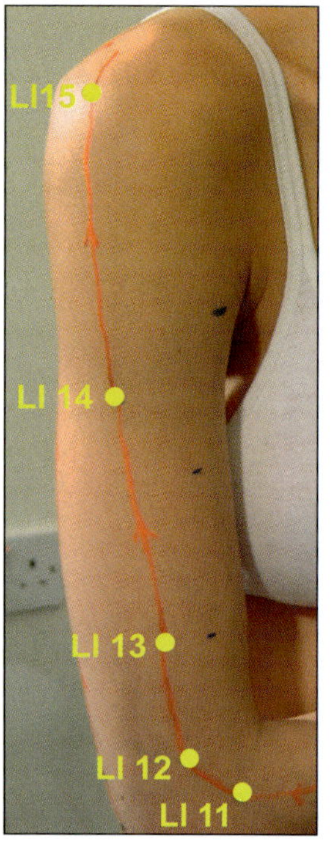

Loc: a) On the lateral aspect of the upper arm.
b) Superior to the lateral epicondyle of the humerus.
c) On the line joining LI 11 and LI 15.
d) Approximately 7 cun proximal to the flexure of the elbow at LI 11.
e) At the insertion('V') of the deltoid into the humerus.

Tip: a) The distance between the transverse cubital crease and the axillary fold is 9 cun (where the upper arm joins the torso).
b) Run your finger from LI 11 proximally along the border of the humerus on the lateral surface of the upper arm towards the shoulder.
c) To expose the deltoid muscle the patients arm needs to be abducted against resistance.
d) The deltoid inserts into the lateral aspect of the humerus at approximately 7 cun proximal to LI 11.

Note: Deadman (1998) locate LI 14 with the upper arm level with the shoulder (transverse) and the lower arm at right angles (vertically downwards). The point is then visible by the insertion of the deltoid muscle and the brachialis muscle. Lavier (1974) measures 7 pouce from the elbow fold to the deltoid 'V'. Katsusuke (1983) locates LI 14 about seven sun above LI 11, on the thumb side of the upper arm, at the place in the upper arm where the triceps muscle gradually narrows to a tendon. Wu (1973) locates CO 14 upon the lateral surface of the arm, seven pouce above the flexure of the elbow and three pouce below the shoulder joint, near the "V" of the deltoid muscle. Shandong (1982) locate Binao (LI 14) on the lateral aspect of the upper arm, slightly anterior to the insertion of the m. deltoideus on the line between Pt. Jianyu (LI 15) and Pt. Quchi (LI 11).

Legge (1999) locates LI 14 anterior and superior to the insertion of the deltoid into the humerus, on the line connecting LI 11 and LI 15. Lotan (2000) locates LI 14 anterior to the deltoid, about 0.5 cun superior (and anterior) ti the (conspicuous) deltoid lower edge. Soulié (1994) locates LI 14 on the lateral aspect of the arm: three FW (Finger Width) below the lower part of the large head of the humerus; six FW below the acromion; on the angle of the anterior edge of the prominence at the mid-length of the humerus and the inferior edge of a transverse insertion (the extremity of the inserton of the pectoralis major, lattisimus dorsi and teres major); between the two bundles of the deltoid muscle; on the upper part of a hollow above the opposed insertions of the deltoid and brachialis anterior; three FW above LI 13; two large FW below and posterior to LI 15; three FW anterior and below TW 12; four FW posterior and below LU 2. Yang (1982) locates LI 14 where the antero-inferior border of the deltoid muscle and the medial border of the humerus meet.

Shanghai (1981) locate LI 14 with the arm hanging freely at the side and the elbow bent, this point may be found slightly anterior to the insertion of the deltoid muscle. So (1985) locates LI 14 on the outside centre line of the arm, three divisions down from LI 15.

Ellis (1991) locate LI 14 on the upper arm, slightly superior to the insertion of the deltoid muscle (m. deltoideus), on the line connecting LI 11 and LI 15. Li (1991) locates LI 14 on the radial side of the humerus, superior to the lower end of m. deltoideus, on the line connecting with LI 11 and LI 15. Masayoshi (1975) locates LI 14 at 3 sun below LI 15 and at the anterior margin of the deltoid muscle.

LI 15 JIAN YU – SHOULDER JOINT

⊥ ***0.5 TO 1.0 CUN*** Δ *7*

- 8 EXTRAORDINARY VESSEL/Coalescent Point of the Yang Heel/Yang Motility Vessel (Yang Qiao Mai)
- RE-UNION/Crossing/Meeting Point of the Large Intestine Channel with the Yang Heel/Yang Motility Vessel – Hand Yang Ming Channel with the Yang Qiao Mai

Pos: Position of patient: supine or seated with the forearm positioned so that the medial surface of the upper arm is against the torso with the elbow flexed at an angle of 90 degrees. Alternatively, with the patient supine, the forearm can be extended and partially pronated so that the radial border of the radius is uppermost.

Loc: a) On the lateral aspect of the shoulder.
b) Inferior to the acromion.
c) Between the acromion process of the scapula bone and the greater tuberosity of the humerus.
d) At the centre of the upper portion of the deltoid muscle.

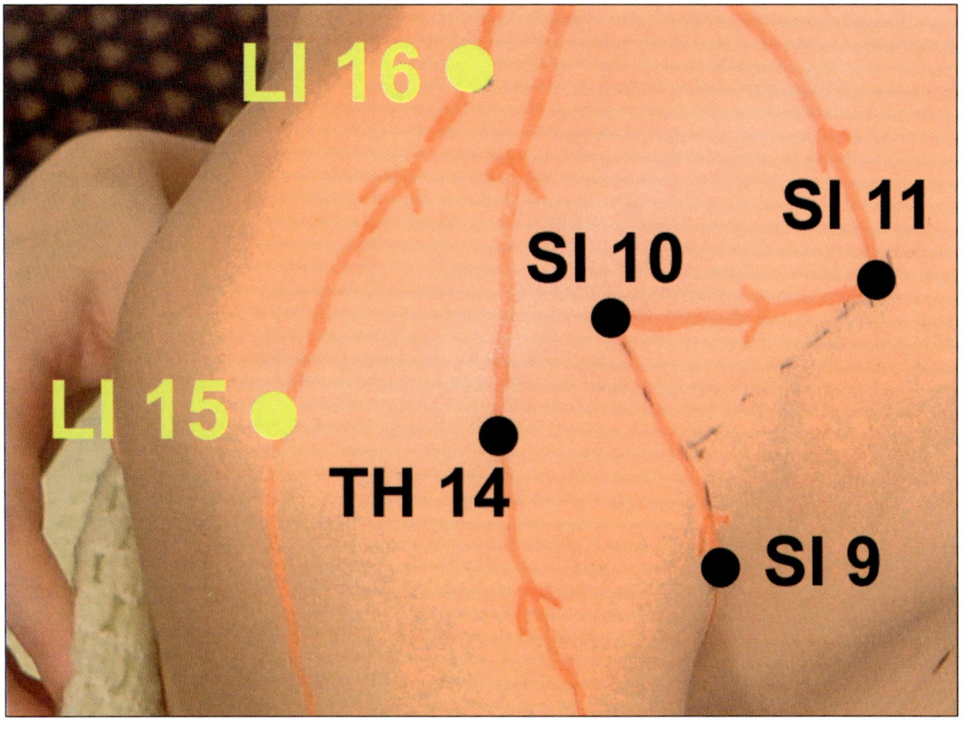

Tip:
a) Run your finger from LI 11 proximally along the border of the humerus on the lateral surface of the upper arm into the centre of the deltoid muscle towards the shoulder.
b) The patients arm needs to be abducted to expose the depression between the acromion and the greater tuberosity of the humerus.
c) LI 15 is located in the depression found in the gap formed when the am is abducted and adducted (the gap will increase and decrease on abduction and adduction).
d) The deltoid muscle becomes more flaccid when the arm is supported at the elbow, making it more easy to feel the underlying bone structure.
e) Ensure that the patients arm is in a relaxed position when needling this point.
f) SI 10, TH 14 and LI 15 are located in relation to the acromion process of the scapula. The acromion forms a scallop shape and these three points lie inferior to it.
g) LI 15 is the most lateral point with TH 14 located approximately 1 cun posterior to this point and SI 10 located approximately 1 cun medial to TH 14, (these points are approximately equidistant to each other).
h) SI 10 is inferior to the neck of the acromion, TH 14 is located on the inferolateral corner of the acromion process, at the acromion angle. LI 15 is inferior to the acromion, betweenthe acromion and the greater tuberosity of the humerus.

Note: Voisin (1974) locates LI 15 on the middle of the deltoid, between four bony prominences: acromion, clavicle, coracoid process and head of humerus. Katsusuke (1983) locates LI 15 at the depression between the tip of the shoulder and the triceps muscle when the arm is held outstretched in a horizontal position. Thumb side of the upper arm at the tip of the acromion process. Legge (1999) locates LI 15 anterior and inferior to the acromion, between the anterior and medial portions of the deltoid. When the arm is adducted, the point is in the anterior of the two depressions appearing lateral to the acromion process. Lotan (2000) locates LI 15 about 0.3 cun inferior to the acromion anteror corner.

Soulié (1994) locates LI 15 on the anterior shoulder; in the hollow between the anterior edge of the clavicle, on the upper medial edge of the humerus, lateral and superior to the prominence of the coracoid process; just in the angle of the apophysis of the humerus; two large FW (Finger Width) above and anterior (medial) to LI 14; three large FW medial and anterior to TW 13; four FW lateral to LU 1. Shanghai (1981) locate LI 15 in the middle of the upper part of the deltoid muscle at the shoulder, between the acromion and greater tubercle of the humerus.

When the arm is abducted parallel to the ground, this point can be found in a distinct depression just in front of the shoulder. Ellis (1991) locate LI 15 inferior to the acromion, and slightly anterior to the middle of the upper portion of the deltoid muscle (m. deltoideus). When the arm is in full abduction, the point is anterior of the two depressions appearing at the border of the acromiohumeral junction.

Li (1991) locates LI 15 in the middle of the upper portion of m. deltoideus. When the arm is in full abduction, the point is in the anterior of the two depressions which appear at the anterior border of the acrmioclavicular joint. The point in the posteior depression is SJ 14. When the arm is lowered, LI 15 will be just inferior to the anterior border of the acromion.

LI 16 JU GU – GREAT BONE

⊥ ***0.5 TO 0.7 CUN*** △ ***3 TO 7***

- 8 EXTRAORDINARY VESSEL/Coalescent Point of the Yang Heel/Yang Motility Vessel (Yang Qiao Mai)
- RE-UNION/Crossing/Meeting Point of the Large Intestine Channel with the Yang Heel/Yang Motility Vessel – Hand Yang Ming Channel with the Yang Qiao Mai

Pos: Position of patient: supine or seated with the arms at their side.

Loc: a) On the superior aspect of the shoulder.
b) In the depression between the acromial extremity of the clavicle and the scapular spine.

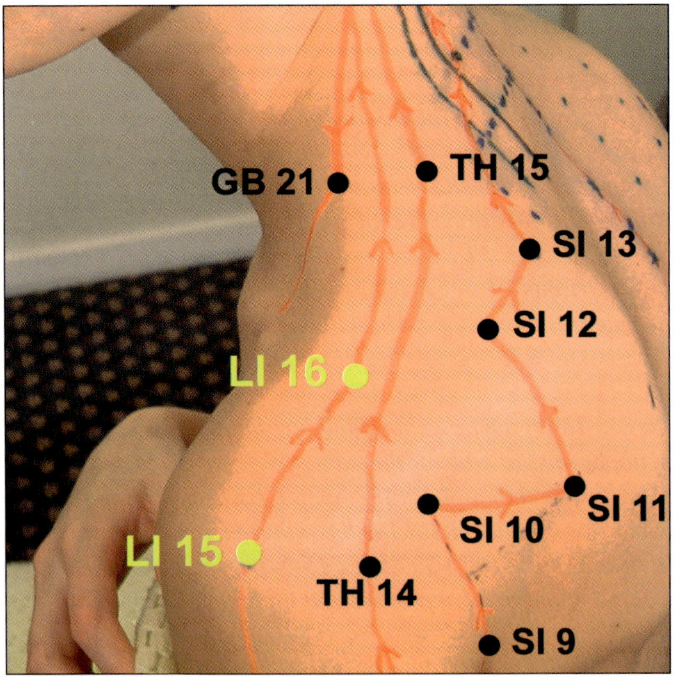

Tip: a) An angle is formed on the superior aspect of the shoulder by the acromial extremity of the clavicle and the scapular spine.
b) To locate this angle feel along either the superior border of the clavicle from the sternal end to the acromial end, or to feel the superior border of the scapular spine at the lateral end.
c) The point is located where the acromial extremity of the clavicle and the scapular spine meet.

LI 17-18 are on the lateral aspect of the neck. To locate the channel with the patient lying down, expose the posterior border of the sternocleidomastoid muscle by asking the patient to lift their head. With the patient sitting up, to expose the posterior border of the sternocleidomastoid on one side, ask the patient to rotate the head against resistance on the opposite side.

LI 17 TIAN DING – HEAVENLY VESSEL

⊥ ***0.3 TO 0.5 CUN*** △ ***3 TO 7***

Pos: Position of patient: supine or seated.

Loc:
a) On the lateral aspect of the neck.
b) Superior to the supraclavicular fossa.
c) Just below the level of the prominence of the laryngeal cartilage.
d) On the posterior border of the clavicular head of the sternocleidomastoid muscle.
e) Approximately 1 cun inferior to LI 18.

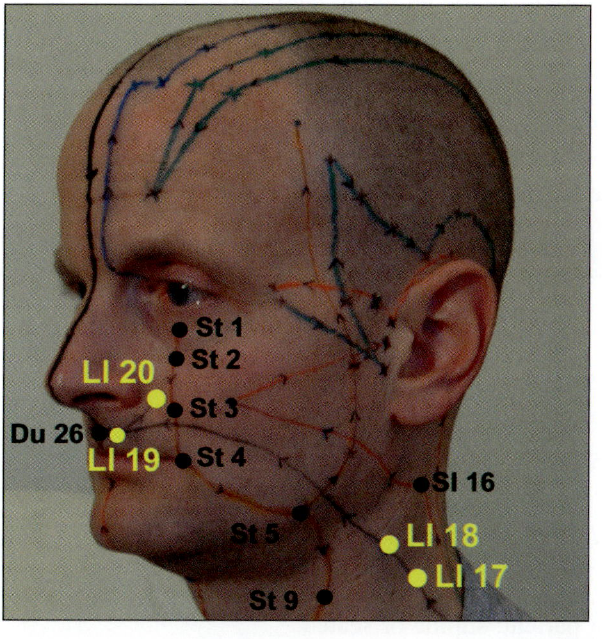

Tip:
a) Follow the contour of the channel from LI 16 (at the angle formed by the acromial end of the clavicle and the lateral end of the spine of the scapular) towards the neck, crossing the anterior border of the trapezius.
b) To locate the posterior border of the clavicular head of the sternocleidomastoid muscle, ask the patient to lift their head if supine. If seated ask them to rotate their head against resistance which is applied to the opposite side of the face.
c) The most important guide for locating this point is to gently palpate along the posterior border of the clavicular head of the sternocleidomastoid muscle. The point is located approximately 1 cun inferior to the level of LI 18 in the seam between the sternal and clavicular heads of the sternocleidomastoid muscle.

Note: Voisin (1974) locates LI 17 at the sternocleidomastoid: at the level of the middle of the thyroid cartilage. Katsusuke (1983) locates LI 17 at three sun to the side of the Adam's apple and one sun downward. or to the outer edge of the sternomastoid muscle. Wu (1973) locates CO 17 at the base of the neck, behind the stern-cleido-mastoid muscle. Soulié (1994) locates LI 17 on the lateral side of the neck; about three FW (Finger Width) under the bony prominence behind the ear (mastoid process); on the anterior and superior edge of a small round deep prominence (the lateral point of the third cervical vertebra); between two muscles; four FW under LI 18; two FW under and before SI 16; three FW under and a little more in front of TW 16. Shanghai (1981) locate LI 17 midway between LI 18 and S 12, at the posterior margin of the sternocleidomastoid muscle.

So (1985) locates LI 17, starting at the tip of the Adam's apple (CV 23), go lateral to the outer edge of the larynx (this is ST 9); then go down one division to the outer edge of the thyroid; this is the point. Shanghai (1993) locate LI 17 on the lateral side of the neck, above the supraclavicular fossa, below LI 18, on the posterior border of the sternocleidomastoid muscle, at the midpoint between the level of the superior thyroid notch and the upper border of the sternoclavicular articulation. Eachou (1995) locates LI 17 in a seated position, above the midpoint of the supraclavicular fossa 0.5 inch posteror to the posterior margin of the sternocleidomastoid muscle, at the midpoint between LI 18 and ST 12, or 1 inch below LI 18. Ellis (1991) locate LI 17 on the anterior lateral aspect of the neck, superior to the midpoint of the supraclavicular fossa, on the posterior border of the sternocleidomastoid muscle (m. sternocleidomastoideus). Huang (1993) locates LI 17 (in the neck) above the supraclavicular fossa directly below Probruberance Assistant (LI 18) and one cun and five fen posterior to Qi Abode (St 11). Masayoshi (1975) locates LI 17 on the side of the neck & posterior margin of the lower 1/4th of the sternocleidomastoid muscle.

LI 18 FU TU – SUPPORT AND RUSH OUT

⊥ ***0.3 TO 0.5 CUN*** Δ ***3***

- WINDOW OF THE SKY/Window of Heaven

Pos: Position of patient: supine or seated.

Loc:
a) On the lateral aspect of the neck.
b) Superior to the supraclavicular fossa.
c) In the the seam between the sternal and clavicular heads of the sternocleidomastoid muscle.
d) At the level of the prominence of the laryngeal cartilage.
e) Approximately 1 cun superior to LI 17.

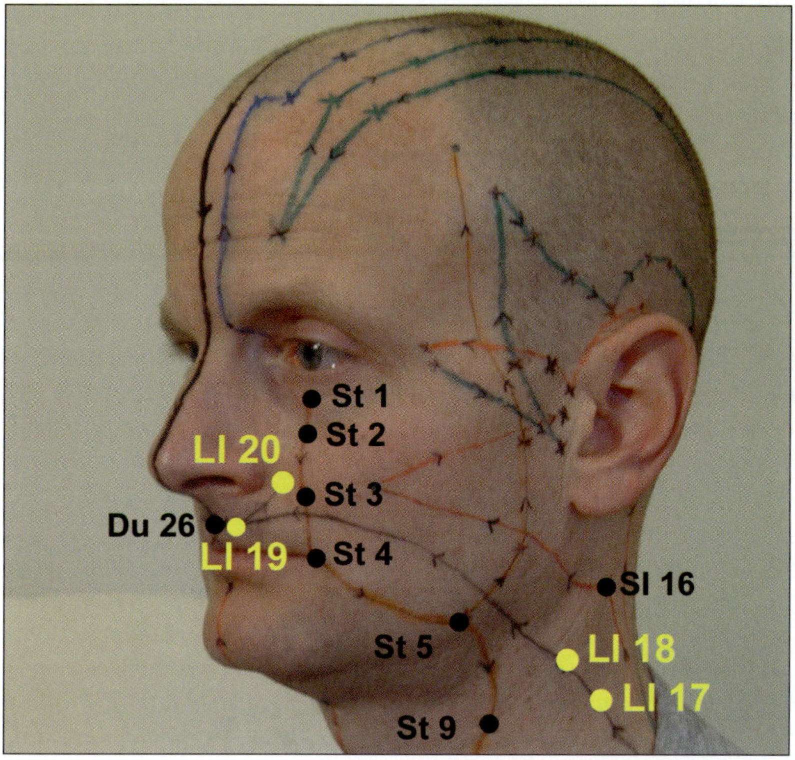

Tip:
a) To expose the sternocleidomastoid muscle, ask the patient to lift their head if supine. If seated ask them to rotate their head against resistance applied to the opposite side of the face.
b) The sternocleidomastoid muscle can be palpated as two distinct insertions at the level of the superior borders of the sternum and clavicle, (one into the sternal notch and the other at the medial third of the clavicle).
c) To locate the seam between the sternal and clavicular heads of the sternocleidomastoid muscle, place a finger in the space between these two insertions and run it superiorly towards the mastoid process. Although there is no longer a space between the two heads at this level, the seam between these two parts of the sternocleidomastoid should be still palpable.
d) The level at which this point can be located is approximately level to the prominence of the laryngeal cartilage (Adam's Apple) following the curved contour of the neck.
e) Imagine the line a choker chain follows when it is worn at this level of the neck. This contour at the approximate level of the prominence of the laryngeal cartilage links St 9, LI 18 and SI 16, LI 18 is between St 9 and SI 16.

Note: Traditionally 3 cun lateral to the mid-point of the laryngeal prominence of the thyroid cartilage. Academy (1975) locates LI 18 at 3 cun lateral to the thyroid cartilage, between the sternal and clavicular heads of the sternocleidomastoid muscle. Voisin (1974) locates LI 18 on the anterior border of the sternocleidomastoid, at the level of the upper border of the thyroid cartilage. Wu (1973) locates CO 18 at one pouce above CO 17 (which is located at the base of the neck, behind the sterno-cleido-mastoid muscle). Jayasuriya (1982) locates LI 18 at 3 cun lateral to the prominence of the thyroid cartilage (Adam's apple). Shandong (1982) locate Futu (LI 18) on the posterior border of the m, sterno-cleido-mastoideus, at the level of the prominentia leryngea.

Soulié (1994) locates LI 18 on the superior lateral side of the neck just under the inferoposterior angle of the lower jaw; in the angle of the anterior edge of the muscle on the slant (sternocleidomastoid), and on the superior edge of a narrow transverse muscle (belly of the digastric muscle); four FW (Finger Width) above and anterior to LI 17; two FW anterior and under SI 17; three FW under ST 6; two FW above and posterior to ST 9; two FW in front of SI 16. Qiu (1996) locates LI 18 at 3 cun lateral to the tip of the Adam's apple, between the sternal head and clavicular head of the m. sternocleidomastoideus. Shanghai (1981) locate LI 18 at 3 units beside the larymgeal prominence, lateral to S 9 and in the posterior margin of the sternocleidomastoid muscle. So (1985) locates LI 18 one division (the foreneck is divided into 3 divisions) above LI 17 slanting up the outer edge of the thyroid gland.

Shanghai (1993) locate LI 18 on the lateral side of the neck, about two finger breadth lateral to ST 9 of the Stomach Meridian, between the anterior and posterior borders of the sternocleidomastoid muscle and at the level of the thyroid cartilage. Eachou (1995) locates LI 18 in a seated or supine position, on the lateral side of the neck in between the sternal and clavicular heads of the sternocleidomastoid muscle, and 3 inches lateral to the apex of the Adam's apple. Li (1991) locates LI 18 at the midpoint of the m. sternocleidomastoideus, 3 cun lateral to Adam's apple. Huang (1993) locates LI 18 one cun and five fen lateral to Man's Prognosis (St 9).

LI 19-20 are on the face.

LI 19 HE LIAO – GRAIN BONE

⊥ ***0.1 TO 0.3 CUN*** ∆ ***FORBIDDEN TO MOXA***

Pos: Position of patient: Supine.

Loc:
a) On the face.
b) Between the superior border of the upper lip and the inferior border of the nostril.
c) Inferior to the lateral margin of the nostril.
d) Level with and 0.5 cun lateral to Du 26 which is located one third of the distance down the philtrum from the nasal spine to the vermilion border of the upper lip.

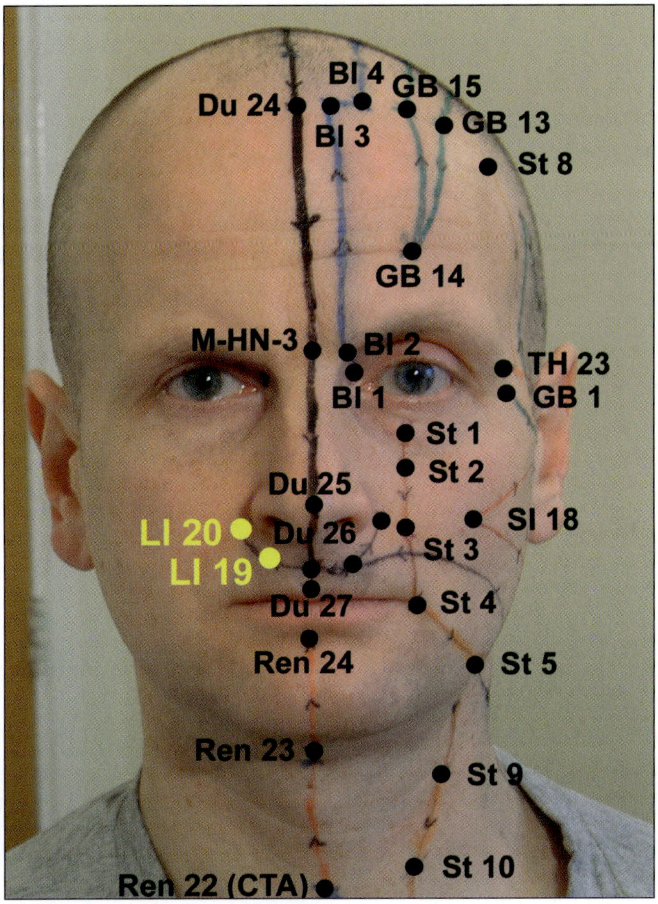

Tip: a) The description of this point refers to the lateral margin of the nostril. The point is to lateral if located directly inferior to the lateral margin of the nostril.

b) The actual location places this point nearer to the midline at 0.5 cun lateral to Du 26.

c) Du 26 is located in the centre of the groove which runs between the nasal spine and the vermilion border of the upper lip (the philtrum).

d) The level of Du 26 is one third of the length of the philtrum, inferior to the nasal spine.

e) To measure one third of the distance down the philtrum, mark a line at the inferior border of the nasal spine and another line at the vermilion border of the upper lip, then divide the distance between these two lines into three.

Note: Some Schools and texts locate LI 19 on the opposite side of the face via Du 26, some locate it on the same side of the face. The College of Traditional Acupuncture locate LI 19 and LI 20 on the opposite side of the face, therefore the left hand channel ends on the right side of the face, and the right channel ends on the left side of the face. Wu (1973) locates LI 19 below the nose at one half pouce from the nasolabial sulcus midway between the inferior edge of the ala of the nose and the edge of the upper lip. Worsley (1982) locates X 19 half-way between the inferior border of the nose and the edge of the upper lip, one half ACI medial to the nasolabial fold. Voisin (1974) locates LI 19 on the upper lip: 1.5 fb (finger breadth) medially to the centre of the nasolabial fold. Soulié (1994) locates LI 19 on the upper lip; one half FW (Finger Width) inferior and lateral to the inferior edge of the nostril; at the angle of the upper edge of the obicularis muscle of the lips and the medial edge of the elevator of the upper lip; in a hollow; two FW inferior and posterior to LI 20; at the same level and lateral to GV 26 (Du 26); two FW anterior (medial) to ST 3; three FW anterior and superior to ST 4, which the large intestine crosses. Li (1991) locates LI 19 at the medial side of the ala nasi, 0.5 cun lateral to Du 26.

LI 20 YING XIANG – WELCOME FRAGRANCE

⊥ ***0.1 TO 0.3 CUN*** △ ***FORBIDDEN TO MOXA***

- EXIT
- RE-UNION/Crossing/Meeting Point of the Large Intestine Channel with the Stomach Channel – Hand Yang Ming Channel with the Foot Yang Ming Channel

Pos: Position of patient: Supine.

Loc:
a) On the face.
b) Level with the lateral part of the nasal wing of the nostril.
c) In the nasolabial groove (the laughter line).
d) Superior to the root of the canine tooth.

Tip:
a) Feel for the most lateral part of the nasal wing of the nostril and drop into the bony crevice.
b) This point usually lies on the nasolabial groove but occasionally this groove is more lateral than the location of the point.
c) Palpation in this area will locate the gap in the bone which is found between the lateral margin of the nasal wing of the nostril and the skin overlying the apex of the root of the upper canine tooth

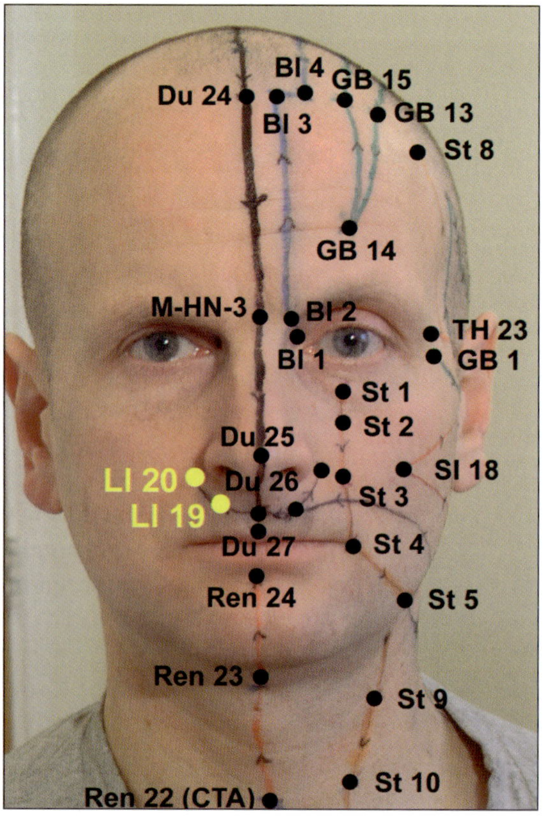

Note: Some Schools and texts locate LI 20 on the opposite side of the face via Du 26 and LI 19, some locate it on the same side of the face. The College of Traditional Acupuncture locate LI 19 and LI 20 on the opposite side of the face, therefore the left hand channel ends on the right side of the face, and the right channel ends on the left side of the face. The distance from the nostril has traditionally varied for this point, for example being located at the mid-point of a horizontal line drawn between the outermost point of the ala nasi and the nasolabial groove. Hyodo (1975) locates LI 20 at the exterior side of the nasal wing.

Worsley (1982) locates LI 20 on the face, at the inferior edge of the alum, 1 fen (0.1 cun) lateral to the alum. Voisin (1974) locates LI 20 on the cheek: lower part of the fold formed with the ala nasi. Jayasuriya (1982) locates LI 20 at the midpointof a horizontal line drawn between the outermost point of the ala nasi and the naso-labial groove.

Wu (1973) locates CO 20 upon the face, within the fold of the cheek at the height of the inferior edge of the ala nasi. Shandong (1982) locate Yingwiang (LI 20) between the nasolabial groove and the midpoint of the lateral border of the alae nasi. Lotan (2000) locates LI 20 in the nasolabial groove, level with the midpoint of the nasal ala lateral border.

Soulié (1994) locates LI 20 beside the nose: one half FW (Finger Width) lateral to the mid-height of the nostril; at the angle of the inferior edge of the bony horizontal edge and the anterior (medial) edge of the canine and elevator of the upper lip; in a hollow; two FW above LI 19. Qiu (1996) locates LI 20 in the nasolabial groove, at the level of the midpoint of the lateral border of the ala nasi. Shanghai (1981) locate LI 20 at 0.5 unit lateral to the nostril, in the nasolabial sulcus.

So (1985) locates LI 20 at 0.5 eye division from the outer side of nostril on the "smile line" at the level of the bottom of the nostril. Shanghai (1993) locate LI 20 at the upper segment of the nasolabial groove of the face, at the level of the middle part of the nasal ala, 1 cun superior and lateral to LI 19. Eachou (1995) locates LI 20 in a supine position, on the superior part of the nasolabial groove 0.5 inches lateral to the midpoint of the lateral border of the ala nasi, or 1 inch superior and lateral to LI 19. Ellis (1991) locate LI 20 in the nasolabial groove, at the level of the midpoint of the lateral border of ala nasi. Li (1991) locates LI 20 in the nasolabial groove, at the level of the midpoint of the lateral border of the ala nasi.

REFERENCES FOR THE LARGE INTESTINE CHANNEL

Huang-fu Mi. Trans: Yang Shou-zhong and Charles Chace 1993 The Systematic Classic of Acupuncture & Moxibustion – LI 1: 177; LI 8: 179; LI 9: 179; LI 10: 179; LI 11: 179; LI 17: 152; LI 18: 151

Ellis, Wiseman, Boss 1991 Fundamentals of Chinese Acupuncture – LI 1 (Classical Location): 93; LI 4: 106; LI 11: 99; LI 14: 101; LI 15: 102; LI 17: 104; LI 20: 106

Soulié De Morant, George. 1994 Chinese Acupuncture – LI 4: 350; LI 6: 351; LI 7: 352; LI 8: 352; LI 9: 353; LI 10: 354; LI 11: 354; LI 12: 355; LI 13: 356; LI 14: 356; LI 15: 356; LI 17: 357; LI 18: 358; LI 19: 358; LI 20: 359

Masayoshi Hyodo 1975 Ryodoraku Treatment – LI 1: 43; LI 6: 43; LI 7: 43; LI 8: 43; LI 9: 43; LI 11: 43; LI 12: 42; LI 14: 42; LI 17: 42; LI 20: 42

So, James Tin Yau (Dr) 1985 The Book of Acupuncture Points: LI 1: 115; LI 4: 115; LI 7: 180; LI 8: 181; LI 11: 118; LI 12: 182; LI 14: 119; LI 17: 183; LI 18: 183; LI 20: 29

Lawson-Wood, D&J 1973 Acupuncture Handbook – X 2: 32; X 4: 40; X 7: 63; X 11: 24

Worsley, J R 1982 Traditional Chinese Acupuncture Volume 1 – Meridians and Points. X 2: 195; X 4: 195; X 7: 197; X 11: 199; X 12: 201; X 13: 201; X 19: 203; X 20: 203

Jayasuriya, Anton 1982 Clinical Acupuncture – LI 4: 388; LI 11: 388; LI 12: 388; LI 19: 389; LI 20: 389

Cheng Xinnong (Editor) 1987 Chinese Acupuncture and Moxibustion – LI 4: 132; LI 11: 134; LI 12: 134

Deadman, Peter; Al-Khafaji, Mazin; Baker, Kevin 1998 Manual of Acupuncture, An – LI 6: 108; LI 13: 115; LI 14: 115

Academy of Traditional Chinese Medicine, The. 1975 – Outline of Chinese Acupuncture, An. LI 4: 102; LI 6: 102; LI 13: 104; LI 18: 106

Shandong Medical College and Shandong College of Traditional Chinese Medicine 1982 Anatomical Atlas of Chinese Acupuncture Points – Hegu (LI 4): 11; Yangxi (LI 5): 11; Binao (LI 14): 12; Futu (LI 18): 12; Yingxiang (LI 20): 12

Legge, David 1999 Acupuncture Points and Meridians – LI 4: 23; LI 10: 24; : LI 11: 24; LI 14: 24; LI 15: 24

Lotan Alon (2000) – LI 4: 25; LI 11: 25; LI 14: 29; LI 15: 29; LI 20: 31

Qiu Mao-Liang 1996 Chinese Acupuncture and Moxibustion – LI 4: 68; LI 11: 70; LI 12: 70; LI 18: 71; LI 20: 72

Shanghai College of Traditional Chinese Medicine 1993 Applied Anatomical Charts of Acupuncture – LI 4: 10; LI 11: 14; LI 17: 16; LI 18: 16/17; LI 20: 18

Eachou Chen 1995 Cross-sectional Anatomy of Acupoints – LI 4: 37/38; LI 10: 20; LI 11: 17; LI 17: 137; LI 18: 131; LI 20: 118

Li Ding (Prof.). 1991. Acupuncture, Meridian Theory and Acupuncture Points – LI 4: 124; LI 7: 126; LI 8: 126; LI 9: 127; LI 11: 129; LI 14: 130; LI 15: 130/131; LI 18: 132; LI 19: 133; LI 20: 134

Voisin, Dr. H 1974 Essentials of Acupuncture – LI 6: 74; LI 7: 74; LI 8: 74; LI 9: 74; LI 10: 74; LI 12: 74; LI 13: 74; LI 15: 74; LI 17: 74; LI 18: 74; LI 19: 74; LI 20: 74

Lavier, Dr. J 1974 Points of Chinese Acupuncture – CO 7: 19; Upper Arm Pouce Measurement: 12/13; CO 13: 13

Wu, Wei-P'ing 1973 Chinese Acupuncture – CO 7: 63; CO 8: 63; CO 9: 63; CO 10: 64; CO 12: 64; CO 13: 64; CO 14: 64; CO 17: 65; CO 18: 65; CO 19: 65; CO 20: 65

Katsusuke Serizawa 1983 Tsubo – Vital Points for Oriental Therapy – LI 7: 115; LI 10: 103; LI 11: 85; LI 14: 123; LI 15: 122; LI 17: 125

Shanghai College of Traditional Medicine 1981 Acupuncture – A Comprehensive Text – LI 11: 230; LI 14: 227; LI 15: 222; LI 17: 309; LI 18: 165; LI 20: 153

Yang Jiasan (Prof) 1982 The Way to Locate Acu-Points – LI 14: 31

THE STOMACH CHANNEL OF THE FOOT (YANG MING)

Primary Channel

The Stomach channel starts on the face at LI 20, ascends the side of the nose to the anterior median line at the bridge of the nose and to Bl 1, then turns downwards to St 1-3. At St 3 the channel goes to Du 26, back to St 4 and down to Ren 24, encircling the mouth. The channel continues to St 5, and round to St 8 at the temporal hairline, (via the cheek, angle of the mandible and zygomatic arch, crossing GB 3 in front of the ear, and GB 6/5/4), finally reaching the forehead at Du 24.

(Some texts mention another deep channel passing through the eyes and into the brain.)

A branch emerges at St 5 and continues down the throat to St 12, where a deep channel travels alongside the superficial channel through the chest and diaphragm to Ren 13, enters the stomach and connects to the spleen, continues to Ren 12 and on down to St 30, where it rejoins the superficial channel. From St 12 the main channel travels straight down the chest, passing through the nipple, and descends the abdomen to St 30. Yet another branch travels from St 11 to Du 14 on the posterior torso.

The rejoined channel now runs down the leg to St 36. At St 36 a tibia branch runs lateral to the main channel and ends at the lateral nail point of the third digit, while the channel continues through points 35 to 45 at the lateral side of the second digit.

Another branch runs from St 42 to link with Sp 1 at the medial side of the first digit.

Divergent Channel

Leaving the primary channel on the thigh this enters the abdomen, connects with the stomach, and disperses through the spleen. It then ascends through the heart, and follows the oesophagus to the mouth. It continues up beside the nose to connect with the eye, then rejoins the primary channel.

Connecting Channel

Leaving the primary channel at St 40 on the lower leg, this connects with the Spleen channel. One branch follows the lateral margin of the tibia up across the thigh and trunk to the top of the head to converge with the other Yang channels. A second branch diverges in the neck and connects with the throat.

Muscle Channel

This originates at the second, third and fourth digits, binds at the dorsum of the foot, and slants upwards along the lateral aspect of the leg, binding at the lateral aspect of the knee. This branch then crosses and binds at the hip and lower ribs before circling behind the body to connect with the spine.

A second branch divides from the first above the ankle, following the tibia to bind at the knee. A sub branch crosses to the head of the fibula to join with the Gallbladder channel. From the knee, the channel ascends the thigh and binds again in the pelvic region, where it joins with the reproductive organs.

It then continues up the abdomen and chest to bind with the clavicle (St 12), then passes up the neck and around the mouth, binding at the inferior border of the nose. Above, it joins the Bladder muscle channel to form a muscular net around the eye. A sub branch separates at the jaw and crosses the face, binding in front of the ear.

THE STOMACH CHANNEL OF THE FOOT

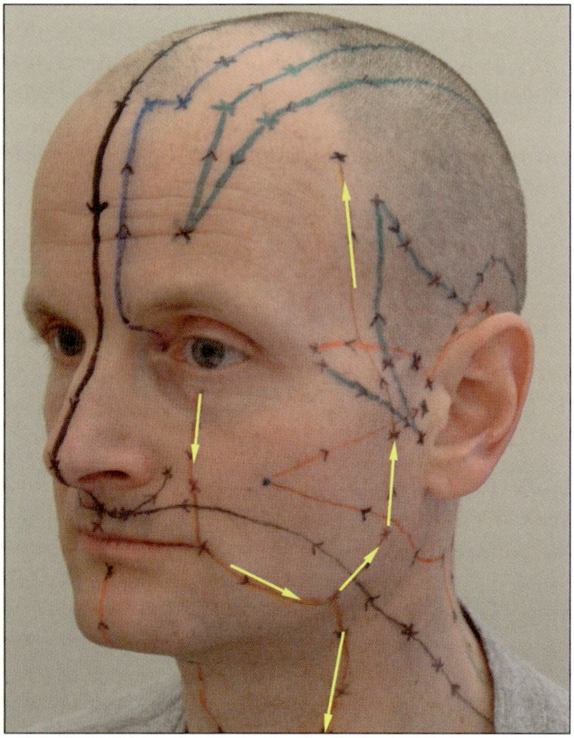

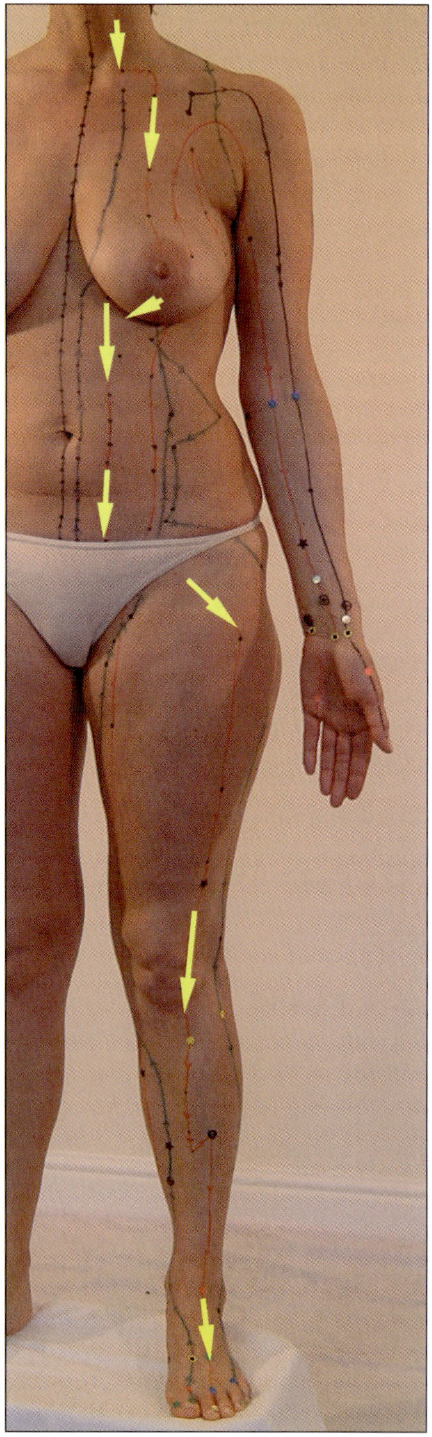

Points of the Stomach Channel – Foot Yang Ming (St/ST/S/XI)

St 1-7 are on the face, St 8 at the corner of the forehead.

The distance between the two corners of the forehead is measured as 9 cun.

St 1 CHENG QI – RECEIVE TEARS

⊥ ***0.1 TO 0.3 CUN*** ***Δ FORBIDDEN TO MOXA***

- ENTRY
- 8 EXTRAORDINARY VESSEL/Coalescent Point of Yang Heel/Yang Motility Vessel (Yang Qiao Mai)
- 8 EXTRAORDINARY VESSEL/Coalescent Point of Ren Mai (Conception/Directing Vessel)
- RE-UNION/Crossing/Meeting Point of the Stomach Channel with the Ren Mai and Yang Heel/Yang Motility Vessels – Foot Yang Ming Channel with the Conception/Directing Vessel and Yang Qiao Mai

Pos: Position of patient: supine.

Loc: a) On the face.
b) Inferior to the centre of the pupil with the eyes looking straight forward.
c) Between the eyeball and the infraorbital margin formed by the zygomatic bone and maxilla bone (these two bones form the inferior border of the orbit).
d) Superior to the zygomaxillary notch.
e) Traditionally 0.7 cun below the pupil.

Tip: a) Feel for the edge of the infraorbital margin of the zygomatic and maxilla bones.
b) Often you will be able to feel a palpable notch on the edge of the bone. This notch is where the zygomatic and the maxilla bones meet (zygomaxillary suture).
c) Once established, ask the patient to look directly ahead, draw a mark at the zygomaxillary notch.
d) The point is located immediately superior to the notch, in the space between the infraorbital margin and the eyeball.
e) Ensure that you angle the needle towards St 2.
f) To prevent the bone being clipped, ensure that the needle is not inserted too close to the infraorbital margin.

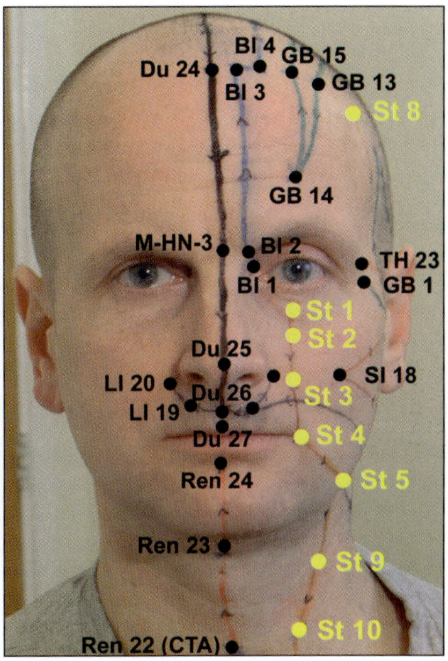

Note: Voisin (1974) numbers this point S 4, located on the cheek: straight below the pupil, slightly below the lower border of the orbit. Soulié (1994) locates ST 4 (our St 1) lateral to the lateral corner of the eye, a little lateral to the angle of the lateral edge of the orbital arch and the superior edge of the zygomatic arch, just at the superior edge of the suture of the zygomatic arch and the cheekbone; three FW (Finger Width) just under ST 8; one FW lateral and a little above ST 2; separated from SI 18 by the zygomatic arch; two FW anterior and below GB 1. Worsley (1982) locates XI 1 on the cheek, immediately superior to the infra-orbital foramen, on the inferior border of the orbit, in the line with the centre of the pupil with the eye looking straight ahead.

St 2 SI BAI – FOUR WHITES

⊥ ***0.1 TO 0.3 CUN*** ***Δ 3 TO 5***

Pos: Position of patient: supine.

Loc: a) On the face.
b) In the infraorbital foramen of the maxilla bone.
c) Inferior to St 1, and inferior to the centre of the pupil of the eye (traditionally 1 cun below the pupil).

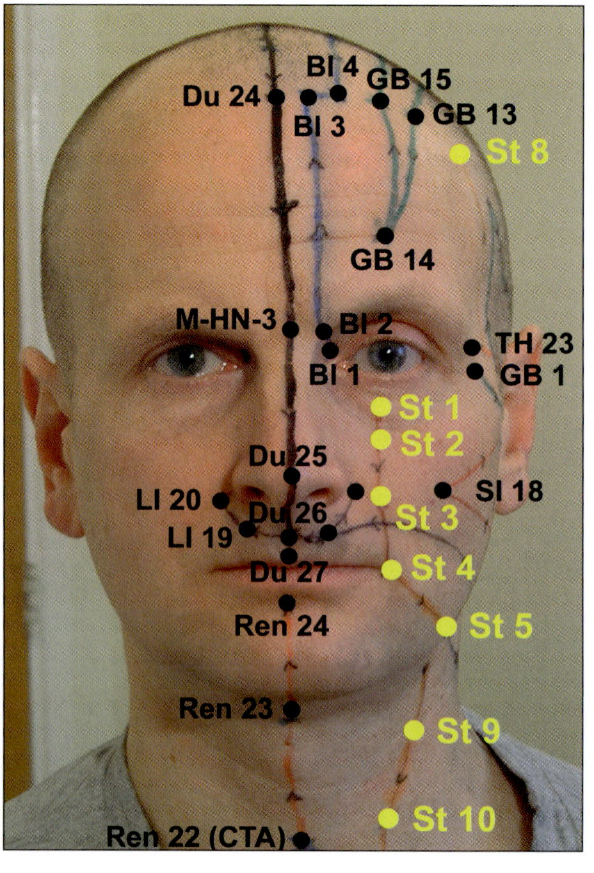

Tip: a) There is a palpable depression in the infraorbital foramen of the maxilla bone. The point is located in this foramen.
b) This foramen is inferior to St 1 (and the centre of the pupil when the person is looking directly ahead).
c) To locate this point palpate along the infraorbital margin for the notch where the zygomatic and maxilla bones meet at St 1.
d) When the location of this notch is established, run your finger inferiorly just over the curve of the maxilla bone. The foramen is sensitive and will be felt as a large depression.

Note: Voisin (1974) numbers this point S 5, located on the cheek: straight below the pupil, at 0.5 fb (finger breadth) below S 4 (our St 1). Soulié (1994) locates ST 5 (our St 2) on the face, under the middle of the eye, on the superior edge of the cheekbone, at the point where it turns forward, on the bone of the orbital arch, under a notch on its superior edge; one FW (Finger Width) in front of and below ST 1; one large FW lateral and above ST 3; one FW in front and above SI 18. Wu (1973) locates ST 2 at 3 fen (0.3 cun) below ST 1. Worsley (1982) locates XI 2 on the cheek, in the depression of the infra-orbital foramen, 3 fen (0.3 cun) inferior to the inferior edge of the orbit.

St 3 JU LIAO – GREAT CHEEKBONE

⊥ ***0.1 TO 0.5 CUN*** Δ 5

- 8 EXTRAORDINARY VESSEL/Coalescent Point of the Yang Heel/Yang Motility Vessel (Yang Qiao Mai)
- RE-UNION/Crossing/Meeting Point of the Stomach Channel with the Yang Heel/Yang Motility Vessel – Foot Yang Ming Channel with the Yang Qiao Mai

Pos: Position of patient: supine.

Loc: a) On the face.
b) On the maxilla bone.
c) Directly inferior to the centre of the pupil of the eyes when the person is looking directly ahead.
d) Inferior to St 1, and St 2,
e) Level with the inferior border of the nostrils.

Tip: a) Draw a vertical line from St 1 (or the centre of the pupil when the person is looking straight ahead).
b) Draw a horizontal line level with the inferior border of the nostrils.
c) The point is located approximately where these two lines intersect.
d) Palpating around this area will give a more accurate point location.

Note: Traditionally located directly below St 2, at the level of the lower border of the nostrils (alum or ala nasi), on the lateral side of the nasolabial groove. Eachou (1995) locates St 3 about 0.8 inches lateral to the nostril directly below the pupils. Huang (1993) locates this point 8 fen lateral to the nostrils, directly below the pupils of the eyes. Some texts refer to the inferior border of the nostrils as the alum or ala nasi of the nose. Voisin (1974) numbers this point S 6, located on the cheek: straight below the pupil, at the level of the lower part of the ala nasi. Wu (1973) locates ST 3 upon the cheek bone at 8 fen (0.8 cun) outside the ala nasi.

Soulié (1994) locates ST 6 (our St 3) on the cheek, in the angle of the anterior (or medial) edge of the cheek bone and of the inferior edge of the large prominence of the orbital arch; in a hollow; one large FW (Finger Width) above and in front of ST 2; three little FW above and anterior (medial) to LI 20; one large FW under and lateral to BL 1. Worsley (1982) locates XI 3 on the zygomatic bone, directly inferior to the infra-orbital foramen, at the level of the inferior border of the alum of the nose.

St 4 DI CANG – EARTH GRANARY

⊥ ***0.1 TO 0.4 CUN*** Δ **5**

- 8 EXTRAORDINARY VESSEL/Coalescent Point of the Yang Heel/Yang Motility Vessel (Yang Qiao Mai)
- RE-UNION/Crossing/Meeting Point of the Stomach Channel with the Large Intestine Channel, the Ren Mai and Yang Heel/Yang Motility Vessels – Foot Yang Ming Channel with the Hand Yang Ming Channel, Conception/Directing Vessel and Yang Qiao Mai

Pos: Position of patient: supine.

Loc: a) On the face.
b) Inferior to the centre of the pupil of the eye when the person is looking directly ahead.
c) Inferior to St 1, St 2 and St 3.
d) Level with the corner of the mouth.
e) Traditionally 0.4 cun lateral to the corner of the mouth.

Tip: a) Draw a vertical line from St 1 (or the centre of the pupil when the person is looking straight ahead).
b) Draw a horizontal line, laterally from the corner of the mouth.
c) The point is located where the two lines intersect.
d) Palpating around this area will give a more accurate point location.

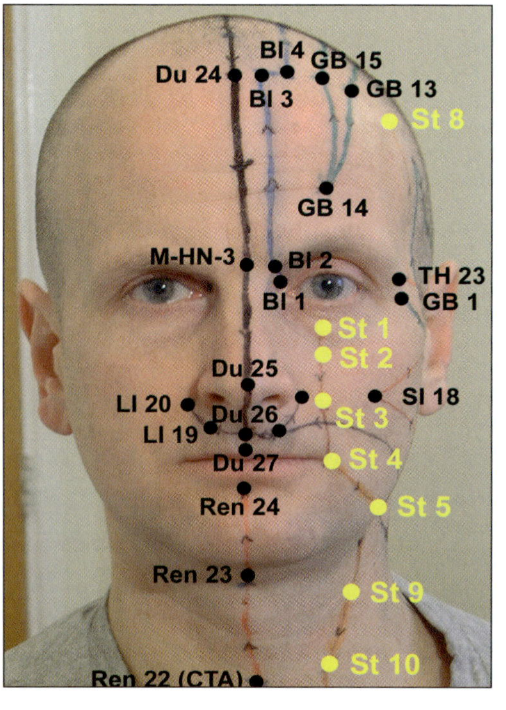

Note: Voisin (1974) numbers this point S 7, located on the cheek, at 1 fb (finger breadth) lateral to the commisure of the lips. Wu (1973) locates ST 4 at 4 fen (0.4 cun) outside the angle of the mouth, upon the facial artery. Huang (1993) also locates St 4 at 4 fen lateral to the corners of the mouth. Soulié (1994) locates ST 7 (our St 4) on the cheek: at one FW (Finger Width) lateral to the corner of the mouth.; in the angle of the anterior and inferior edge of the large muscle (masseter), and of the lateral edge of the vertical artery (facial artery); three FW below ST 3; two FW above and a little medial to ST 5. The meridian of the large intestine passes through "dicang" (ST 4).

St 5 DA YING – GREAT WELCOME

⊥ ***0.3 TO 0.5 CUN*** Δ ***3 TO 5***

- RE-UNION/Crossing/Meeting Point of Stomach and Gall Bladder Channels – Foot Yang Ming and Foot Shao Yang Channels

Pos: Position of patient: supine.

Loc:
a) On the face.
b) On the mandible bone (lower jaw).
c) In the groove on the anterior border of the masseter muscle when the teeth are clenched.

Tip:
a) Following the lower jaw line, run your finger from the anterior median line of the mandible (lower jaw) towards the ear.
b) Ask the patient to clench their teeth to expose the masseter muscle.
c) It may be difficult to expose the anterior border of the masseter muscle when it is relaxed, therefore ask the patient to keep clenching and relaxing their jaw.
d) The pulse of the facial artery, which is located on the anterior border of the masseter muscle, can sometimes be felt.
e) St 5 is located directly on the anterior border of the masseter muscle.
f) The patient should not clench their teeth when the point is needled.

Note: Traditionally 1.3 cun anterior to the angle of the mandible, where the pulse of the facial artery is palpable. Voisin (1974) numbers this point S 8, located on the neck: lower border of the mandible, 2 fb (finger breadth) in front of its angle. Wu (1973) locates ST 5 upon the inferior edge of the mandible before the gonion in the hollow of the facial artery.

Soulié (1994) locates ST 8 (our St 5) on the jaw, two FW (Finger Width) in front of the inferior, posterior angle, at the angle of the of the inferior edge of the jaw and the anterior edge of the the vertical artery (facial artery); deep on the myohyoidus muscle.; about two FW below and lateral to ST 4 under the corner of the mouth; four FW superior and medial to LI 18. The meridian of the large intestine passes through daying (ST 5). Huang (1993) locates St 5 in a depression that is one cun and two fen to the lower border of the mandible where vessels beat. Shandong (1982) locate Daying at 0.5 cun below Pt. Jiache (St 6), a groove appears when the mouth is closed and the cheeks are blown

St 6 JIA CHE – MANDIBLE WHEEL

⊥ ***0.3 TO 0.5 CUN*** Δ ***3 TO 7***

- SUN SI-MIAO GHOST (Gui) – Ghost Point Name: Gui Chuang – Ghost's Bed or Ghost Forest

Pos: Position of patient: supine.

Loc:
a) On the face.
b) On the mandible bone (lower jaw).
c) On the prominence of the masseter muscle when the teeth are clenched.
d) One finger breadth or 0.8 cun anterior and superior to the angle of the mandible bone.

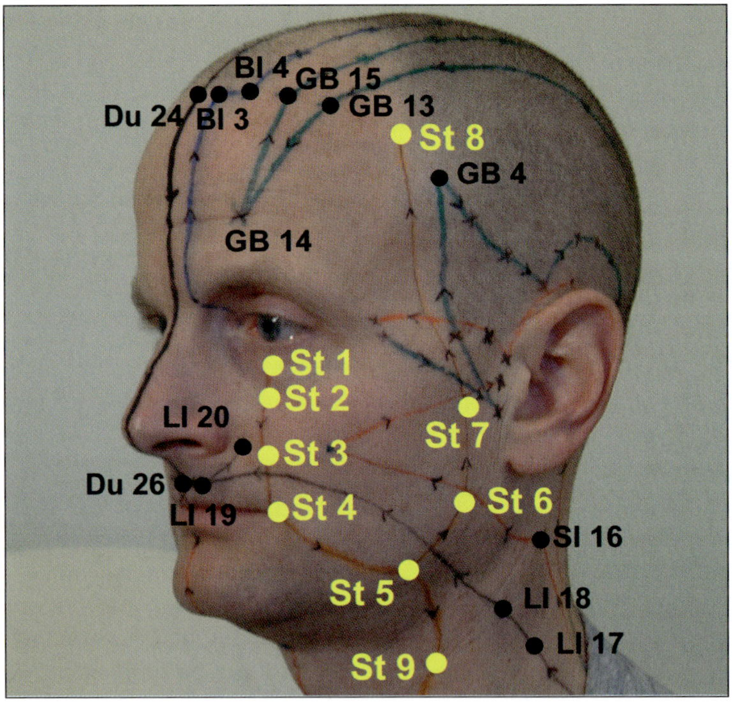

Tip:
a) Following the lower jaw line, run your finger from the anterior median line of the mandible (lower jaw) towards the ear.
b) Ask the patient to clench their teeth to expose the masseter muscle.
c) It may be difficult to expose the anterior border of the masseter muscle when it is relaxed, therefore ask the patient to keep clenching and relaxing their jaw.
d) The point is located at the prominence of the masseter muscle.
e) Make sure the patient's teeth are unclenched when palpating to facilitate accurate location for this point.
f) The patient should not clench their teeth when the point is needled.

Note: Worsley (1982) locates XI 6 at 4 fen (0.4 cun) anterior and superior to the angle of the mandible, in the depression between the two bellies of the masseter. Wu (1973) locates ST 6 at the angle of the mandible between the insertions of the massester muscle. Voisin (1974) numbers this point S 3, located on the cheek: in front of the angle of the mandible, on the posterior border of the masseter. Soulié (1994) locates ST 3 (our St 6) on the inferior, posterior cheek, just in the anterior angle of the posterior rise of the rising branch of the protrusion of the inferior posterior point of the maxillary bone.

Between the two insertions of the large muscle which hardens by clenching the teeth (masseter muscle); in a hollow; three FW (Finger Width) lateral to ST 4; two FW lateral and a little above ST 5; two FW under GB 2. Huang (1993) locates St 6 at the angle of the lower jaw where a hole appears when the mouth is opened. Shandong (182) locate Jiache one finger width anterior and superior to the angle of the lower jaw, at the prominence of the m. masseter during mastication.

St 7 XIA GUAN – LOWER PASSAGE

⊥ ***0.3 TO 0.5 CUN*** ***Δ FORBIDDEN TO MOXA***

- RE-UNION/Crossing/Meeting Point of the Stomach Channel with the Gall Bladder Channel – Foot Yang Ming Channel with the Foot Shao Yang Channel

Pos: Position of patient: supine.

Loc: a) On the face.
b) Inferior to the zygomatic arch of the temporal bone.
c) Anterior to the condyle of the mandible bone (when the mouth is closed).
d) Directly superior to St 6.

Tip: a) Locate St 6 and ask the patient to clench their teeth.
b) Run your finger directly superior to St 6 until it reaches the inferior border of the zygomatic arch.
c) Ask the patient to open their mouth to locate the condyle of the mandible.
d) Ask the patient to close their mouth when actually locating the point, which is in a hollow formed by the condyle of the mandible when the mouth is opened.
e) St 7 is located anterior to the condyle of the mandible bone, inferior to the zygomatic arch and directly superior to St 6 (the prominence of the masseter bone).
f) Palpating around this area will give a more accurate point location.

Note: Voisin (1974) numbers this point S 2, located at the lower border of the zygomatic arch, slightly behind the posterior border of the masseter. Soulié (1994) locates ST 2 (our St 7) on the cheek, in the angle of the lateral inferior edge of the cheekbone and of the inferior edge of the large muscles (masseter); in a hollow; three FW below ST 1; three narrow FW above ST 4.

Huang (1993) locates St 7 at the lower border of the zygomatic arch, anterior to the auricle and near the pulsating vessel where a hole appears when the mouth is shut but disappears when the mouth is open. Wu (1973) locates ST 7 before the ear under the zygomatic arch in front of the condyle of the mandible, in the hollow which fills upon opening the mouth. Shandong (1982) locate Xiaguan in the depression formed by arcus zygomaticus and incisura mandibulae.

Legge (1999) locates St 7 anterior to the temperomandibular joint, in the depression at the inferior border of the zygomatic arch. Lotan (2000) locates St 7 when the mouth is closed, in the depression, vertically inferior to the vertical slit on the zygomatic arch inferior border, level with the condylar process; level with the tragus inferior notch and GB 2.

St 8 TOU WEI – HEAD TIED

⊥ ***0.3 TO 0.5 CUN*** *∆ **FORBIDDEN TO MOXA***

- 8 EXTRAORDINARY VESSEL/Coalescent Point of Yang Linking Vessel (Yang Wei Mai) – see note
- RE-UNION/Crossing/Meeting Point of the Stomach Channel with the Gall Bladder Channel and the Yang Linking Vessel – Foot Yang Ming Channel with the Foot Shao Yang Channel and the Yang Wei Mai

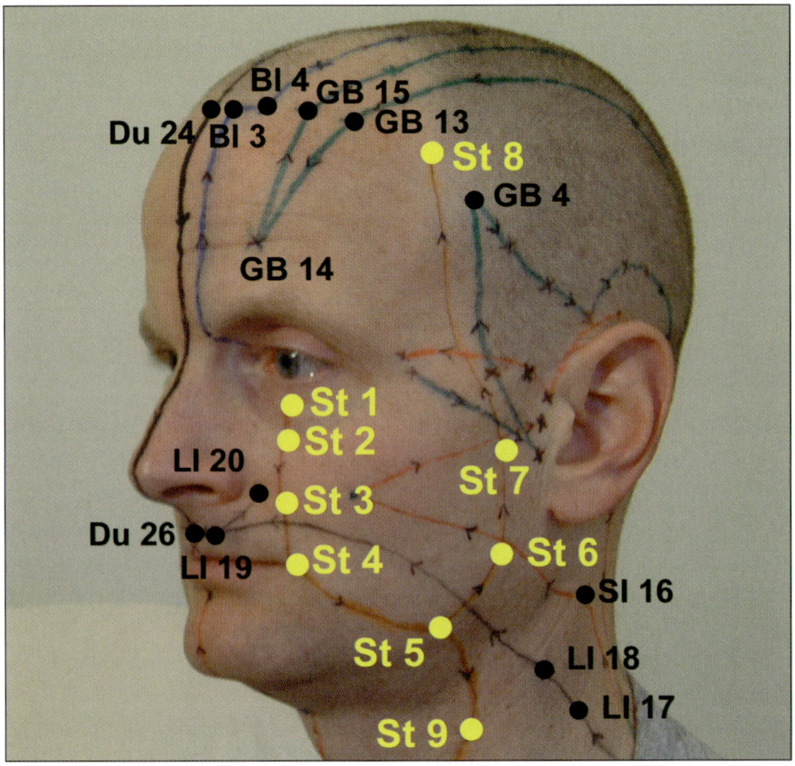

Pos: Position of patient: supine.

Loc:
a) On the head.
b) At the corner of the forehead.
c) In a groove formed by the frontal bone of the skull and the medial border of the temporalis muscle.
d) On a vertical line directly superior to the lateral canthus of the eye.
e) 0.5 cun posterior to the natural anterior hairline.
f) 4.5 cun lateral to the anterior median line.
g) At the level of Du 24.

Tip:
a) The corner of the forehead is the meeting point of the most lateral, anterior and superior aspects of the head (like the corner of a box).
b) Often a groove runs up the anterolateral aspect of the forehead towards the natural anterior hairline. The groove is formed by the frontal bone and the medial border of the temporalis muscle which becomes more obvious when the patient clenches their teeth.
c) If the groove is located, St 8 is just posterior to the natural anterior hairline and level with Du 24 (which is on the anterior median line of the head 0.5 cun posterior to the natural anterior hairline).
d) Palpate on a vertical line directly superior from the lateral canthus of the eye to the corner of the head.
e) Palpate just posterior to the natural anterior hairline at the corner of the forehead.
f) If the hairline has receded especially on men, the point may lie anterior to their current hairline. There may be a change in the skin texture on the head indicating the original position of the hairline.
g) If you were to place one end of a pen at the lateral aspect of the nasal wing, and the other end of the pen on the lateral corner of the eyebrow (this is not where the eyebrow ends but where the anterior and lateral aspects of the frontal bone meet) the line of the pen will give you the angle at which St 8 will be located.
h) The distance between the lateral corners of the forehead (or between the points of St 8) is 9 cun, but the point should be located using anatomical landmarks.
i) When needling this point the patients' jaw should be relaxed (teeth not clenched).

Note: Voisin (1974) numbers this point S 1, and is the beginning of the Stomach channel, located on the forehead at the normal hairline, 2 fb (finger breadth) above and lateral to the lateral extremity of the eyebrow. Wu (1973) locates ST 8 upon the cranium, at 4 pouces horizontally from Du 24, somewhat ahead of the frontal parietal suture. Soulié (1994) numbers this point as ST 1 (our St 8), located on the anterior part of the upper temple; at the angle of the lateral inferior edge of the frontal bulge, at the lateral edge of the vertical ridge of the frontal crest and at the inferior edge of the horizontal relief (superior temporal crest); two FW (Finger Width) in anterior to GB 16; one large FW above and anterior to TW 23.

Note: In some texts St 8 is listed as an 8 EXTRAORDINARY VESSEL/Coalescent Point of Yang Wei Mai (Yang Linking Vessel), whereas in others it is omitted.

St 9-11 are on the anterolateral aspect of the neck.

To display the sternocleidomastoid muscle, raise the head halfway off the couch. To expose it on one side, place the flat of the hand against the cheek on the opposite side and ask the patient to push towards and against the hand.

St 9 REN YING – PEOPLE WELCOME

⊥ *0.2 TO 0.5 CUN* *∆ FORBIDDEN TO MOXA*

- WINDOW OF THE SKY/Window of Heaven
- A POINT OF THE SEA OF QI (There are two other Sea of Qi Points: Ren 17 and Bl 10 – see note)
- RE-UNION/Crossing/Meeting Point of the Stomach Channel with the Gall Bladder Channel – Foot Yang Ming Channel with the Foot Shao Yang Channel

Pos: Position of patient: supine or seated.

Loc:
a) On the anterior aspect of the neck.
b) On the anterior border of the sternocleidomastoid muscle.
c) In the the seam between the sternal head of the sternocleidomastoid muscle and the prominence of the laryngeal cartilage.
d) Approximately at the level of the prominence of the laryngeal cartilage.
e) On a contour between the prominence of the laryngeal cartilage and SI 16.

Tip:
a) If supine ask the patient to lift their head to expose the sternocleidomastoid muscle, If seated ask them to rotate their head against resistance applied to the opposite side of the face.
b) The sternal head of the sternocleidomastoid muscle can be palpated as a distinct insertion into the suprasternal notch located at the level of the superior border of the sternum.
c) To locate the seam between the sternal head of the sternocleidomastoid muscle and the prominence of the laryngeal cartilage, place the flat of the finger on the medial border of the sternal insertion of the sternocleidomastoid muscle and palpate up the anterior border of the muscle.
d) The location of the point is approximately level with the prominence of the laryngeal cartilage (Adam's Apple).

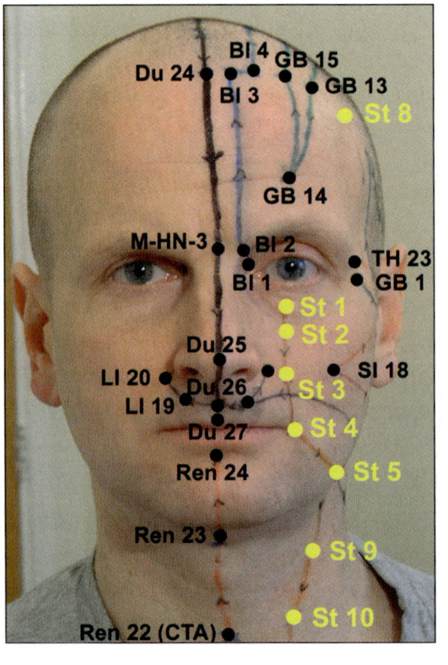

e) Imagine the line a choker necklace follows when it is worn on the neck. This line is approximately level with the prominence of the laryngeal cartilage and links St 9, LI 18 and SI 16. St 9 is anterior to LI 18 and SI 16.
f) The carotid artery pulse may be felt on or in the proximity of the point, but palpation will give you an accurate location for St 9.
g) If you run your finger down from St 5 on to the neck you should automatically fall in to the seam between the lateral border of the laryngeal cartilage and the anterior border of the sternocleidomastoid muscle.
h) The Stomach channel runs from St 5 on to the neck towards St 9 and another channel runs along the mandible (jaw) from St 5 and on to the head at St 8.
i) St 8 does not directly connect to St 9.

Note: Traditionally 1.5 cun lateral to the prominence of the laryngeal cartilage, on the carotid artery. Many other locations for this point put it between the lateral border of the laryngeal cartilage and the carotid artery. Lavier (1974) in an illustration and Wu (1973) both locate St 9 upon the lateral surface of the neck, below the mandible in front of the stern-cleido-mastoid muscle upon the external carotid artery. Voisin (1974) locates S 9 on the neck: upper lateral corner of the thyroid cartilage. Masayoshi (1975) locates ST 9 at the height of the superior margin of the thyroid cartilage.

So (1985) locates ST 9 at 1 and a half divisions lateral to the centre of the Adam's apple. Katsusuke (1983) locates this point at 1 sun and 5 bu on either side of the Adam's apple. Huang (1993) locates St 9 at the major pulsating vessel in the neck which may be palpated on either side of the throat knot. Soulié (1994) locates ST 9 on the front of the neck; two FW (Finger Width) on either side of the medial line; at the level of the upper point of the thyroid cartilage (larynx); at the angle of the anterior edge (medial) of the large muscle (sternocleidomastoid); dee, the strong artery (carotid artery) and on the superior lateral edge of the thyroid cartilage; in a hollow; four FW below ST 5; two above ST 10; two FW on either side of CV 23 (Ren 23). Shandong (1982) locate Renyang at 1.5 cun lateral of the prominentia laryngea, on the anterior border of the m. sterno-cleido mastoideus, at the pulsation of a. carotis communis (avoid puncturing the blood vessel).

Note: The Ling Shu (Spiritual Pivot) Chapter 33 describes areas where the Seas are located rather than point numbers. Ren 17 and St 9 locations seem to have universal agreement as Seas of Qi, but the other Sea of Qi point(s) in the region of the neck, Bl 10 or Du 14/Du 15 seem to have differences of opinion. The College of Traditional Acupuncture favours using Bl 10 as they classify Du 15 as a Sea of Marrow Point.

St 10 SHUI TU – WATER RUSHING OUT

⊥ ***0.2 TO 0.5 CUN*** **Δ *FORBIDDEN TO MOXA***

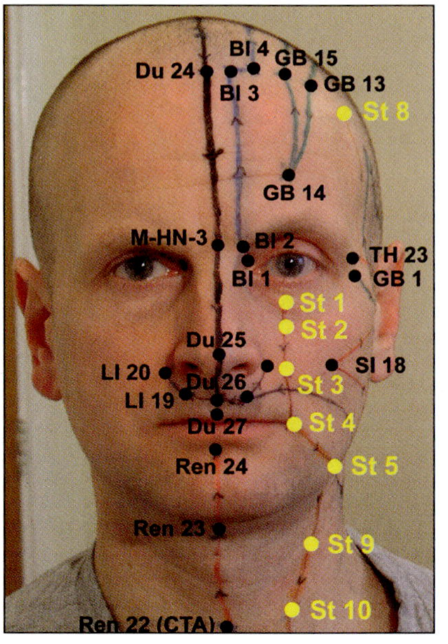

Pos: Position of patient: supine or seated.

Loc:
a) On the anterior aspect of the neck.
b) On the anterior border of the sternocleidomastoid muscle.
c) In the the seam between the sternal head of the sternocleidomastoid muscle and the cricoid cartilage.
d) At the level of the cricoid cartilage.
e) Midway between St 9 and St 11 (see separate descriptions).

Tip:
a) If supine ask the patient to lift their head to expose the sternocleidomastoid muscle. If seated ask them to rotate their head against resistance applied to the opposite side of the face.
b) The sternal head of the sternocleidomastoid muscle can be palpated as a distinct insertion into the suprasternal notch located at the level of the superior border of the sternum.
c) To locate the seam between the sternal head of the sternocleidomastoid muscle and the prominence of the laryngeal cartilage, place the flat of the finger on the medial border of the sternal insertion of the sternocleidomastoid muscle and palpate up the anterior border of the muscle.
d) The point is located in the seam approximately level to the cricoid cartilage which is felt as the first broad band of cartilage on the trachea from the suprasternal notch upwards.
e) If you run your finger down from St 5 (separate location) on to the neck you should automatically fall in to the seam between the lateral border of the laryngeal and cricoid cartilages and the anterior border of the sternocleidomastoid muscle.

Note: The origin of St 10 at 1 ACI inferior to St 9 may be of Japanese origin. Worsley (1982) locates XI 10 on the anterior border of the strnocleidomastoid, at the level of the cricoid cartilage, approximatley 1 ACI inferior to XI 9. Wu (1973) locates ST 10 upon the anterior edge of the sterno-cleido-mastoid muscle, two pouce below ST 9, Lavier (1974) in an illustration clearly shows ST 10 at the mid-point of ST 9-11, Wu and Lavier locate ST 9 just inferior to the mandible. Voisin (1974) locates S 10 on the neck: lower lateral corner of the thyroid cartilage. Masayoshi (1975) locates ST 10 at the height of the inferior margin of the thyroid cartilage. Soulié (1994) locates ST 10 on the front of the neck: about two FW (Finger Width) from the medial line, at the level of the joints of the thyroid cartilage (larynx) and cricoid cartilage (sublaryngeal); at the angle of the anterior edge of the muscle (sternocleidomastoid muscle); deep, with the cricoid artery and at the superior edge of the transverse bulge; in a hollow; two FW below ST 9; four FW above and anterior (medial) to ST 12.

St 11 QI SHE – QI COTTAGE

⊥ ***0.3 CUN*** Δ ***3***

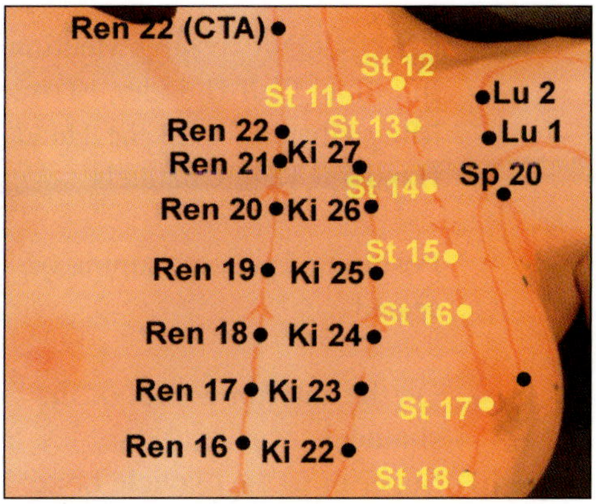

Pos: Position of patient: supine or seated.

Loc: a) On the anterior aspect of the neck.
b) At the root of the neck.
c) On the superior border of the sternal end of the clavicle.
d) Between the sternal and clavicular heads of the sternocleidomastoid muscle.
e) Just lateral to the insertion of the sternal head of the sternocleidomastoid muscle (on to the sternal end of the clavicle).

Tip: a) St 11 can be located easier by having the patient supine. Ask the patient to lift their head to expose the sternal and clavicular heads of the sternocleidomastoid muscle.
b) To locate and mark this point you need to have both hands free.
c) With the patient seated, pushing their forehead against resistance will expose the sternal and clavicular heads of the sternocleidomastoid muscle.
d) You should be able to see the sternal and clavicular heads of the sternocleidomastoid muscle as well as being able to see the superior border of the sternal end of the clavicle. If you palpate at this location you should be able to feel a palpable groove on the clavicle, and the point is located on the superior border just lateral to the sternal head insertion of the sternocleidomastoid muscle.

Note: Traditionally this point is directly inferior to St 9. Huang (1993) locates St 11 directly inferior to St 9 and lateral to CV 22 (Ren 22). Worsley (1982) locates XI 11 as in the location description above. He also measures the point at 2 ACI (Anatomical Chinese Inch) lateral to the median line. Wu (1973) locates St 11 above the clavicle, at one and one half pouce from the median line.

Soulié (1994) locates ST 11 on the lower neck: just at the lateral superior edge of the point (horn) of the sternum (manubrium); in the angle of the superior medial edge of the insertion of the sternocleidomastoid muscle and at the point of the bone; deep, on the sternohyoideus; in a hollow; two FW (Finger Width) below ST 10; on either side of CV 22 (Ren 22). Voisin (1974) locates S 11 on the neck: upper border of the clavicle, just lateral to its sternal extremity.

Eachou (1995) locates ST 11 at 1.5 inches lateral to CV 22 and at the superior margin of the medial clavicle, between the sternal and clavicular heads of the sternocleidomastoid muscle. Katsusuke (1983) locates ST 11 at one sun and five bu on either side of the central point in the front of the neck, also at the inner tip of the clavicles and upper tip of the sternum. So (1985) locates ST 11 at 1 division directly below ST 10, on the tip of the clavicle behind a tendon, one half a division higher than CV 22.

St 12 QUE PEN – BROKEN BOWL

⊥ ***0.3 CUN*** Δ ***3***

- RE-UNION/Crossing/Meeting Point of the Stomach Channel with the Large Intestine, Gall Bladder, Triple Heater and Small Intestine Channels – Foot Yang Ming Channel with the Hand Yang Ming, Foot Shao Yang, Hand Shao Yang and Hand Tai Yang Channels

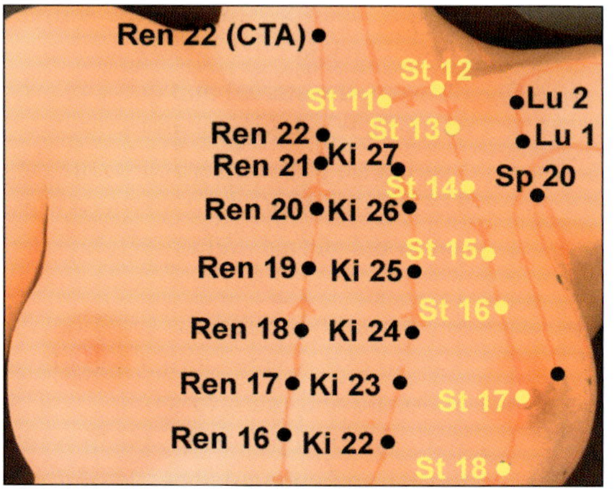

Pos: Position of patient: supine or seated.

Loc:
- a) On the anterior aspect of the shoulder.
- b) Superior to the clavicle bone.
- c) In the centre of the supraclavicular fossa.
- d) In a palpable notch.
- e) 4 cun lateral to the anterior median line (Ren channel).

Cun:
- a) The transverse cun measurements for the upper jiao (chest) includes the Kidney, Stomach, Spleen and Lung channels (lateral to the anterior median line). The cun measurements are as follows:
  Ki 22 to Ki 27 = 2 cun; St 13 to St 18 = 4 cun; Sp 17 to Sp 20 = 6 cun and Lu 1 to Lu 2 = 6 cun.
- b) The transverse measurement for the upper jiao is calculated using the anterior median line and the mid point of the clavicle.
- c) Identify the mid point of the clavicle by locating the medial end of the clavicle at the sterno-clavicular joint and the lateral end at the acromioclavicular joint and divide the distance into two.
- d) The distance from the anterior median line to the mid point of the clavicle is 4 cun.
- e) St 12 is not listed in a) because it is not classed as a chest point. Chest points are inferior to the clavicle. St 12 is superior to the clavicle at the same cun measurement, (4 cun lateral tothe anterior median line) as the Stomach chest points.

Tip:
- a) Locate 4 cun measurement lateral to the anterior median line (this measurement is often referred to as being on the mamillary line).
- b) The Stomach channel follows the contours of the chest, especially the curvature of the breast on a woman as it travels down towards the nipple. The more 'flat chested' a person is the lesser the curvature is.
- c) Ask the patient to shrug their shoulders to identify the supraclavicular fossa. The supraclavicular fossa is formed by the anterior border of the trapezius muscle, the superior border of the clavicle and the sternocleidomastoid muscle.
- d) It is possible to see the superior border of the clavicle at approximately 4 cun lateral to the anterior median line. You should be able to feel a palpable groove on the

clavicle, and the point is located just superior to this groove in the centre of the supraclavicular fossa.

e) The apex of the lungs are near to the surface of the skin, in the proximity of St 12. Do not needle deeper than 0.3 cun and make sure you are superior enough so that you do not 'nick' the clavicle with the tip of the needle.

Note: The mamillary line, or paramedian nipple line is used to describe the 4 cun line that passes through the nipples. 8 cun is commonly measured from the anterior median line to the acromial end of the clavicle (at its lateral border). Soulié (1994) locates ST 12 on the anterior lateral neck; three large FW (Finger Width) lateral to the swelling of the clavicle (horn of the sternum); just above (behind) the clavicle; in the angle of the deep; superior edge of the first rib and of the lateral edge of the hard muscle (anterior scalenus) with the strong artery (carotid); in a hollow; four FW lateral to St 11 and two FW medial and above ST 13. Wu (1973) locates ST 12 above the clavicle at four pouce from the median line.

Voisin (1974) locates S 12 on the neck: upper border of the clavicle, 2 fb (finger breadth) lateral to its sternal extremity. Legge (1999) locates St 12 in the supraclavicular fossa, just behind the clavicle, directly above the nipple (4 cun lateral to the Ren Channel). Lotan (2000) locates St 12 superior to the clavicle, 4 cun lateral to the front midline; in the supraclavicular fossa; vertically superior to the midpoint between the armpit anterior crease (axillary fold) and the front midline.

The distance between the anterior median line and the contour linking the mid-point of the clavicle with the centre of the nipple is 4 cun. The Stomach channel is located at 4 cun lateral to the anterior median line.

The transverse measurement for the chest (upper jiao) is calculated as 8 cun from the anterior median line to the tip of the acromion process.

The transverse distance between the two nipples is 8 cun. The distance between the bilateral Stomach channels at St 12 is also 8 cun, and can be used as a substitute measurement. (St 12 is just superior to the clavicle, in a palpable notch, at the mid-point of the supraclavicular fossa.)

The transverse cun measurements for the upper jiao (chest) which includes the Kidney, Stomach, Spleen and Lung channels (lateral to the anterior median line) are as follows:

Ki 22 to Ki 27 = 2 cun
St 13 to St 18 = 4 cun
Sp 17 to Sp 20 = 6 cun
Lu 1 to Lu 2 = 6 cun

The longitudinal measurements of the anterior torso are:

9 cun from the xiphisternal joint to the suprasternal fossa (with the space between 2 ribs measuring approximately 1.6 cun in the lower chest, and 1 cun in the upper chest)
8 cun from the centre of the umbilicus to the xiphisternal joint.

For the descriptions relating to the channels in the middle jiao, the longitudinal cun measurements are given from the centre of the umbilicus superiorly or from the xiphisternal joint inferiorly , depending on the direction of the flow of the channel.

5 cun from the centre of the umbilicus to the superior border of the symphysis pubis bone.

For the descriptions relating to the channels in the lower jiao, the longitudinal cun measurements are given from the centre of the umbilicus inferiorly or from the superior border of the symphysis pubis bone superiorly, depending on the direction of the flow of the channel.

St 13-30 are on the anterior torso, (St 13-18 in the upper jiao, St 19-25 in the middle jiao, St 26-30 in the lower jiao).

St 13-18 all lie in the pectoralis major muscle.

St 13 QI HU – QI DOOR

⊥ *0.3 CUN* Δ 5

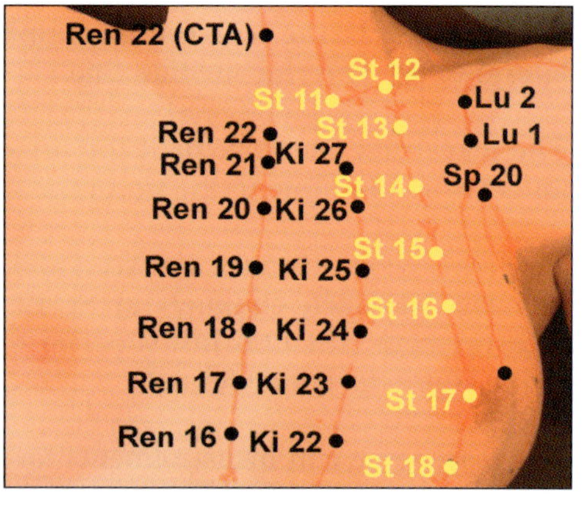

Pos: Position of patient: supine or seated.

Loc:
a) On the anterior aspect of the torso.
b) On the chest (in the upper jiao).
c) Just inferior to the clavicle, in a palpable notch.
d) In the pectoralis major muscle.
e) Directly inferior to St 12 (see separate description).
f) 4 cun lateral to the anterior median line (Ren channel).

Cun:
a) The transverse cun measurements for the upper jiao (chest) includes the Kidney, Stomach, Spleen and Lung channels (lateral to the anterior median line). The cun measurements are as follows:
Ki 22 to Ki 27 = 2 cun; St 13 to St 18 = 4 cun; Sp 17 to Sp 20 = 6 cun and Lu 1 to Lu 2 = 6 cun.
b) The transverse measurement for the upper jiao is calculated using the anterior median line and the mid point of the clavicle.
c) Identify the mid point of the clavicle by locating the medial end of the clavicle at the sterno-clavicular joint and the lateral end of the acromioclavicular joint, and divide the distance by half.

d) The distance from the anterior median line to the mid point of the clavicle is 4 cun.
e) The transverse distance between the two nipples (on a man) is 8 cun, thus the distance from the anterior median line to the nipple is 4 cun.

Tip: a) Locate 4 cun lateral to the anterior median line (this measurement is also referred to being located on the mamillary line).
b) The Stomach channel follows the contours of the chest, especially the curvature of the breast on a woman as it travels down towards the nipple. The more 'flat chested' a person is the lesser the curvature.
c) Place your finger between the first and second ribs which is the first intercostal space and run it laterally to the 4 cun measurement. Your finger should be in the deepest part of the intercostal space. As you run your finger laterally the intercostal space begins to curve upwards.
d) The inferior border of the clavicle is at the superior aspect of the first intercostal space, (not in the deepest part of it). The point is just inferior to the border at 4 cun lateral to the anterior median line. Make sure you are not palpating the point in the deepest part of the intercostal space otherwise you will be palpating St 14.
e) Palpation will locate the point accurately.

Note: The mamillary line, or paramedian nipple line is used to describe the 4 cun line that passes through the nipples. 8 cun is commonly measured from the anterior median line to the acromial end of the clavicle (at its lateral border). Soulié (1994) locates ST 13 at the lateral superior thorax just under the clavicle: three FW (finger width) lateral to the sternoclavicular angle; at the the angle of the inferior edge of the clavicle and the lateral edge of the clavicular insertion of the pectoralis major; two FW inferior and lateral to ST 12; two FW superior and medial to ST 14; three FW lateral to KI 27; three FW medial to LU 1. Wu (1973) locates ST 13 in the subclavicular hollow at two pouce caudal to ST 12.

Eachou (1995) locates ST 13 at 4 inches lateral to the anterior midline and in the infraclavicular fossa. Voisin (1974) locates S 13 on the breast at the infraclavicular fossa and slightly medial to the mamillary line. Shanghai (1993) locates ST 13 at the lower border of the midpoint of the clavicle and at 4 cun lateral to the anterior median line or Ren 21. Huang (1993) locates St 13 under the clavicle 2 cun lateral to Ki 27. Shandong (1982) locate Qihu inferior to the loer border of the middle point of the clavicula, 4 cun lateral to Pt. Xuanji (Ren 21). Lotan (2000) locates St 13 in the gap between the clavicle and the 1st rib, 4 cun lateral to the front midline

St 14 KU FANG – STOREHOUSE

⊥ ***0.3 CUN*** Δ ***5***

Pos: Position of patient: supine or seated.

Loc:
a) On the anterior aspect of the torso.
b) On the chest (in the upper jiao).
c) Inferior to the clavicle.
d) In the first intercostal space.
e) In the pectoralis major muscle.
f) 4 cun lateral to the anterior median line (Ren channel).

Cun:
a) The transverse cun measurements for the upper jiao (chest) includes the Kidney, Stomach, Spleen and Lung channels (lateral to the anterior median line). The cun measurements are as follows:
Ki 22 to Ki 27 = 2 cun; St 13 to St 18 = 4 cun; Sp 17 to Sp 20 = 6 cun and Lu 1 to Lu 2 = 6 cun.
b) The transverse measurement for the upper jiao is calculated using the anterior median line and the mid point of the clavicle.
c) Identify the mid point of the clavicle by locating the medial end of the clavicle at the sterno-clavicular joint and the lateral end of the acromioclavicular joint, and divide the distance by half.
d) The distance from the anterior median line to the mid point of the clavicle is 4 cun.
e) The transverse distance between the two nipples (on a man) is 8 cun, thus the distance from the anterior median line to the nipple is 4 cun.

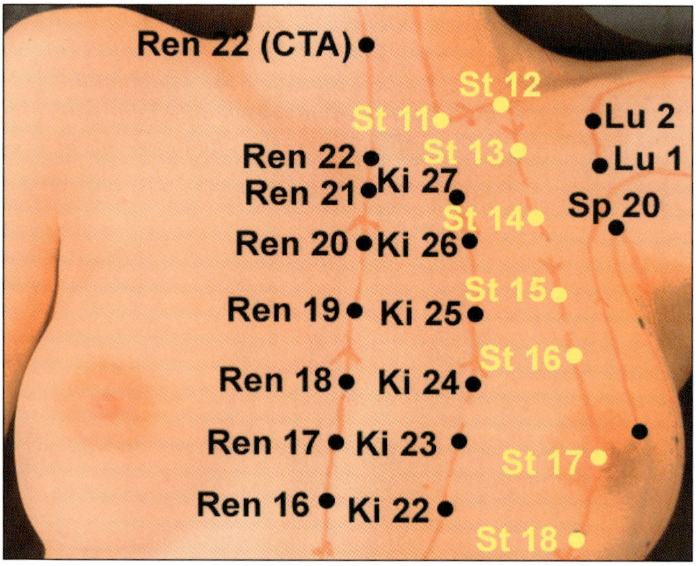

Tip:
a) Locate 4 cun lateral to the anterior median line (this measurement is also referred to being located on the mamillary line).
b) The Stomach channel follows the contours of the chest, especially the curvature of the breast on a woman as it travels down towards the nipple. The more 'flat chested' a person is the lesser the curvature.
c) Place your finger in the first intercostal space between the first and second ribs and run laterally 4 cun. As you run your finger laterally the intercostal space begins to curve upwards and you should be in the deepest part of the intercostal space
d) The inferior border of the clavicle is at the superior aspect of the first intercostal space, (not in the deepest part of it). The point is just inferior to the border at 4 cun lateral to the anterior median line. Make sure you are palpating the point in the deepest part of the intercostal space otherwise you could be palpating St 13 (which is more superior).
e) Palpation will locate the point accurately.
f) An easy way to remember which Stomach point lies in which intercostal space is to remember the formula: Stomach point X minus 13 equals intercostal space X. For example, St 14 – 13 = 1st intercostal space; St 18 – 13 = 5th intercostal space; etc.

Note: The mamillary line, or paramedian nipple line is used to describe the 4 cun line that passes through the nipples. 8 cun is commonly measured from the anterior median line to the acromial end of the clavicle (at its lateral border). Academy (1975) locates St 14 in the first intercostal space at 4 cun lateral to Ren 20.

Shanghai (1993) locates ST 14 in the first intercostal space and at 4 cun lateral to the anterior median line or Ren 20. Huang (1993) locates St 14 at 1 cun and 6 fen below St 13.

Soulié (1994) locates ST 14 on the lateral superior thorax: two FW (Finger Width) lateral to the angle of the sternum and the second rib; in the angle of the edge under the extremity of the first rib of the inferior edge of the oblique muscle (clavicular fascia of the pectoralis major); one large FW under the clavicle; in a hollow; two FW below ST 13; two FW above ST 15; two FW lateral to KI 26; two FW medial to LU 1.

Legge (1999) locates St 14 in the first intercostal space, about 1 cun below St 13, directly above the nipple.

St 15 WU YI – ROOM SCREEN

⊥ ***0.3 CUN*** Δ ***3 TO 5***

Pos: Position of patient: supine or seated.

Loc:
a) On the anterior aspect of the torso.
b) On the chest (in the upper jiao).
c) In the second intercostal space.
d) In the pectoralis major muscle.
e) 4 cun lateral to the anterior median line (Ren channel).

Cun:
a) The transverse cun measurements for the upper jiao (chest) includes the Kidney, Stomach, Spleen and Lung channels (lateral to the anterior median line). The cun measurements are as follows:
Ki 22 to Ki 27 = 2 cun; St 13 to St 18 = 4 cun; Sp 17 to Sp 20 = 6 cun and Lu 1 to Lu 2 = 6 cun.
b) The transverse measurement for the upper jiao is calculated using the anterior median line and the mid point of the clavicle.
c) Identify the mid point of the clavicle by locating the medial end of the clavicle at the sterno-clavicular joint and the lateral end of the acromioclavicular joint, and divide the distance by half.
d) The distance from the anterior median line to the mid point of the clavicle is 4 cun.
e) The transverse distance between the two nipples (on a man) is 8 cun, thus the distance from the anterior median line to the nipple is 4 cun.

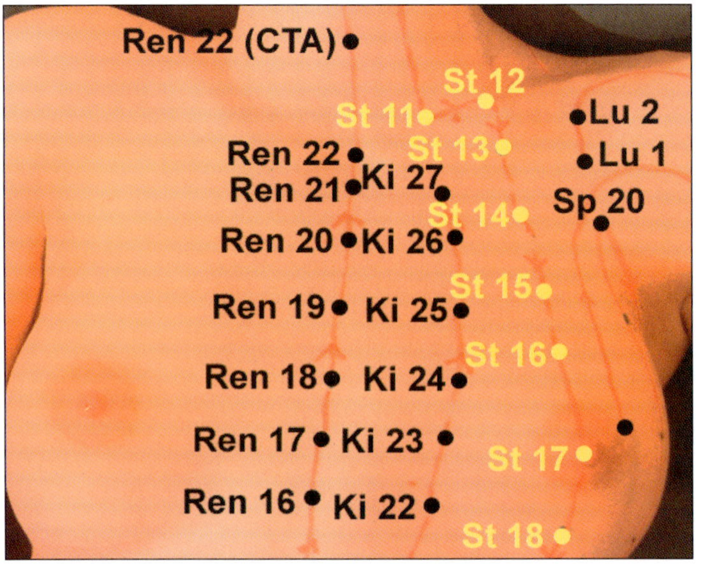

Tip:
a) Locate 4 cun measurement lateral to the anterior median line (this measurement is often referred to as being on the mamillary line).
b) The Stomach channel follows the contours of the chest, especially the curvature of the breast on a woman as it travels down towards the nipple. The more 'flat chested' a person is the lesser the curvature is.
c) The second rib is easier to locate than the first rib which articulates with the sternal angle located at the level of the sternum.
d) Place your finger in the second intercostal space between the second and third ribs and run laterally 4 cun. As you run your finger laterally the intercostal space begins to curve upwards and you should be in the deepest part of the intercostal space
e) Palpation will locate the point accurately.
f) An easy way to remember which Stomach point lies in which intercostal space is to remember the formula: Stomach point X minus 13 equals intercostal space X. For example, St 15 – 13 = 2nd intercostal space; St 18 – 13 = 5th intercostal space; etc.

Note: Some traditions use a mamillary line, or a paramedian nipple line to describe the 4 cun line that passes through the nipples. There are also traditions that measure 8 cun from the anterior median line to the tip of the acromion process of the scapula.

Shanghai (1993) locates ST 15 in the second intercostal space and at 4 cun lateral to the anterior median line or Ren 19. Academy (1975) locates St 15 in the second intercostal space at 4 cun lateral to Ren 19. Huang (1993) locates St 15 at 1 cun and 6 fen below St 14.

Soulié (1994) locates ST 15 on the anterior superior thorax: two large FW (Finger Width) lateral to the angle of the sternum and the second rib; in the angle of the inferior edge of the second rib (first under the clavicle) and of the superior edge of the sternal fascia of the pectoralis major; under the clavicular fascia; in a hollow; two FW below and slightly medial to ST 14; three tightened fingers above ST 16; three FW lateral to LI 25; three FW medial to HT 1.

Legge (1999) locates St 15 in the 2nd intercostal space, directly above the nipple.

St 16 YING CHUANG – BREAST WINDOW

⊥ ***0.3 CUN*** Δ **5**

Pos: Position of patient: supine or seated.

Loc:
a) On the anterior aspect of the torso.
b) On the chest (in the upper jiao).
c) In the third intercostal space.
d) In the pectoralis major muscle.
e) 4 cun lateral to the anterior median line (Ren channel).

Cun:
a) The transverse cun measurements for the upper jiao (chest) includes the Kidney, Stomach, Spleen and Lung channels (lateral to the anterior median line). The cun measurements are as follows:
Ki 22 to Ki 27 = 2 cun; St 13 to St 18 = 4 cun; Sp 17 to Sp 20 = 6 cun and Lu 1 to Lu 2 = 6 cun.
b) The transverse measurement for the upper jiao is calculated using the anterior median line and the mid point of the clavicle.
c) Identify the mid point of the clavicle by locating the medial end of the clavicle at the sterno-clavicular joint and the lateral end of the acromioclavicular joint, and divide the distance by half.
d) The distance from the anterior median line to the mid point of the clavicle is 4 cun.
e) The transverse distance between the two nipples (on a man) is 8 cun, thus the distance from the anterior median line to the nipple is 4 cun.

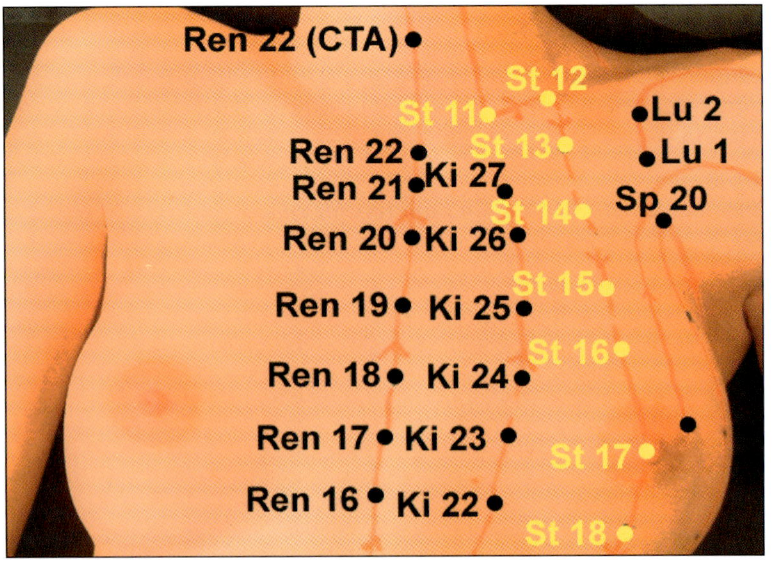

Tip:
a) Locate 4 cun measurement lateral to the anterior median line (this measurement is often referred to as being on the mamillary line).
b) The Stomach channel follows the contours of the chest, especially the curvature of the breast on a woman as it travels down towards the nipple. The more 'flat chested' a person is the lesser the curvature is.
c) Place your finger in the third intercostal space between the third and fourth ribs and run laterally 4 cun. As you run your finger laterally the intercostal space begins to curve upwards and you should be in the deepest part of the intercostal space
d) Palpation will locate the point accurately.
e) It can be difficult to locate the third intercostal space onwards as the pectoralis major muscle covers the surface of the ribs. To assist with point location place a finger in both the first and second intercostal space.
f) Your fingers are now a "rib space" apart. If you place one finger in the second intercostal space, your other finger should then give you a good approximation of the position of the third intercostal space (intercostal spaces are approximately of equal width). You can continue with this method of locating the intercostal spaces. The spaces become more lateral at the level of the fourth intercostal space. At this level the costal cartilages of the lower ribs can merge together to attach to the sternum rather than having individual articulations with the sternum. The intercostal spaces are therefore only easily palpable more laterally.
g) Note that the nipples on men or 'flat chested' women are generally located at the fourth intercostal space.
h) An easy way to remember which Stomach point lies in which intercostal space is to remember the formula: Stomach point X minus 13 equals intercostal space X. For example, St 16 – 13 = 3rd intercostal space; St 18 – 13 = 5th intercostal space; etc.

Note: Some traditions use a mamillary line, or a paramedian nipple line to describe the 4 cun line that passes through the nipples. There are also traditions that measure 8 cun from the anterior median line to the tip of the acromion process of the scapula. Shanghai (1993) locates ST 16 in the third intercostal space and at 4 cun lateral to the anterior median line or Ren 18. Academy (1975) locates St 16 in the third intercostal space at 4 cun lateral to Ren 18. Huang (1993) locates St 16 at 1 cun and 6 fen below St 15.

Soulié (1994) locates ST 16 on the chest; two large FW (Finger Width) lateral to the sternum; two FW just above the nipple (men); at the angle of the inferior edge of the third rib (second under the clavicle in this place) and of the lateral (external) edge of the intercostal ligament; in a hollow; on the pectoralis major; three FW under ST 15; two FW above ST 17; three FW lateral to KI 24; two FW medial to PC 1. Legge (1999) locates St 16 in the third intercostal space, directly above the nipple.

St 17 RU ZHONG – CENTRE OF THE BREASTS

⊥ ***FORBIDDEN TO NEEDLE*** Δ ***FORBIDDEN TO MOXA***

Pos: Position of patient: supine (for reference purposes only as this point is forbidden to needle and moxa).

Loc: a) On the anterior aspect of the torso.
b) On the chest (in the upper jiao).
c) In the fourth intercostal space.
d) On the pectoralis major muscle.
e) 4 cun lateral to the anterior median line (Ren channel).
f) In the centre of the nipple.

Cun: a) The transverse cun measurements for the upper jiao (chest) includes the Kidney, Stomach, Spleen and Lung channels (lateral to the anterior median line). The cun measurements are as follows:
Ki 22 to Ki 27 = 2 cun; St 13 to St 18 = 4 cun; Sp 17 to Sp 20 = 6 cun and Lu 1 to Lu 2 = 6 cun.
b) The transverse measurement for the upper jiao is calculated using the anterior median line and the mid point of the clavicle.
c) Identify the mid point of the clavicle by locating the medial end of the clavicle at the sterno-clavicular joint and the lateral end of the acromioclavicular joint, and divide the distance by half.
d) The distance from the anterior median line to the mid point of the clavicle is 4 cun.
e) The transverse distance between the two nipples (on a man) is 8 cun, thus the distance from the anterior median line to the nipple is 4 cun.

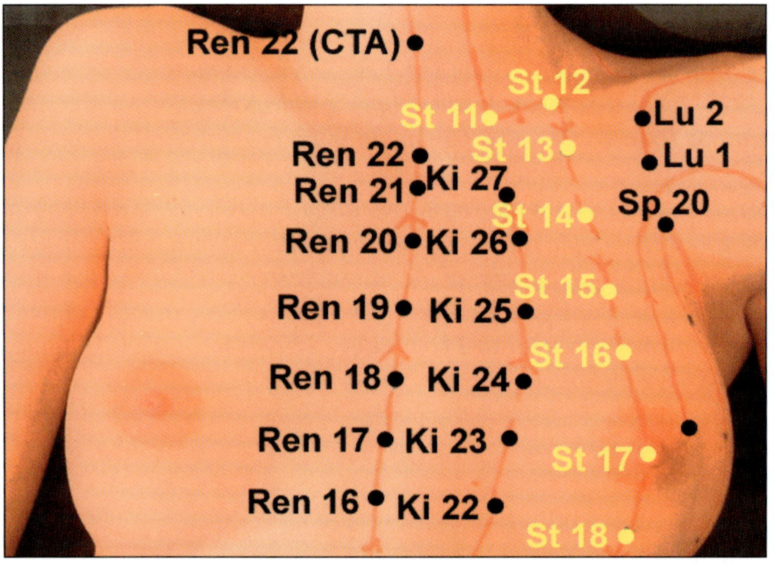

Tip:
a) The tips below are for the use of landmarks only as this point should not be needled or moxaed.
b) Locate 4 cun measurement lateral to the anterior median line (this measurement is often referred to as being on the mamillary line).
c) The Stomach channel follows the contours of the chest, especially the curvature of the breast on a woman as it travels down towards the nipple. The more 'flat chested' a person is the lesser the curvature is.
d) Place your finger in the fourth intercostal space between the fourth and fifth ribs and run laterally 4 cun. As you run your finger laterally the intercostal space begins to curve upwards and you should be in the deepest part of the intercostal space
e) Palpation will locate the point accurately.
f) It can be difficult to locate the third intercostal space onwards as the pectoralis major muscle covers the surface of the ribs. To assist with point location place a finger in both the first and second intercostal space.
g) Your fingers are now a "rib space" apart. If you place one finger in the second intercosta space, your other finger should then give you a good approximation of the position of the third intercostal space (intercostal spaces are approximately of equal width). You can continue with this method of locating the intercostal spaces. The spaces become more lateral at the level of the fourth intercostal space. At this level the costal cartilages of the lower ribs can merge together to attach to the sternum rather than having individual articulations with the sternum. The intercostal spaces are therefore only easily palpable more laterally.
h) Note that the nipples on men or 'flat chested' women are generally located at the fourth intercostal space.
i) An easy way to remember which Stomach point lies in which intercostal space is to remember the formula: Stomach point X minus 13 equals intercostal space X.
For example, St 17 – 13 = 4th intercostal space; St 18 – 13 = 5th intercostal space; etc.

Note: Some traditions use a mamillary line, or a paramedian nipple line to describe the 4 cun line that passes through the nipples. There are also traditions that measure 8 cun from the anterior median line to the tip of the acromion process of the scapula. Academy (1975) locates St 17 in the fourth intercostal space, midline of the clavicle.

St 18 RU GEN – ROOT OF THE BREASTS

⊥ ***0.3 CUN*** Δ ***3 TO 5***

Pos: Position of patient: supine.

Loc: a) On the anterior aspect of the torso.
b) On the chest (in the upper jiao).
c) In the fifth intercostal space.
d) 4 cun lateral to the anterior median line.

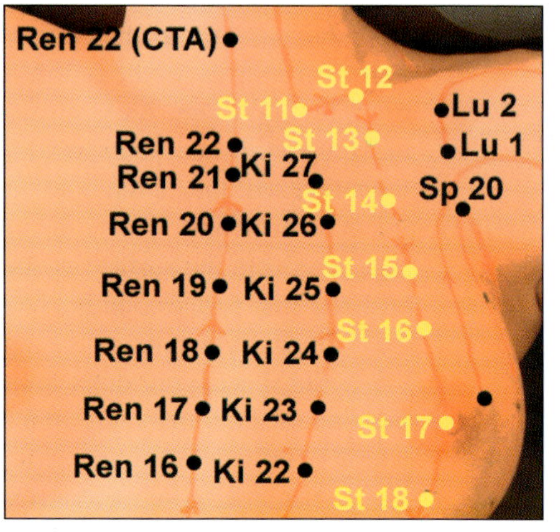

Cun: a) The transverse cun measurements for the upper jiao (chest) includes the Kidney, Stomach, Spleen and Lung channels (lateral to the anterior median line). The cun measurements are as follows:
Ki 22 to Ki 27 = 2 cun; St 13 to St 18 = 4 cun; Sp 17 to Sp 20 = 6 cun and Lu 1 to Lu 2 = 6 cun.
b) The transverse measurement for the upper jiao is calculated using the anterior median line and the mid point of the clavicle.
c) Identify the mid point of the clavicle by locating the medial end of the clavicle at the sterno-clavicular joint and the lateral end of the acromioclavicular joint, and divide the distance by half.
d) The distance from the anterior median line to the mid point of the clavicle is 4 cun.
e) The transverse distance between the two nipples (on a man) is 8 cun, thus the distance from the anterior median line to the nipple is 4 cun.

Tip: a) Locate 4 cun measurement lateral to the anterior median line (this measurement is often referred to as being on the mamillary line).
b) The Stomach channel follows the contours of the chest, and especially the curvature of the breast on a woman as it travels down towards the nipple. The more the person is 'flat chested' the less curvature there is going to be to the nipple for the Stomach channel.
c) Place your finger between the fifth and sixth ribs which is the fifth intercostal space and run it laterally to the 4 cun measurement.Your finger should be in the deepest part of the intercostal space. As you run your finger laterally the intercostal space begins to curve upwards.
d) Palpation in this area should reveal the accurate location for this point.
e) On women the point lies inferior to the breast tissue at the root of the breast, hence its name.
f) You may have problems feeling for the intercostal spaces from the third intercostal space downwards, because of the pectoralis major muscle covering the surface of the ribs. To help you with this you can usually feel the first and second intercostal spaces quite easily from the sternal end of the ribs by placing two of your fingers in the first and second intercostal spaces.

g) Your fingers are now a "rib space" apart, so if you place one finger in the second intercostal space, your other finger should then give you a good approximation of the position of the third intercostal space as the intercostal spaces are of approximately equal width. You can continue with this procedure of working your way down the intercostal spaces, but as you go down past the fourth intercostal space you will need to feel for the spaces more laterally. This is because at this level the costal cartilages of the lower ribs can merge together to attach to the sternum rather than having individual articulations with the sternum. The intercostal spaces are therefore only easily palpable more laterally, and will curve upwards as you palpate laterally from the sternum.

h) Note that the nipples on men or 'flat chested' women are generally located at the fourth intercostal space.

i) An easy way to remember which Stomach point lies in which intercostal space is to remember the formula: Stomach point X minus 13 equals intercostal space X. For example, St 18 – 13 = 5th intercostal space; St 14 – 13 = 1st intercostal space; etc.

Note: Some traditions use a mamillary line, or a paramedian nipple line to describe the 4 cun line that passes through the nipples. There are also traditions that measure 8 cun from the anterior median line to the tip of the acromion process of the scapula. Shanghai (1993) locates ST 18 in the first intercostal space and at 4 cun lateral to the anterior median line or Ren 16. Huang (1993) locates St 18 at 1 cun and 6 fen below the breast.

Soulié locates ST 18 under the breast (men), two FW (Finger Width) under the nipple; at the angle between the inferior edge of the fifth rib (the nipple is on the bottom of the fourth) and the lateral edge of an intercostal ligament; in a hollow; two FW just below ST 17; two FW above and slightly lateral to ST 19; three FW lateral to KI 22; two FW medial to LR 14. Legge (1999) locates St 18 in the intercostal space (the 5th) below the nipple.

The transverse measurement for the middle and lower abdomen (middle and lower jiao) is calculated as 2 cun, between the anterior median line (at the centre of the umbilicus) and the lateral border of the rectus abdominis muscle (St 25).

The lateral border of the rectus abdominis muscle is not the actual edge of the muscle but the most prominent surface of the muscle before it begins to 'slope' in to the torso. By visualising the corner of an inverted 'L', the point is located on the antero-lateral edge of the muscle. To locate this muscle ask the patient to slightly raise their head. The lateral border of the rectus abdominis muscle is on the most lateral part of the palpable curve which is more medial than the actual edge of the muscle.

The transverse cun measurements for the middle and lower abdomen (middle and lower jiao) includes the Kidney, Stomach, Spleen, Gall Bladder and Liver channels (lateral to the anterior median line) as follows:

Ki 11 to Ki 21 = 0.5 cun
St 19 to St 30 = 2 cun
Sp 13 to Sp 16 = 6 cun (Sp 12 = 3.5 cun)
GB 24 = 4 cun
Liv 14 = 4 cun

Ki 16, St 25 and Sp 15 are all transversely level with the centre of the umbilicus and are used as reference points for marking the respective channel cun measurements.

The longitudinal measurements of the anterior torso are:

9 cun from the xiphisternal joint to the suprasternal fossa (measuring approximately 1.6 cun in the lower chest intercostal spaces, and 1 cun in the upper chest intercostal spaces)

8 cun from the centre of the umbilicus to the xiphisternal joint. For the descriptions relating to the channels in the middle jiao, the longitudinal cun measurements are given from the centre of the umbilicus superiorly or from the xiphisternal joint inferiorly, depending on the direction of the flow of the channel.

5 cun from the centre of the umbilicus to the superior border of the symphysis pubis bone. For the descriptions relating to the channels in the lower jiao, the longitudinal cun measurements are given from the centre of the umbilicus inferiorly or from the superior border of the symphysis pubis bone superiorly, depending on the direction of the flow of the channel.

Note: The mid and lower abdomen (middle and lower jiao) transverse distances between the anterior median line (Ren Mai/Conception Vessel) and the Kidney channel, and the anterior median line (Ren Mai/Conception Vessel) and the Stomach channel have varied markedly in Acupuncture literature. The Stomach channel is given as 2/2.5/3 cun from the anterior median line (Ren Mai/Conception Vessel) in different texts. The currently accepted measurement is 2 cun from the anterior median line to the Stomach channel, which is the space between the centre of the umbilicus and the lateral border of the rectus abdominis muscle.

St 19 BU RONG – NOT AT EASE

⊥ *0.3 TO 0.5 CUN* ∆ *3 TO 7*

FORBIDDEN TO NEEDLE AND MOXA THIS POINT DURING PREGNANCY

Pos: Position of patient: supine.

Loc: a) On the anterior aspect of the torso.
b) On the mid-abdomen (in the middle jiao).
c) On the lateral border of the rectus abdominis muscle.
d) 2 cun lateral to the anterior median line.
e) 6 cun superior to the level of the centre of the umbilicus.
f) 2 cun inferior to the level of the xiphisternal joint.
g) Level with Ren 14 .

Cun: a) The transverse measurement for the middle and lower abdomen (middle and lower jiao) is 2 cun between the anterior median line (at the centre of the umbilicus) and the lateral border of the rectus abdominis muscle (at St 25).

b) The lateral border of the rectus abdominis muscle is not the actual edge of the muscle but the most prominent surface of the muscle before it begins to 'slope' in to the torso. By visualising the corner of an inverted 'L', the point is located on the antero-lateral edge of the muscle. To locate this muscle ask the patient to slightly raise their head. The lateral border of the rectus abdominis muscle is on the most lateral part of the palpable curve which is more medial than the actual edge of the muscle.

c) Another way to mark out the transverse cun measurements at the level of the umbilicus is to locate the medial border of the anterior superior iliac spine (part of the iliac crest). To locate the 4 cun line of the Spleen channel, place a pen longitudinally on the medial border of the anterior superior iliac spine approximately halfway between the centre of the umbilicus and the superior border of the symphysis pubis bone. For the Stomach channel divide the 4 cun measurement in half to get 2 cun. The edge of the rectus abdominis muscle is measured as 4 cn. Once established you can then divide the 4 cun into other cun measurements for use on the Stomach and Kidney and Spleen channels etc.

d) The transverse cun measurements for the middle and lower abdomen (middle and lower jiao) includes the Kidney, Stomach, Spleen, Gall Bladder and Liver channels (lateral to the anterior median line): Ki 11 to Ki 21 = 0.5 cun; St 19 to St 30 = 2 cun; Sp 12 = 3.5 cun; Sp 13 to Sp 16 = 4 cun; GB 24 = 4 cun; Liv 14 = 4 cun.

e) Ki 16, St 25 and Sp 15 are all transversely level with the centre of the umbilicus and used as reference points for marking their channels cun measurements.

f) The longitudinal measurement of the mid abdomen is 8 cun from the centre of the umbilicus to the xiphisternal joint (Ren 16).

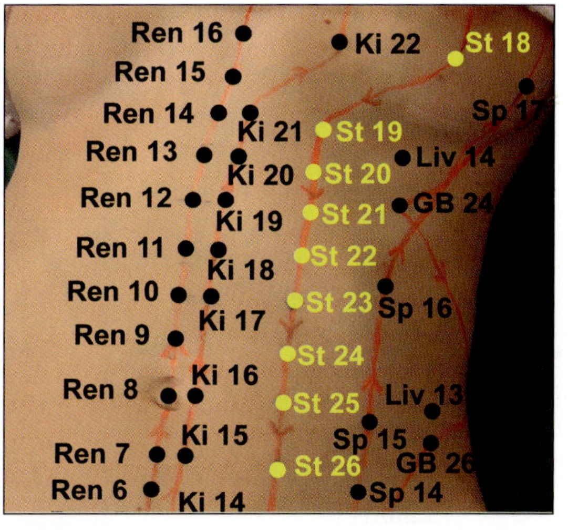

Tip: a) Locate the 2 cun measurement level with the centre of the umbilicus and lateral to the anterior median line (St 25).

b) The Stomach channel follows the curved ridge of the rectus abdominis muscle as it travels down towards the groin.

c) Place your finger on the anterior median line, (Ren 14) 6 cun superior to the level of the umbilicus, and run laterally 2 cun and palpate for the point.

d) You could mark 2 cun lateral to the anterior median line first, and then palpate with the flow of the Stomach channel to 2 cun inferior to the level of the xiphisternal joint.

e) If the patient has a long xiphoid process then palpate for the point level with the cun measurement rather than with the Ren point (the length of the xiphoid affects only the Ren channel).

Note: Some acupuncture schools have used different transverse cun measurements at the level of the umbilicus: the Kidney channel has been put at 1.5 pouce/ACI, the Stomach channel at 2.5 or 3 pouce/ACI and the Spleen channel at 4 or 4.5 pouce/ACI. A few schools still do use these transverse measurements, but they still mainly have the same longitudinal measurements for their point locations as the majority use.

Wu (1973) locates ST 19 at 3 pouce from the median line and also on a horizontal line that passes through the fossa of the xiphoid process. Worsley (1982) locates XI 19 on the thorax, 3 ACI (Anatomical Chinese Inch) lateral to the median line, 6 ACI superior to the level of the umbilicus and at the level of XIII 14 (Ren 14).

Soulié (1994) locates ST 19 at four FW (Finger Width) directly below the nipple. three tightened FW lateral to the sternum and in the angle that is between the superior edge of the aixth rib and the lateral edge of a vertical intercostal ligament; two FW below ST 18; two FW above ST 20; two large FW lateral to KI 21; three FW medial to SP 17.

Voisin (1974) locates S 19 on the abdomen on the cartilage between the 6th and 7th ribs. Lavier (1974) in an illustration locates ST 19 at 3 pouce lateral to the median line, medial to the rib cage and 6 pouce superior to the level of the umbilicus with the longitudinal measurement for the middle abdomen taken as 7 pouce from the level of the umbilicus and the tip of the xiphoid process. Katsusuke (1983) locates ST 19 on either side of the diaphragm at the front edges of the 8th ribs. Huang (1993) locates St 19 at 1 cun and 5 fen lateral to Ki 21 and at 2 cun bilateral to the Conception Vessel, or 4 cun from the tip of the 4th rib.

St 20 CHENG MAN – RECEIVING FULLNESS

⊥ ***0.5 TO 0.8 CUN*** **Δ *3 TO 7***
FORBIDDEN TO NEEDLE AND MOXA THIS POINT DURING PREGNANCY

Pos: Position of patient: supine.

Loc:
a) On the anterior aspect of the torso.
b) On the mid-abdomen (in the middle jiao).
c) On the lateral border of the rectus abdominis muscle.
d) 2 cun lateral to the anterior median line.
e) 5 cun superior to the level of the centre of the umbilicus.
f) 3 cun inferior to the level of the xiphisternal joint.
g) Level with Ren 13.

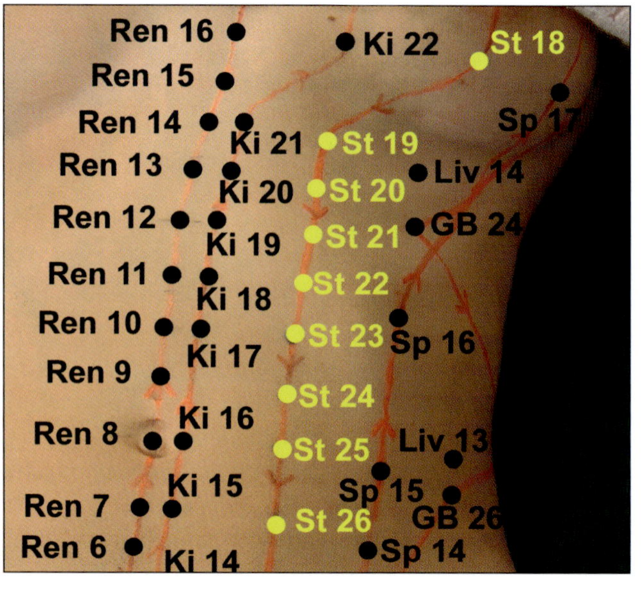

Cun: a) The transverse measurement for the middle and lower abdomen (middle and lower jiao) is 2 cun between the anterior median line (at the centre of the umbilicus) and the lateral border of the rectus abdominis muscle (at St 25).

b) The lateral border of the rectus abdominis muscle is not the actual edge of the muscle but the most prominent surface of the muscle before it begins to 'slope' in to the torso. By visualising the corner of an inverted 'L', the point is located on the antero-lateral edge of the muscle. To locate this muscle ask the patient to slightly raise their head. The lateral border of the rectus abdominis muscle is on the most lateral part of the palpable curve which is more medial than the actual edge of the muscle.

c) Another way to mark out the transverse cun measurements at the level of the umbilicus is to locate the medial border of the anterior superior iliac spine (part of the iliac crest). To locate the 4 cun line of the Spleen channel, place a pen longitudinally on the medial border of the anterior superior iliac spine approximately halfway between the centre of the umbilicus and the superior border of the symphysis pubis bone. For the Stomach channel divide the 4 cun measurement in half to get 2 cun. The edge of the rectus abdominis muscle is measured as 4 cun. Once established you can then divide the 4 cun into other cun measurements for use on the Stomach and Kidney and Spleen channels etc.

d) The transverse cun measurements for the middle and lower abdomen (middle and lower jiao) includes the Kidney, Stomach, Spleen, Gall Bladder and Liver channels (lateral to the anterior median line): Ki 11 to Ki 21 = 0.5 cun; St 19 to St 30 = 2 cun; Sp 12 = 3.5 cun; Sp 13 to Sp 16 = 4 cun; GB 24 = 4 cun; Liv 14 = 4 cun.

e) Ki 16, St 25 and Sp 15 are all transversely level with the centre of the umbilicus and used as reference points for marking their channels cun measurements.

f) The longitudinal measurement of the mid abdomen is 8 cun from the centre of the umbilicus to the xiphisternal joint (Ren 16).

Tip: a) Locate the 2 cun measurement level with the centre of the umbilicus and lateral to the anterior median line (St 25).

b) The Stomach channel follows the curved ridge of the rectus abdominis muscle as it travels down towards the groin.

c) Place your finger on the anterior median line, (Ren 13) 5 cun superior to the level of the umbilicus, and run laterally 2 cun and palpate for the point.

d) You could mark 2 cun lateral to the anterior median line first, and then palpate with the flow of the Stomach channel to 3 cun inferior to the level of the xiphisternal joint.

e) If the patient has a long xiphoid process then palpate for the point level with the cun measurement rather than with the Ren point (the length of the xiphoid affects only the Ren channel).

Note: Some acupuncture schools have used different transverse cun measurements at the level of the umbilicus: the Kidney channel has been put at 1.5 pouce/ACI, the Stomach channel at 2.5 or 3 pouce/ACI and the Spleen channel at 4 or 4.5 pouce/ACI. A few schools still do use these transverse measurements, but they still mainly have the same longitudinal measurements for their point locations as the majority use.Wu (1973) locates ST 20 at 3 pouce from the median line and at 1 pouce below ST 19. Worsley (1982) locates XI 20 on the abdomen, 3 ACI (Anatomical Chinese Inch) lateral to the median line, 5 ACI superior to the level of the umbilicus and level of XIII 13 (Ren 13). Soulié (1994) locates ST 20 on the mid-thorax: vertical from the nipple; at the level of the inferior extremity of the sternum; in the angle between the inferior edge of the sixth rib (the seventh being joined to the sternum) and the lateral edge of one tendon (insertion of the rectus abdominus); two FW (Finger Width) below ST 19; two FW above ST 21 and three FW lateral to CV 15 (Ren 15). Voisin (1974) locates S 20 on the abdomen on the cartilage between the 7th and 8th ribs. Lavier (1974) in an illustration locates ST 20 at 3 pouce lateral to the median line, and 5 pouce superior to the level of the umbilicus with the longitudinal measurement for the middle abdomen taken as 7 pouce from the level of the umbilicus and the tip of the xiphoid process.

St 21 LIANG MEN – BRIDGE GATE

⊥ ***0.5 TO 0.8 CUN*** **Δ** ***5 TO 15***
FORBIDDEN TO NEEDLE AND MOXA THIS POINT DURING PREGNANCY

Pos: Position of patient: supine.

Loc:
a) On the anterior aspect of the torso.
b) On the mid-abdomen (in the middle jiao).
c) On the lateral border of the rectus abdominis muscle.
d) 2 cun lateral to the anterior median line.
e) 4 cun superior to the level of the centre of the umbilicus.
f) 4 cun inferior to the level of the xiphisternal joint.
g) Level with Ren 12.

Cun:
a) The transverse measurement for the middle and lower abdomen (middle and lower jiao) is 2 cun between the anterior median line (at the centre of the umbilicus) and the lateral border of the rectus abdominis muscle (at St 25).
b) The lateral border of the rectus abdominis muscle is not the actual edge of the muscle but the most prominent surface of the muscle before it begins to 'slope' in to the torso. By visualising the corner of an inverted 'L', the point is located on the antero-lateral edge of the muscle. To locate this muscle ask the patient to slightly raise their head. The lateral border of the rectus abdominis muscle is on the most lateral part of the palpable curve which is more medial than the actual edge of the muscle.
c) Another way to mark out the transverse cun measurements at the level of the umbilicus is to locate the medial border of the anterior superior iliac spine (part of the iliac crest). To locate the 4 cun line of the Spleen channel, place a pen longitudinally on the medial border of the anterior superior iliac spine approximately halfway between the centre of the umbilicus and the superior border of the symphysis pubis bone. For the Stomach channel divide the 4 cun

measurement in half to get 2 cun. The edge of the rectus abdominis muscle is measured as 4 cun. Once established you can then divide the 4 cun into other cun measurements for use on the Stomach and Kidney and Spleen channels etc.

d) The transverse cun measurements for the middle and lower abdomen (middle and lower jiao) includes the Kidney, Stomach, Spleen, Gall Bladder and Liver channels (lateral to the anterior median line): Ki 11 to Ki 21 = 0.5 cun; St 19 to St 30 = 2 cun; Sp 12 = 3.5 cun; Sp 13 to Sp 16 = 4 cun; GB 24 = 4 cun; Liv 14 = 4 cun.

e) Ki 16, St 25 and Sp 15 are all transversely level with the centre of the umbilicus and used as reference points for marking their channels cun measurements.

f) The longitudinal measurement of the mid abdomen is 8 cun from the centre of the umbilicus to the xiphisternal joint (Ren 16).

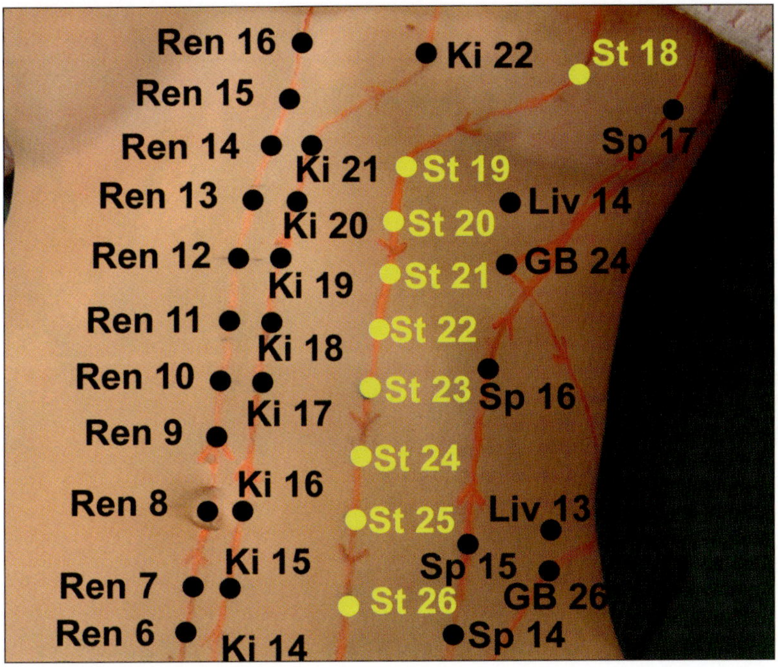

Tip: a) Locate the 2 cun measurement level with the centre of the umbilicus and lateral to the anterior median line (St 25).

b) The Stomach channel follows the curved ridge of the rectus abdominis muscle as it travels down towards the groin.

c) Place your finger on the anterior median line, (Ren 12) 4 cun superior to the level of the umbilicus, and run laterally 2 cun and palpate for the point.

d) You could mark 2 cun lateral to the anterior median line first, and then palpate with the flow of the Stomach channel to 4 cun inferior to the level of the xiphisternal joint.

Note: Some acupuncture schools have used different transverse cun measurements at the level of the umbilicus: the Kidney channel has been put at 1.5 pouce/ACI, the Stomach channel at 2.5 or 3 pouce/ACI and the Spleen channel at 4 or 4.5 pouce/ACI. A few schools still do use these transverse measurements, but they still mainly have the same longitudinal measurements for their point locations as the majority use.Wu (1973) locates ST 21 at 3 pouce from the median line and at 2 pouce below ST 19.

Worsley (1982) locates XI 21 on the abdomen, 3 ACI (Anatomical Chinese Inch) lateral to the median line, 4 ACI superior to the level of the umbilicus, at the level of XIII 12 (Ren 12). Soulié (1994) locates ST 21 on the thorax: approximately vertical from the nipple; on the inferior edge of the seventh rib (the last joint on the sternum); on the lateral edge of one intercostal ligament; in a hollow; at two FW (Finger Width) below ST 20; two FW above ST 22.

Voisin (1974) locates S 21 on the abdomen on the cartilage between the 8th and 9th ribs. Lavier (1974) in an illustration locates ST 21 at 3 pouce lateral to the median line, and 4 pouce superior to the level of the umbilicus with the longitudinal measurement for the middle abdomen taken as 7 pouce from the level of the umbilicus and the tip of the xiphoid process.

St 22 GUAN MEN – BORDER GATE

⊥ ***0.8 TO 1.0 CUN*** **Δ *5 TO 15***
FORBIDDEN TO NEEDLE AND MOXA THIS POINT DURING PREGNANCY

Pos: Position of patient: supine.

Loc: a) On the anterior aspect of the torso.
b) On the mid-abdomen (in the middle jiao).
c) On the lateral border of the rectus abdominis muscle.
d) 2 cun lateral to the anterior median line.
e) 3 cun superior to the level of the centre of the umbilicus.
f) 5 cun inferior to the level of the xiphisternal joint.
g) Level with Ren 11.

Cun: a) The transverse measurement for the middle and lower abdomen (middle and lower jiao) is 2 cun between the anterior median line (at the centre of the umbilicus) and the lateral border of the rectus abdominis muscle (at St 25).
b) The lateral border of the rectus abdominis muscle is not the actual edge of the muscle but the most prominent surface of the muscle before it begins to 'slope' in to the torso. By visualising the corner of an inverted 'L', the point is located on the antero-lateral edge of the muscle. To locate this muscle ask the patient to slightly raise their head. The lateral border of the rectus abdominis muscle is on the most lateral part of the palpable curve which is more medial than the actual edge of the muscle.
c) Another way to mark out the transverse cun measurements at the level of the umbilicus is to locate the medial border of the anterior superior iliac spine (part of the iliac crest). To locate the 4 cun line of the Spleen channel, place a pen longitudinally on the medial border of the anterior superior iliac spine approximately halfway between the centre of the umbilicus and the superior border

of the symphysis pubis bone. For the Stomach channel divide the 4 cun measurement in half to get 2 cun. The edge of the rectus abdominis muscle is measured as 4 cun. Once established you can then divide the 4 cun into other cun measurements for use on the Stomach and Kidney and Spleen channels etc.

d) The transverse cun measurements for the middle and lower abdomen (middle and lower jiao) includes the Kidney, Stomach, Spleen, Gall Bladder and Liver channels (lateral to the anterior median line): Ki 11 to Ki 21 = 0.5 cun; St 19 to St 30 = 2 cun; Sp 12 = 3.5 cun; Sp 13 to Sp 16 = 4 cun; GB 24 = 4 cun; Liv 14 = 4 cun.

e) Ki 16, St 25 and Sp 15 are all transversely level with the centre of the umbilicus and used as reference points for marking their channels cun measurements.

f) The longitudinal measurement of the mid abdomen is 8 cun from the centre of the umbilicus to the xiphisternal joint (Ren 16).

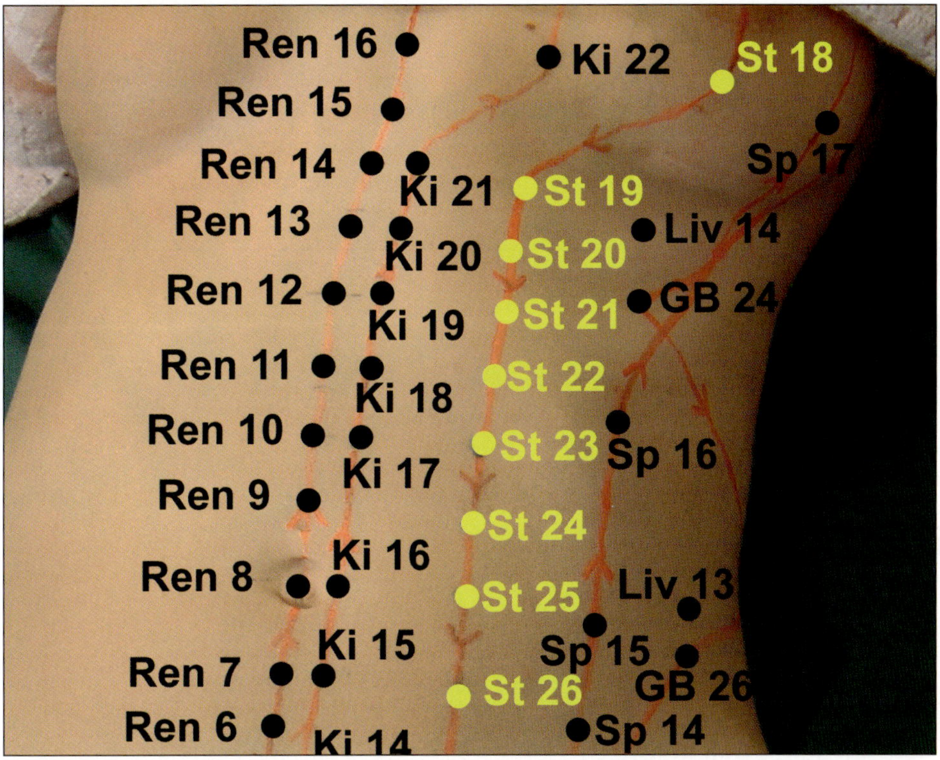

Tip: a) Locate the 2 cun measurement level with the centre of the umbilicus and lateral to the anterior median line (St 25).

b) The Stomach channel follows the curved ridge of the rectus abdominis muscle as it travels down towards the groin.

c) Place your finger on the anterior median line, (Ren 11) 3 cun superior to the level of the umbilicus, and run laterally 2 cun and palpate for the point.

d) You could mark 2 cun lateral to the anterior median line first, and then palpate with the flow of the Stomach channel to 5 cun inferior to the level of the xiphisternal joint.

Note: Some acupuncture schools have used different transverse cun measurements at the level of the umbilicus: the Kidney channel has been put at 1.5 pouce/ACI, the Stomach channel at 2.5 or 3 pouce/ACI and the Spleen channel at 4 or 4.5 pouce/ACI. A few schools still do use these transverse measurements, but they still mainly have the same longitudinal measurements for their point locations as the majority use. Wu (1973) locates ST 22 at 3 pouce from the median line and at 3 pouce below ST 19.

Worsley (1982) locates XI 22 on the abdomen, 3 ACI (Anatomical Chinese Inch) lateral to the median line, and 3 ACI superior to the level of the umbilicus at the level of XIII 11 (Ren 11). Soulié (1994) locates ST 22 on the lower lateral thorax: one large FW (Finger Width) lateral to the angle of the eighth and ninth ribs; approximately vertical from the nipple; in the angle between the inferior edge of the eighth rib and the anterior (medial) edge of an intercostal ligament; in a hollow; at two FW (Finger Width) below ST 21; two FW above and lateral to ST 23; about at the level of KI 20;

Voisin (1974) locates S 22 on the abdomen at 1.5 fb (finger breadth) below S 21. Lavier (1974) in an illustration locates ST 22 at 3 pouce lateral to the median line, and 3 pouce superior to the level of the umbilicus with the longitudinal measurement for the middle abdomen taken as 7 pouce from the level of the umbilicus and the tip of the xiphoid process.

St 23 TAI YI – GREAT ONENESS

⊥ ***0.7 TO 1.0 CUN*** Δ ***5 TO 10***
FORBIDDEN TO NEEDLE AND MOXA THIS POINT DURING PREGNANCY

Pos: Position of patient: supine.

Loc: a) On the anterior aspect of the torso.
b) On the mid-abdomen (in the middle jiao).
c) On the lateral border of the rectus abdominis muscle.
d) 2 cun lateral to the anterior median line.
e) 2 cun superior to the level of the centre of the umbilicus.
f) 6 cun inferior to the level of the xiphisternal joint.
g) Level with Ren 10.

Cun: a) The transverse measurement for the middle and lower abdomen (middle and lower jiao) is 2 cun between the anterior median line (at the centre of the umbilicus) and the lateral border of the rectus abdominis muscle (at St 25).
b) The lateral border of the rectus abdominis muscle is not the actual edge of the muscle but the most prominent surface of the muscle before it begins to 'slope' in to the torso. By visualising the corner of an inverted 'L', the point is located on the antero-lateral edge of the muscle. To locate this muscle ask the patient to slightly raise their head. The lateral border of the rectus abdominis muscle is on the most lateral part of the palpable curve which is more medial than the actual edge of the muscle.

c) Another way to mark out the transverse cun measurements at the level of the umbilicus is o locate the medial border of the anterior superior iliac spine (part of the iliac crest). To locate the 4 cun line of the Spleen channel, place a pen longitudinally on the medial border of the anterior superior iliac spine approximately halfway between the centre of the umbilicus and the superior border of the symphysis pubis bone. For the Stomach channel divide the 4 cun measurement in half to get 2 cun. The edge of the rectus abdominis muscle is measured as 4 cun. Once established you can then divide the 4 cun into other cun measurements for use on the Stomach and Kidney and Spleen channels etc.

d) The transverse cun measurements for the middle and lower abdomen (middle and lower jiao) includes the Kidney, Stomach, Spleen, Gall Bladder and Liver channels (lateral to the anterior median line): Ki 11 to Ki 21 = 0.5 cun; St 19 to St 30 = 2 cun; Sp 12 = 3.5 cun; Sp 13 to Sp 16 = 4 cun; GB 24 = 4 cun; Liv 14 = 4 cun.

e) Ki 16, St 25 and Sp 15 are all transversely level with the centre of the umbilicus and used as reference points for marking their channels cun measurements.

f) The longitudinal measurement of the mid abdomen is 8 cun from the centre of the umbilicus to the xiphisternal joint (Ren 16).

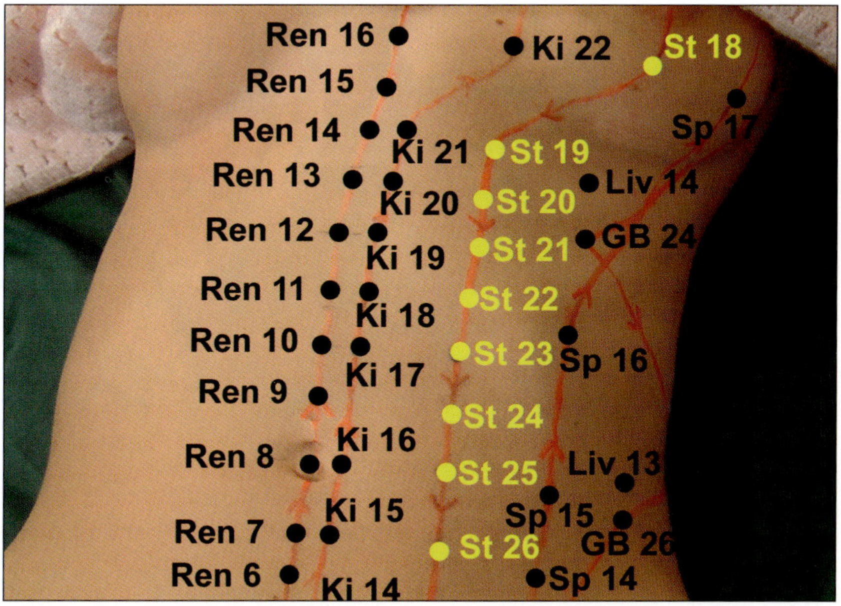

Tip: a) Locate the 2 cun measurement level with the centre of the umbilicus and lateral to the anterior median line (St 25).

b) The Stomach channel follows the curved ridge of the rectus abdominis muscle as it travels down towards the groin.

c) Place your finger on the anterior median line, (Ren 10) 2 cun superior to the level of the umbilicus, and run laterally 2 cun and palpate for the point.

d) You could mark 2 cun lateral to the anterior median line first, and then palpate with the flow of the Stomach channel to 6 cun inferior to the level of the xiphisternal joint.

Note: Some acupuncture schools have used different transverse cun measurements at the level of the umbilicus: the Kidney channel has been put at 1.5 pouce/ACI, the Stomach channel at 2.5 or 3 pouce/ACI and the Spleen channel at 4 or 4.5 pouce/ACI. A few schools still do use these transverse measurements, but they still mainly have the same longitudinal measurements for their point locations as the majority use.Wu (1973) locates ST 23 at 3 pouce from the median line and at 4 pouce below ST 19. Worsley (1982) locates XI 23 on the abdomen, 3 ACI (Anatomical Chinese Inch) lateral to the median line and 2 ACI superior to the level of the umbilicus, at the level of XIII 10 (Ren 10).

Soulié (1994) locates ST 23 on the epigastrium; on the edge of the ribs; just at the medial (anterior) edge of the union of the tenth rib, on the ninth rib; on the rectus abdominis; in a hollow; at two FW (Finger Width) below and medial ST 22; approximately two FW below and lateral to ST 24; two FW medial the SP 16; four FW medial to LR 13; one FW lateral and superior to KI 18; about at the level of CV 10 (Ren 10) .Voisin (1974) locates S 23 on the abdomen: 2.5 fb (finger breadth) below S 21. Lavier (1974) in an illustration locates ST 23 at 3 pouce lateral to the median line, and 2 pouce superior to the level of the umbilicus with the longitudinal measurement for the middle abdomen taken as 7 pouce from the level of the umbilicus and the tip of the xiphoid process.

St 24 HUA ROU MEN – LUBRICATION FOOD GATE

⊥ ***0.7 TO 1.0 CUN*** ***Δ 5 TO 15***
FORBIDDEN TO NEEDLE AND MOXA THIS POINT DURING PREGNANCY

Pos: Position of patient: supine.

Loc: a) On the anterior aspect of the torso.
b) On the mid-abdomen (in the middle jiao).
c) On the lateral border of the rectus abdominis muscle.
d) 2 cun lateral to the anterior median line.
e) 1 cun superior to the level of the centre of the umbilicus.
f) 7 cun inferior to the level of the xiphisternal joint.
g) Level with Ren 9 (which is on the anterior median line, at 1 cun superior to the level of the centre of the umbilicus).

Cun: a) The transverse measurement for the middle and lower abdomen (middle and lower jiao) is 2 cun between the anterior median line (at the centre of the umbilicus) and the lateral border of the rectus abdominis muscle (at St 25).
b) The lateral border of the rectus abdominis muscle is not the actual edge of the muscle but the most prominent surface of the muscle before it begins to 'slope' in to the torso. By visualising the corner of an inverted 'L', the point is located on the antero-lateral edge of the muscle. To locate this muscle ask the patient to slightly raise their head. The lateral border of the rectus abdominis muscle is on the most lateral part of the palpable curve which is more medial than the actual edge of the muscle.

c) Another way to mark out the transverse cun measurements at the level of the umbilicus is to locate the medial border of the anterior superior iliac spine (part of the iliac crest). To locate the 4 cun line of the Spleen channel, place a pen longitudinally on the medial border of the anterior superior iliac spine approximately halfway between the centre of the umbilicus and the superior border of the symphysis pubis bone. For the Stomach channel divide the 4 cun measurement in half to get 2 cun. The edge of the rectus abdominis muscle is measured as 4 cun. Once established you can then divide the 4 cun into other cun measurements for use on the Stomach and Kidney and Spleen channels etc.

d) The transverse cun measurements for the middle and lower abdomen (middle and lower jiao) includes the Kidney, Stomach, Spleen, Gall Bladder and Liver channels (lateral to the anterior median line): Ki 11 to Ki 21 = 0.5 cun; St 19 to St 30 = 2 cun; Sp 12 = 3.5 cun; Sp 13 to Sp 16 = 4 cun; GB 24 = 4 cun; Liv 14 = 4 cun.

e) Ki 16, St 25 and Sp 15 are all transversely level with the centre of the umbilicus and used as reference points for marking their channels cun measurements.

f) The longitudinal measurement of the mid abdomen is 8 cun from the centre of the umbilicus to the xiphisternal joint (Ren 16).

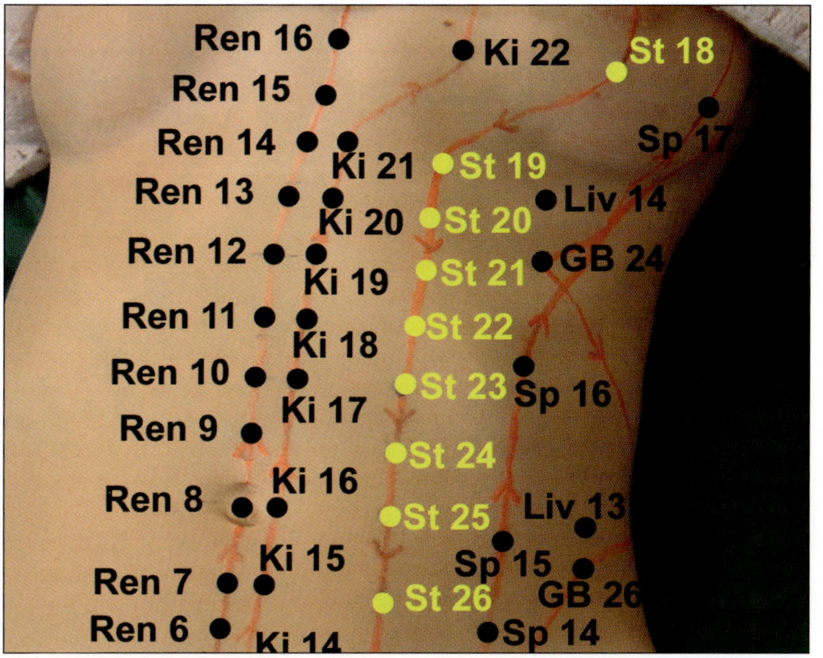

Tip: a) Locate the 2 cun measurement level with the centre of the umbilicus and lateral to the anterior median line (St 25).

b) The Stomach channel follows the curved ridge of the rectus abdominis muscle as it travels down towards the groin.

c) Place your finger on the anterior median line, (Ren 9) 1 cun superior to the level of the umbilicus, and run laterally 2 cun and palpate for the point.

d) You could mark 2 cun lateral to the anterior median line first, and then palpate with the flow of the Stomach channel to 7 cun inferior to the level of the xiphisternal joint.

Note: Some acupuncture schools have used different transverse cun measurements at the level of the umbilicus: the Kidney channel has been put at 1.5 pouce/ACI, the Stomach channel at 2.5 or 3 pouce/ACI and the Spleen channel at 4 or 4.5 pouce/ACI. A few schools still do use these transverse measurements, but they still mainly have the same longitudinal measurements for their point locations as the majority use.Wu (1973) locates ST 24 at 3 pouce from the median line and at 5 pouce below ST 19. Worsley (1982) locates XI 24 on the abdomen, 3 ACI (Anatomical Chinese Inch) lateral to the median line, and 1 ACI superior to the level of the umbilicus, at the level of XIII 9 (Ren 9).

Soulié (1994) locates ST 24 on the abdomen: at the level of one large FW (Finger Width) above the navel, at the inferior edge of the tenth rib and at the point of the eleventh rib; approximately vertical to the nipple; two FW under the anterior angle of the union of the tenth on the ninth rib; at the lateral edge of the rectus abdominus; in a hollow; two FW below ST 23; one large FW above ST 25; about two FW lateral to KI 17; four FW from CV 9 (Ren 9). Voisin (1974) locates S 24 on the abdomen at 4 fb (finger breadth) from the midline and at 3 fb below the costal border. Lavier (1974) in an illustration locates ST 24 at 3 pouce lateral to the median line, and 1 pouce superior to the level of the umbilicus with the longitudinal measurement for the middle abdomen taken as 7 pouce from the level of the umbilicus and the tip of the xiphoid process.

St 25 TIAN SHU – HEAVENLY PIVOT

⊥ ***0.5 TO 0.8 CUN*** Δ ***3 TO 20***
FORBIDDEN TO NEEDLE AND MOXA THIS POINT DURING PREGNANCY

- A Seven Internal Dragons (I.D's) Point (the other points are Ren 15 "Master", St 32 and St 41)
- ALARM/Front Collecting/ Front Mu/Herald Point of Large Intestine
- RE-UNION/Crossing/ Meeting Point of Stomach and Large Intestine Channels- Foot Yang Ming Hand and Yang Ming Channels

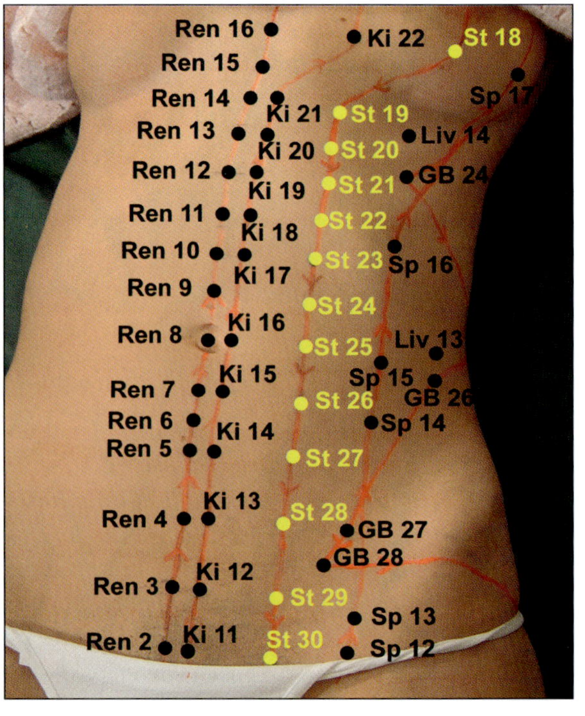

Pos: Position of patient: supine.

Loc: a) On the anterior aspect of the torso.
b) In between the mid-abdomen and lower abdomen (in between the middle and lower jiao).

c) On the lateral border of the rectus abdominis muscle.
d) 2 cun lateral to the anterior median line.
e) Level with the centre of the umbilicus.
f) 8 cun inferior to the level of the xiphisternal joint.
g) Level with Ren 8 (which is in the centre of the umbilicus).

Cun: a) The transverse measurement for the middle and lower abdomen (middle and lower jiao) is 2 cun between the anterior median line (at the centre of the umbilicus) and the lateral border of the rectus abdominis muscle (at St 25).
b) The lateral border of the rectus abdominis muscle is not the actual edge of the muscle but the most prominent surface of the muscle before it begins to 'slope' in to the torso. By visualising the corner of an inverted 'L', the point is located on the antero-lateral edge of the muscle. To locate this muscle ask the patient to slightly raise their head. The lateral border of the rectus abdominis muscle is on the most lateral part of the palpable curve which is more medial than the actual edge of the muscle.
c) Another way to mark out the transverse cun measurements at the level of the umbilicus is to locate the medial border of the anterior superior iliac spine (part of the iliac crest). To locate the 4 cun line of the Spleen channel, place a pen longitudinally on the medial border of the anterior superior iliac spine approximately halfway between the centre of the umbilicus and the superior border of the symphysis pubis bone. For the Stomach channel divide the 4 cun measurement in half to get 2 cun. The edge of the rectus abdominis muscle is measured as 4 cun. Once established you can then divide the 4 cun into other cun measurements for use on the Stomach and Kidney and Spleen channels etc.
d) The transverse cun measurements for the middle and lower abdomen (middle and lower jiao) includes the Kidney, Stomach, Spleen, Gall Bladder and Liver channels (lateral to the anterior median line): Ki 11 to Ki 21 = 0.5 cun; St 19 to St 30 = 2 cun; Sp 12 = 3.5 cun; Sp 13 to Sp 16 = 4 cun; GB 24 = 4 cun; Liv 14 = 4 cun.
e) The longitudinal measurement of the lower abdomen is 5 cun from the centre of the umbilicus to the superior border of the symphysis pubis bone.
f) Ki 16, St 25 and Sp 15 are all transversely level with the centre of the umbilicus and used as reference points for marking their channels cun measurements.
g) The longitudinal measurement of the mid abdomen is 8 cun from the centre of the umbilicus to the xiphisternal joint (Ren 16). The longitudinal measurement of the lower abdomen is 5 cun from the superior border of the symphysis pubis bone to the centre of the umbilicus.

Tip: a) Locate the 2 cun measurement level with the centre of the umbilicus and lateral to the anterior median line (at St 25).
b) The Stomach channel follows the curved ridge of the rectus abdominis muscle as it travels down towards the groin.
c) Place your finger on the lateral edge of the umbilicus and run it laterally to 2 cun and then palpate the area s to reveal the accurate location of this point.
d) You could also mark 2 cun lateral to the anterior median line first, and then palpate with the flow of the Stomach channel to the level of the centre of the umbilicus.

Note: Some acupuncture schools have used different transverse cun measurements at the level of the umbilicus: the Kidney channel has been put at 1.5 pouce/ACI, the Stomach channel at 2.5 or 3 pouce/ACI and the Spleen channel at 4 or 4.5 pouce/ACI. A few schools still do use these transverse measurements, but they still mainly have the same longitudinal measurements for their point locations as the majority use. Worsley (1982) locates XI 25 on the abdomen, 3 ACI (Anatomical Chinese Inch) lateral to the median line, at the level of the centre of the umbilicus (XIII 8 /Ren 8/ CV 8), on the lateral edge of the rectus abdominis. Voisin (1974) locates St 25 on the abdomen, 4 fb (finger breadth) lateral to the umbilicus. Wu (1973) locates ST 25 at the level of the umbilicus, and at 3 pouce from the median line. Lavier (1973) illustrates ST 25 as being located on a level with the umbilicus, at 3 pouce lateral to the anterior median line.

Soulié (1994) locates ST 25 on the abdomen; at the level of and about three FW (finger width) lateral to the umbilicus, at the lateral edge of the vertical muscle (rectus abdominus); on the aponeurosis of the union with the external oblique muscle; in a hollow; one large FW below ST 24; one large FW above ST 26; two FW lateral to KI 16; one large FW medial to SP 15.

The transverse measurement for the middle and lower abdomen (middle and lower jiao) is calculated as 2 cun, between the anterior median line (at the centre of the umbilicus) and the lateral border of the rectus abdominis muscle (at St 25). Alternatively the cun measurements between the anterior median line (at the centre of the umbilicus) and the medial border of the anterior superior iliac spine which is part of the iliac crest of the ilium (one of three parts of the in nominate or hip bone) is 4 cun.

The lateral border of the rectus abdominis muscle is not the actual edge of the muscle but the most prominent surface of the rectus abdominis muscle before it begins to 'slope' in to the torso, eg. the corner of an inverted 'L', just before you go on to the lateral aspect from the anterior surface. When the muscle is contracted by asking your patient to raise their head slightly, the muscle forms a curved ridge that can be palpated. The lateral border of the rectus abdominis muscle is on the most lateral part of the palpable curve which makes it more medial than the actual edge of the muscle.

The transverse cun measurements for the middle and lower abdomen (middle and lower jiao) which includes the Kidney, Stomach, Spleen, Gall Bladder and Liver channels (lateral to the anterior median line) are as follows:

Ki 11 to Ki 21 = 0.5 cun
St 19 to St 30 = 2 cun
Sp 13 to Sp 16 = 4 cun (Sp 12 = 3.5 cun)
GB 24 = 4 cun
Liv 14 = 4 cun

Note: Some acupuncture schools have used different transverse cun measurements at the level of the umbilicus: the Kidney channel has been put at 0.5, 1 and 1.5 pouce/ACI, the Stomach channel at 2.5 or 3 pouce/ACI and the Spleen channel at 4 or 4.5 pouce/ACI. A few schools still do use these transverse measurements, but they still mainly have the same longitudinal measurements for their point locations as the majority use.

Ki 16, St 25 and Sp 15 are all transversely level with the centre of the umbilicus and are used as reference points for marking their channels cun measurements.

The longitudinal measurements of the anterior torso are:

> **9 cun from the xiphisternal joint to the suprasternal fossa (with the space between 2 ribs measuring approximately 1.6 cun in the lower chest, and 1 cun in the upper chest)**
>
> **8 cun from the centre of the umbilicus to the xiphisternal joint. For the descriptions relating to the channels in the middle jiao, the longitudinal cun measurements are given from the centre of the umbilicus superiorly or from the xiphisternal joint inferiorly, depending on the direction of the flow of the channel.**
>
> **5 cun from the centre of the umbilicus to the superior border of the symphysis pubis bone. For the descriptions relating to the channels in the lower jiao, the longitudinal cun measurements are given from the centre of the umbilicus inferiorly or from the superior border of the symphysis pubis bone superiorly, depending on the direction of the flow of the channel.**

St 26 WAI LING – OUTSIDE MOUND

⊥ *0.7 TO 1.0 CUN* Δ 5
FORBIDDEN TO NEEDLE AND MOXA THIS POINT DURING PREGNANCY

Pos: Position of patient: supine.

Loc:
a) On the anterior aspect of the torso.
b) On the lower abdomen (in the lower jiao).
c) On the lateral border of the rectus abdominis muscle.
d) 2 cun lateral to the anterior median line.
e) 1 cun inferior to the level of the centre of the umbilicus.
f) Level with Ren 7.

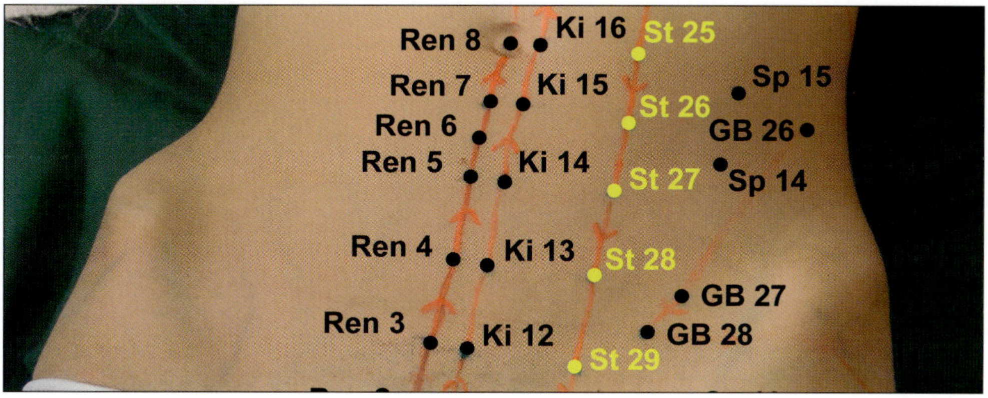

Cun: a) The transverse measurement for the middle and lower abdomen (middle and lower jiao) is 2 cun between the anterior median line (at the centre of the umbilicus) and the lateral border of the rectus abdominis muscle (at St 25).

b) The lateral border of the rectus abdominis muscle is not the actual edge of the muscle but the most prominent surface of the muscle before it begins to 'slope' in to the torso. By visualising the corner of an inverted 'L', the point is located on the antero-lateral edge of the muscle. To locate this muscle ask the patient to slightly raise their head. The lateral border of the rectus abdominis muscle is on the most lateral part of the palpable curve which is more medial than the actual edge of the muscle.

c) Another way to mark out the transverse cun measurements at the level of the umbilicus is to locate the medial border of the anterior superior iliac spine (part of the iliac crest). To locate the 4 cun line of the Spleen channel, place a pen longitudinally on the medial border of the anterior superior iliac spine approximately halfway between the centre of the umbilicus and the superior border of the symphysis pubis bone. For the Stomach channel divide the 4 cun measurement in half to get 2 cun. The edge of the rectus abdominis muscle is measured as 4 cun. Once established you can then divide the 4 cun into other cun measurements for use on the Stomach and Kidney and Spleen channels etc.

d) The transverse cun measurements for the middle and lower abdomen (middle and lower jiao) includes the Kidney, Stomach, Spleen, Gall Bladder and Liver channels (lateral to the anterior median line): Ki 11 to Ki 21 = 0.5 cun; St 19 to St 30 = 2 cun; Sp 12 = 3.5 cun; Sp 13 to Sp 16 = 4 cun; GB 24 = 4 cun; Liv 14 = 4 cun.

e) The longitudinal measurement of the lower abdomen is 5 cun from the centre of the umbilicus to the superior border of the symphysis pubis bone.

Tip: a) Locate the 2 cun measurement level with the umbilicus and lateral to the anterior median line (St 25).

b) The Stomach channel follows the curved ridge of the rectus abdominis muscle as it travels down towards the groin.

c) Mark out 5 equal cun measurements longitudinally from the superior border of the symphysis pubis bone to the centre of the umbilicus at the anterior median line.

d) If you cannot feel the superior border of the symphysis pubis bone, ask the patient to semi-flex their legs, this should soften the abdominal muscles to enable you to palpate the superior border of the symphysis pubis.

e) Place your finger on the anterior median line, (Ren 7) 1 cun inferior to the level of the centre of the umbilicus, and run it laterally to 2 cun and then palpate for the point.

f) You could mark 2 cun lateral to the anterior median line first, and palpate with the flow of the Stomach channel from the level of the umbilicus (St 25) to 1 cun inferior to it.

Note: Some acupuncture schools have used different transverse cun measurements at the level of the umbilicus: the Kidney channel has been put at 1.5 pouce/ACI, the Stomach channel at 2.5 or 3 pouce/ACI and the Spleen channel at 4 or 4.5 pouce/ACI. A few schools still do use these transverse measurements, but they still mainly have the same longitudinal measurements for their point locations as the majority use. Voisin (1974) doesn't give this point a location but gives a point name instead, "McBurney's point". Worsley (1982) locates XI 26 on the abdomen, 3 ACI (Anatomical Chinese Inch) lateral to the median line and 1 ACI inferior to the level of the umbilicus, and at the level of XIII 7 (Ren 7). Wu (1973) locates ST 26 at 1 pouce below ST 25, and at 3 pouce from the median line. Lavier (1973) illustrates ST 26 as being located 1 pouce below ST 25, at 3 pouce lateral to the anterior median line. Soulié (1994) locates ST 26 on the abdomen; at the level of one FW (finger width) under the umbilicus; approximately three large FW from the median line, on the lateral edge of the rectus abdominus; a little medial to the vertical rise of the external oblique muscle; in a hollow; one large FW under ST 25; two FW above ST 27; two FW lateral to KI 15; approximately three large FW from CV 7 (Ren 7).

St 27 DA JU – GREAT MIGHT

⊥ ***0.7 TO 1.0 CUN*** **Δ** ***5 TO 10***
FORBIDDEN TO NEEDLE AND MOXA THIS POINT DURING PREGNANCY

Pos: Position of patient: supine.

Loc: a) On the anterior aspect of the torso.
b) On the lower abdomen (in the lower jiao).
c) On the lateral border of the rectus abdominis muscle.
d) 2 cun lateral to the anterior median line.
e) 2 cun inferior to the level of the centre of the umbilicus.
f) Level with Ren 5.

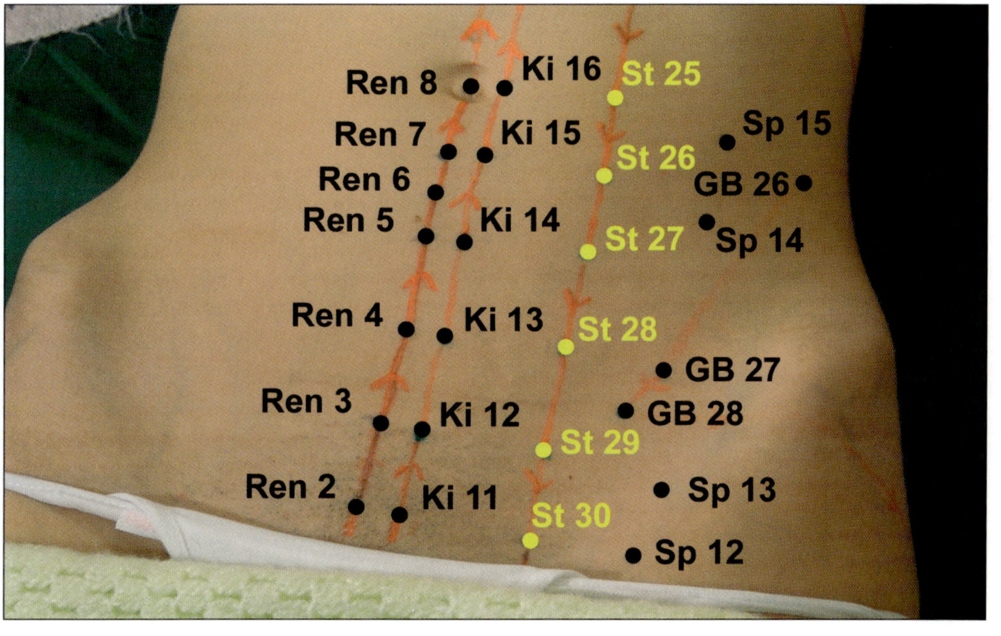

Cun: a) The transverse measurement for the middle and lower abdomen (middle and lower jiao) is 2 cun between the anterior median line (at the centre of the umbilicus) and the lateral borde of the rectus abdominis muscle (at St 25).

b) The lateral border of the rectus abdominis muscle is not the actual edge of the muscle but the most prominent surface of the muscle before it begins to 'slope' in to the torso. B visualising the corner of an inverted 'L', the point is located on the antero-lateral edge of the muscle. To locate this muscle ask the patient to slightly raise their head. The lateral border of the rectus abdominis muscle is on the most lateral part of the palpable curve which is more medial than the actual edge of the muscle.

c) Another way to mark out the transverse cun measurements at the level of the umbilicus is to locate the medial border of the anterior superior iliac spine (part of the iliac crest). To locate the 4 cun line of the Spleen channel, place a pen longitudinally on the medial border of the anterior superior iliac spine approximately halfway between the centre of the umbilicus and the superior border of the symphysis pubis bone. For the Stomach channel divide the 4 cun measurement in half to get 2 cun. The edge of the rectus abdominis muscle is measured as 4 cun. Once established you can then divide the 4 cun into other cun measurements for use on the Stomach and Kidney and Spleen channels etc.

d) The transverse cun measurements for the middle and lower abdomen (middle and lower jiao) includes the Kidney, Stomach, Spleen, Gall Bladder and Liver channels (lateral to the anterior median line): Ki 11 to Ki 21 = 0.5 cun; St 19 to St 30 = 2 cun; Sp 12 = 3.5 cun; Sp 13 to Sp 16 = 4 cun; GB 24 = 4 cun; Liv 14 = 4 cun.

e) The longitudinal measurement of the lower abdomen is 5 cun from the centre of the umbilicus to the superior border of the symphysis pubis bone.

Tip: a) Locate the 2 cun measurement that is level with the umbilicus and lateral to the anterior median line (St 25).

b) The Stomach channel follows the curved ridge of the rectus abdominis muscle as it travels down towards the groin.

c) Mark out 5 equal cun measurements longitudinally from the superior border of the symphysis pubis bone to the centre of the umbilicus at the anterior median line.

d) If you cannot feel the superior border of the symphysis pubis bone, ask your patient to semi-flex their legs, this should soften the abdominal muscles so you can palpate the superior border of the symphysis pubis.

e) Place your finger on the anterior median line, (Ren 5) 2 cun inferior to the level of the centre of the umbilicus, and run it laterally to 2 cun and then palpate for the point.

f) You can mark 2 cun lateral to the anterior median line first, and then palpate with the flow of the Stomach channel from the level of the umbilicus (St 25) 2 cun inferior to it.

Note: Some acupuncture schools have used different transverse cun measurements at the level of the umbilicus: the Kidney channel has been put at 1.5 pouce/ACI, the Stomach channel at 2.5 or 3 pouce/ACI and the Spleen channel at 4 or 4.5 pouce/ACI. A few schools still do use these transverse measurements, but they still mainly have the same longitudinal measurements for their point locations as the majority use. Voisin (1974) locates S 27 on the abdomen at 1.5 fb (finger breadth) below "McBurney's point" (St 26) and slightly medially.

Worsley (1982) locates XI 27 on the abdomen, 3 ACI (Anatomical Chinese Inch) lateral to the median line and 2 ACI inferior to the level of the umbilicus, and at the level of XIII 5 (Ren 5). Wu (1973) locates ST 27 at 2 pouce below ST 25, and at 3 pouce from the median line. Lavier (1973) illustrates ST 27 as being located 2 pouce below ST 25, at 3 pouce lateral to the anterior median line. Soulié (1994) locates ST 27 on the abdomen; at the level of half the distance from the umbilicus to the pelvis; approximately three large FW (Finger Width) from the midline, on the lateral edge of the rectus abdominus; a little medial to the vertical rise of the external oblique muscle; in a hollow; two FW below ST 26; one large FW above ST 28; about two FW lateral to KI 14; three or four large FW from CV 5 (Ren 5).

St 28 SHUI DAO – WATER PATH

⊥ ***0.7 TO 1.0 CUN*** ∆ ***5 TO 10***
FORBIDDEN TO NEEDLE AND MOXA THIS POINT DURING PREGNANCY

Pos: Position of patient: supine.

Loc: a) On the anterior aspect of the torso.
b) On the lower abdomen (in the lower jiao).
c) On the lateral border of the rectus abdominis muscle.
d) 2 cun lateral to the anterior median line.
e) 3 cun inferior to the level of the centre of the umbilicus.
f) Level with Ren 4.

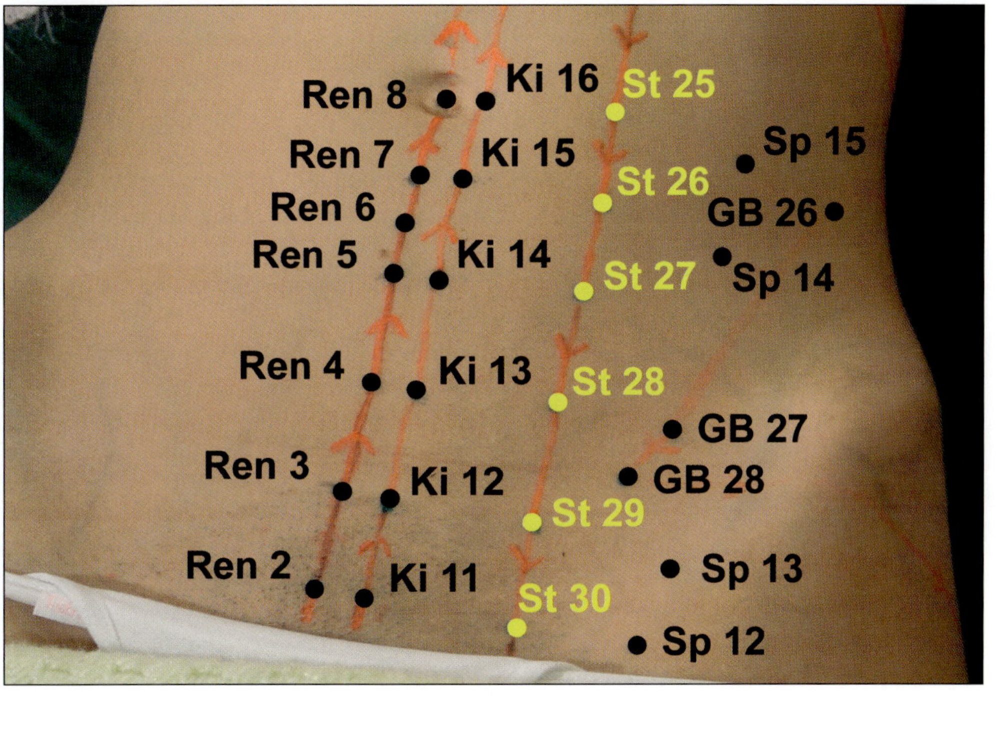

Cun: a) The transverse measurement for the middle and lower abdomen (middle and lower jiao) is 2 cun between the anterior median line (at the centre of the umbilicus) and the lateral border of the rectus abdominis muscle (at St 25).

b) The lateral border of the rectus abdominis muscle is not the actual edge of the muscle but the most prominent surface of the muscle before it begins to 'slope' in to the torso. By visualising the corner of an inverted 'L', the point is located on the antero-lateral edge of the muscle. To locate this muscle ask the patient to slightly raise their head. The lateral border of the rectus abdominis muscle is on the most lateral part of the palpable curve which is more medial than the actual edge of the muscle.

c) Another way to mark out the transverse cun measurements at the level of the umbilicus is to locate the medial border of the anterior superior iliac spine (part of the iliac crest). To locate the 4 cun line of the Spleen channel, place a pen longitudinally on the medial border of the anterior superior iliac spine approximately halfway between the centre of the umbilicus and the superior border of the symphysis pubis bone. For the Stomach channel divide the 4 cun measurement in half to get 2 cun. The edge of the rectus abdominis muscle is measured as 4 cun. Once established you can then divide the 4 cun into other cun measurements for use on the Stomach and Kidney and Spleen channels etc.

d) The transverse cun measurements for the middle and lower abdomen (middle and lower jiao) includes the Kidney, Stomach, Spleen, Gall Bladder and Liver channels (lateral to the anterior median line): Ki 11 to Ki 21 = 0.5 cun; St 19 to St 30 = 2 cun; Sp 12 = 3.5 cun; Sp 13 to Sp 16 = 4 cun; GB 24 = 4 cun; Liv 14 = 4 cun.

e) The longitudinal measurement of the lower abdomen is 5 cun from the centre of the umbilicus to the superior border of the symphysis pubis bone.

Tip: a) Locate the 2 cun measurement level with the umbilicus and lateral to the anterior median line (St 25).

b) The Stomach channel follows the curved ridge of the rectus abdominis muscle as it travels down towards the groin.

c) Mark out 5 equal cun measurements longitudinally from the superior border of the symphysis pubis bone to the centre of the umbilicus at the anterior median line.

d) If you cannot feel the superior border of the symphysis pubis bone, ask your patient to semi-flex their legs, this should soften the abdominal muscles so you can palpate the superior border of the symphysis pubis.

e) Place your finger on the anterior median line, (Ren 4) 3 cun inferior to the level of the centre of the umbilicus, run laterally to 2 cun and palpate for the point.

f) You can mark 2 cun lateral to the anterior median line first, and then palpate with the flow of the Stomach channel from the level of the umbilicus (St 25) 3 cun inferior to it.

Note: Some acupuncture schools have used different transverse cun measurements at the level of the umbilicus: the Kidney channel has been put at 1.5 pouce/ACI, the Stomach channel at 2.5 or 3 pouce/ACI and the Spleen channel at 4 or 4.5 pouce/ACI. A few schools still do use these transverse measurements, but they still mainly have the same longitudinal measurements for their point locations as the majority use. Voisin (1974) locates S 28 on the abdomen, on the lateral border of the rectus abdominis and at 3 fb (finger breadth) above the pubis.

Worsley (1982) locates XI 28 on the abdomen, 3 ACI (Anatomical Chinese Inch) lateral to the median line, 3 ACI inferior to the level of the umbilicus, and at the level of XIII 4 (Ren 4). Wu (1973) locates ST 28 at 3 pouce below ST 25, and at 3 pouce from the median line. Lavier (1973) illustrates ST 28 as being located 3 pouce below ST 25, at 3 pouce lateral to the anterior median line. Soulié (1994) locates ST 28 on the abdomen; at the level of three FW (finger width) above the pelvis (one below the pelvic-umbilical midpoint); about three large FW from the median line, on the lateral edge of the rectus abdominus; a little medial to the rise of the external oblique muscle; one large FW below ST 27; one large FW above ST 29; two FW lateral from KI 13; three FW lateral from CV 4 (Ren 4).

St 29 GUI LAI – THE RETURN

⊥ ***0.5 TO 1.0 CUN*** **Δ** ***5 TO 7***
FORBIDDEN TO NEEDLE AND MOXA THIS POINT DURING PREGNANCY

Pos: Position of patient: supine.

Loc:
a) On the anterior aspect of the torso.
b) On the lower abdomen (in the lower jiao).
c) On the lateral border of the rectus abdominis muscle.
d) 2 cun lateral to the anterior median line.
e) 4 cun inferior to the level of the centre of the umbilicus.
f) Level with Ren 3.

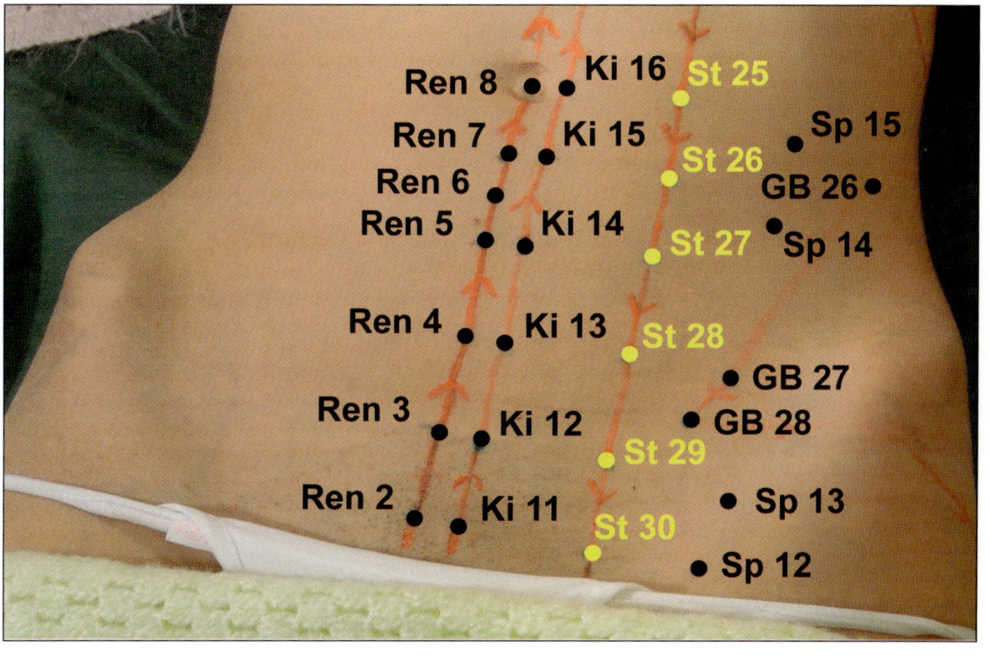

Cun: a) The transverse measurement for the middle and lower abdomen (middle and lower jiao) is 2 cun between the anterior median line (at the centre of the umbilicus) and the lateral border of the rectus abdominis muscle (at St 25).

b) The lateral border of the rectus abdominis muscle is not the actual edge of the muscle but the most prominent surface of the muscle before it begins to 'slope' in to the torso. By visualising the corner of an inverted 'L', the point is located on the antero-lateral edge of the muscle. To locate this muscle ask the patient to slightly raise their head. The lateral border of the rectus abdominis muscle is on the most lateral part of the palpable curve which is more medial than the actual edge of the muscle.

c) Another way to mark out the transverse cun measurements at the level of the umbilicus is to locate the medial border of the anterior superior iliac spine (part of the iliac crest). To locate the 4 cun line of the Spleen channel, place a pen longitudinally on the medial border of the anterior superior iliac spine approximately halfway between the centre of the umbilicus and the superior border of the symphysis pubis bone. For the Stomach channel divide the 4 cun measurement in half to get 2 cun. The edge of the rectus abdominis muscle is measured as 4 cun. Once established you can then divide the 4 cun into other cun measurements for use on the Stomach and Kidney and Spleen channels etc.

d) The transverse cun measurements for the middle and lower abdomen (middle and lower jiao) includes the Kidney, Stomach, Spleen, Gall Bladder and Liver channels (lateral to the anterior median line): Ki 11 to Ki 21 = 0.5 cun; St 19 to St 30 = 2 cun; Sp 12 = 3.5 cun; Sp 13 to Sp 16 = 4 cun; GB 24 = 4 cun; Liv 14 = 4 cun.

e) The longitudinal measurement of the lower abdomen is 5 cun from the centre of the umbilicus to the superior border of the symphysis pubis bone.

Tip: a) Locate the 2 cun measurement level with the umbilicus and lateral to the anterior median line (St 25).

b) The Stomach channel follows the curved ridge of the rectus abdominis muscle as it travels down towards the groin.

c) Mark out 5 equal cun measurements longitudinally from the superior border of the symphysis pubis bone to the centre of the umbilicus at the anterior median line.

d) If you cannot feel the superior border of the symphysis pubis bone, ask your patient to semi-flex their legs, this should soften the abdominal muscles so you can palpate the superior border of the symphysis pubis.

e) Place your finger on the anterior median line, (Ren 3) 4 cun inferior to the level of the centre of the umbilicus, run laterally to 2 cun and palpate for the point.

f) You can mark 2 cun lateral to the anterior median line first, and then palpate with the flow of the Stomach channel from the level of the umbilicus (St 25) 4 cun inferior to it.

Note: Some acupuncture schools have used different transverse cun measurements at the level of the umbilicus: the Kidney channel has been put at 1.5 pouce/ACI, the Stomach channel at 2.5 or 3 pouce/ACI and the Spleen channel at 4 or 4.5 pouce/ACI. A few schools still do use these transverse measurements, but they still mainly have the same longitudinal measurements for their point locations as the majority use. Huang (1993) locates St 29 at 2 cun below St 28.

Voisin (1974) locates S 29 on the abdomen, on the lateral border of the rectus abdominis and at 2 fb (finger breadth) above the pubis.

Worsley (1982) locates XI 29 on the abdomen, 3 ACI (Anatomical Chinese Inch) lateral to the median line and 4 ACI inferior to the level of the umbilicus, at the level of XIII 3 (Ren 3). Wu (1973) locates ST 29 at 4 pouce below ST 25, and at 3 pouce from the median line. Lavier (1973) illustrates ST 29 as being located 4 pouce below ST 25, at 3 pouce lateral to the anterior median line. Soulié (1994) locates ST 29 on the abdomen; at the level of one FW (finger width) above the pelvis; about three FW from the median line, on the lateral edge of the rectus abdominus; a little medial to the vertical rise of the external oblique muscle; in a hollow; one FW under ST 28; one FW above ST 30; about two FW lateral from KI 12; about three FW lateral to CV 3 (Ren 3).

St 30 QI CHONG – QI RUSHING

⊥ ***0.3 TO 0.5 CUN*** **Δ *3 TO 7***
FORBIDDEN TO NEEDLE AND MOXA THIS POINT DURING PREGNANCY

- 8 EXTRAORDINARY VESSEL/Coalescent Point of Penetrating Vessel (Chong Mai) – see note
- RE-UNION/Crossing/Meeting Point of the Stomach Channel with the Penetrating Vessel – Foot Yang Ming with the Chong Mai
- A POINT OF THE SEA OF NOURISHMENT (Waters and Grains) (There is one other Sea of Nourishment Point: St 36)

Pos: Position of patient: supine.

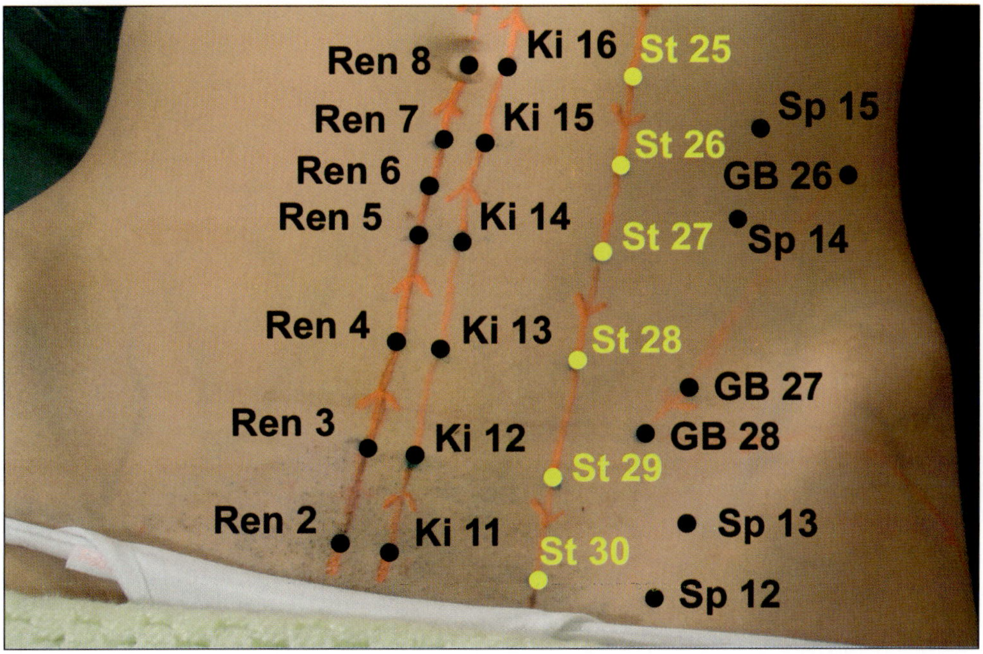

Loc: a) On the anterior aspect of the torso.
b) On the lower abdomen (in the lower jiao).
c) On the lateral border of the rectus abdominis muscle.
d) Level with the superior border of the symphysis pubis bone.
e) 2 cun lateral to the anterior median line.
f) 5 cun inferior to the level of the centre of the umbilicus.
g) Level with Ren 2 (which is on the anterior median line, at 5 cun inferior to the level of the centre of the umbilicus.

Cun: a) The transverse measurement for the middle and lower abdomen (middle and lower jiao) is 2 cun between the anterior median line (at the centre of the umbilicus) and the lateral border of the rectus abdominis muscle (at St 25).
b) The lateral border of the rectus abdominis muscle is not the actual edge of the muscle but the most prominent surface of the muscle before it begins to 'slope' in to the torso. B visualising the corner of an inverted 'L', the point is located on the antero-lateral edge of th muscle. To locate this muscle ask the patient to slightly raise their head. The lateral border of the rectus abdominis muscle is on the most lateral part of the palpable curve which is more medial than the actual edge of the muscle.
c) Another way to mark out the transverse cun measurements at the level of the umbilicus is to locate the medial border of the anterior superior iliac spine (part of the iliac crest). To locate the 4 cun line of the Spleen channel, place a pen longitudinally on the medial border of the anterior superior iliac spine approximately halfway between the centre of the umbilicus and the superior border of the symphysis pubis bone. For the Stomach channel divide the 4 cun measurement in half to get 2 cun. The edge of the rectus abdominis muscle is measured as 4 cun. Once established you can then divide the 4 cun into other cun measurements for use on the Stomach and Kidney and Spleen channels etc.
d) The transverse cun measurements for the middle and lower abdomen (middle and lower jiao) includes the Kidney, Stomach, Spleen, Gall Bladder and Liver channels (lateral to the anterior median line): Ki 11 to Ki 21 = 0.5 cun; St 19 to St 30 = 2 cun; Sp 12 = 3.5 cun; Sp 13 to Sp 16 = 4 cun; GB 24 = 4 cun; Liv 14 = 4 cun.
e) The longitudinal measurement of the lower abdomen is 5 cun from the centre of the umbilicus to the superior border of the symphysis pubis bone.

Tip: a) Locate the 2 cun measurement level with the umbilicus and lateral to the anterior median line (St 25).
b) The Stomach channel follows the curved ridge of the rectus abdominis muscle as it travels down towards the groin.
c) The rectus abdominis muscle narrows as it runs down towards the groin, and it inserts at the pubic tubercles. Therefore St 30 may be nearer to the actual edge of the rectus abdominis muscle than the lateral border of it, and may be just slightly less than the 2 cun transverse measurement.
d) Mark out 5 equal cun measurements longitudinally from the superior border of the symphysis pubis bone to the centre of the umbilicus at the anterior median line.

e) If you cannot feel the superior border of the symphysis pubis bone, ask your patient to semi-flex their legs, this should soften the abdominal muscles so you can palpate the superior border of the symphysis pubis.
f) Place your finger on the anterior median line, (Ren 2) 5 cun inferior to the level of the centre of the umbilicus, run laterally to 2 cun and palpate for the point.
g) You can mark 2 cun lateral to the anterior median line first, and then palpate with the flow of the Stomach channel from the level of the umbilicus (St 25) 5 cun inferior to it.

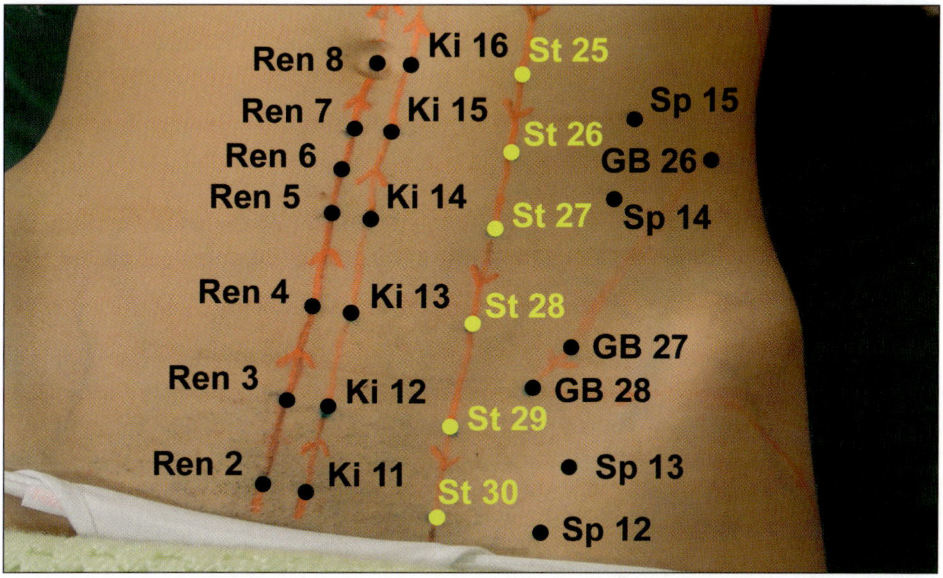

Note: Some acupuncture schools have used different transverse cun measurements at the level of the umbilicus: the Kidney channel has been put at 1.5 pouce/ACI, the Stomach channel at 2.5 or 3 pouce/ACI and the Spleen channel at 4 or 4.5 pouce/ACI. A few schools still do use these transverse measurements, but they still mainly have the same longitudinal measurements for their point locations as the majority use. Huang (1993) locates St 30 below St 29, at 1 cun above the groin, where a pulsating vessel is palpable. Voisin (1974) locates S 30 on the pubis: upper border of the pubis, at 3 fb (finger breadth) from the midline.

Worsley (1982) locates XI 30 on the abdomen, 3 ACI (Anatomical Chinese Inch) lateral to the median line, at the level of the superior edge of the pubic symphysis, at the level of XIII 2 (Ren 2). Wu (1973) locates ST 30 at 5 pouce below ST 25, and at 3 pouce from the median line. Lavier (1973) illustrates ST 30 as being located 5 pouce below ST 25, at 3 pouce lateral to the anterior median line. Soulié (1994) locates ST 30 on the abdomen, lower lateral; in the angle of the superior edge of the apparant extremity of the transverse bone (pubis) and the medial edge of the muscle passing above the pubis (psoas); in a hollow. The medial branch of an artery; one FW below ST 29; the meridian goes towards the exterior and at two FW crosses SP 12 in order to go four finger widths on the lateral adge of the sartorius muscle, at ST 31; two FW from KI 11; about four FW from CV 2 (Ren 2).

Shandong (1982) locate Qichong latero-superior to the tuberculum pubicum, 2 cun lateral to the midline, upper portion of inguinal region, medial to the artery. Legge (1999) locates St 30 at the level of the superior border of the symphysis pubis, 2 cun lateral the the anterior median line (Qugu (Ren 2)), superior to the inguinal ligament. The pulse of the femoral artery can be felt lateral to this point.

Note: In some texts St 30 is listed as an 8 EXTRAORDINARY VESSEL/Coalescent Point of Chong Mai (Penetrating Vessel), whereas in others it is omitted. The Chong Mai originates here.

Cun Measurements of the Upper Leg

The distance from a line drawn transversely between the gluteal groove and the medial root of the lower limb (at the level of the lower border of the pubic symphysis where the medial side of the upper leg joins the torso), to the medial popliteal crease (flexure of the knee) is 14 cun.

The distance between the popliteal crease (flexure of the knee) to the superior border of the greater trochanter of the femur, when the leg is abducted, is measured as 19 cun. There seems to be great discrepancies with other descriptions of the anatomy that have used the 19 cun measurement, eg. 19 cun from the popliteal crease to the superior and inferior borders of the pubic symphysis and 19 cun from the popliteal crease to the prominence or inferior border of the greater trochanter of the femur.

14 cun is the accepted bone proportional measurement of the thigh.

Note: Wu (1973) gives St 31/St 32 as "13 and 7 pouce above the flexure", whereas St 33 is "3 pouce above the upper edge of the patella" and St 34 is "1 pouce below St 33". Lavier (1974) shows the total longitudinal measurement of the thigh to be 13 pouce, with St 31/32/33/34 at 13/7/5/4 pouce respectively. Worsley (1982) uses 13 ACI from the medial extremity of the knee crease to the medial extremity of the groin and locates St 31/32/33/34 at 13/7/5/4 ACI proximal to the flexure of the knee. Shanghai (1993) locates ST 30 lateral and superior to the pubis tubercle, 2 cun lateral to the anterior midline, above the inguinal groove and on the medial side of the artery. Shandong (1982) locates Qichong (St 30) laterao-superior to the tuberculum pubicum, 2 cun lateral to the midline, upper portion of inguinal region, medial to the artery.

St 31-34 are on the anterior surface of the thigh, on a line connecting the anterior superior iliac spine of the ilium (one of three parts of the innominate or hip bone) and the superolateral corner of the patella bone.

St 31 BI GUAN – THIGH BORDER

⊥ ***0.5 TO 1.0 CUN*** **Δ** ***3 TO 7***

Pos: Position of patient: supine.

Loc: a) On the anterior surface of the upper thigh.
b) On a line connecting the anterior superior iliac spine of the ilium bone and the superolateral corner of the patella bone.
c) Directly inferior to the anterior superior iliac spine of the ilium bone.
d) On the lateral border of the sartorius muscle.
e) In the seam between the rectus femoris and vastus lateralis muscles.
f) Level with a line drawn between the lower border of the symphysis pubis bone and the gluteal groove, approximately 14 cun proximal to the popliteal crease (flexure of the knee).

Tip: a) Mark out the level of the inferior border of the symphysis pubis bone (where the medial side of the upper leg joins the torso) and the gluteal groove (and join the marks up).
b) This line is 14 cun proximal to the popliteal crease (flexure of the knee).
c) Flex and extend the knee to expose the seam between the rectus femoris and the vastus lateralis muscles. The vastus lateralis muscle usually disappears at this level, if not, the point will be located between the lateral border of the rectus femoris and the medial border of the vastus lateralis muscles instead.
d) By flexing and extending the knee you should be able to palpate the lateral border of the sartorius muscle at 14 cun.
e) The sartorius muscle is a relatively narrow band of muscle that originates from the anterior superior iliac spine (ASIS) of the ilium and runs medially down to the thigh to attach itself to the upper part of the medial surface of the shaft of the tibia bone.
f) Run your finger down from the anterior superior iliac spine of the ilium and directly inferior to this you should feel the seam of the vastus lateralis and the rectus femoris muscles at approximately 14 cun. Palpation should reveal a good depression for the point.

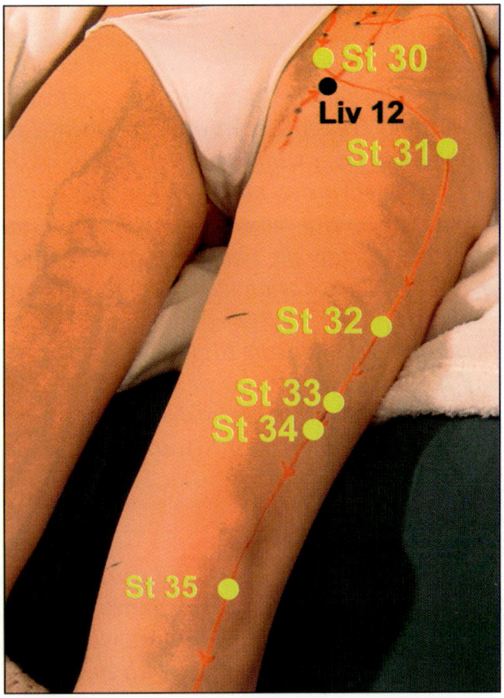

Note: Worsley (1982) Wu (1973) and Lavier (1974) use 13 pouce/ACI (Anatomical Chinese Inch) from the medial extremity of the knee crease to the medial extremity of the groin or the great trochanter. Worsley (1982) locates St 31/32/33/34 at 13/7/5/4 ACI proximal to the flexure of the knee. Wu (1973) gives St 31/St 32 as "13 and 7 pouce above the flexure", whereas St 33 is "3 pouce above the upper edge of the patella" and St 34 is "1 pouce below St 33". Lavier (1974) shows the total longitudinal measurement of the thigh to be 13 pouce, with St 31/32/33/34 at 13/7/5/4 pouce respectively. Huang (1993) locates St 31 above the knee and proximal to St 32 in the parting of the flesh. Lavier (1974) illustrates the point as being level with the greater trochanter of the femur and in a seam that is formed by the sartorius, rectus femoris and vastus lateralis muscles.

Worsley (1982) locates XI 31 on the anterior surface of the thigh, 13 ACI (Anatomical Chinese Inch) proximal to the flexure of the knee, between the vastus lateralis and the rectus femoris. Soulié (1994) locates ST 31 on the anterior face of the thigh: about four FW (Finger Width) below the inguinal crease; about at the mid-width of the thigh; on the medial edge of the large lateral muscle (tensor facia lata muscle); on the lateral edge of the oblique muscle (sartorius); in a hollow; four FW above ST 32. Voisin (1974) locates S 31 at "Scarpa's Triangle", at the medial border of the sartorius, at the level of the lower part of the greater trochanter.

Wu (1973) locates ST 31 upon the anterior surface of the thigh at thirteen pouces above the flexure of the popliteus, between the sartorius and the tensor fasciae latae. Cheng (1987) locates S 31 at the crossing point of a line drawn directly down from the anterior superior iliac spine and the line level with the lower border of the symphysis pubis, in the depression on the lateral side of the sartorius muscle when the thigh is flexed. Shanghai (1993) locates ST 31 directly below the anterior superior iliac spine, at the level of the perineum. Shanghai (1981) locates S 31 directly below the anterior superior iliac spine and level with the perineum. Hyodo (1975) locates ST 31 in a triangular depression made by muscles.

Shandong (1982) locate Biguan at the junction of a line between the spina iliac anterior-superior and lateral upper border of the patella and horizontal line of the perineum. Academy (1975) locates St 31 directky below the anterior superior iliac spine, in a line level with the lower border of the pubic symphysis. Jayasuriya (1982) locates St 31 at the meeting point of the vertical line from the anterior superior iliac spine and the horizontal line from the lower border of the pubic symphysis.

Legge (1999) locates St 31 inferior to the anterior superior iliac spine (ASIS), about 3 cun below the level of the inferior border of the symphysis pubis. In the depression on the lateral side of the sartorius which bulges when the thigh is actively flexed. Lotan (2000) locates St 31 lateral to the sartorius, level with the pubis inferior border; level with the greater trochanter tip; on the rectus femoris.

St 32 FU TU – PROSTRATE HARE

⊥ ***0.5 TO 1.0 CUN*** ∆ ***3 TO 7***

- A Seven Internal Dragons (I.D's) Point (the other points are Ren 15 "Master", St 25 and St 41)

Pos: Position of patient: supine.

Loc: a) On the anterior surface of the thigh.
b) On a line connecting the anterior superior iliac spine of the ilium and the superolateral corner of the patella bone.
c) In the seam between the rectus femoris and the vastus lateralis muscles.
d) 8 cun proximal to the popliteal crease (flexure of the knee).

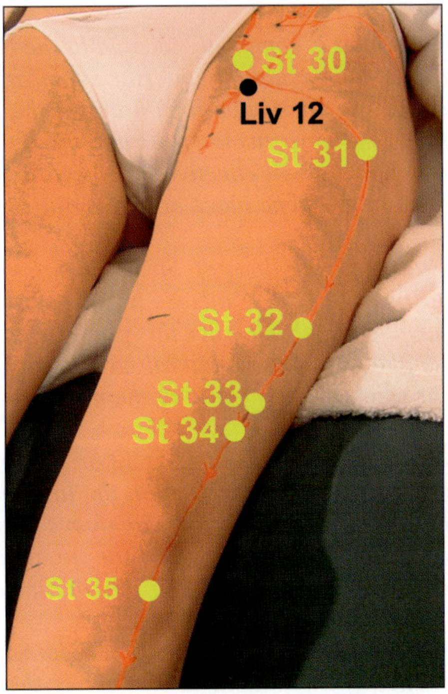

Tip: a) The distance at the level of the inferior border of the symphysis pubis bone (where the medial side of the upper leg joins the torso) and the gluteal groove to the popliteal crease (the flexure of the knee) is approximately 14 cun.
b) To expose the seam between the rectus femoris and the vastus lateralis muscles, flex and extend the knee.
c) Run your finger down from the anterior superior iliac spine (ASIS), which is part of the iliac crest of the ilium. Directly inferior to this you should feel the seam formed by the lateral border of the rectus femoris muscle and the medial border of the vastus lateralis muscle at approximately 14 cun. If you run your finger along this seam down the thigh to 8 cun, you should be able to palpate a clear depression for the point.
d) Alternatively, for anatomy purposes (as you will be going against the flow of the channel), place your finger on the lateral edge of the patella bone and ask your patient to raise their leg in the extended position a seam should appear.
e) After locating the seam superior to the patella bone, ask your patient to relax their leg again. You should be able to palpate for the point by running your finger along the seam towards 8 cun.

Note: Chinese Acupuncture texts give the cun for ST 32/33/34 as 6/3/2 cun respectively above the laterosuperior border of the patella. There is no discrepancy with the above locations, as the distance from the lateral aspect of the popliteal crease (at the flexure of the knee) to the laterosuperior border of the patella is equivalent to 2 cun, therefore many texts use 6 cun proximal to the superior border of the patella as opposed to 8 cun from the flexure of the knee. Worsley (1982) Wu (1973) and Lavier (1974) use 13 pouce/ACI (Anatomical Chinese Inch) from the medial extremity of the knee crease to the medial extremity of the groin or the great trochanter. Worsley (1982) locates St 31/32/33/34 at 13/7/5/4 ACI proximal to the flexure of the knee.

Wu (1973) gives St 31/St 32 as "13 and 7 pouce above the flexure", whereas St 33 is "3 pouce above the upper edge of the patella" and St 34 is "1 pouce below St 33". Lavier (1974) shows the total longitudinal measurement of the thigh to be 13 pouce, with St 31/32/33/34 at 13/7/5/4 pouce respectively.

This point is commonly located in the belly of the rectus femoris muscle, or simply located on a line connecting the anterior superior iliac spine and lateral border of the patella, at 6 cun above the laterosuperior border of the patella. When this point is needled either in the seam between the vastus lateralis and the rectus femoris muscle or in the belly of the rectus femoris muscle, you will effectively be needling the same point as the angles you needle them at will meet in the same place at their required needle depth.

Huang (1993) locates St 32 at 6 cun above the knee on a prominence of the the flesh. Jayasuriya (1982) locates St 32 at 6 cun above the midpoint of the superior border of the patella. He also locates this point by using the tip of the middle finger. With the patient seated he places his contralateral wrist crease on the middle of the knee cap and the fingers along the thigh. Where the tip of the middle finger is placed on the thigh is where St 32 is located.

Shanghai (1981) locates St 32 on the thigh at 6 cun above the lateral margin of the knee cap. Qiu (1996) locates ST 32 on the line joining the anterior superior iliac spine and the lateral border of the patella, at 6 cun above the laterosuperior border of the patella. So (1985) locates ST 32 at 6 divisions above the proximal border of the kneecap, also at 3 divisions directly above ST 33, a little to the side of the centre of the thigh.

Cheng (1987) locates S 32 on the line connecting the anterior superior iliac spine and lateral border of the patella, 6 cun above the laterosuperior border of the patella in the m. rectus femoris. Shanghai (1993) locates St 32 when the knee is extended, on the line connecting the superior iliac spine and ST 35, 6 cun above the upper border of the patella. Li (1991) locates this point at 6 cun above the laterosuperior border of the patella.

Eachou (1995) locates ST 32 in a seated or supine position, on the anterior thigh on a line between the anterior superior spine of the ilium and the lateral patellar bone, 6 inches above the lateral superior margin of the patella. Another way he locates this point is to place the proximal skin crease of the palm on the middle of the patella and to put the fingers together on the front thigh. The point is then located at the tip of the middle finger. Worsley (1982) locates XI 32 on the anterior surface of the thigh, 7 ACI (Anatomical Chinese Inch) proximal to the flexure of the knee, between the vastus lateralis and the rectus femoris.

Wu (1973) locates ST 32 on the anterior surface of the thigh at 7 pouce above the level of the flexure of the popliteus, between the rectus femoris and vastus lateralis. Lavier (1974) in an illustration locates St 32 in a seam between the vastus lateralis and rectus femoris muscles, at 7 pouce proximal to the flexure of the knee.

Voisin (1974) locates S 32: vastus lateralis, midway between the pubis and patella. Deadman (1998) locates ST 32 on a line drawn from the lateral border of the patella to the anterior superior iliac spine, at 6 cun proximal to the superior border of the patella. Soulié (1994) locates ST 32 on the thigh: anterior, external face, eight FW (Finger Width) above the patella, on the lateral face of the femur; in the angle between the lateral edge of the rectus anterior and the superior edge of the transverse bulge, on the vastus lateralis; in a hollow; four FW below ST 31; four FW above ST 33; four FW anterior to GB 32.

Shandong (1982) locate Femur-Futu (St 32) at 6 cun above the superior border of the patella, on the line between the spina iliac anterior superior and latero-superior border of the patella. Academy (1975) locates St 32 at 6 cun above the superior border of the patella. By placing the middle of the 1st wrist crease on the middle of the knee with the fingers close together, the point is where the middle finger rests. Ellis (1991) locates ST 32 at 6 inches above the laterosuperior border of the patella, on the line connecting the anterior superor iliac spine and the lateral border of the patella.

Lotan (2000) locates St 32 on the line connecting the patella's lateral-superior corner with the ASIS, 6 cun superior to the patella; 8 cun superior to the knee fold (popliteal crease); the patella height. Legge (1999) locates St 32 at 6 cun above the lateral corner of the superior border of the patella, on the line connecting the anterior superior iliac spine and the lateral border of the patella.

St 33 YIN SHI – YIN MARKET

⊥ ***0.3 TO 0.7 CUN*** △ ***3 TO 5***

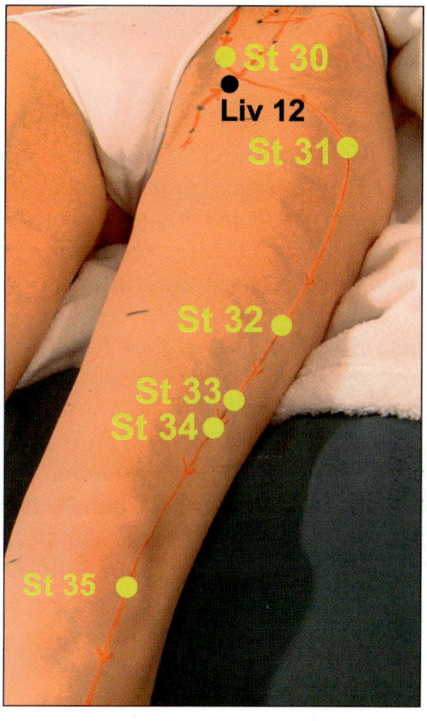

Pos: Position of patient: supine.

Loc:
a) On the anterior surface of the thigh.
b) On a line connecting the anterior superior iliac spine of the ilium and the superolateral corner of the patella bone.
c) In the seam between the rectus femoris and the vastus lateralis muscles.
d) 5 cun proximal to the popliteal crease (flexure of the knee).

Tip:
a) The distance at the level of the inferior border of the symphysis pubis bone (where the medial side of the upper leg joins the torso) and the gluteal groove to the popliteal crease (the flexure of the knee) is approximately 14 cun.
b) To expose the seam between the rectus femoris and the vastus lateralis muscles, flex and extend the knee.

c) Run your finger down from the anterior superior iliac spine (ASIS), which is part of the iliac crest of the ilium. Directly inferior to this you should feel the seam of the rectus femoris and the vastus lateralis muscles at approximately 14 cun. If you run your finger along this seam down the thigh to 5 cun, you should be able to palpate a clear depression for the point.

d) Alternatively, for anatomy purposes (as you will be going against the flow of the channel), place your finger on the lateral edge of the patella bone and ask your patient to raise their leg in the extended position a seam should appear.

e) After locating the seam superior to the patella bone, ask your patient to relax their leg again. You should be able to palpate for the point by running your finger along the seam towards 5 cun.

Note: Chinese Acupuncture texts give the cun for ST 32/33/34 as 6/3/2 cun respectively above the laterosuperior border of the patella. There is no discrepancy with the above locations, as the distance from the lateral aspect of the popliteal crease (at the flexure of the knee) to the laterosuperior border of the patella is equivalent to 2 cun, therefore many texts use 3 cun proximal to the superior border of the patella as opposed to 5 cun from the flexure of the knee. Worsley (1982) Wu (1973) and Lavier (1974) use 13 pouce/ACI (Anatomical Chinese Inch) from the medial extremity of the knee crease to the medial extremity of the groin or the great trochanter. Worsley (1982) locates St 31/32/33/34 at 13/7/5/4 ACI proximal to the flexure of the knee. Wu (1973) gives St 31/St 32 as "13 and 7 pouce above the flexure", where as St 33 is "3 pouce above the upper edge of the patella" and St 34 is "1 pouce below St 33". Lavier (1974) shows the total longitudinal measurement of the thigh to be 13 pouce, with St 31/32/33/34 at 13/7/5/4 pouce respectively.

Many descriptions simply say that St 33. is simply at 3 cun above the laterosuperior border of the patella, on the line connecting the anteror superior iliac spine and the laterosuperior corner of the patella, making no reference to the vastus lateralis and the rectus femoris muscles.

Wu (1973) locates ST 33 upon the anterior surface of the thigh between the rectus femoris and the vastus lateralis, at three pouce above the upper edge of the patella. Voisin (1974) locates S 33 at 4 fb (finger breadth) above the patella, straight over the lateral upper corner. Soulié (1994) locate ST 33 on the anterior lateral face of the thigh: four FW (Finger Width) above the patella. Anterior lateral face of the femur: in the angle between the external edge of the large anterior tendon (triceps) and the inferior edge of a transverse bulge; on the vastus lateralis; in a hollow; four FW below ST 32; three large FW above ST 34; four FW anterior and above GB 33.

Shandong (1982) locate Yinshi at 3 cun above the latero-superior border of the patella, between m. rectus femoris and m. vastus lateralis. Legge (1999) locates St 33 at 3 cun above the superior border of the patella on the line connecting the anterior superior iliac spine and lateral border of the patella. Lotan (2000) locates St 33 with the patients' leg bent, on the line connecting the patella lateral-superior corner with the ASIS, 3 cun proximal to the patella; between the rectus femoris and the vastus lateralis.

St 34 LIANG QIU – BEAM MOUND

⊥ ***0.3 TO 0.5 CUN*** Δ ***3 TO 5***

- ACCUMULATION/Xi Cleft/Gueki
- COUSIN in association with Bl 10

Pos: Position of patient: supine.

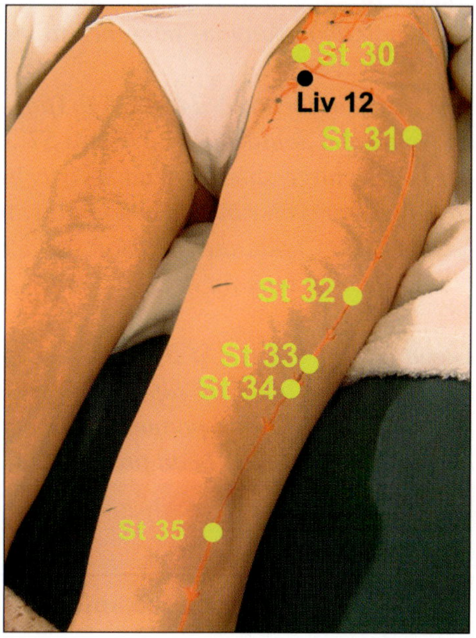

Loc: a) On the anterior surface of the thigh.
b) On a line connecting the anterior superior iliac spine of the ilium and the superolateral corner of the patella.
c) In the seam between the rectus femoris and the vastus lateralis muscles.
d) 4 cun proximal to the popliteal crease (flexure of the knee).

Tip: a) The distance at the level of the inferior border of the symphysis pubis bone (where the medial side of the upper leg joins the torso) and the gluteal groove to the popliteal crease (the flexure of the knee) is approximately 14 cun.
b) To expose the seam between the rectus femoris and the vastus lateralis muscles, flex and extend the knee.
c) Run your finger down from the anterior superior iliac spine (ASIS), which is part of the iliac crest of the ilium. Directly inferior to this you should feel the seam of the rectus femoris and the vastus lateralis muscles at approximately 14 cun. If you run your finger along this seam down the thigh to 4 cun, you should be able to palpate a clear depression for the point.
d) Alternatively, for anatomy purposes (as you will be going against the flow of the channel), place your finger on the lateral edge of the patella bone and ask your patient to raise their leg in the extended position a seam should appear.
e) After locating the seam superior to the patella bone, ask your patient to relax their leg again. You should be able to palpate for the point by running your finger along the seam towards 4 cun.

Note: Chinese Acupuncture texts give the cun for ST 32/33/34 as 6/3/2 cun respectively above the laterosuperior border of the patella. There is no discrepancy with the above locations, as the distance from the lateral aspect of the popliteal crease (at the flexure of the knee) to the laterosuperior border of the patella is equivalent to 2 cun, therefore many texts use 2 cun proximal to the superior border of the patella as opposed to 4 cun from the flexure of the knee. Worsley (1982) Wu (1973) and Lavier (1974) use 13 pouce/ACI (Anatomical Chinese Inch) from the medial extremity of the knee crease to the medial extremity of the groin or the great trochanter. Worsley (1982) locates St 31/32/33/34 at 13/7/5/4 ACI proximal to the flexure of the knee. Wu (1973) gives St 31/St 32 as "13 and 7 pouce above the flexure", whereas St 33 is "3 pouce above the upper edge of the patella" and St 34 is "1 pouce below St 33". Lavier (1974) shows the total longitudinal measurement of the thigh to be 13 pouce, with St 31/32/33/34 at 13/7/5/4 pouce respectively.

Many descriptions simply say that St 34 is at 2 cun above the laterosuperior border of the patella, on the line connecting the anteror superior iliac spine and the laterosuperior corner of the patella making no reference to the vastus lateralis and the rectus femoris muscles.

Voisin (1974) locates S 34 at 1.5 fb (finger breadth) above the patella, straight over the lateral upper corner. Soulié (1994) locates ST 34 on the knee: In the angle between the upper lateral edge of the large anterior tendon (triceps) and deep on the top edge of the femur; on the lower edge of a transverse bulge; in a hollow; three large FW (Finger Width) below ST 33. Wu (1973) locates ST 34 upon the anterior surface of the thigh, at one pouce below ST 33. Shandong (1982) locate Liangqiu at 2 cun above the supra-lateral border of the patella.

Legge (1999) locates St 34 at 2 cun above the superior border of the patella, on the line connecting the anterior superior iliac spine and lateral border of the patella. Lotan (2000) locates St 34 with the patients' leg bent, on the line connecting the patella superior-lateral corner with the ASIS, 2 cun proximal to the patella; between the rectus femoris and the vastus lateralis.

St 35 is on the anterolateral aspect of the flexure of the knee.

St 35 DU BI – CALF NOSE

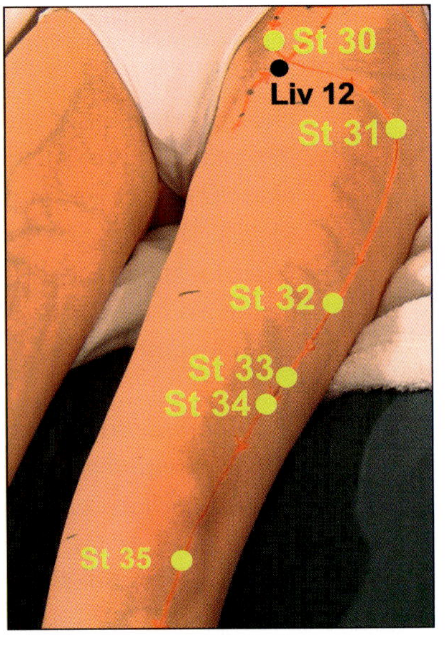

⊥ ***0.3 TO 0.7 CUN*** Δ 3

Pos: Position of patient: supine with the knee flexed.

Loc:
a) On the leg.
b) On the anterolateral aspect of the flexure of the knee.
c) At the inferolateral corner of the patella.
d) On the lateral border of the patellar ligament.
e) In the joint between the tibia and femur bones.

Tip:
a) By flexing the knee a depression is formed by the inferolateral corner of the patella, the patellar ligament, and the joint formed by the tibia and femur bones.

b) Palpation should enable you to feel for the deepest part of the depression.
c) Always mark and subsequently needle the point with the knee in the flexed position.
d) This point is known as one of the "Eyes of the Knee – Xi Yan".

Note: Wu (1973) locates ST 35 outside the rotular tendon, above the plateau of the tibia. Soulié (1994) locates ST 35 on the anterior lateral knee: in the angle between the lateral edge of the anterior patellar-tibial tendon and the superior edge of the head of the tibia; one FW (Finger Width) below and lateral to the inferior edge of the patella; in a hollow; five FW below ST 24; three FW above ST 36.

The distance between the popliteal crease to the prominence of the lateral malleolus is measured as 16 cun.

St 36-40 are on the anterolateral aspect of the lower limb.

St 36 ZU SAN LI – LEG THREE MILES

⊥ ***0.5 TO 1.0 CUN*** **Δ** ***3 TO 20***

- EARTH
- HORARY from 7 a.m. to 9 a.m.
- SEASONAL HORARY – Late Summer
- A POINT OF THE SEA OF NOURISHMENT (Waters and Grains) (There is one other Sea of Nourishment Point: St 30)
- GREATER INFLUENTIAL /Greater Assembling Point of the Stomach and Abdomen.
- HE – SEA/Shu – Transporting/Antique
- LOWER HE-SEA point of the Stomach
- COUSIN in association with LI 4
- ONE OF THE HEAVENLY STAR POINTS OF MA DAN-YANG (the others are: Lu 7, LI 4, LI 11, St 44, Bl 40, Bl 57, Bl 60, Ht 5, GB 34, GB 39 and Liv 3)

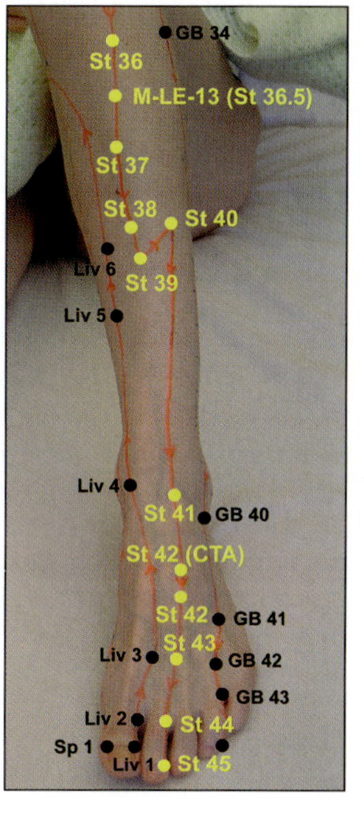

Pos: Position of patient: supine.

Loc: a) On the anterolateral aspect of the lower leg.
b) Lateral to the anterior crest of the tibia bone.
c) Just inferior to the inferior border of the tibial tuberosity of the tibia bone.
d) On the medial border of the tibialis anterior muscle.
e) Approximately 13 cun proximal to the prominence of the lateral malleolus.
f) Approximately 1 cun inferior to the level of GB 34 .
g) Approximately 3 cun below St 35.

Tip:
a) Flex, extend and invert the foot to expose the tibialis anterior muscle to locate the point on the medial border.
b) The emphasis should be placed on the anatomical descriptions, rather than the cun measurements. The cun measurement is not always accurate due to the variation in size of the tibial tuberosity of the tibia bone.
c) The tibial tuberosity of the tibia bone is where the patellar ligament attaches to the bone. You should feel a bony prominence when palpating along this ligament from the patella bone to where it attaches to the tibia bone.
d) St 36 is located inferior to the inferior border of the tibial tuberosity of the tibia bone and lateral to the anterior crest of the tibia bone.
e) Palpation will give you the accurate location of this point
f) To semi-flex the knee place a support under the knee, this will enable you to feel a seam between the medial border of the tibialis anterior muscle and the tibia bone as the tibialis anterior muscle falls slightly away from the bone. St 36 is located by palpating for the contour of the tibia bone.
g) If you prefer to use 13 cun as a guide, mark 16 cun from the popliteal crease on the lateral side of the knee flexure and the prominence of the lateral malleolus.
h) Another method of locating this point is to ask the patient to place their thumb on the middle of their knee cap, and then with their four fingers closed against each other, the end of their middle finger should give you an approximation of St 36, (lateral to the anterior crest of the tibia). Note: Right hand on the right leg, left hand on the left leg.
i) Palpate for accurate location.

Note: Traditionally St 36-St 39 are given as one finger-breadth lateral to the anterior crest of the tibia bone. Voisin (1974) locates S 36 on the leg, at 1.5 fb (finger breadth) lateral to the tibial crest, at the level of the fibular neck. Wu (1973) locates ST 36 upon the anterior surface of the leg, between the tibialis anterior and the tibia, at three pouce below the patella.

Soulié (1994) locates ST 36 on the inferior lateral knee; one FW (Finger Width) anterior to the round head of the fibula; in the angle between the deep inferior edge of the head of the fibula and the tendinous edge of the large muscle along the tibia (anterior tibialis); on the anterior edge of a narrow muscle along the head of the fibula (extensor longus); in a hollow; three FW below ST 35; three FW above ST 37; one FW anterior to GB 34.

Eachou (1995) locates ST 36 with a flexed knee or in a supine position, ask the patient put the thumb on the middle of the patella with the remaining four fingers closed together and placed on the lateral side of the patella. The point is located at the tip of the middle finger. Alternative method: the point is located in a fossa 1 finger breadth lateral to the anterior margin of the tibia, and 3 inches inferior to Dubi (ST 35).

Shandong (1982) locate Zusanli at 6 cun below Pt Dubi (St 35), one finger width lateral to the crista anterior tibiae. Legge (1999) locates St 36 at 3 cun below the inferior border of the patella, one finger-breadth lateral to the edge of the tibia. There is often a small notch in the tibia at this level.

Lotan (2000) locates St 36 with the patients' leg slightly bent, in the depression, level with the tibial tuberosity inferior border, 1 fingerbreadth (3rd finger) lateral to the anterior sharp crest of the tibia; about 3 cun inferior to the patella's lateral-inferior corner.

(St 36.5) M-LE-13 LAN WEI XUE – APPENDIX POINT

⊥ ***0.3 TO 0.8 CUN*** **Δ** ***3 TO 7***

- A Seven Internal Dragons (I.D's) Point with Depression (the other points are Ren 15 "Master", St 32 and St 41)

Pos: Position of patient: supine.

Loc:
a) On the anterior aspect of the lower leg.
b) Lateral to the anterior crest of the tibia bone.
c) On the medial border of the tibialis anterior muscle.
e) Approximately 11.5 to 12 cun proximal to the prominence of the lateral malleolus.
f) Approximately half way between St 36 and St 37.

Tip:
a) Flex, extend and invert the foot to expose the tibialis anterior muscle to locate the point on the medial border.
b) To semi-flex the knee place a support under the knee, this will enable you to feel a seam between the medial border of the tibialis anterior muscle and the tibia bone as the tibialis anterior muscle falls slightly away from the bone. The point is located by palpating for the contour of the tibia bone.
c) If you prefer to use 11.5 to 12 cun as a guide, mark 16 cun from the popliteal crease on the lateral side of the knee flexure and the prominence of the lateral malleolus.
d) Divide 16 cun in to four equal measurements of 4 cun. Palpate for the point which is approximately between 11.5 and 12 cun proximal to the prominence of the lateral malleolus.
e) To help with the location of this point, run your finger with the flow of the channel down the leg from the tibial tuberosity of the tibia bone and along the lateral border of the tibial crest.

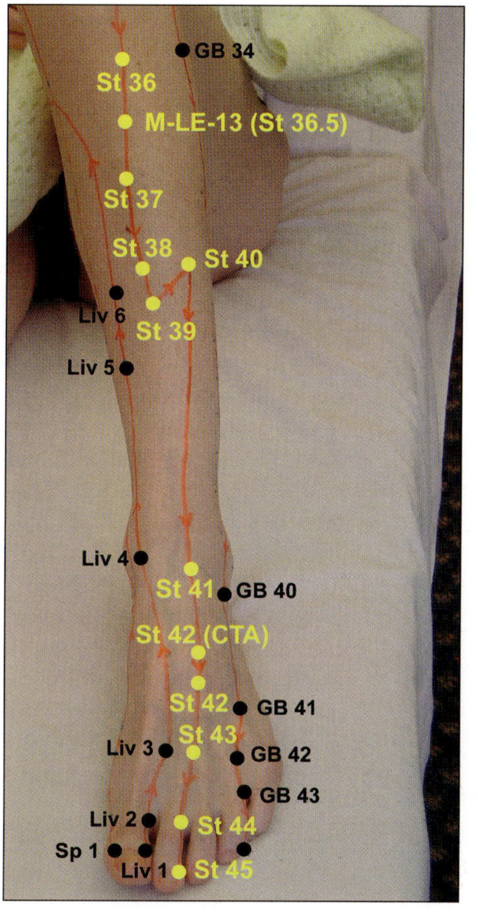

St 37 SHANG JU XU – UPPER GREAT VOID

⊥ ***0.3 TO 0.8 CUN*** Δ ***3 TO 7***

- LOWER POINT OF THE SEA OF BLOOD (There are two Lower Sea of Blood Points, the other is St 39. There is also an Upper Sea of Blood Point: Bl 11)
- LOWER HE-SEA point of the Large Intestine

Pos: Position of patient: supine.

Loc: a) On the anterior aspect of the lower leg.
b) Lateral to the anterior crest of the tibia bone.
c) On the medial border of the tibialis anterior muscle.
e) Approximately 10 cun proximal to the prominence of the lateral malleolus.
f) Approximately 3 cun inferior to St 36.

Tip: a) Flex, extend and invert the foot to expose the tibialis anterior muscle to locate the point on the medial border.
b) To semi-flex the knee place a support under the knee, this will enable you to feel a seam between the medial border of the tibialis anterior muscle and the tibia bone as the tibialis anterior muscle falls slightly away from the bone. St 37 is located by palpating for the contour of the tibia bone.
c) If you prefer to use 10 cun as a guide, mark 16 cun from the popliteal crease on the lateral side of the knee flexure and the prominence of the lateral malleolus.
d) To help with the location of this point, run your finger with the flow of the channel down the leg from the tibial tuberosity of the tibia bone and along the lateral border of the tibial crest.
e) Palpate for accurate location.

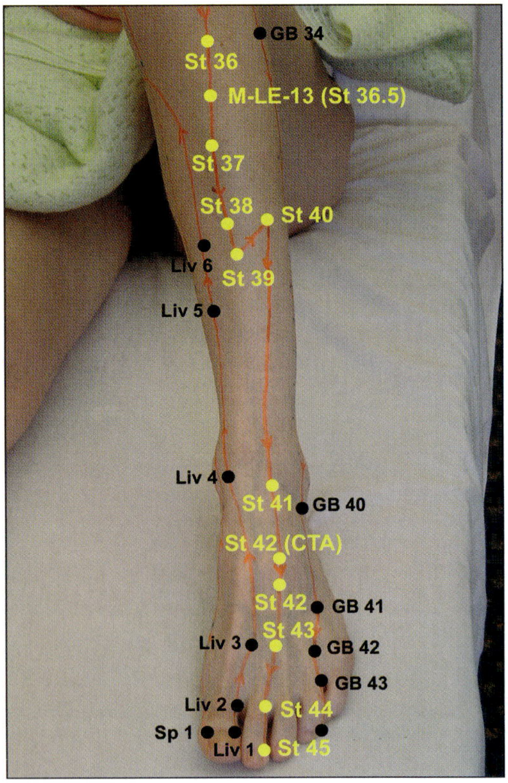

Note: Traditionally St 36-St 39 are given as one finger-breadth lateral to the anterior crest of the tibia bone. Voisin (1974) locates S 37 on the leg, at 3 fb (finger breadths) below S 36. Ellis (1991) locates ST 37 at 6 inches below ST 35 and at a finger's breadth lateral to the anterior crest of the tibia. Academy (1975) and Legge (1999) locate this point at 6 cun below St 35 and at a finger's breadth lateral to the anterior crest of the tibia. Soulié (1994) locates ST 37 on the anterior lateral lower leg: three FW (Finger Width) below the head of the fibula; in the angle

between the inferior edge of a transverse membrane (aponeurosis of the leg) and the anterior edge of the extensor longus, which runs along the fibula; posterior edge of a large muscle running along the fibula (tibialis anterior); in a hollow; three FW below ST 36; three FW above ST 38. Lotan (2000) locates St 37 at 6 cun inferior to the patella, 1 finger breadth lateral to the anterior crest of the tibia, on the tibialis anterior muscle. Eachou (1995) locates ST 37 at 6 inches below the knee, 1 finger width lateral to the tibia, on the tibialis anterior muscle and between the tibia and fibula. Wu (1973) locates ST 37 at three pouce below ST 36, between the muscle and the tibia.

St 38 TIAO KOU – BRANCH OPENING

⊥ ***0.5 TO 0.8 CUN*** **Δ** ***3 TO 7***

Pos: Position of patient: supine.

Loc:
a) On the anterior aspect of the lower leg.
b) Lateral to the anterior crest of the tibia bone.
c) On the medial border of the tibialis anterior muscle.
e) Approximately 8 cun proximal to the prominence of the lateral malleolus.
f) Approximately 2 cun inferior to St 37.
g) Approximately halfway between St 35 and St 41.

Tip:
a) Flex, extend and invert the foot to expose the tibialis anterior muscle to locate the point on the medial border.
b) To semi-flex the knee place a support under the knee, this will enable you to feel a seam between the medial border of the tibialis anterior muscle and the tibia bone as the tibialis anterior muscle falls slightly away from the bone. St 38 is located by palpating for the contour of the tibia bone.
c) If you prefer to use 8 cun as a guide, mark 16 cun from the popliteal crease on the lateral side of the knee flexure and the prominence of the lateral malleolus and divide into half.
d) To help with the location of this point, run your finger with the flow of the channel down the leg from the tibial tuberosity of the tibia bone and along the lateral border of the tibial crest.
e) Palpate for accurate location.

Note: Traditionally St 36-St 39 are given as one finger-breadth lateral to the anterior crest of the tibia bone. Voisin (1974) locates S 38 on the leg, at 5 fb (finger breadths) below S 36. Ellis (1991) locates ST 38 at 8 inches below ST 35 and 2 inches below ST 37, at the midpoint between ST 35 and ST 41, near the edge of the tibia. Academy (1975) locates St 38 at 8 cun below the knee. Legge (1999) locates this point at 8 cun below St 35, between St 35 and St 41, where there is often a notch in the tibia.

Soulié (1994) locates ST 38 on the anterior, lateral face of the lower leg: six FW (Finger Width) under the heads of the tibia and fibula; in the angle between the inferior edge of a transverse bulge in a hollow, and the anterior edge of the extensor longus, which runs along the fibula; on the posterior edge of the large muscle (tibialis anterior); three FW under ST 37; three FW above ST 39; one large FW above and anterior to GB 35. Huang (1993) locates St 38 at 1 cun above the Lower Ridge (St 39)

Deadman (1998) locates ST 38 midway between the tibio-femoral joint and the prominence of the lateral malleolus. Wu (1973) locates ST 38 at five pouce below ST 36, between the muscle and tibia. Lotan (2000) locates St 38 at 8 cun inferior to the patella, 1 fingerbreadth lateral to the anterior crest of the tibia, on the tibialis anterior muscle. Shanghai (1981) locates S 38 at 2 units below S 37 or 8 units below the knee. Academy (1975) locates St 38 at 8 cun below the knee and at 2 cun below St 37. Eachou (1995) locates ST 38 at 8 inches below ST 35, at the midpoint between ST 35 and ST 41, 1 finger breadth lateral to the anterior tibial crest. Shandong (1982) locate Tiaokou at 8 cun above the lateral condyle of the ankle, one finger width lateral to the crista anterior tibiae. Legge (1999) locates St 38 at 8 cun below Dubi St 35, halfway between Dubi (St 35) and Liexi (St 41), There is often a small notch in the tibia at this level.

St 39 XIA JU XU – LOWER GREAT VOID

⊥ ***0.3 TO 0.8 CUN*** Δ ***3 TO 7***

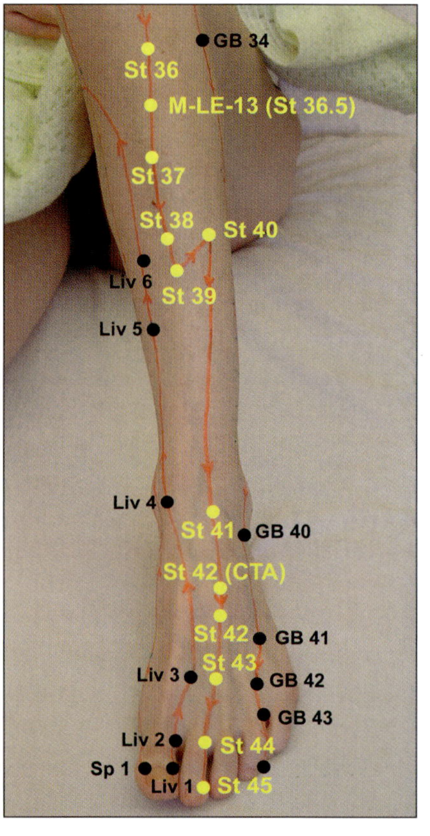

- LOWER POINT OF THE SEA OF BLOOD (There are two Lower Sea of Blood Points, the other is St 37. There is also an Upper Sea of Blood Point: Bl 11)
- LOWER HE-SEA point of the Small Intestine

Pos: Position of patient: supine.

Loc: a) On the anterior aspect of the lower leg.
b) Lateral to the anterior crest of the tibia bone.
c) On the medial border of the tibialis anterior muscle.
d) Approximately 7 cun proximal to the prominence of the lateral malleolus.
e) Approximately 3 cun inferior to St 37.
f) Approximately 1 cun inferior to St 38.

Tip: a) Flex, extend and invert the foot to expose the tibialis anterior muscle to locate the point on the medial border.
b) To semi-flex the knee place a support under the knee, this will enable you to feel a seam

between the medial border of the tibialis anterior muscle and the tibia bone as the tibialis anterior muscle falls slightly away from the bone. St 39 is located by palpating for the contour of the tibia bone.

c) If you prefer to use 7 cun as a guide, mark 16 cun from the popliteal crease on the lateral side of the knee flexure and the prominence of the lateral malleolus and divide into half.
d) To help with the location of this point, run your finger with the flow of the channel down the leg from the tibial tuberosity of the tibia bone and along the lateral border of the tibial crest.
e) Palpate for accurate location.

Note: Traditionally St 36-St 39 are given as one finger-breadth lateral to the anterior crest of the tibia bone.

Soulié (1994) locates ST 39 on the anterior, lateral face of the leg; six FW (Finger Width) above the external malleolus, on the posterior edge of the large muscle (tibialis anterior); in the angle of the upper edge of the transverse bulge; in a hollow; on the anterior edge of the muscle running along the fibula (extensor longus). Wu (1973) locates ST 39 at six pouce below ST 36, between the muscle and the tibia.

Shanghai (1993) locates ST 39 at 1 cun below the centre of the anteriolateral side of the leg, between the tibia and fibula, about 0.5 cun from the anterior crest of the tibia, 9 cun below ST 35 and 1 cun below ST 38.

Voisin (1974) locates S 39 on the leg, at 6 fb (finger breadths) below S 36. Lotan (2000) locates St 39 at 9 cun inferior to the patella, 1 finger breadth lateral to the anterior crest of the tibia, on the tibialis anterior muscle.

Shanghai (1981) locates S 39 at 3 units below S 37 or 9 units below the knee. Eachou (1995) locates ST 39 at 9 inches below ST 35, 1 finger breadth lateral to the anterior tibial crest. Shandong (1982) locate Xiajuxu at 1 cun below Pt. Tiaokou (St 38). Legge (1999) locates St 39 at 1 cun below Tiaokou (St 38), 7 cun above Jiexi (St 41), about one finger-breadth lateral to the edge of the tibia.

St 40 FENG LONG – ABUNDANT SPLENDOUR

⊥ ***0.3 TO 0.5 CUN*** Δ ***3 TO 5***

- JUNCTION/Luo/Connecting/Passage/Lo/Lê
- RE-UNION/Crossing/Meeting Point of the Stomach Channel with the Spleen Channel – Foot Yang Ming Channel with the Foot Tai Yin Channel
- HOST/GUEST COMBINATION – Source Point with the Junction Point of its Paired Official/Organ Therefore St 40 is combined with Sp 3

Pos: Position of patient: supine.

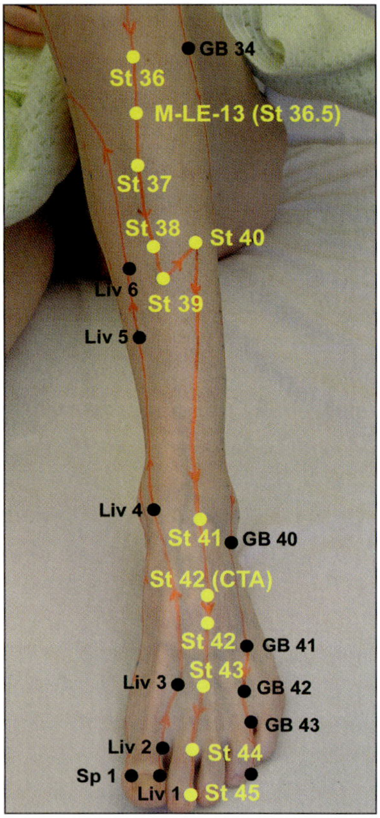

Loc: a) On the anterolateral aspect of the lower leg.
b) On the lateral border of the tibialis anterior muscle.
c) Approximately 8 cun proximal to the prominence of the lateral malleolus.
d) Approximately 1 cun lateral to St 38 (anatomy takes precedence).

Tip: a) Flex, extend and invert the foot to expose the tibialis anterior muscle to locate the media and lateral borders.
b) To semi-flex the knee place a support under the knee, this will enable you to feel the medial and lateral border of the tibialis anterior muscle. St 38 and St 40 are located by palpating the medial and lateral borders of the tibialis anterior muscle respectively.
c) Although the location of St 40 is 1 cun lateral to St 38, anatomy takes precedence where you should palpate for the lateral border of the muscle. The width of this muscle varies from person to person depending on the development of their leg muscles. In this case it may make the measurement more than 1 cun. Footballers in particular have well developed tibialis anterior muscles.
d) If you prefer to use the 8 cun measurement as a guide for St 38 and St 40, mark 16 cun from the popliteal crease on the lateral side of the knee flexure and the prominence of the lateral malleolus and divide into half.
e) Run your finger with the flow of the channel down the leg from the tibial tuberosity of the tibia bone and along the medial border of the tibial crest to the level of St 38. Palpate laterally to the lateral border of the muscle for St 40.
f) Palpate for accurate location.
g) The most common error when locating this point is that it is located too laterally, making the point very close to the Gall Bladder channel which is anterior to the anterior border of the fibula bone.

Note: St 40 is traditionally 2 finger breadths from the anterior crest of the tibia, or 1 finger breadth lateral to St 38. Eachou (1995) locates ST 40 midway between the inferior margin of the patella and the skin crease of the ankle joint (or 8 inches above the lateral malleolus), 1.5 inches lateral to the anterior margin of the tibia or one finger's breadth lateral to ST 38, between the tibia and fibula. Legge (1999) locates St 40 at 8 cun superior and anterior to the external malleolus, about 1 finger breadth posterior to St 38, about halfway between St 35 and the malleolus. Lawson-Wood (1973) locates XI 40 on the antero-extern of the leg, anterior edge of the fibula, 2cm above the middle of a line drawn from the external malleolus to the anterior tuberosity of the tibia.

Voisin (1974) locates S 40 on the leg, at 6 fb (finger breadth) above the lateral malleolus, just in front of the anterior border of the fibula. On an illustration it clearly shows that S 40 is almost on a level with S 39 and not S 38. Wu (1973) locates ST 40 on the outer surface of the leg, behind the tibialis anterior, at the level of ST 38. Soulié (1994) locates ST 40 on the lateral, anterior face of the leg, five FW (finger width) above the external malleolus; in the lower angle of two muscles which narrow (the posterior edge of the tibialis anterior, which runs along the tibia and the anterior edge of the extensor longus, which runs along the fibula); in a hollow. Lotan (2000) locates St 40 at 8 cun inferior to the patella, 2 fingerbreadths (2nd and 3rd finger) lateral to the anterior sharp crest of the tibia; 1 fingerbreadth lateral to St 38; level with the midpoint between the knee joint and the lateral malleolus peak.

St 41 is on the anterior aspect of the flexure of the ankle.

St 41 JIE XI – RELEASED STREAM

⊥ ***0.5 CUN*** **Δ** ***3 TO 7***

- A Seven Internal Dragons (I.D's) Point (the other points are Ren 15 "Master", St 25 and St 32)
- FIRE
- TONIFICATION/Reinforcing
- MOTHER
- JING – RIVER/Shu – Transporting/Antique

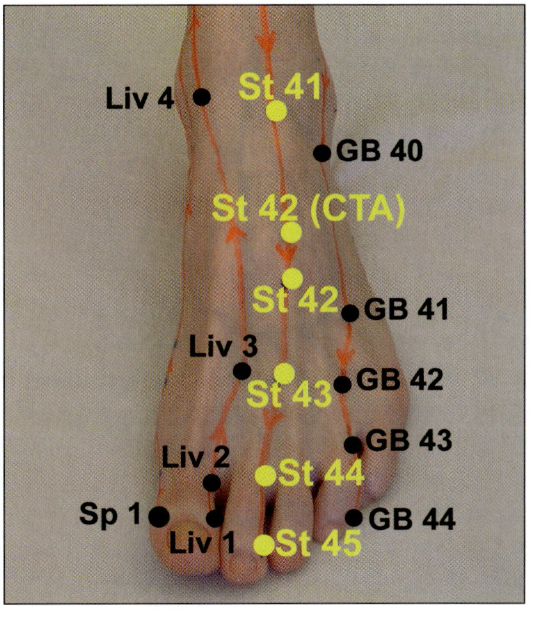

Pos: Position of patient: supine.

Loc: a) On the anterior aspect of the lower limb.
b) On the anterior aspect of the flexure of the ankle.
c) Between the tendons of the extensor digitorum longus and extensor hallucis longus muscles.

Tip: a) Actively flex and extend the foot to expose the tendons of the tibialis anterior, extensor digitorum longus and extensor hallucis longus muscles. You will need to experiment with the positioning of the foot to see which position demonstrates the tendons most clearly.
b) Of the three tendons the tibialis anterior muscle is the most medial and prominent tendon.
c) Draw a line at the flexure of the ankle.
d) Put your finger on the medial malleolus bone.
e) Run your finger anteriorly from the medial malleolus to the lateral border of the tendon of the tibialis anterior muscle. You are now between the tendons of the tibialis anterior and the extensor hallucis longus muscles.
f) Palpate laterally from the lateral border of the extensor hallucis longus muscle until you feel a depression between the tendons of the extensor hallucis longus and the extensor digitorum muscles. The location of the point is at the flexure of the ankle between these two tendons.
g) Palpate for accurate location.

Note: Traditionally located at the level of the tip of the external malleolus. Huang (1993) locates St 41 at 1 cun and 5 fen proximal to St 42, in a depression at the ankle. Wu (1973) locates ST 41 upon the instep in the centre of the malleolar flexure, between two tendons. Voisin (1974) locates S 41 on the foot, dorsum: at the centre of the dorsiflexion fold, just below the tibia. Lawson-Wood (1973) locates XI 41 on the dorsum of the foot, above the scaphoid and cuboid, below the tibia. Soulié (1994) locates ST 41 on the anterior and superior arch, midway between the internal and external malleolus; in the angle between the upper edge of the deep transverse bone (astragalus) and the lateral edge of the large middle tendon (of the tibialis anterior); in a hollow; on the medial edge of the extensor longus.

St 42-45 are on the dorsal surface of the foot

St 42 CHONG YANG – RUSHING YANG

⊥ ***0.3*** Δ ***3 TO 5***

- SOURCE/Yuan/Regulator/Primary
- EXIT
- RE-UNION/Crossing/Meeting Point of the Stomach Channel with the Spleen Channel – Foot Yang Ming Channel with the Foot Tai Yin Channel
- ORIGINAL (for specific symptoms)
- HOST/GUEST COMBINATION – Source Point with the Junction Point of its Paired Official/Organ Therefore St 42 is combined with Sp 4

Pos: Position of patient: supine.

Loc **Location 1 – Preferred by The College of Traditional Acupuncture**

a) On the dorsum of the foot
b) Between the tendons of the extensor digitorum longus and hallucis muscle.
c) In the hollow between the navicular bone, the intermediate cuniform bone and the lateral cuniform bone. This description is more proximal to the other common location – See next page.
d) On a line drawn approximately halfway between St 41 (at the ankle flexure) and St 43 (which is just distal to the flare at the base of the second metatarsal bone).
e) In a hollow that is exposed when the foot and digits are dorsiflexed.

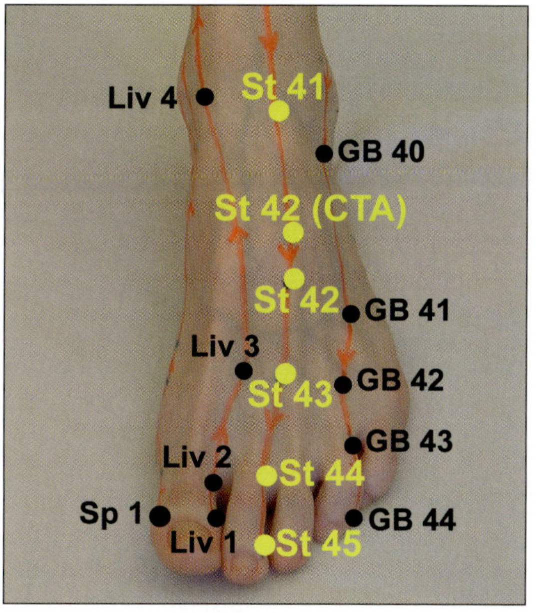

Tip. a) Run your finger with the flow of the channel from St 41, between the tendons of the extensor hallucis longus and extensor digitorum longus muscle on to the dorsal surface of the foot.
b) Your finger should follow the natural curvature of the foot which demonstrates that the channel is not a plumb line, as it appears on some two dimensional illustrations. Three dimensional images of the foot have a slight curvature that runs laterally before flowing medially as it travels towards the lateral aspect of the second digit.
c) Draw the channel line from the flexure of the ankle at St 41 to the lateral aspect of the second digit.
d) From the flexure of the ankle at St 41 run your finger on the dorsum of the foot, until you feel an indentation formed by three bones, the navicular bone, the lateral cuneiform bone and the intermediate cuneiform bone.
e) Palpate for accurate location.
f) If you are having problems palpating the point, feel for the distal corner of the navicular bone on the medial side of the foot (where Ki 2 is located) and palpate for the gap between the navicular bone and the medial cuneiform bone on the dorsal surface of the foot.
g) Draw a transverse line across the dorsal surface of the foot.
h) Where your longitudinal channel line and transverse line intersect with each other, this will give you an approximate area in which to accurately palpate for the point.
i) Another way of locating the point is to halve the distance between St 41 and St 43, this will give you a ball park area in which to palpate for the point on the channel line.

St 42 CHONG YANG – RUSHING YANG

⊥ ***0.3*** Δ ***3 TO 5***

- SOURCE/Yuan/Regulator/Primary
- EXIT
- RE-UNION/Crossing/Meeting Point of the Stomach Channel with the Spleen Channel – Foot Yang Ming Channel with the Foot Tai Yin Channel
- ORIGINAL (for specific symptoms)
- HOST/GUEST COMBINATION – Source Point with the Junction Point of its Paired Official/Organ Therefore St 42 is combined with Sp 4

Pos: Position of patient: supine.

Loc: **Location 2 (Alternative):**

a) On the dorsum of the foot.
b) At the highest point of the dorsum of the foot.
c) Between the bases of the second and third metatarsal bones, and the intermediate and lateral cuneiform bones (this location is more distal to the other common location).
d) The dorsalis pedis artery is sometimes palpable beneath this point.
e) On a line drawn from St 43 (between the second and third metatarsal bones), to St 41 (at the ankle flexure),
f) In a hollow exposed when the foot and digits are dorsiflexed.

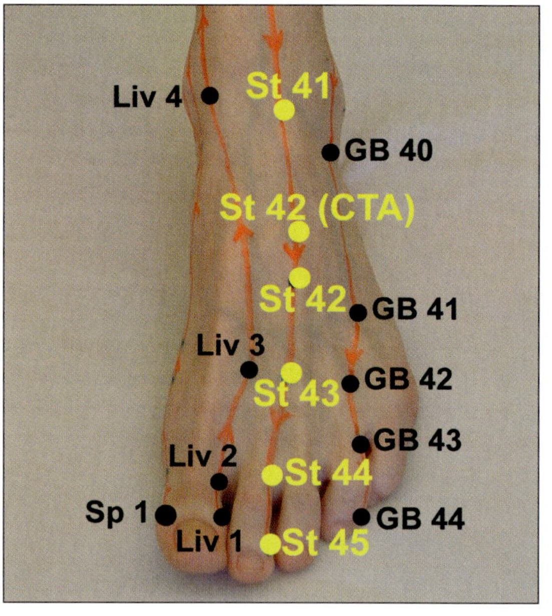

Tip: a) Run your finger with the flow of the channel from St 41, between the tendons of the extensor hallucis longus and extensor digitorum longus muscles on to the dorsal surface of the foot.

b) Your finger should follow the natural curvature of the foot which demonstrates that the channel is not a plumb line, as appears on some two dimensional illustrations. Three dimensional images of the foot have a slight curvature that runs laterally before flowing medially as it travels towards the lateral aspect of the second digit.

c) Draw the channel line from the flexure of the ankle at St 41 to the lateral aspect of the second digit.

d) From the flexure of the ankle at St 41 run your finger on the dorsum of the foot, until you feel an indentation formed by four bones, the bases of the second and third metatarsals, the distal borders of the lateral and intermediate cuneiform bones.
e) Palpate for accurate location.

St 42 Note: Acupuncture texts vary enormously as to where this point is located, and there are contradictory anatomical references given. It is said that St 42 is on the dome of the instep of the foot, where the pulsation of the dorsalis pedis artery is palpable. Also that it is 1.5 cun proximal to St 43, and 1.5 cun distal to St 41, (which would put it approximately at the meeting of the navicular and the cuneiform bones).

Other texts refer to it being in a depression between the bases of the second and third metatarsal bones and the cuneiform bones. This is further complicated by the fact that Low (1988) locates Extra points (dorsal points 18/19) on the line between Stomach 41-43. Wu (1973) locates ST 42 upon the dorsal surface of the foot, at five pouce above ST 44. Lavier (1974) illustrates St 42 as being between the navicular bone, and the lateral and intermediate cuneiform bones.

Worsley (1982) locates St 42 on the dorsal surface of the foot, in the concavity in the meeting of the navicular, lateral cuneiform and intermediate cuneiform bones. Lawson-Wood (1973) locates St 42 on the dorsum of the foot (instep) at the meeting of the scaphoid and the second and third cuneiforms. Voisin (1974) describes and illustrates St 42 as being located on the foot, dorsum: in the cuneonavicular joint, 1 fb (finger breadth) distal to St 41. Cheng's (1987) location is distal to St 41 at the highest point of the dorsum of the foot, in between the second and third metatarsal bones and the cuneiform bone. Eachou (1995) locates St 42 at the highest point of the dorsum of the foot, 1.5 inches below St 41 between the base of the second and third metatarsals and the cuneiform. Yang (1982) locates St 42 1.3 cun below St 41, on the pulse of the dorsal artery. Academy (1975) locates St 42 1.5 cun distal to St 41, at the highest spot of the dorsum of the foot where the artery can be palpated.

Qiu (1996) locates St 42 distal to St 41 between the tendons of the m. extensor digitorum longus and hallucis longus, between the second and third metatarsal bones and the cuneiform bone, where the drosal artery of the foot throbs. Huang's (1993) location is translated as being on the instep 5 cun (to the second toe) at a pulsating vessel 3 cun proximal to St 43. Legge (1999) locates St 42 in the joint between the 2nd and 3rd metatarsal bones and the cuneiform bone, about halfway between St 41 and St 43, where a small pulse can be felt. Shanghai (1993) locates this point at the highest point of the dorsum of the foot, between the tendons of the long extensor muscle of the great toe and long extensor muscle of the toes, at the throbbing point of the dorsal pedis artery. Li (1991) locates St 42 1.3 cun down from St 40 where the pulse is palpable. Soulié (1994) locates St 42 on the dorsal aspect of the foot. In the angle of the anterior edge of the transverse bone (scaphoid) and the medial edge of the extensors. In a hollow behind the articulation of the second and third cuneiforms; three tight FW (Finger Width) in front of ST 41; two FW behind ST 43.

Lotan (2000) locates St 42 at the joint of three bones, the cuneiform and the 2nd and 3rd metatarsals, on the highest part of the dorsal aspect of the foot, lateral to the dorsalis pedis artery. So (1985) locates ST 42 1 and 1/2 divisions distal to ST 41, between the second and third metatarsal bones. There is a pulse at this point. Ellis (1991) locates ST 42 at the highest point of the dorsum of the foot, in the depression between the 2nd and 3rd metatarsal bones and the cuneiform bone. Shanghai (1981) locates S 42 at 1.5 units below S 41 at the hump on the dorsum of the foot and to the side of the dorsalis pedis artery. Jayasuriya (1982) locates St 42 1.5 cun distal to St 41, at the highest point of the dorsum of the foot, in the depression between the 2nd and 3rd metatarsal bones and the cuneiform bone.

Masayoshi (1975) locates St 42 anterior to the junction of the 2nd and 3rd metatarsal bones. Shandong (1982) locate Chongyang anterior inferior to Pt. Jiexi (St 41), at the highest spot of the dorsum of the foot.

Note: Although some location descriptions state that the point lies beneath the dorsalis pedis artery, the artery actually travels between the two heads of the first dorsal interosseous muscle which is between the first and second metatarsal bones. McMinn (1977) clearly illustrates this with photgraphic evidence and a description of where the artery passes. The location of the point makes the artery more lateral than it actually is, so this brings up the question of whether you are able to palpate for the artery or not. The description also states that St 42 is at the highest point of the dorsum of the foot, this appears to make the point more proximal than at the junction of the second and third metatarsal bones and the intermediate and lateral cuneiform bones.

St 43 XIAN GU – SINKING VALLEY

⊥ ***0.3 TO 0.5 CUN*** Δ ***3***

- WOOD
- SHU – STREAM/Shu – Transporting/Antique

Pos: Position of patient: supine.

Loc: a) On the dorsum of the foot.
b) At the junction of the second and third metatarsal bones.
c) Just distal to the flare at the base of the second metatarsal bone.

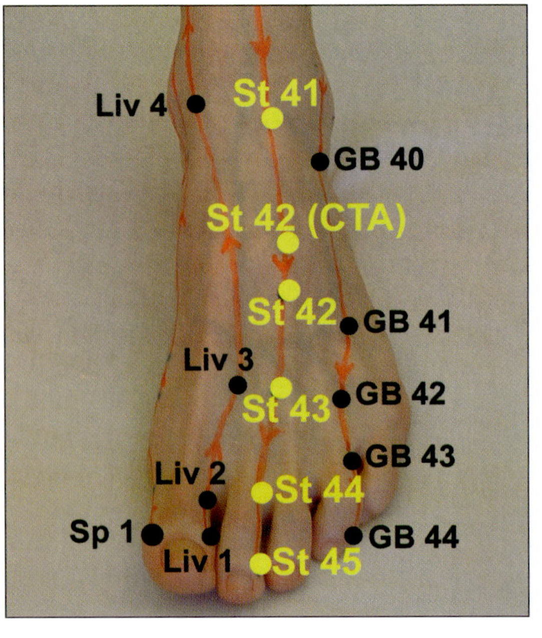

Tip: a) Run your finger from St 41, at the anterior ankle flexure, on to the dorsum of the foot towards the lateral aspect of the second metatarsal bone.

b) You should be able to feel your finger go into the junction between the second and third bases of the metatarsal bones.

c) It may be easier to palpate Liv 3 first as the depression between the flares of the bases of the first and second metatarsal bones are greater than the flares of the bases of the second and third metatarsal bones.

d) Run your finger laterally from Liv 3 to the junction between the bases of the second and third metatarsal bones, St 43 is at the same level or slightly proximal to Liv 3.

e) If you cannot feel the junction then you may need to feel for the second and third metatarsophalangeal joints. To feel these, press your fingers in to the plantar surface of the foot at the level of these metatarso-phalangeal joints, this will demonstrate the second and third metatarsal bones on the dorsum surface of the foot.

f) On the dorsum of the foot, run your fingers proximally from the metatarso-phalangeal joints until you feel the bones flare at the base of the second and third metatarsal bones. The point is located just distal to the flare at the base of the second metatarsal bone.

g) Palpate for the hollow to accurately locate the point.

Note: The traditional location of this point is distal to the junction of the second and third metatarsal bones, but there other descriptions for this point as well. Deadman (1998) locates St 43 between the second and third metatarsal bones, 1 cun proximal to St 44. Eachou (1995) locates St 43 between the second and third metatarsal bones, 2 inches above the toe web. Lotan (2000) locates St 43 between the 2nd and 3rd metatarsals, proximal to the bone heads, level with Sp 3 and Liv 3. Huang (1993) locates St 43 on the lateral border of the (second) toe, in a depression proximal to the base joint of the proximal phalanx, 2 cun proximal to St 44.

Soulié (1994) locates ST 43 on the dorsum of the foot; two FW (Finger Width) behind the articulation of the base of the second and third toes. In the angle of the posterior (superior) head and the body of the long bone of the third toe (third metatarsal). In a hollow. Between the bone and the interdigital artery, vein and nerve; two FW in front of ST 42; approximately two FW behind ST 44; one FW medial to GB 42; two FW lateral to LR 3. Shanghai (1981) locates S 43 between the 2nd and 3rd metatarsal bones, directly above the lateral side of the 2nd toe. Shandong (1982) locate Chongyang anterior inferior to Pt. Jiexi (St 41), at the highest spot of the dorsum of the foot. Legge (1999) locates St 43 in the depression found between the 2nd and 3rd metatarsal bones.

St 44 NEI TING – INNER COURTYARD

⊥ ***0.3 CUN*** Δ ***3***

- WATER
- YING – SPRING/Shu – Transporting/Antique
- ONE OF THE HEAVENLY STAR POINTS OF MA DAN-YANG (the others are: Lu 7, LI 4, LI 11, St 36, Bl 40, Bl 57, Bl 60, Ht 5, GB 34, GB 39 and Liv 3)

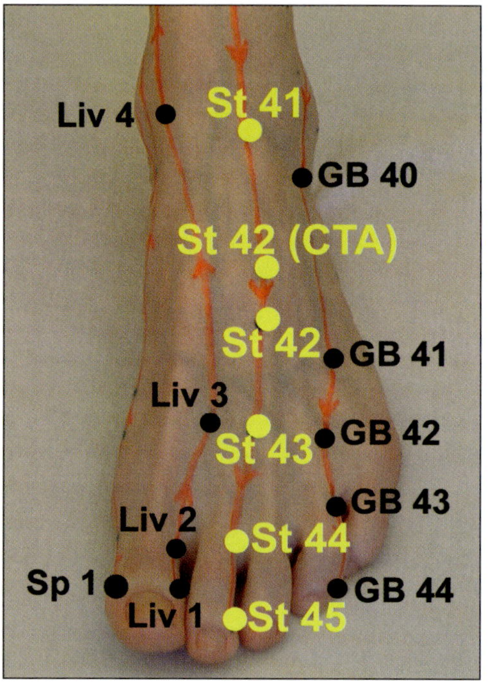

Pos: Position of patient: supine.

Loc:
a) On the dorsum of the foot.
b) Between the second and third digits.
c) Proximal to the web margin.
d) Distal to the metatarso-phalangeal joint of the second digit.
e) Just distal to the flare of the base of the proximal phalanx of the second digit.

Tip:
a) To help demonstrate the metatarso-phalangeal joint, push the pads of your fingers gently in to the plantar surface of the foot directly underneath the base of the second digit. You should be able to feel the metatarso-phalangeal (knuckle) joint on the dorsal surface of the foot as the bones have been pushed upwards and the tendons are more relaxed.
b) In the direction of the flow of the channel palpate from St 41 (at the ankle flexure) along the lateral aspect of the second metatarso-phalangeal joint towards the proximal phalanx of the second digit
c) St 44 is located by palpating over the distal aspect of the second metatarso-phalangeal joint. You should be able to feel the flare which is proximal to the web margin formed between the second and third digits (and distal to the base of the proximal phalanx of the second digit),.
d) Palpate for accurate location.

Note: Traditionally this point is proximal to the web margin in between the second and third digits. Li (1991), Jayasuriya (1982), Academy (1975) and Deadman (1998) all describe this point as being at the traditional location but use 0.5 cun proximal to the web margin. Lotan (2000) locates St 44 between the 2nd and 3rd toes, midway between the web margin and the 2nd metatarsophalangeal joint. Legge (1999) locates this point in the web between the 2nd and 3rd toes, between the web margin and the metatarso-phalangeal joints.

So (1985) locates ST 44 between the second and third toes, halfway between the metatarsophalangeal joint and the web of the toes. Wu (1973) locates ST 44 on the dorsal surface of the foot, posterior to the articulation of the metatarsal phalange of the second toe, on the lateral side of the metatarsal.

Soulié (1994) locates ST 44 on the dorsum of the foot: at the articulation of the second and third toes, in the angle between the anterior head and body of the third metatarsal (of the third toe), towards the second toe; in a hollow; between the vessel and nerve; two FW (Finger Width) approximately in front of ST 43; one FW medial to GB 43; one large FW lateral to LR 2.

St 45 LI DUI – HARD BARGAIN

⊥ ***0.1 CUN*** Δ ***1 TO 3***

- METAL
- SEDATION/Reducing/Dispersing
- CHILD
- JING – WELL/Shu – Transporting/Antique

Pos: Position of patient: supine.

Loc: a) On the foot.
b) The lateral nail point of the second digit.
c) Approximately 0.1 cun proximal to the corner of the nail.
d) Just distal to the flare of the distal phalanx.

Tip: a) The point is level with the nail bed (where the nail attaches to the skin) rather than the cuticle.
b) Draw a horizontal line across the nail bed.
c) Draw a vertical line from the lateral border of the nail towards the nail bed.
d) The lines drawn from b) and c) (vertical and horizontal) form an intersection. This is approximately where the point is located.

Note: Ellis (1991) – the classical location for ST 45 is on the outer side of the end of the toe next to the great toe, the breadth of a Chinese leek leaf from the corner of the nail (The Great compendium). Huang (1993) locates St 45 at the tip of the toe, next to the big one, the distance of a leak leaf from the corner of the nail. Soulié (1994) locates ST 45 on the foot: third toe, ungual phalanx, about mid-width from the medial face (towards the second toe); in the angle between the swelling and the body of the bone, on the dorsal edge of the palmar tendon (flexor); in a hollow.

REFERENCES FOR THE STOMACH CHANNEL

Wu, Wei-P'ing 1973 Chinese Acupuncture – ST 2: 66; ST 3: 66; ST 4: 66; ST 5: 67; ST 6: 67; ST 7: 67; ST 8: 67; ST 9: 67; ST 10: 68; ST 11: 68; ST 12: 68; ST 13: 68; ST 19: 69; ST 20: 69; ST 21: 69; ST 22: 69; ST 23: 70; ST 24: 70; ST 25: 70; ST 26: 70; ST 27: 70; ST 28: 70; ST 31: 71; ST 32: 71; ST 33: 71; ST 34: 71; ST 35: 72; ST 36: 72; ST 37: 72; ST 38: 72; ST 39: 73; ST 40: 73; ST 41: 73; ST 42: 73; ST 44: 73

Voisin, Dr. H 1974 Essentials of Acupuncture – S 1 (St 8): 88; S 2 (St 7): 88; S 3 (St 6): 88; S 4 (St 1): 88; S 5 (St 2): 88; S 6 (St 3): 88; S 7 (St 2): 88; S 8 (St 1): 88; S 9: 88 ; S 10: 88; S 11: 88; S 12: 88; S 13: 88; S 19: 88; S 20: 88; S 21: 88; S 22: 88; S 23: 88; S 24: 88; S 25: 90; S 26: 90; S 27: 90; S 28: 90; S 29: 90; S 30: 90; S 31: 90; S 32: 90; S 33: 90; S 34: 90; S 36: 90; S 37: 90; S 38: 90; S 39: 90; S 40: 90/91; S 41: 90; S 42: 90/91

Soulié De Morant, George. 1994 Chinese Acupuncture – ST 1 (St 8): 360; ST 2 (St 7): 361; ST 3 (St 6): 361; ST 4 (St 1): 361; ST 5 (St 2): 362; ST 6 (St 3): 362; ST 7 (St 4) 363; ST 8 (St 5): 363; ST 9: 363/364; ST 10: 364; ST 11: 365; ST 12: 365; ST 13: 366; ST 14: 366; ST 15: 367; ST 16: 367; ST 18: 368 ST 19: 368/369; ST 20: 369; ST 21: 369; ST 22: 370; ST 23: 370; ST 24: 371; ST 25: 371; ST 26: 372; ST 27: 372; ST 28: 373; ST 29: 373; ST 30: 374; ST 31: 374; ST 32: 375; ST 33: 375; ST 34: 376; ST 35: 376; ST 37: 378; ST 38: 378; ST 39: 379; ST 40: 379; ST 41: 380; ST 42: 380; ST 43: 381; ST 44: 381; ST 45: 382

Eachou Chen 1995 Cross-sectional Anatomy of Acupoints – ST 3: 118; ST 11: 161; ST 13: 161/162; ST 32: 57; ST 36: 68; ST 37: 71/72; ST 38: 74; ST 39: 76; ST 40: 73; ST 42: 90; ST 43: 93

Huang-fu Mi. Trans: Yang Shou-zhong and Charles Chace 1993 The Systematic Classic of Acupuncture & Moxibustion – St 3: 146; St 4: 148; St 5: 148; St 6: 148; St 7: 149; St 11: 151; St 13: 157; St 14: 147; St 15: 147; St 16: 158; St 18: 158; St 19: 165; St 29: 167; St 31: 192; St 32: 192; St 41: 190; St 42: 190; St 45: 190

Worsley, J R 1982 Traditional Chinese Acupuncture Volume 1 – Meridians and Points. XI 1: 215; XI 2: 215; XI 3: 215; XI 6: 217; XI 10: 217; XI 11: 219; XI 19: 221; XI 20: 221; XI 21: 221; XI 22: 221; XI 23: 223; XI 24: 223; XI 25: 223; XI 26: 225; XI 27: 225; XI 28: 225; XI 29: 225; XI 30: 225; Thigh ACI measurements: 12; XI 31: 225; XI 32: 227; XI 33: 227; XI 34: 227; XI 42: 231

Legge, David 1999 Acupuncture Points and Meridians – St 7: 29; St 12: 30; St 14: 30; St 15: 30; St 16: 30; St 18: 30; St 30: 31; St32: 32; St 33: 32; St 34: 32; St 36: 32; St 37: 32; St 38: 32; St 39: 32; St 40: 33; St 42: 33; St 44: 33

Lotan, Alon 2000 Acupoint Location Guide – St 7: 35; St 12: 39; St 13: 39; St 32: 45; St 33: 45; St 34: 45; St 36: 47; St 37: 47; St 38: 47; St 39: 47; St 40: 47; St 42: 49; St 43: 49; St 44: 49

Lavier, Dr. J 1974 Points of Chinese Acupuncture – ST 9: 63; ST 10: 63; ST 19: 51; ST 20: 51; ST 21: 51; ST 22: 51; ST 23: 51; ST 24: 51; ST 25: 51; ST 26: 53; ST 27: 53; ST 28: 53; ST 29: 53; ST 30: 53; ST 31: 25; ST 32: 25; ST 33: 25; ST 34: 25; ST 42: 43

Masayoshi Hyodo 1975 Ryodoraku Acupuncture – ST 9: 67; ST 10: 67; ST 31: 64; ST 42: 65

Katsusuke Serizawa 1983 Tsubo – Vital Points for Oriental Therapy – ST 9: 135; ST 11: 147; ST 19: 67

So, James Tin Yau (Dr) 1985 The Book of Acupuncture Points: ST 9: 215; ST 11: 216; ST 32: 220; ST 42: 152; ST 44: 152

Shanghai College of Traditional Chinese Medicine. 1993 Applied Anatomical Charts of Acupuncture and Moxibustion – ST 13: 26; ST 14: 26; ST 15: 26; ST 16: 26; ST 17: 28; ST 18: 28; ST 30: 32; ST 31: 34; ST 32: 220; ST 39: 38; ST 42: 40

Academy of Traditional Chinese Medicine, The. 1975 – Outline of Chinese Acupuncture, An. St 14: 112; St 15: 113; St 16: 113; St 17: 113; St 31: 115; St 32: 116; St 37: 117; St 38; 117; St 42: 119; St 44: 120

Shandong Medical College and Shandong College of Traditional Chinese Medicine 1982 Anatomical Atlas of Chinese Acupuncture Points – Daying (St 5): 15; Jiache (St 6): 15; Xiaguan (St 7): 15; Renying (St 9): 16; Qihu (St 13): 16; Qichong (St 30): 17; Biguan (St 31): 17; Femur-Futu (St 32): 17; Yinshi (St 33): 17; Liangqiu (St 34): 17; Zusanli (St 36): 17; Tiaokou (St 38): 18; Xiajuxu (St 39): 18; Chongyang (St 42): 18

Shanghai College of Traditional Medicine 1981 Acupuncture – A Comprehensive Text – S 31: 268; S 32: 269; S 38: 315; S 39: 315; S 42: 315; S 43: 315

Cheng Xinnong (Editor) 1987 Chinese Acupuncture and Moxibustion – S 31: 144; S 32: 145; S 42: 147

Jayasuriya, Anton 1982 Clinical Acupuncture – St 31: 391; St 32: 391; St 42: 391; St 44: 391

Qiu Mao-Liang 1996 – Chinese Acupuncture and Moxibustion – ST 32: 80/81; ST 42: 83

Deadman, Peter; Al-Khafaji, Mazin; Baker, Kevin 1998 Manual of Acupuncture, An – ST 32: 155; ST 38: 163; ST 42: 169; ST 43: 170

Li Ding (Prof.). 1991. Acupuncture, Meridian Theory and Acupuncture Points – St 32: 199; St 42: 206

Ellis, Wiseman and Boss. 1991 Fundamentals of Chinese Acupuncture – ST 32: 130; ST 37:134; ST 38: 134; ST 42: 137; ST 45 (Classical Location): 139

Low, Royston. 1988 The Non-Meridial Points of Acupuncture – St 42:

Lawson – Wood 1973 Acupuncture Handbook – XI 40: 50; XI 41: 26; XI 42: 42

Yang Jiasan (Prof) 1982 The Way to Locate Acu-Points – St 42: 37

McMinn, R M H and Hutchings, R T. 1977 Colour Atlas of Human Anatomy, A. – Dorsalis Pedis Artery: 322

THE SPLEEN CHANNEL OF THE FOOT (TAI YIN)

Primary Channel

The Spleen channel begins at a superficial level at Sp 1 on the medial aspect of the first digit, runs up the medial aspects of the foot and leg, and enters the lower abdomen at Sp 12/13, where the channel crosses to Ren 3 and Ren 4. The channel continues to Sp 14/15, entering the spleen and pancreas and connecting with the stomach above Ren 10.

One deep branch travels from the stomach (at Ren 10) through the diaphragm and onwards to the heart, to link with the Heart Channel. The main branch goes to Sp 16, then ascends through the diaphragm (passing GB 24 and Liv 14) and chest to end at Sp 21.

From Sp 20 a deep channel passes centrally across the chest, past Lu 1 and through the neck and oesophagus to the root of the tongue, where it radiates around the back of the tongue and sublingual areas.

Divergent Channel

Leaving the primary channel on the thigh, this converges with the Divergent channel of the Stomach and passes up to the throat, then enters the tongue.

Connecting Channel

This leaves the primary channel at Sp 4 on the medial aspect of the foot and connects with the Stomach channel. A branch ascends to the abdomen to connect with the stomach and intestines.

Muscle Channel

This originates on the medial side of the first digit and ascends the foot to bind with the medial malleolus. It passes up to bind with the medial aspect of the knee, then traverses the medial aspect of the thigh to bind with the hip and join the reproductive organs. It crosses the abdomen, binds with the umbilicus, enters the abdominal cavity, binds with the ribs and finally disperses through the chest. An internal branch binds to the spine.

THE SPLEEN CHANNEL OF THE FOOT

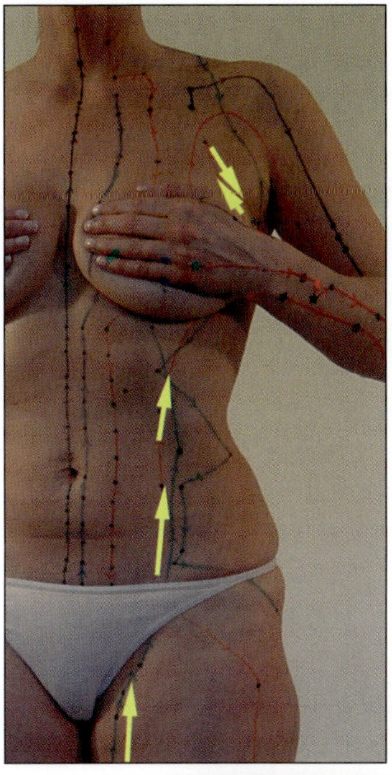

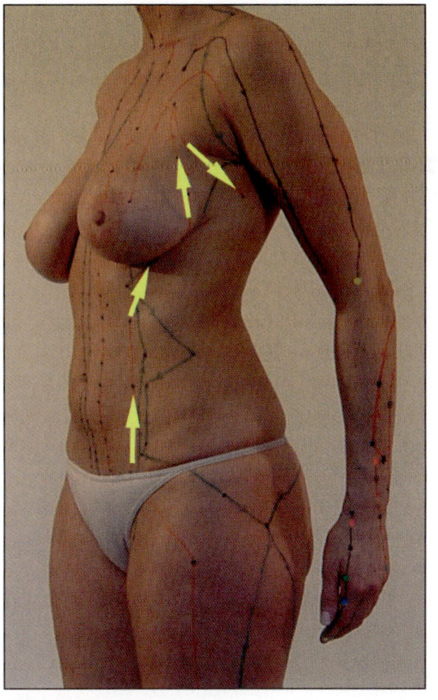

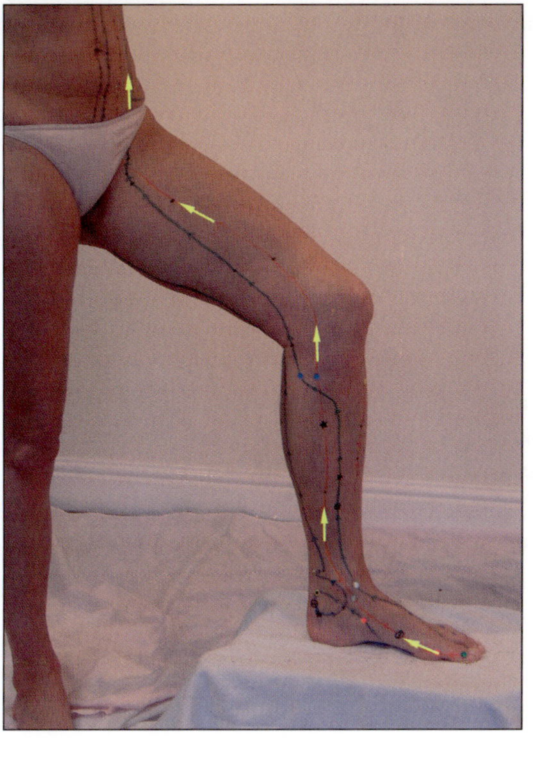

Points of the Spleen Channel – Foot Tai Yin (Sp/SP/XII)

Sp 1-2 are on the medial aspect of the first digit, Sp 3-4 on the medial border of the foot, Sp 5 on the medial aspect of the flexure of the ankle.

Sp 1 YIN BAI – RETIRED WHITE

⊥ ***0.1 TO 0.2 CUN*** Δ ***3 TO 5***

- WOOD
- ENTRY
- JING – WELL/Shu – Transporting/Antique
- RE-UNION/Crossing/Meeting Point of the Spleen Channel with the Stomach Channel – Foot Tai Yin Channel with the Foot Yang Ming Channel
- SUN SI-MIAO GHOST (Gui) – Ghost Point Name: Gui Lei – Ghost Fortress, Ghost Pile or Ghost Eye

Pos: Position of patient: supine.

Loc:
a) On the foot.
b) On the dorsal aspect of the first digit (big toe).
c) The medial nail point of the first digit.
d) Approximately 0.1 cun proximal to the corner of the nail.
e) Just distal to the flare of the distal phalanx.

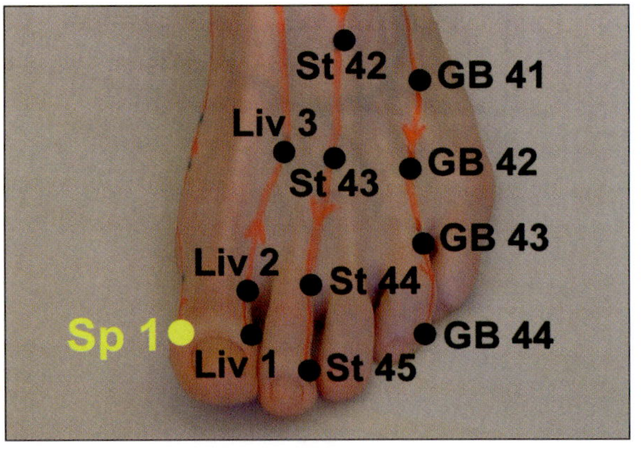

Tip:
a) The point is level with the nail bed (where the nail attaches to the skin) rather than the cuticle.
b) Draw a horizontal line across the nail bed.
c) Draw a vertical line from the medial border of the nail towards the nail bed.
d) The lines drawn from b) and c) (vertical and horizontal) form an intersection. This is approximately where the point is located.
e) This point may lie approximately halfway between the corner of the nail and the interphalangeal joint (the joint between the distal and proximal phalanges of the big toe).

Note: Ellis (1991) – the classical location for SP 1 is on the inner side of the big toe, the width of a Chinese leek leaf from the corner of the nail (The Great Compendium). Huang (1993) locates Sp 1 at the tip of the medial aspect of the big toe, the distance of a Chinese leek leaf from the corner of the nail.

Sp 2 DA DU – GREAT CAPITAL

⊥ ***0.1 TO 0.3 CUN*** Δ ***3 TO 5***

- FIRE
- TONIFICATION/Reinforcing
- MOTHER
- YING – SPRING/Shu – Transporting/Antique

Pos: Position of patient: supine.

Loc: a) On the medial surface of the foot.
b) On the medial surface of the first digit (big toe).
c) Distal to the first metatarsophalangeal joint.
d) Just distal to the flare of the base of the first proximal phalanx.
e) Approximately at the junction of the change in skin colour.

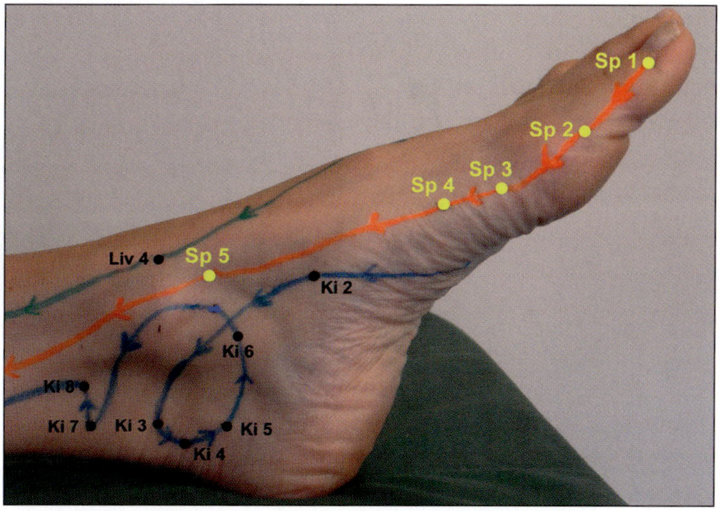

Tip: a) Sp 2 is on the bone (first proximal phalanx) of the big toe.
b) Place your finger on Sp 1 (the nail point) and run your finger along the Spleen channel towards the first metatarsophalangeal joint (knuckle of the big toe).
c) As you are running your finger towards the first metatarsophalangeal joint the channel begins to flow towards the medial surface of the first digit and you should be able to feel the contour of the first proximal phalanx bone begin to flare.
d) The point should be palpated with your finger just distal to the flare of the base of the first proximal phalanx. Sometimes the point can be located on the most medial aspect of the toe or just inferior to the flare of the base of the proximal phalanx.
e) The point will be on the medial surface of the first digit and often at the junction of the change in skin colour.

Note: Traditionally this point is distal and inferior to the flare of the base of the first proximal phalanx.

Sp 3 TAI BAI – SUPREME WHITE

⊥ ***0.3 CUN*** Δ ***3 TO 5***

- SOURCE/Yuan/Regulator/Primary
- EARTH
- HORARY from 9 a.m. to 11 a.m.
- SEASONAL HORARY – Late Summer
- SHU – STREAM/Shu – Transporting/Antique
- HOST/GUEST COMBINATION – Source Point with the Junction Point of its Paired Official/Organ Therefore Sp 3 is combined with St 40

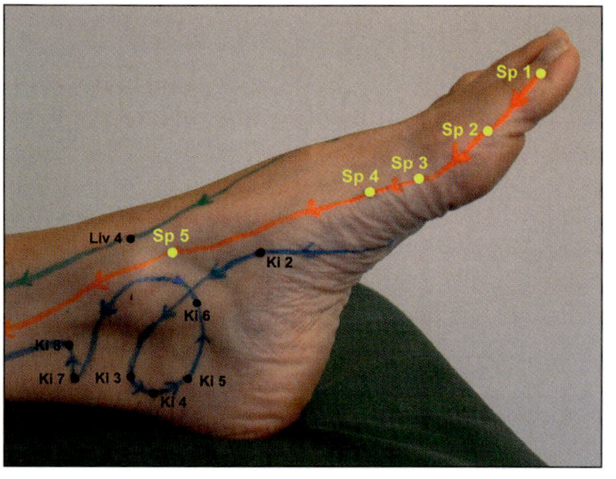

Pos: Position of patient: supine.

Loc: a) On the medial surface of the foot.
b) Proximal to the first metatarsophalangeal joint.
c) Proximal and inferior to the flare of the head of the first metatarsal bone.

Tip: a) Place your finger on Sp 1 (the nail point) and run your finger along the Spleen channel towards the first metatarsophalangeal joint (knuckle of the big toe).
b) Run your finger with the flow of the channel towards the first metatarsophalangeal joint where the channel begins to flow towards the medial surface of the first digit. You should be able to feel the contour of the first proximal phalanx where it begins to flare.
c) Run your finger over the first metatarsophalangeal joint until you are proximal to the flare of the joint (which is proximal to the head of the first metatarsal bone).
d) Just proximal to the flare of the head of the first metatarsal bone on the medial surface of the foot, the channel runs inferior to the head of the first metatarsal bone, sometimes at the junction of the change in skin colour.
e) The point should be palpated just proximal and inferior to the flare of the head of the first metatarsal bone.

Note: Traditionally at the junction of the change in skin colour. Lotan (2000) locates Sp 3 inferior and proximal to the 1st metatarsal bone head; proximal and inferior to the metatarsophalangeal joint; between the abductor hallucis tendon and the bone.

Sp 4 GONG SUN – PRINCE'S GRANDSON / GRANDFATHER GRANDSON

⊥ ***0.3 CUN*** Δ ***3***

- JUNCTION/Luo/Connecting/Passage/Lo/Lê
- 8 EXTRAORDINARY CHANNELS CONFLUENT/8 Extraordinary Meridians Confluent/8 Extraordinary Vessels Opening/Master Point of the Penetrating Vessel (Chong Mai)
- 8 EXTRAORDINARY VESSEL/Coupled Point of the Yin Linking Vessel (Yin Wei Mai)
- RE-UNION/Crossing/Meeting Point of the Spleen Channel with the Stomach Channel – Foot Tai Yin Channel with the Foot Yang Ming Channel
- HOST/GUEST COMBINATION – Source Point with the Junction Point of its Paired Official/Organ Therefore Sp 4 is combined with St 42

Pos: Position of patient: supine.

Loc: a) On the medial surface of the foot.
b) Distal and inferior to the base of the first metatarsal bone.
c) Just distal to the flare of the base of the first metatarsal bone.
d) Approximately 1 cun proximal to Sp 3.

Tip: a) Run your finger with the flow of the channel from the medial nail point of the big toe over the medial surface of the first metatarsophalangeal joint until you are proximal to the flare of the joint (which is proximal to the head of the first metatarsal bone).
b) The channel runs inferior from the head to the base of the first metatarsal bone before flowing over and on to bone again.
c) To locate the point palpate from the flare of the head of the first metatarsal bone along the medial surface of the foot just inferior to the first metatarsal bone towards the flare of the base of the first metatarsal bone.
d) The point should be palpated just proximal and inferior to the flare of the head of the first metatarsal bone, sometimes at the junction of the change in skin colour.
e) The point is not always at 1 cun therefore the anatomy should always take precedence over the cun measurement.
f) A common mistake is to locate the point in the joint formed by the base of the first metatarsal bone and the distal border of the medial cuneiform bone. If you are in this joint you have palpated past the flare of the metatarsal bone.
g) As the flare of the base of the first metatarsal bone is sometimes hard to locate, it can be easier to locate the joint formed by the base of the first metatarsal bone and the distal border of the medial cuneiform bone.
h) Palpate along the channel on the medial surface of the foot and feel the anatomy running distal to the joint, this will reduce the possibility of locating the point too proximal and in the joint.

Note: Traditionally at the junction of the change in skin colour. Soulié (1994) locates SP 4 on the foot: medial edge (medially facing the other foot), mid-length; in the inferior angle between the foint of the first metatarsal and the first cuneiform bone; in a hollow; two FW (Finger Width) posterior and lateral to SP 3; two large FW ahead of SP 5; two large FW medial to ST 42. Lotan (2000) locates Sp 4 inferior to the 1st metatarsal bone, distal to the bone base; on the borderline between the sole skin and pigmented skin; about 1.2 cun proximal to Sp 3; between the abductor hallucis tendon and the bone.

Sp 5 SHANG QIU – MERCHANT MOUND

⊥ ***0.3 CUN*** Δ ***3 TO 7***

- METAL
- SEDATION/Reducing/Dispersing
- CHILD
- JING – RIVER/Shu – Transporting/Antique
- RE-UNION/Crossing/Meeting Point of the Veins

Pos: Position of patient: supine.

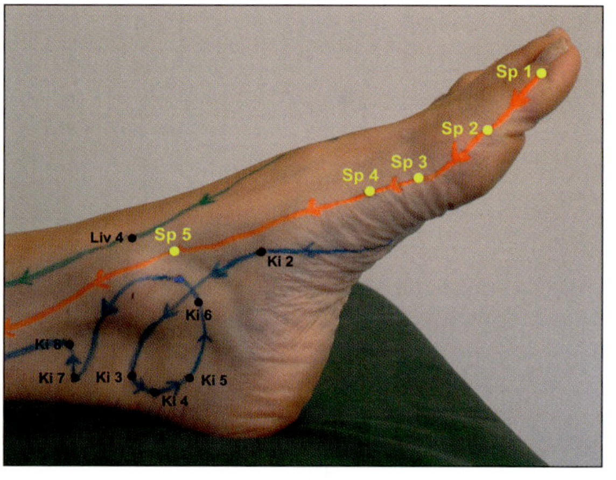

Loc: a) On the medial aspect of the ankle.
b) Anterior and inferior to the medial malleolus bone.
c) Medial to the tendon of the tibialis anterior muscle.

Tip: a) The point lies in the deepest part of the hollow formed by the medial malleolus bone and the medial border of the tendon of the tibilais anterior muscle.
b) Dorsiflex and invert the foot to demonstrate the tendon of the tibialis anterior muscle which in turn exposes the hollow where the point is located.
c) If you were to have the foot in a relaxed position and to place your two index fingers anterior and inferior to the lateral and medial malleoli and wiggle the foot from side to side, your fingers should fall in to two hollows. Your fingers would look like a bolt going straight through from one side to the other. The two points in these hollows are Sp 5 (medial surface hollow) and GB 40 (lateral surface hollow).
d) The point is located at the intersection of lines drawn from the anterior and inferior borders of the medial malleolus.

Note: Traditionally the point is located midway between the tuberosity of the navicular bone and the prominence of the medial malleolus. Voisin (1974) locates Sp 5 on the dorsum of the foot, 1.5 fb (finger breadth) distal and slightly below the medial malleolus, against the medial border of the tendon of the extensor hallucis longus. Wu (1973) locates SP 5 in front and above the medial malleolus, between two tendons.

Soulié (1994) locates SP 5 on the foot, medial edge, one small FW (Finger Width) in front of the medial malleolus, in the angle between the posterior edge of one transverse bone (scaphoid) and the bone under the malleolus of the talus; in a hollow; under the tendon of the tibialis anterior; two large FW above and behind SP 4; five FW under SP 6; one large FW medial to ST 41; separated by the tibia and malleolus from KI 4.

Lawson-Wood (1973) locates XII 5 about 4cm below and in front of the internal malleolus, in the hollow between the navicular and cuneiform. Lotan (2000) locates Sp 5 in the depression, level with the medial malleolus inferior border, vertically inferior to the medial malleolus anterior border; midway between the navicular tuberosity and the medial malleolus peak.

Lotan also has an alternate location for Sp 5 (which is the same as the main location above): in the depression, level with the medial malleolus inferior border, posterior to the tibialis anterior; 0.5 cun anterior to the meeting of two imaginary lines: the vertical line anterior to the medial malleolus and the horizontal line, inferior to the same malleolus.

Cun Measurements of the Medial Aspect of the Leg

The distance from the prominence of the medial malleolus to the popliteal crease on the medial side of the knee flexure is measured as 15 cun. This must be measured with the patient in a supine position with the leg flat. This method may seem more user friendly than using the 13 cun measurement as it should be easier to divide the 15 cun measurement in to 3 sections of 5 and then to divide the 5 in to 1 cun measurements.

The distance from the prominence of the medial malleolus to the inferior border of the medial condyle of the tibia bone (Sp 9) is measured as 13 cun. This must be measured with the patient in a seated position with the knee bent at 90 degrees. The difficulty of measuring 13 cun is not just dividing 13 cun in to equal 1 cun measurements but to accurately mark the inferior border of the medial condyle of the tibia where Sp 9 is located can be difficult.

Note: There are approximately 2 cun between the inferior border of the medial condyle of the tibia and the popliteal crease on the medial flexure of the knee, If you were to measure 13 cun in the supine position and measure 2 cun to the popliteal crease of the medial flexure of the knee, the 2 cun measurement would seem greater compared when locating the cun measurments in the seated position.

Sp 6-9 are on the medial aspect of the lower leg.

Sp 6 SAN YIN JIAO – THREE YIN CROSSING

⊥ *0.3 TO 0.5 CUN* Δ *3 TO 10*
ALWAYS FORBIDDEN TO NEEDLE AND MOXA THIS POINT IN PREGNANCY

- RE-UNION/Crossing/Meeting Point of the Three Yin (Leg) Channels: Spleen, Kidney and Liver – Foot Tai Yin, Foot Shao Yin and Foot Jue Yin Channels

Pos: Position of patient: supine (at 15 cun), or in a seated position with the leg bent at 90 degrees (at 13 cun).

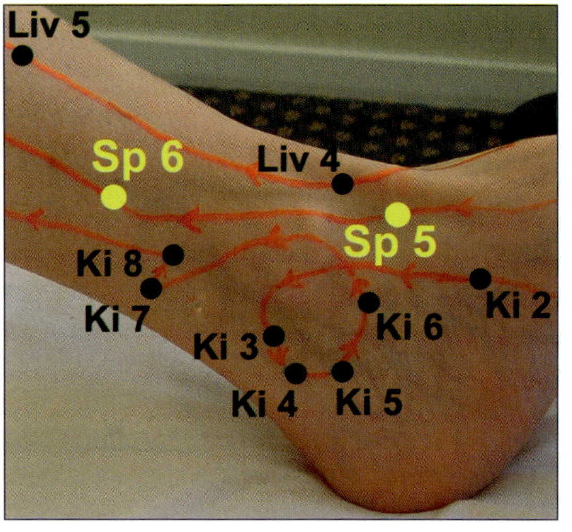

Loc: a) On the lower leg.
b) On the medial aspect of the lower leg.
c) On the posterior border of the medial aspect of the tibia bone.
d) Between the tibia bone and the soleus muscle.
e) 3 cun proximal to the prominence of the medial malleolus.

Cun: a) The distance from the prominence of the medial malleolus (ankle) bone to the popliteal crease on the medial side of the knee flexure is measured as 15 cun.
b) 15 cun is measured with the patient in a supine position with the leg flat.
c) This method may seem more user friendly than using the 13 cun measurement as it should be easier to divide 15 cun in to 3 sections of 5 and then to divide the 5 in to 1 cun measurements.
d) 13 cun is measured with the patient's leg bent at 90 degrees. It is measured from the prominence of the medial malleolus to the inferior border of the medial condyle of the tibia bone, please refer to Sp 9 cun measurements sections c) to g).

Tip: a) Place a rolled towel under the knee so that the leg is slightly bent but supported. This will ensure that the soleus and gastrocnemius muscles falls away from the tibia bone, and identify the medial border of the tibia bone.
b) When locating this point it is important to make sure that you are not on the bone as the posterior border of the medial aspect of the tibia curves slightly.
c) Run the flat of your finger along the posterior border of the medial aspect of the tibia bone from the flexure of the ankle at Sp 5 towards the knee crease (popliteal crease).
d) Palpation will reveal the accurate location of this point which is approximately 3 cun proximal to the medial malleolus.

Note: Historically there have been various cun locations for Sp 6. Wu (1973) locates SP 6 at 4 pouce, behind the tibia. Lavier (1974) in an illustration measures SP 6 at 4 pouce. His pouce measurement for the medial aspect of the leg is 15 pouce from the tip of the internal malleolus to the popliteal crease. From his illustration it looks like it is at the inferior edge of the medial malleolus and not at the prominence of it.

Soulié (1994) locates SP 6 on the medial surface of the lower leg: four FW (Finger Width) below the bone of the ankle (medial malleolus); just on the lateral edge of the narrow relief of the posterior side; in a hollow; on the inferior edge of a bulge; at the level of the top of the relief, mid-width; five FW above SP 5; two large FW below SP 7; one FW ahead and above KI 8; three FW above and a little posterior to LR 5. Worsley (1982) locates XII 6 on the medial surface of the leg, 4 ACI (Anatomical Chinese Inch) proximal to the prominence of the medial malleolus, posterior to the edge of the tibia.

Lavier and Worsley both place the Spleen and Liver channels together at the same location on the posterior border of the medial aspect of the tibia. An explanation for this could be that the Liver and Spleen channels flow to the surface at their points and therefore they do not flow into each other, instead they only share the same anatomical features.

Sp 7 LOU GU – LEAKY VALLEY

⊥ ***0.3 TO 0.5 CUN*** **Δ 3**

Pos: Position of patient: supine (at 15 cun), or in a seated position with the leg bent at 90 degrees (at 13 cun).

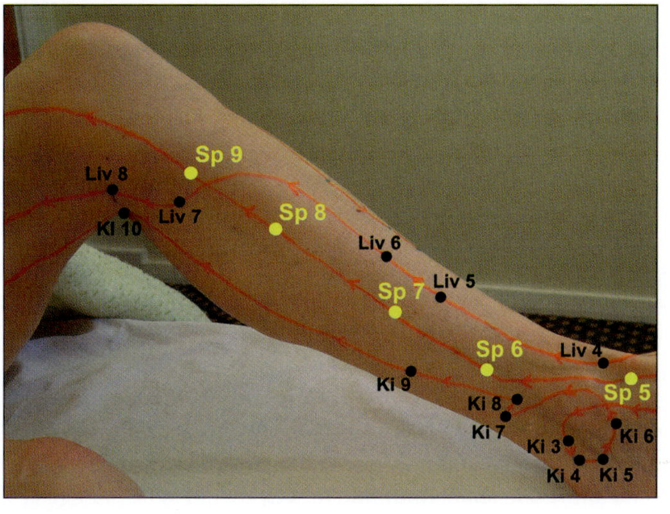

Loc: a) On the lower leg.
b) On the medial aspect of the lower leg.
c) On the posterior border of the medial aspect of the tibia.
d) Between the tibia bone and the soleus muscle.
e) 6 cun proximal to the prominence of the medial malleolus.
f) 3 cun superior to Sp 6

Cun: a) The distance from the prominence of the medial malleolus (ankle) bone to the popliteal crease on the medial side of the knee flexure is measured as 15 cun.
b) 15 cun is measured with the patient in a supine position with the leg flat.
c) This method may seem more user friendly than using the 13 cun measurement as it should be easier to divide 15 cun in to 3 sections of 5 and then to divide the 5 in to 1 cun measurements.
d) 13 cun is measured with the patient's leg bent at 90 degrees. It is measured from the prominence of the medial malleolus to the inferior border of the medial condyle of the tibia bone, please refer to Sp 9 cun measurements sections c) to g).

Tip: a) Place a rolled towel under the knee so that the leg is slightly bent but supported. This will ensure that the soleus and gastrocnemius muscles falls away from the tibia bone, and identify the medial border of the tibia bone.
b) When locating this point it is important to make sure that you are not on the bone as the posterior border of the medial aspect of the tibia curves slightly.
c) Run the flat of your finger along the posterior border of the medial aspect of the tibia bone from the flexure of the ankle at Sp 5 towards the knee crease (popliteal crease).
d) As the tibia curves slightly, Sp 7 is approximately one finger width posterior to the posterior border of the tibia.
e) Palpation will reveal the accurate location of this point which is approximately 6 cun proximal to the medial malleolus.

Note: Historically there have been various cun locations for Sp 7. Wu (1973) locates SP 7 upon the medial surface of the leg behind the tibia, at 7 pouce and behind the tibia. Lavier (1974) in an illustration locates SP 7 at 7 pouce. Soulié (1994) locates SP 7 on the medial lower leg; seven FW (Finger width) above the medial malleolus; on the tibia; just on the lateral edge of the narrow relief of the posterior side; on the inferior edge of a bulge; two large FW above SP 6; two FW under SP 8; one FW posterior and a little above LR 6; two FW above and anterior to KI 9.

Lavier's pouce measurement for the medial aspect of the leg is measured as 15 pouce from the tip of the internal malleolus to the popliteal crease. From his illustration it looks like it is at the inferior edge of the medial malleolus and not at the prominence of it. Worsley (1982) locates XII 7 on the medial surface of the leg, 7 ACI (Anatomical Chinese Inch) proximal to the prominence of the medial malleolus, posterior to the edge of the tibia.

Lavier and Worsley both place the Spleen and Liver channels together at the same location, on the posterior border of the medial aspect of the tibia. An explanation for this could be that the Liver and Spleen channels flow to the surface at their points and therefore they do not flow into each other, they only share the same anatomical features instead. Legge (1999) locates the point at 6 cun above the tip of the medial malleolus and also inferior to the belly of the gastrocnemius.

Shanghai (1993) locates SP 7 on the middle part of the medial side of the leg, 6 cun above the medial malleolus, at the junction of the anterior third and middle third between the medial border of the tibia and the posterior midline of the leg.

Sp 8 DI JI – EARTH MOTIVATOR

⊥ ***0.3 TO 0.5 CUN*** Δ ***3 TO 7***

- ACCUMULATION/Xi Cleft/Gueki

Pos: Position of patient: supine (at 15 cun), or in a seated position with the leg bent at 90 degrees (at 13 cun).

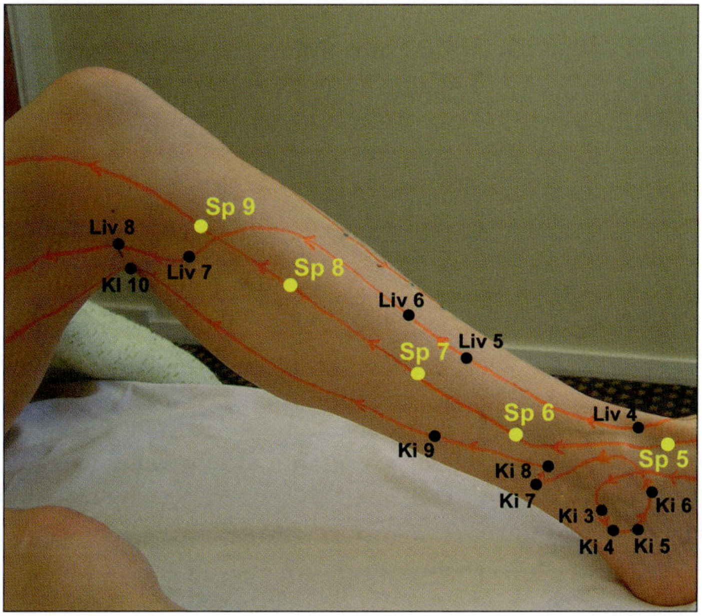

Loc:
a) On the lower leg.
b) On the medial aspect of the lower leg.
c) On the posterior border of the medial aspect of the tibia.
d) Between the tibia bone and the soleus muscle.
e) 10 cun proximal to the prominence of the medial malleolus.
f) 3 cun distal to Sp 9.
g) 4 cun proximal to Sp 7.

Cun:
a) The distance from the prominence of the medial malleolus to the popliteal crease on the medial side of the knee flexure is measured as 15 cun.
b) 15 cun is measured with the patient in a supine position with the leg flat.
c) This method may seem more user friendly than using the 13 cun measurement as it should be easier to divide 15 cun in to 3 sections of 5 and then to divide the 5 in to 1 cun measurements.
d) 13 cun is measured with the patient's leg bent at 90 degrees. It is measured from the prominence of the medial malleolus to the inferior border of the medial condyle of the tibia, please refer to Sp 9 cun measurements sections c) to g).

Tip: a) Place a rolled towel under the knee so that the leg is slightly bent but supported. This will ensure that the soleus and gastrocnemius muscles falls away from the tibia, and identify the medial border of the tibia.

b) When locating this point it is important to make sure that you are not on the bone as the posterior border of the medial aspect of the tibia curves slightly.

c) Run the flat of your finger along the posterior border of the medial aspect of the tibia from the flexure of the ankle at Sp 5 towards the popliteal crease.

d) As the tibia curves slightly, Sp 8 is approximately one finger width posterior to the posterior border of the tibia.

e) Palpation will reveal the accurate location of this point which is approximately 10 cun proximal to the medial malleolus.

Note: Historically there have been various cun locations for Sp 8. Wu (1973) locates SP 8 upon the internal surface of the leg at 6 pouce below the articular flexure of the knee, and 9 pouce above the medial malleolus. Lavier (1974) illustrates Sp 9 at 9 pouce. Lavier (1974), the pouce measurement for the medial aspect of the leg is measured as 15 pouce from the tip of the internal malleolus to the popliteal crease. From his illustration it looks like it is at the inferior edge of the medial malleolus and not at the prominence of it.

Worsley (1982) locates XII 8 on the medial surface of the leg, 9 ACI (Anatomical Chinese Inch) proximal to the prominence of the medial malleolus, posterior to the edge of the tibia. Lavier and Worsley both place the Spleen and Liver channels together at the same location on the posterior border of the medial aspect of the tibia. An explanation for this could be that the Liver and Spleen channels flow to the surface at their points and therefore they do not flow into each other, they only share the same anatomical features instead.

Voisin (1974) locates Sp 8 on the posterior border of the tibia, 4 fb (finger breadth) below the tibial plateau. Soulié (1994) locates SP 8 on the medial face of the lower leg, three FW (Finger Width) under the head of the tibia, on the tibia at the posterior edge; in the angle between the inferior posterior edge of the tibia and the inferior edge of the transverse bulge; at the level of a notch it the bone; in a hollow; two FW above SP 7.

Shanghai (1993) locates SP 8 on the medial side of the tibia, between the posterior border of the tibia and the soleus muscle, 5 cun below the medial side of the knee, 3 cun below SP 9 and 4 cun above SP 7. Legge (1999) locates Sp 8 at 3 cun below Yinlingquan (Sp9), about a finger's breadth posterior to the border of the tibia.

Sp 9 YIN LING QUAN – YIN MOUND SPRING

⊥ ***0.5 TO 0.8 CUN*** **Δ 3**

- WATER
- HE – SEA/Shu – Transporting/Antique
- COUSIN in association with GB 34

Pos: Position of patient: supine with the leg slightly flexed (at 15 cun), or in a seated position with the leg bent at 90 degrees (at 13 cun).

Loc:
a) On the lower leg.
b) On the medial aspect of the lower leg.
c) On the posterior border of the medial aspect of the tibia.
d) On the inferior border of the medial condyle of the tibia.
e) Between the tibia bone and the gastrocnemius muscle.
f) Level with the tuberosity of the tibia bone and GB 34 (see separate description).
g) 13 cun proximal to the prominence of the medial malleolus.

Cun:
a) In the supine position, the distance from the prominence of the medial malleolus to the popliteal crease on the medial side of the knee flexure is measured as 15 cun.
b) 15 cun is measured with the patient in a supine position with the leg flat.
c) This method may seem more user friendly than using the 13 cun measurement as it should be easier to divide 15 cun in to 3 sections of 5 and then to divide the 5 in to 1 cun measurements.
d) 13 cun is measured with the patient's leg bent at 90 degrees. It is measured from the prominence of the medial malleolus to the inferior border of the medial condyle of the tibia, so it is important that Sp 9 is accurately located.
e) Sp 9 is used as a landmark when locating the Spleen, Liver and Kidney channel points.
f) 13 cun can be split in to equal cun measurements by using the width of 4 fingers held close together which measures 3 cun. You will need the patient's own fingers to give guidance as to the width used as their fingers may be a different size than your own. The measurement for the width of the fingers are taken from the joint that is formed by the proximal and intermediate (middle) phalanges.
g) Once the width of the fingers is established, place one edge of your fingers on the prominence of the medial malleolus, then on the other edge of your finger draw a mark on the leg to give you 3 cun.
h) From the 3 cun mark to the inferior border of the medial condyle of the tibia at Sp 9 there are 10 cun, therefore it should be easier for you to divide 10 cun in half to give two 5 cun divisions, and then divide again in to 5 equal measurements to give 1 cun divisions.

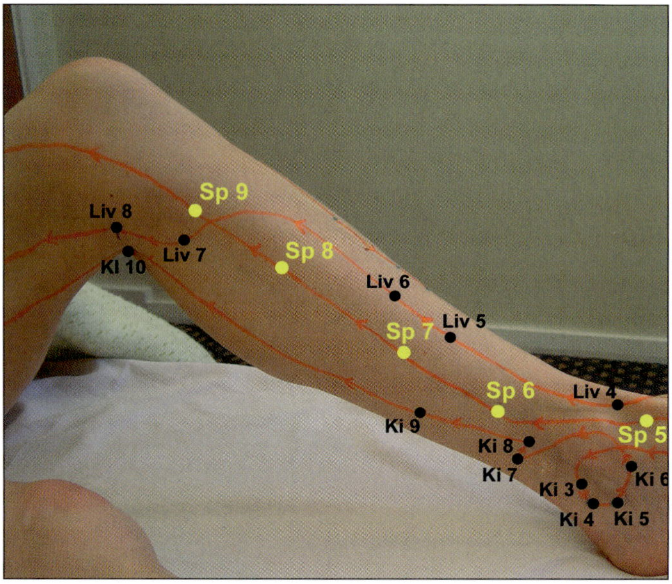

Tip:

a) Place a rolled towel under the knee so that the leg is slightly bent but supported. This will ensure that the soleus and gastrocnemius muscles falls away from the tibia, and identify the medial border of the tibia.

b) Run the flat of your finger from the flexure of the ankle towards the popliteal crease along the posterior border of the medial aspect of the tibia until your finger begins to curve with the contour of the bone. The bone contour changes when you are feeling the inferior border of the medial condyle of the tibia.

c) 13 cun is located at the level where the tibia begins to curve or flare at the tibial tubersosity.

d) The point can be accurately palpated between the inferior border of the medial condyle of the tibia and the gastrocnemius muscle. This will also give you a reference point for 13 cun.

e) Also as a guide, Sp 9 is approximately on a level with the anterior and inferior border of the fibula, where GB 34 is located. Imagine a bolt going through Sp 9, to meet GB 34 and vice versa.

Cun Measurements of the Upper Leg

The distance from a line drawn transversely between the gluteal groove and the medial root of the lower limb (at the level of the lower border of the pubic symphysis where the medial side of the upper leg joins the torso), to the medial popliteal crease (flexure of the knee) is 14 cun.

The distance between the popliteal crease (flexure of the knee) to the superior border of the greater trochanter of the femur, when the leg is abducted, is measured as 19 cun. There seems to be great discrepancies with other descriptions of the anatomy that have used the 19 cun measurement, eg. 19 cun from the popliteal crease to the superior and inferior borders of the pubic symphysis and 19 cun from the popliteal crease to the prominence or inferior border of the greater trochanter of the femur.

<u>14 cun is the accepted bone proportional measurement of the thigh.</u>

Sp 10 XUE HAI – SEA OF BLOOD

⊥ ***0.3 TO 0.5 CUN*** Δ ***3 TO 10***

Pos: Position of patient; supine.

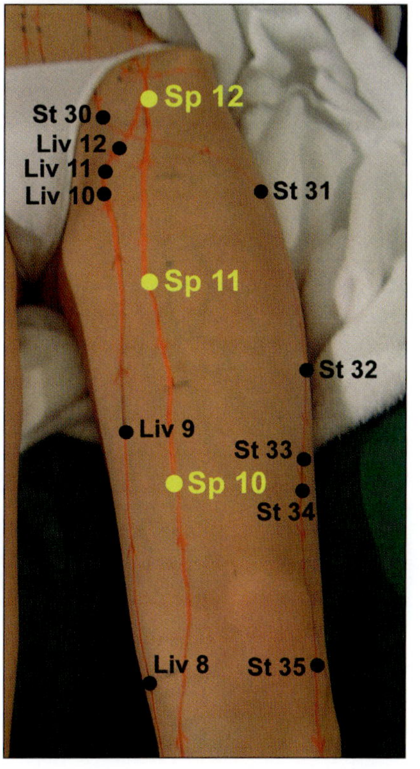

Loc:
a) On the medial aspect of the upper thigh.
b) On the vastus medialis muscle (which is one of the four quadriceps muscles).
c) On the prominence of the vastus medialis muscle (in the centre) when the foot is flexed.
d) 4 cun proximal to the medial popliteal crease (flexure of the knee).

Tip:
a) Mark out the level of the inferior border of the symphysis pubis bone (where the medial side of the upper leg joins the torso) and the medial popliteal crease (flexure of the knee).
b) There are 14 cun between these two marks.
c) Flex and extend the knee to expose the vastus medialis muscle. Once you have identified the muscle make sure you locate the point with the patient's leg is relaxed.
d) The point is located on the prominence of the vastus medialis muscle approximately 4 cun proximal to the medial popliteal crease (flexure of the knee).
e) There are four ways of checking the cun measurements: see f), g), h) and i).
f) Mark out 14 cun proximal to the medial popliteal crease, as explained in a) and b) and mark 4 cun proximal to the popliteal crease.
g) The longitudinal measurement of the patella is 2 cun, therefore double this to give 4 cun. Use this measurement from the popliteal crease or the inferior border of the patella bone to get the approximate location on the prominence of the vastus medialis muscle.
h) With the knee flexed place the heel of your hand on the inferior border of the patella so the middle part of your palm encases or cups the patella. Depending on which leg you are marking, you should always have your thumb placed on the medial side of the leg on the prominence of the vastus medialis muscle. Make sure your index finger and thumb are at an angle of 45 degrees from each other. The point should lie approximately at the tip of your thumb.
i) Use the following method if you don't want to mark out 14 cun from the inferior border of the symphysis pubis to the medial popliteal crease. The superior border of the patella to the inferior border of the symphysis pubis measures 12 cun, which

can be divided in to equal cun measurements by using the width of 4 fingers held close together which measures 3 cun. You will need the patient's own fingers to give guidance as to the width used as their fingers may be a different size than your own. The measurement for the width of the fingers are taken from the joint that is formed by the proximal and intermediate (middle) phalanges.

j) Sp 10 is palpated with the flow of the channel from the inferior border of the medial condyle of the tibia (Sp 9) to the vastus medialis (at 4 cun proximal to the popliteal crease).

Note: Traditionally, the location for Sp 10 is 2 cun superior to the superior medial corner of the patella on the bulge of the vastus medialis muscle. Worsley (1982) locates XII 10 on the anterior surface of the thigh, 3 ACI (Anatomical Chinese Inch) proximal to the flexure of the knee, in the middle of the belly of the vastus medialis muscle. Wu (1973) locates SP 10 at the antero-medial surface of the thigh, at 3 pouce above the articular flexure of the knee, posterior to the sartorius. Lavier (1974) illustrates the total longitudinal measurement of the thigh to be 13 pouce, with SP 10 at 3 pouce proximal to the flexure of the knee. Voisin (1974) locates Sp 10 on the thigh, medial aspect, at 3 fb (finger breadth) above the posterior border of the medial femoral condyle, and on the posterior border of the sartorius.

Soulié (1994) locates SP 10 on the medial face of the superior part of the knee; slightly above the angle between the posterior edge of the femur and the large inferior head (medial condyle); in the superior part of the hollow; in the angle of the femur and the lower edge of an oblique muscle (vastus medialis); seven large FW above SP 9; two large FW below SP 11. Worsley (1982) Wu (1973) and Lavier (1974) use 13 ACI/pouce from the medial extremity of the knee crease to the medial extremity of the groin or the great trochanter.

Shandong (1982) locate xuehai at 2 cun above the antero-superior border of the patella, when the knee is flexed.

Lotan (2000) locates Sp 10 with the leg flexed, in the depression, 2 cun proximal to the patella medial-superior corner; The depression can be felt in the corner of the bulge that is formed when the knee is flexed; Medial to the vastus medialis midline.

Sp 11 JI MEN – BASKET GATE

⊥ ***0.3 TO 0.5 CUN*** Δ ***3***

Pos: Position of patient: supine.

Loc: a) On the medial aspect of the upper thigh.
b) In a groove between the medial border of the sartorius muscle and the gracilis muscle.
c) 10 cun proximal to the medial popliteal crease (flexure of the knee).
d) 6 cun proximal to Sp 10.
e) On a line drawn from Sp 10 to Sp 12.

Tip: a) Mark out the level of the inferior border of the symphysis pubis bone (where the medial side of the upper leg joins the torso) and the medial popliteal crease (flexure of the knee).
b) There are 14 cun between these two marks.
c) Mark out 10 cun proximal to the medial popliteal crease.
d) Sp 10 is at 4 cun proximal to the medial popliteal crease (see Sp 10 tips f) to i)). Double 4 cun to give you 8 cun, then take the longitudinal length of the patella which is 2 cun and add this length on to the 8 cun to get 10 cun.
e) One other way of marking the cun is to use 6 cun proximal to Sp 10.
f) An easier method of locating this point is to run your finger from Sp 10 (on the prominence of the vastus medialis muscle) towards the groin, at 10 cun you should eventually feel a seam between the sartorius muscle and the gracilis muscle.
g) Note that on some people this point may be between the sartorius muscle and vastus medialis muscle depending on the anatomy of the sartorius muscle at the level of 10 cun proximal to the medial popliteal crease, therefore palpation is of utmost importance.

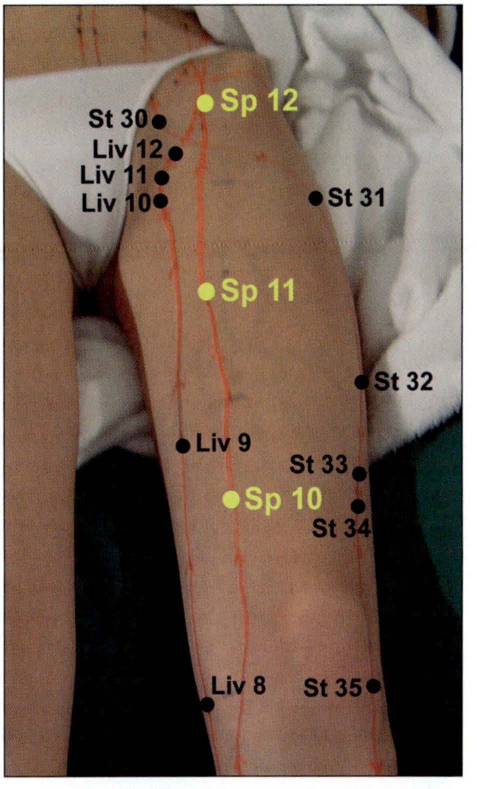

Note: There are schools that locate Sp 11 at approximately the same level (10 cun), but at the medial/posterior/anterior aspect of the sartorius muscle. The traditional location simply locates Sp 11 on a line drawn from Sp 10 to Sp 12 without using any anatomy, therefore palpation is of utmost importance when locating this point. Lavier (1974) illustrates Sp 11 to be at 8 pouce and at the medial aspect of the sartorius muscle, with 13 pouce measured between the greater trochanter of the femur and the popliteal crease of the knee. Worsley (1982) locates XII 11 on the anterior surface of the thigh, 9 ACI (Anatomical Chinese Inch) proximal to the flexure of the knee, on the anterior border of the sartorius.

Voisin (1974) locates Sp 11 on the medial aspect of the thigh, 5 fb (finger breadths) above the preceding point (Sp 10). Wu (1973) locates SP 11 on the medial surface of the thigh, posterior to the sartorius and at the start of the abductor brevis, upon the femoral artery (no measurement is given here). Soulié (1994) locates SP 11 on the medial thigh, about mid-width: three FW (Finger Width) above the protruberance of the lower head of the femur (medial condyle); in the angle between the posterior edge of the tibia and the lower edge of the transverse mass; in a hollow; between the bone and the semimembranosus muscle; two large FW above SP 10; one FW above and posterior to LR 9.

Eachou (1995) and Shanghai (1981) locates SP 11 medial to the sartorius muscle, 6 inches/units above SP 10. Masayoshi (1975) locates SP 11 at the inner side of the front of the thigh at the intersection of the rectus femoris and sartorius muscles. Worsley (1982) Wu (1973) and Lavier (1974) use 13 ACI/pouce from the medial extremity of the knee crease to the medial extremity of the groin or the greater trochanter. Shandong (1982) locate Jimen at 6 cun above Pt. Xuehai (Sp 10). Legge (1999) locates Sp 11 ay 6 cun above Sp 10, on the line drawn from Sp 10 to Sp 12, on the anterior border of the sartorius.

The transverse measurement for the middle and lower abdomen (middle and lower jiao) is calculated as 2 cun, between the anterior median line (at the centre of the umbilicus) and the lateral border of the rectus abdominis muscle (St 25).

The lateral border of the rectus abdominis muscle is not the actual edge of the muscle but the most prominent surface of the muscle before it begins to 'slope' in to the torso. By visualising the corner of an inverted 'L', the point is located on the antero-lateral edge of the muscle. To locate this muscle ask the patient to slightly raise their head. The lateral border of the rectus abdominis muscle is on the most lateral part of the palpable curve which is more medial than the actual edge of the muscle.

The transverse cun measurements for the middle and lower abdomen (middle and lower jiao) includes the Kidney, Stomach, Spleen, Gall Bladder and Liver channels (lateral to the anterior median line) as follows:

Ki 11 to Ki 21 = 0.5 cun
St 19 to St 30 = 2 cun
Sp 13 to Sp 16 = 6 cun (Sp 12 = 3.5 cun)
GB 24 = 4 cun
Liv 14 = 4 cun

Ki 16, St 25 and Sp 15 are all transversely level with the centre of the umbilicus and are used as reference points for marking the respective channel cun measurements.

The longitudinal measurements of the anterior torso are:

9 cun from the xiphisternal joint to the suprasternal fossa (measuring approximately 1.6 cun in the lower chest intercostal spaces, and 1 cun in the upper chest intercostal spaces)

8 cun from the centre of the umbilicus to the xiphisternal joint
For the descriptions relating to the channels in the middle jiao, the longitudinal cun measurements are given from the centre of the umbilicus superiorly or from the xiphisternal joint inferiorly, depending on the direction of the flow of the channel.

5 cun from the centre of the umbilicus to the superior border of the symphysis pubis bone.

For the descriptions relating to the channels in the lower jiao, the longitudinal cun measurements are given from the centre of the umbilicus inferiorly or from the superior border of the symphysis pubis bone superiorly, depending on the direction of the flow of the channel.

Note: The mid and lower abdomen (middle and lower jiao) transverse distances between the anterior median line (Ren Mai/Conception Vessel) and the Kidney channel, and the anterior median line (Ren Mai/Conception Vessel) and the Stomach channel have varied markedly in Acupuncture literature. The Stomach channel is given as 2/2.5/3 cun from the anterior median line (Ren Mai/Conception Vessel) in different texts. The currently accepted measurement is 2 cun from the anterior median line to the Stomach channel, which is the space between the centre of the umbilicus and the lateral border of the rectus abdominis muscle.

Sp 12-Sp 21 are on the anterior torso. (Sp 12-Sp 14 in the lower jiao, Sp 15 and Sp 16 in the middle jiao, Sp 17-Sp 21 in the upper jiao.)

Sp 12 CHONG MEN – RUSHING GATE

⊥ ***0.5 TO 0.7 CUN*** ***Δ 5***
FORBIDDEN TO NEEDLE AND MOXA THIS POINT DURING PREGNANCY

- 8 EXTRAORDINARY VESSEL/Coalescent Point of Yin Linking Vessel (Yin Wei Mai) – see note
- RE-UNION/Crossing/Meeting Point of the Spleen Channel with the Liver Channel and the Yin Linking Vessel – Foot Tai Yin Channel with the Foot Jue Yin Channel and the Yin Wei Mai

Pos: Position of patient: supine.

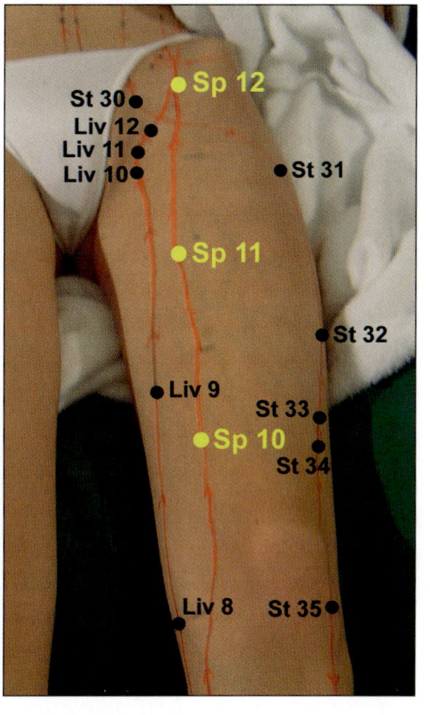

Loc: a) On the anterior torso.
b) On the lower abdomen (lower jiao)
c) Level with the superior border of the symphysis pubis bone (at Ren 2).
d) On the lateral edge of the femoral artery.
e) Superior to the lateral end of the inguinal groove.
f) 3.5 cun lateral to the anterior median line.

Cun: a) The transverse measurement for the middle and lower abdomen (middle and lower jiao) is 2 cun between the anterior median line (at the centre of the umbilicus) and the lateral border of the rectus abdominis muscle (at St 25). You will need to double this cun measurement to give you 4 cun lateral to the anterior median line, and then to palpate approximately 0.5 cun medially to give the cun measurement for Sp 12 (at the level of Ren 2).

b) The lateral border of the rectus abdominis muscle is not the actual edge of the muscle bu the most prominent surface of the muscle before it begins to 'slope' in to the torso. By visualising the corner of an inverted 'L', the Stomach channel is located on the antero-lateral edge of the muscle. To locate this muscle ask the patient to slightly raise their head. The lateral border of the rectus abdominis muscle is on the most lateral part of the palpable curve which is more medial than the actual edge of the muscle. Once the antomy has been identified to give the Stomach channel, double this measurement to give 4 cun lateral to the anterior median line, the Spleen channel. At the level of Ren 2 (just superior to the superior border of the symphysis pubis) palpate approximately 0.5 cun medial to 4 cun , this should locate Sp 12.

c) Another way to mark out the transverse cun measurements at the level of the umbilicus is to locate the medial border of the anterior superior iliac spine (part of the iliac crest). To locate the 4 cun line of the Spleen channel, place a pen longitudinally on the medial border of the anterior superior iliac spine approximately halfway between the centre of the umbilicus and the superior border of the symphysis pubis bone. The edge of the rectus abdominis muscle is measured as 4 cun. Once established divide 4 cun into other cun divisions for use on the Stomach and Kidney channels etc.

d) The transverse cun measurements for the middle and lower abdomen (middle and lower jiao) includes the Kidney, Stomach, Spleen, Gall Bladder and Liver channels (lateral to the anterior median line): Ki 11 to Ki 21 = 0.5 cun; St 19 to St 30 = 2 cun; Sp 12 = 3.5 cun; Sp 13 to Sp 16 = 4 cun; GB 24 = 4 cun; Liv 14 = 4 cun.

e) The longitudinal measurement of the lower abdomen is 5 cun from the centre of the umbilicus to the superior border of the symphysis pubis bone.

Tip: a) First locate the superior border of the symphysis pubis bone and draw in a transverse line from the anterior median line.

b) Then palpate for the femoral artery on the transverse line.

c) Palpation for the point on the lateral edge of the femoral artery should be approximately 3.5 cun lateral to the anterior median line. Anatomy takes precedence over the cun measurement for this point. Sp 12 is definately not on the artery.

d) If preferred mark out 3.5 cun then use the cun guidelines section above.

Note: Historically this point has been given as 3/3.5/4/4.5 cun lateral to the anterior median line. Worsley (1982) locates XII 12 on the flexure of the groin, 4 ACI (Anatomical Chinese Inch) lateral to the anterior median line and 4 ACI inferior to the level of the umbilicus, on a level with XIII 3 (Ren 3). Voisin (1974) locates Sp 12 in the inguinal flexion fold, midway between the anterior superior iliac spine and the pubic symphysis.
Masayoshi (1975) locates Sp 12 directly above the central part of the inguinal ligament where you can feel the pulsation of the femoral artery.

Wu (1973) locates SP 12 upon the crease of the groin, at four and one half pouce from the anterior median line. Lavier (1974) in an illustration locates this point on the inguinal fold and at four and one half pouce lateral to the anterior median line "VC" (Ren Line). Soulié (1994) locates SP 12 on the groin: mid-distance from the apparent extremity of the pubis to the inferior point of the crest of the hip (anterior superior iliac spine); on the lower edge of the deep oblique rise (iliac bone); in a hollow in the triangle between the medial edge of the iliac muscle on an angle towards the hip (causes the leg to lift and cross) and the lateral edge of the muscle (greater psoas) passing above the iliac bone (and inserted on the lumbar vertebae); deep is the pectineus muscle; in the angle between the psoas and the iliac bone; three large FW (Finger Width) under SP 13; two large FW lateral to ST 30.

Shandong (1982) locate Chongmen at 3.5 cun lateral to the symphysis pubis, on the lateral side of the a. femoralis. Legge (1999) locates Sp 12 at 3.5 cun lateral to the midpoint of the upper border of the symphysis pubis. The pulse of the femoral artery can be felt just medial to the point.

Note: In some texts Sp 12 is listed as an 8 EXTRAORDINARY VESSEL/Coalescent Point of Yin Wei Mai (Yin Linking Vessel), whereas in others it is omitted.

Sp 13 FU SHE – OFFICIAL RESIDENCE

⊥ ***0.5 TO 0.7 CUN*** Δ ***5 TO 10***
FORBIDDEN TO NEEDLE AND MOXA THIS POINT DURING PREGNANCY

- 8 EXTRAORDINARY VESSEL/Coalescent Point of Yin Wei Mai (Yin Linking Vessel)
- RE-UNION/Crossing/Meeting Point of the Spleen Channel with the Liver Channel and the Yin Linking Vessel – Foot Tai Yin Channel with the Foot Jue Yin Channel and the Yin Wei Mai

Pos: Position of patient: supine.

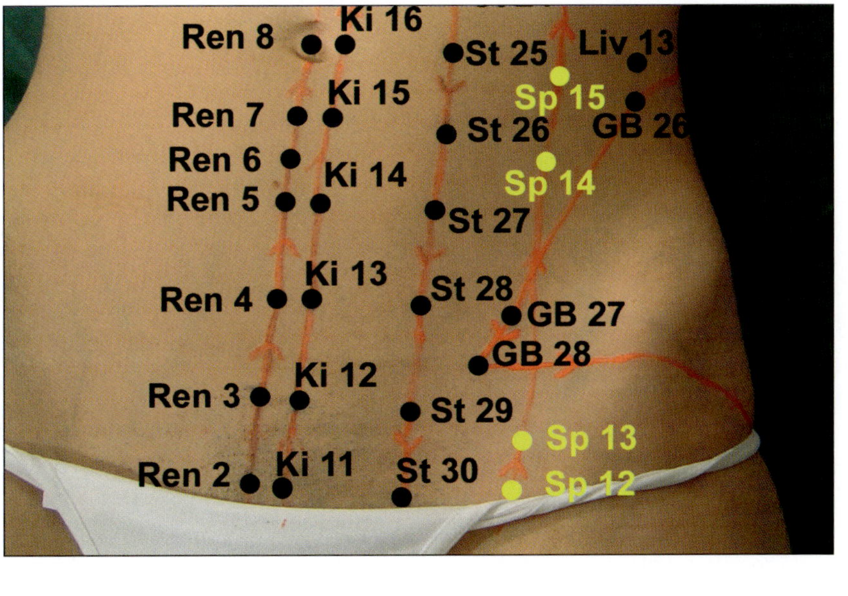

Loc:
a) On the anterior aspect of the torso.
b) On the lower abdomen (in the lower jiao).
c) On the lateral edge of the rectus abdominis muscle.
d) Superior to the inguinal ligament.
e) 4 cun lateral to the anterior median line.
f) 0.5 cun lateral to and 0.7 cun superior to Sp 12.
g) 0.7 cun superior to the superior border of the symphysis pubis bone (at Ren 2)
h) 4.3 cun inferior to the level of the centre of the umbilicus or Sp 15.
i) 3 cun inferior to Sp 14.

Cun:
a) The transverse measurement for the middle and lower abdomen (middle and lower jiao) is 2 cun between the anterior median line (at the centre of the umbilicus) and the lateral border of the rectus abdominis muscle (at St 25). You will need to double this cun measurement to give 4 cun lateral to the anterior median line for the Spleen channel.
b) The lateral border of the rectus abdominis muscle is not the actual edge of the muscle but the most prominent surface of the muscle before it begins to 'slope' in to the torso. By visualising the corner of an inverted 'L', the Stomach channel is located on the antero-lateral edge of the muscle. To locate this muscle ask the patient to slightly raise their head. The lateral border of the rectus abdominis muscle is on the most lateral part of the palpable curve which is more medial than the actual edge of the muscle. Once the anatomy has been identified to give the Stomach channel, double this measurement to give 4 cun lateral to the anterior median line, the Spleen channel.
c) Another way to mark out the transverse cun measurements at the level of the umbilicus is to locate the medial border of the anterior superior iliac spine (part of the iliac crest). To locate the 4 cun line of the Spleen channel, place a pen longitudinally on the medial border of the anterior superior iliac spine approximately halfway between the centre of the umbilicus and the superior border of the symphysis pubis bone. The edge of the rectus abdominis muscle is measured as 4 cun. Once established divide 4 cun into other cun divisions for use on the Stomach and Kidney channels etc.
d) The transverse cun measurements for the middle and lower abdomen (middle and lower jiao) includes the Kidney, Stomach, Spleen, Gall Bladder and Liver channels (lateral to the anterior median line): Ki 11 to Ki 21 = 0.5 cun; St 19 to St 30 = 2 cun; Sp 12 = 3.5 cun; Sp 13 to Sp 16 = 4 cun; GB 24 = 4 cun; Liv 14 = 4 cun.
e) The longitudinal measurement of the lower abdomen is 5 cun from the centre of the umbilicus to the superior border of the symphysis pubis bone.

Tip:
a) Locate 4 cun lateral to the anterior median line, transversely level to the centre of the umbilicus.
b) Mark out 5 equal cun longitudinal measurements on the anterior median line from the superior border of the symphysis pubis bone to the centre of the umbilicus.
c) If you cannot feel the superior border of the symphysis pubis bone, ask the patient to semi-flex their legs, this should soften the abdominal muscles enough in this area to allow palpation of the superior border of the symphysis pubis.

d) Locate Sp 12 by feeling for the superior border of the symphysis pubis bone (at Ren 2) and then palpate laterally until you are able to feel a pulse on the femoral artery. Sp 12 is on the lateral edge of this and just superior to the lateral end of the inguinal groove.
e) Approximately 0.7 cun superior to Sp 12 you should be able to feel a contour on the lower abdomen that takes you laterally from approximately 3.5 cun to 4 cun.
f) The longitudinal measurement for the lower abdomen provides a reference for the location of Sp 13 which is 0.7 cun superior to the superior border of the symphysis pubis bone.
g) The 5 cun longitudinal measurement for the lower abdomen can also be used for locating Sp 13 at 4.3 cun inferior to the level of the centre of the umbilicus (or Sp 15) as the point will be nearer to 4 cun than 5 cun. Note that if you were to palpate with your finger inferiorly from Sp 15 to locate this point you would be palpating against the flow of the Spleen channel. Try palpating from the groin with the flow of the channel to Sp 13 instead.
h) Palpation in this area should reveal the accurate location for this point.

Note: Sp 13 has been given different transverse distances lateral to the median line but current Chinese literature uses 4 cun for Sp 13-16, but there have been instances where the transverse measurement has been given at 3.5 cun because the abdomen can often narrow at this point. Sp 11-16 are also said to be on a vertical line directly below the nipple (i.e. at 4 cun), with the exception to Sp 13 (at 3.5 cun). Some acupuncture schools have used different transverse cun measurements at the level of the umbilicus: the Kidney channel has been located at 0.5 or 1.5 pouce/ACI, the Stomach channel at 2.5 or 3 pouce/ACI and the Spleen channel at 4 or 4.5 pouce/ACI. A few schools still do use these transverse measurements.

Shanghai (1981) locates Sp 13 at 3.5 cun lateral to the anterior median line. Voisin (1974) locates Sp 13 on the abdomen, at 1.5 fb (finger breadth) medially to and below the anterior superior iliac spine. (There are a few longitudinal differences for this point: Lavier (1974) illustrates Sp 13 at 1 pouce superior to the superior border of the symphysis pubis and has the point at 4.5 pouce lateral to the anterior median line "VC" (Ren line). Worsley (1982) locates XII 13 on the abdomen, 4 ACI (Anatomical Chinese Inch) lateral to the median line and 3 ACI inferior to the level of the umbilicus on a level with XIII 4 (Ren 4).

Soulié (1994) locates SP 13 on the inferior lateral abdomen: one half FW (Finger Width) in front of the lower point of the crest of the hip (anterior superior iliac spine) and from the insertion onto it of the sartorius muscle; on the external oblique muscle; above the deep prominence of the iliac bone; in a hollow; on the iliac muscle; three large FW above SP 12; three large FW under SP 14; one small FW lateral to ST 29. Yang (1982) locates Sp 13 at 1 cun above Sp 12. Wu (1973) locates SP 13 upon the abdomen, at four and one half pouce from the anterior median line , and at one pouce above SP 12. Shandong (1982) locate Fushe at 0.7 cun above Pt. Chongmen (Sp 12)

Sp 14 FU JIE – ABDOMEN KNOT

⊥ ***0.5 TO 0.7 CUN*** Δ ***5 TO 15***
FORBIDDEN TO NEEDLE AND MOXA THIS POINT DURING PREGNANCY

Pos: Position of patient: supine.

Loc: a) On the anterior aspect of the torso.
b) On the lower abdomen (in the lower jiao).
c) On the lateral edge of the rectus abdominis muscle.
d) 4 cun lateral to the anterior median line.
e) 3.7 cun superior to Sp 12.
f) 1.3 cun inferior to the level of the centre of the umbilicus or Sp 15 (which is 4 cun lateral to and level with the centre of the umbilicus).

Cun: a) The transverse measurement for the middle and lower abdomen (middle and lower jiao) is 2 cun between the anterior median line (at the centre of the umbilicus) and the lateral border of the rectus abdominis muscle (at St 25). You will need to double this cun measurement to give 4 cun lateral to the anterior median line for the Spleen channel.
b) The lateral border of the rectus abdominis muscle is not the actual edge of the muscle but the most prominent surface of the muscle before it begins to 'slope' in to the torso. By visualising the corner of an inverted 'L', the Stomach channel is located on the antero-lateral edge of the muscle. To locate this muscle ask the patient to slightly raise their head. The lateral border of the rectus abdominis muscle is on the most lateral part of the palpable curve which is more medial than the actual edge of the muscle. Once the anatomy has been identified to give the Stomach channel, double this measurement to give 4 cun lateral to the anterior median line, the Spleen channel.
c) Another way to mark out the transverse cun measurements at the level of the umbilicus is to locate the medial border of the anterior superior iliac spine (part of the iliac crest). To locate the 4 cun line of the Spleen channel, place a pen longitudinally on the medial border of the anterior superior iliac spine approximately halfway between the centre of the umbilicus and the superior border of the symphysis pubis bone. The edge of the rectus abdominis muscle is measured as 4 cun. Once established divide 4 cun into other cun divisions for use on the Stomach and Kidney channels etc.
d) The transverse cun measurements for the middle and lower abdomen (middle and lower jiao) includes the Kidney, Stomach, Spleen, Gall Bladder and Liver channels (lateral to the anterior median line): Ki 11 to Ki 21 = 0.5 cun; St 19 to St 30 = 2 cun; Sp 12 = 3.5 cun; Sp 13 to Sp 16 = 4 cun; GB 24 = 4 cun; Liv 14 = 4 cun.
e) The longitudinal measurement of the lower abdomen is 5 cun from the centre of the umbilicus to the superior border of the symphysis pubis bone.

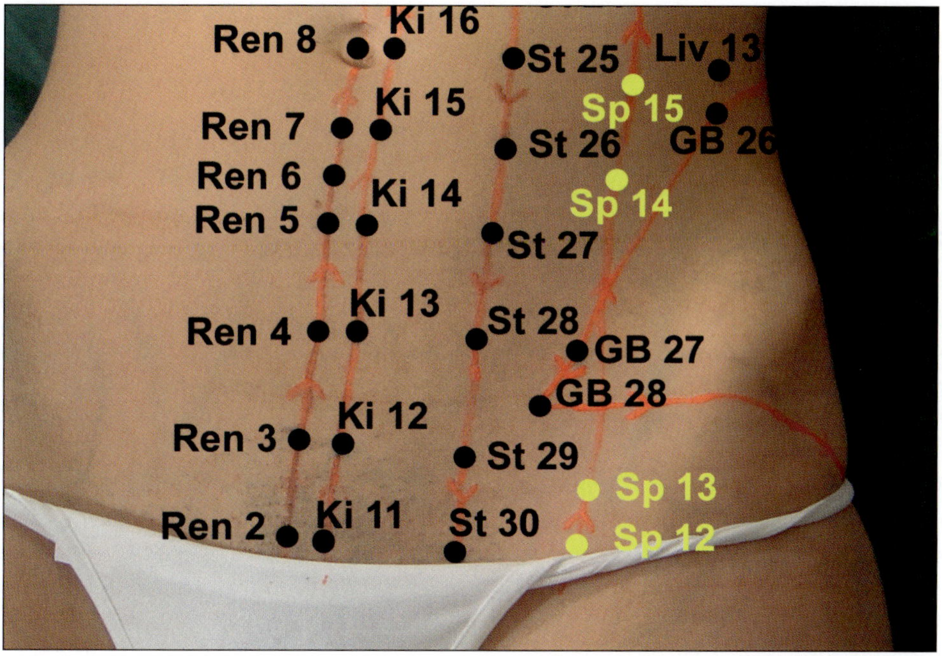

Tip: a) Locate 4 cun lateral to the anterior median line, transversely level to the centre of the umbilicus.

b) Mark out 5 equal cun longitudinal measurements on the anterior median line from the superior border of the symphysis pubis bone to the centre of the umbilicus.

c) If you cannot feel the superior border of the symphysis pubis bone, ask the patient to semi-flex their legs, this should soften the abdominal muscles enough in this area to allow palpation of the superior border of the symphysis pubis.

d) Palpate for Sp 14 between 3 and 4 cun superior to Sp 12 or between 1 and 2 cun inferior to the level of the centre of the umbilicus (Sp 15), 4 cun lateral to the anterior median line where the intersection of the transverse line meets the longitudinal line on the lower abdomen.

d) If using the 3 to 4 cun measurement superior to Sp 12 the location of the point will be nearer to the 4 cun mark than the 3 cun mark (3.7 cun superior to Sp 12).

e) If using the 1 to 2 cun measurement, inferior to the level of the umbilicus, Sp 14 will be located nearer to the 1 cun measurement than the 2 cun measurement (1.3 cun inferior to the level of the centre of the umbilicus or Sp 15). If palpating down the abdomen from the level of the centre of the umbilicus at Sp 15 this will be against the flow of the channel. Try palpating from the groin with the flow of the channel to Sp 14 instead.

f) Palpation in this cun area should reveal the accurate location for this point.

Note: Sp 14 has been given different transverse distances to the median line but current Chinese literature uses 4 cun for Sp 13-16. Sp 11-16 are also said to be on a vertical line directly below the nipple (i.e. at 4 cun), with the exception to Sp 13 (at 3.5 cun). Some acupuncture schools have used different transverse cun measurements at the level of the umbilicus: the Kidney channel has been located at 1.5 pouce/ACI, the Stomach channel at 2.5 or 3 pouce/ACI and the Spleen channel at 4 or 4.5 pouce/ACI. A few schools still do use these transverse measurements.

The longitudinal interspaces given above have been common throughout ancient Chinese texts but there are other measurements given too: Qiu (1993) locates Sp 14 ,3 cun above Sp 13 and 1.3 cun below Sp 15. Shanghai (1981) locates this point at 3 units above Sp 13 and 3.5 units lateral to the anterior median line. Soulié (1994) locates SP 14 on the lateral abdomen; a little anterior and under the anterior and superior angle of the crest of the hip; about mid-distance from the iliac bone and the free end of the eleventh rib. In a hollow of the oblique muscles; about at the level of two FW (Finger Width) under the umbilicus; three large FW above SP 13; two FW under SP 15; three large FW in front of GB 26; one large FW lateral to ST 26. Shanghai (1981) locates Sp 14 at 3.5 units lateral to the median line and 3 units above Sp 13.

Worsley (1982) locates XII 14 on the abdomen, 4 ACI (Anatomical Chinese Inch) lateral to the median line and 1 ACI inferior to the level of the umbilicus, on a level with XIII 7 (Ren 7). Lavier (1974) illustrates Sp 14 being either at 4 pouce superior to SP 12 or 1 pouce inferior to the level of the umbilicus and at 4.5 pouce lateral to the anterior median line VC (Ren line). Voisin (1974) locates Sp 14 on the abdomen, at 2 fb (finger breadth) medially to the anterior superior iliac spine. Wu (1973) locates SP 14 upon the abdomen at four and one half pouce from the anterior median line and at four pouce above SP 12.

Sp 15 DA HENG – GREAT HORIZONTAL

⊥ ***0.7 TO 1.0 CUN*** ***Δ 5 TO 10***
FORBIDDEN TO NEEDLE AND MOXA THIS POINT DURING PREGNANCY

- 8 EXTRAORDINARY VESSEL/Coalescent Point of Yin Linking Vessel (Yin Wei Mai)
- RE-UNION/Crossing/Meeting Point of the Spleen Channel with the Yin Linking Vessel – Foot Tai Yin Channel with the Yin Wei Mai

Pos: Position of patient: supine.

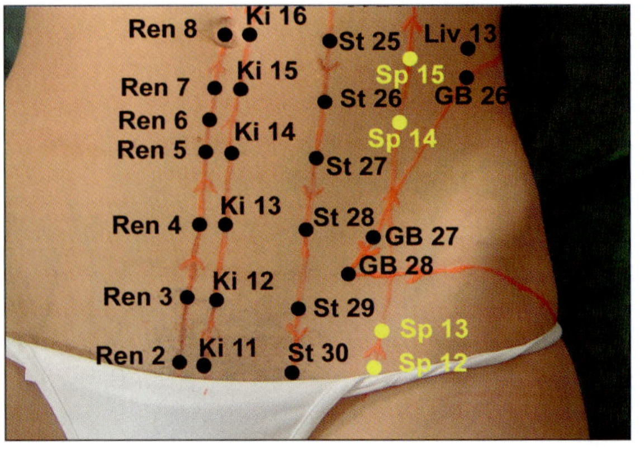

Loc:
a) On the anterior aspect of the torso.
b) In between the mid-abdomen and lower abdomen (in between the middle and lower jiao).
c) On the lateral edge of the rectus abdominis muscle.
d) 4 cun lateral to the anterior median line or 4 cun lateral to the level of the centre of the umbilicus and Ren 8.

Cun: a) The transverse measurement for the middle and lower abdomen (middle and lower jiao) is 2 cun between the anterior median line (at the centre of the umbilicus) and the lateral border of the rectus abdominis muscle (at St 25). You will need to double this cun measurement to give 4 cun lateral to the anterior median line for the Spleen channel.

b) The lateral border of the rectus abdominis muscle is not the actual edge of the muscle but the most prominent surface of the muscle before it begins to 'slope' in to the torso. By visualising the corner of an inverted 'L', the Stomach channel is located on the antero-lateral edge of the muscle. To locate this muscle ask the patient to slightly raise their head. The lateral border of the rectus abdominis muscle is on the most lateral part of the palpable curve which is more medial than the actual edge of the muscle. Once the anatomy has been identified to give you the Stomach channel, double this measurement to give 4 cun lateral to the anterior median line, the Spleen channel.

c) Another way to mark out the transverse cun measurements at the level of the umbilicus is to locate the medial border of the anterior superior iliac spine (part of the iliac crest). To locate the 4 cun line of the Spleen channel, place a pen longitudinally on the medial border of the anterior superior iliac spine approximately halfway between the centre of the umbilicus and the superior border of the symphysis pubis bone. The edge of the rectus abdominis muscle is measured as 4 cun. Once established divide 4 cun into other cun divisions for use on the Stomach and Kidney channels etc.

d) The transverse cun measurements for the middle and lower abdomen (middle and lower jiao) includes the Kidney, Stomach, Spleen, Gall Bladder and Liver channels (lateral to the anterior median line): Ki 11 to Ki 21 = 0.5 cun; St 19 to St 30 = 2 cun; Sp 12 = 3.5 cun; Sp 13 to Sp 16 = 4 cun; GB 24 = 4 cun; Liv 14 = 4 cun.

e) The longitudinal measurement of the lower abdomen is 5 cun from the centre of the umbilicus to the superior border of the symphysis pubis bone.

f) Ki 16, St 25 and Sp 15 are all transversely level with the centre of the umbilicus and used as reference points for marking their channels cun measurements.

g) The longitudinal measurement of the mid abdomen is 8 cun from the centre of the umbilicus to the xiphisternal joint (Ren 16). The longitudinal measurement of the lower abdomen is 5 cun from the superior border of the symphysis pubis bone to the centre of the umbilicus.

Tip: a) Locate 4 cun lateral to the anterior median line, level with the centre of the umbilicus.

b) This point is commonly marked too superiorly or inferiorly, therefore ensure that you are level with the centre of the umbilicus as

c) Palpation in the cun area should reveal the accurate location for the point. Try palpating laterally from the umbilicus to 4 cun and feel for the point.

d) Another method is to lightly place the flat of your finger along the direction of the channel and palpate from the superior border of the symphysis pubis towards the umbilicus until you are at the level of the centre of the umbilicus (at 4 cun lateral to the anterior median line).

Note: Sp 15 has been given different transverse distances to the median line but current Chinese literature uses 4 cun for Sp 13-16. Sp 11-16 are also said to be on a vertical line directly below the nipple (i.e. at 4 cun), with the exception to Sp 13 (at 3.5 cun). Some acupuncture schools have used different transverse cun measurements at the level of the umbilicus: the Kidney channel has been located at 1.5 pouce/ACI, the Stomach channel at 2.5 or 3 pouce/ACI and the Spleen channel at 4 or 4.5 pouce/ACI. A few schools still do use these transverse measurements.Shanghai (1981) locates Sp 15 at 3.5 units lateral to the navel. Soulié (1994) locates SP 15 on the lateral abdomen, at the waist, mid-distance between the iliac crest and the free end of the eleventh rib; at the level of the umbilicus; about at the vertical of the point of the hip; on the oblique and transverse muscles; one large FW (Finger Width) lateral to the rectus abdominus muscle; in a hollow; two FW above SP 14; four FW under SP 16; about two FW lateral to ST 25. Lavier (1974) on an illustration locates the point at 4.5 pouce lateral to the centre of the umbilicus. Wu (1973) locates SP 15 upon the abdomen, at four and one half pouce from the anterior median line above SP 12 and at the level of the umbilicus. Voisin (1974) locates Sp 15 on the abdomen; at 7 fb (finger breadth) lateral to the umbilicus.

Sp 16 FU AI – ABDOMEN SORROW

⊥ ***0.5 TO 0.7 CUN*** **Δ** ***5 TO 10***
FORBIDDEN TO NEEDLE AND MOXA THIS POINT DURING PREGNANCY

- 8 EXTRAORDINARY VESSEL/Coalescent Point of Yin Linking Vessel (Yin Wei Mai)
- RE-UNION/Crossing/Meeting Point of the Spleen Channel with the Yin Linking Vessel – Foot Tai Yin Channel with the Yin Wei Mai

Pos: Position of patient: supine.

Loc:
a) On the anterior aspect of the torso.
b) On the mid-abdomen (in the middle jiao).
c) On the lateral edge of the rectus abdominis muscle.
d) 4 cun lateral to the anterior median line.
e) 3 cun superior to Sp 15.
f) Level with Ren 11 (which is 3 cun superior to the level of the centre of the umbilicus).

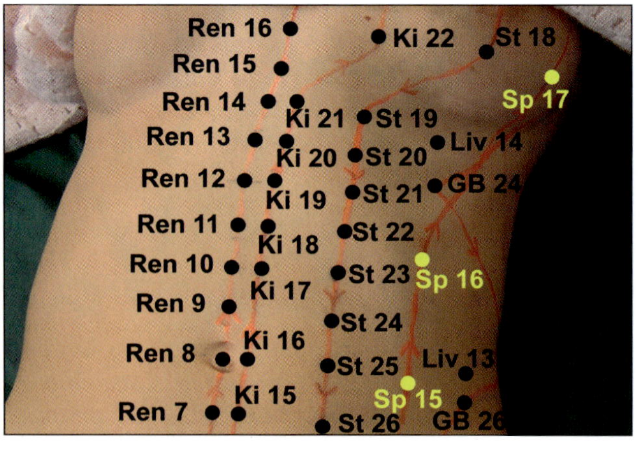

Cun: a) The transverse measurement for the middle and lower abdomen (middle and lower jiao) is 2 cun between the anterior median line (at the centre of the umbilicus) and the lateral border of the rectus abdominis muscle (at St 25). You will need to double this cun measuremento give you 4 cun lateral to the anterior median line for the Spleen channel.

b) The lateral border of the rectus abdominis muscle is not the actual edge of the muscle but the most prominent surface of the rectus abdominis muscle before it begins to 'slope' in to the torso, eg. the corner of an inverted 'L', just before you go on to the lateral aspect from the anterior surface. When the muscle is contracted by asking your patient to raise their head slightly, the muscle forms a curved ridge that can be palpated. The lateral border of the rectus abdominis muscle is on the most lateral part of the palpable curve which makes it more medial than the actual edge of the muscle. Once the anatomy has been identified to give you the Stomach channel, double this measurement to give 4 cun lateral to the anterior median line, the Spleen channel.

c) Another way to mark out the transverse cun measurements at the level of the umbilicus is to locate the medial border of the anterior superior iliac spine (part of the iliac crest). To locate the 4 cun line of the Spleen channel, place a pen longitudinally on the medial border of the anterior superior iliac spine approximately halfway between the centre of the umbilicus and the superior border of the symphysis pubis bone. The edge of the rectus abdominis muscle is measured as 4 cun. Once established divide 4 cun into other cun divisions for use on the Stomach and Kidney channels etc.

d) Often you can feel for the edge (not the border) of the rectus abdominis muscle by asking the patient to raise their head. The edge of the rectus abdominis muscle is measured as 4 cun. Once established divide up the 4 cun in to other cun measurements for use on the Stomach and Kidney channels etc.

e) The transverse cun measurements for the middle and lower abdomen (middle and lower jiao) includes the Kidney, Stomach, Spleen, Gall Bladder and Liver channels (lateral to the anterior median line): Ki 11 to Ki 21 = 0.5 cun; St 19 to St 30 = 2 cun; Sp 12 = 3.5 cun; Sp 13 to Sp 16 = 4 cun; GB 24 = 4 cun; Liv 14 = 4 cun.

f) Ki 16, St 25 and Sp 15 are all transversely level with the centre of the umbilicus and used as reference points for marking their channels cun measurements.

g) The longitudinal measurement of the mid abdomen is 8 cun from the centre of the umbilicus to the xiphisternal joint (Ren 16).

Tip:

a) Locate 4 cun level with the centre of the umbilicus and lateral to the anterior median line.

b) Mark out 8 cun longitudinal measurements.

c) Draw a transverse and longitudinal line. The two lines intersect at 4 cun lateral to the anterior median line, and at 3 cun superior to the centre of the umbilicus. This will give a ball park area where to palpate for the point.

d) The longitudinal measurement is level with Ren 11 (which is 3 cun superior to the centre of the umbilicus) or 3 cun directly superior to Sp 15.

e) Palpation in the cun area should reveal the accurate location for Sp 16. Palpate with the flow of the Spleen channel from the level of the umbilicus (at 4 cun lateral to the anterior median line) and feel for a depression at 3 cun superior to the level of the umbilicus.

f) Alternatively locate Sp 16 by palpating 4 cun laterally from Ren 11 to the lateral edge of the rectus abdominis muscle.

g) The point can be located on the edge of or medial to the rib cage.

Note: Sp 16 has been given different transverse distances to the median line but current Chinese literature uses 4 cun for Sp 13-16. Sp 11-16 are also said to be on a vertical line directly below the nipple (i.e. at 4 cun), with the exception to Sp 13 (at 3.5 cun). Some acupuncture schools have used different transverse cun measurements at the level of the umbilicus: the Kidney channel has been located at 1.5 pouce/ACI, the Stomach channel at 2.5 or 3 pouce/ACI and the Spleen channel at 4 or 4.5 pouce/ACI. A few schools still do use these transverse measurements.

Shanghai (1981) locates Sp 16 at 3 units above Sp 15 and 3.5 units lateral to the midsternal line. Worsley (1982) locates XII 16 on the abdomen, 4 ACI (Anatomical Chinese Inch) lateral to the median line. and 2.5 ACI superior to the level of the umbilicus, at a level half-way between XIII 10 (Ren 10) and XIII 11 (Ren 11), on the paramedian nipple line. Wu (1973) locates SP 16 upon the abdomen, at three pouce above Sp 15 which is also at four and one half pouce lateral to the anterior median line.

Voisin (1974) locates Sp 16 in the ninth intercostal space, and slightly medial to the anterior axillary line. Soulié (1994) locates SP 16 on the inferior lateral thorax between the ninth and tenth ribs, in the lateral angle of the anterior meeting of the ribs; on the inferior edge of the ninth rib; on the anterior edge of a vertical tendon; in a hollow; four FW (finger width) above SP 15; five FW under SP 17; four FW lateral to ST 23; two FW lateral to LR 13 (Liv 13). Lavier (1974) on an illustration locates the point at 4.5 pouce lateral to the anterior median line (VC) and almost level with VC 11 (Ren 11). So (1985) locates SP 16 at 4 divisions lateral to CV 11.

The distance between the anterior median line and the contour linking the mid-point of the clavicle with the centre of the nipple (on a man) is 4 cun. The Spleen channel (Sp 17 to Sp 20) lies at 6 cun lateral to the anterior median line.

The transverse measurement for the chest (upper jiao) is calculated as 8 cun from the anterior median line to the tip of the acromion process.

The transverse distance between the two nipples (on a man) is 8 cun. The distance between the bilateral Stomach channels at St 12 is also 8 cun, and can be used as a substitute measurement. (St 12 is just superior to the clavicle, in a palpable notch, at the mid-point of the supraclavicular fossa.)

The transverse cun measurements for the upper jiao (chest) which includes the Kidney, Stomach, Spleen and Lung channels (lateral to the anterior median line) are as follows:

Ki 22 to Ki 27 = 2 cun
St 13 to St 18 = 4 cun
Sp 17 to Sp 20 = 6 cun
Lu 1 to Lu 2 = 6 cun

The longitudinal measurements of the anterior torso are:

9 cun from the xiphisternal joint to the suprasternal fossa (with the space between 2 ribs measuring approximately 1.6 cun in the lower chest, and 1 cun in the upper chest)

8 cun from the centre of the umbilicus to the xiphisternal joint

For the descriptions relating to the channels in the middle jiao, the longitudinal cun measurements are given from the centre of the umbilicus superiorly or from the xiphisternal joint inferiorly, depending on the direction of the flow of the channel.

5 cun from the centre of the umbilicus to the superior border of the symphysis pubis.

For the descriptions relating to the channels in the lower jiao, the longitudinal cun measurements are given from the centre of the umbilicus inferiorly or from the superior border of the symphysis pubis superiorly, depending on the direction of the flow of the channel.

Sp 17 SHI DOU – FOOD DRAIN

⊥ ***0.3 TO 0.5 CUN*** ***Δ 5***

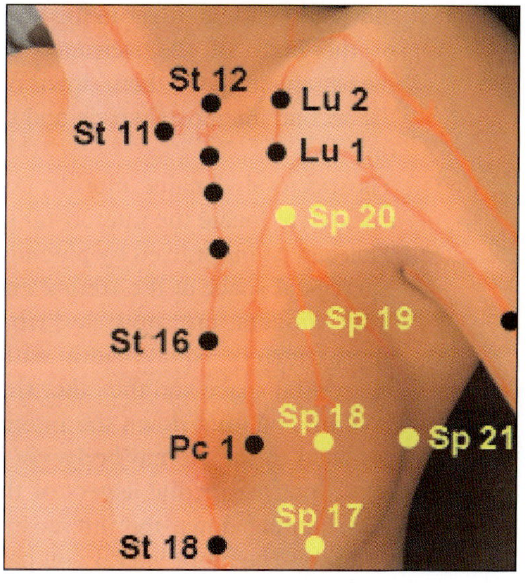

Pos: Position of patient: supine.

Loc:
a) On the anterior aspect of the torso.
b) On the chest (in the upper jiao).
c) In the fifth intercostal space.
d) 6 cun lateral to the anterior median line.
e) 2 cun lateral to the mamillary line.

Cun:
a) The transverse cun measurements for the chest (upper jiao) includes the Kidney, Stomach, Spleen and Lung channels (lateral to the anterior median line). The cun measurements are as follows: Ki 22 to Ki 27 = 2 cun; St 13 to St 18 = 4 cun; Sp 17 to Sp 20 = 6 cun and Lu 1 to Lu 2 = 6 cun.
b) The transverse measurement for the upper jiao is calculated using the anterior median line and the mid point of the clavicle bone.
c) Identify the mid point of the clavicle by locating the medial end of the clavicle at the sterno-clavicular joint and the lateral end of the acromioclavicular joint, and divide the distance by half.
d) The distance from the anterior median line to the mid point of the clavicle is 4 cun. From here divide again to give 2 cun spaces medial and lateral to 4 cun, therefore giving 2 and 6 cun measurements. The Spleen channel is 6 cun lateral to the anterior median line.
e) The transverse distance between the two nipples (on a man) is 8 cun, thus the distance from the anterior median line to the nipple is 4 cun.

Tip:
a) Locate 6 cun lateral to the anterior median line.
b) The Spleen channel follows the contours of the chest, and especially the curvature of the breast on a woman as it travels upwards towards the nipple. The more the person is 'flat chested' the lesser the curvature will be.

c) Place your finger between the fifth and sixth ribs (which is the fifth intercostal space) and palpate laterally to 6 cun. Your finger should be in the deepest part of the intercostal space. As you run your finger laterally the intercostal space begins to curve upwards. On women you may need to ask them to lift their breast (left breast, right hand; right breast, left hand) to access this point at 6 cun lateral to the anterior median line.

d) Palpation in this area should reveal the accurate location for Sp 17. As you are palpating laterally you will eventually feel costal cartilage on each rib. This may make it difficult to feel for the intercostal space, and many practitioners inadvertantly go in to the next intercostal space. Make sure the flat of your finger remains in the intercostal space between the ribs, to eliminate any errors.

e) If there are difficulties feeling for the fifth intercostal space then try feeling for the first and second intercostal spaces which are the easiest to palpate for. Place your index and middle finger in the first and second intercostal spaces on the lateral border of the body of the sternum, then with your two fingers staying at the same measurement move them down one intercostal space so that you have one finger in the second intercostal space and the other finger in the third intercostal space and so on.

f) The pectoralis major muscle covers the surface of the ribs which can make it difficult to locate the intercostal spaces from the third intercostal space downwards. This can be minimised by placing the first and second fingers in the first and second intercostal space at the sternal end of the ribs.

g) Your fingers are now a "rib space" apart. As the intercostal spaces are approximately equal width with each other, placing one finger in the second intercostal space and the other finger should fall into the third intercostal space . As you are counting down the intercostal spaces, the ribs inferior to the sternum are attached to the sternal body via bars of costal or hyaline cartilage. This cartilage opens out the medial aspect of the rib cage more laterally. This means that as you are counting down the intercostal spaces you will need to run your fingers more laterally. The more lateral you palpate the easier the intercostal spaces are to locate. As you palpate laterally from the sternum the intercostal spaces will curve upwards.

h) As a check the fourth intercostal space usually is at the level of the nipple (in a flat chested person).

i) Another way of identifying the intercostal spaces is to count them from the bottom of the rib cage upwards. For the 9th intercostal space (there are 9 intercostal spaces in total) palpate for the inferior border of the rib cage which will be the 10th rib. Place your finger in the intercostal space superior to this rib. You will now be in the 9th intercostal space.

j) When the 9th intercostal space has been established, place the flat of your index or middle finger in the 9th intercostal space and palpate for the 8th intercostal space by feeling for th superior border of the 9th rib. Once you have located the 9th rib, palpate superiorly until you feel a softness, which will be the 8th intercostal space. Use this procedure to palpate and locate the other intercostal spaces.

k) Sp 17 is located in the fifth intercostal space, 6 cun lateral to the anterior median line, or 2 cun lateral to the mamillary line.

l) Palpate laterally from the 5th intercostal space following the contour of the intercostal space until you can feel Sp 17 (at 6 cun lateral to the anterior median line).

m) An easy way to remember which Spleen point lies in which intercostal space is to remember the formula: 22 minus Spleen point X equals intercostal space X.
For example, 22 – Sp 17 = 5th intercostal space; 22 – Sp 20 = 2nd intercostal space; etc.

Note: Voisin (1974) locates Sp 17 at the 6th rib, upper border, at 3 fb (finger breadth) lateral to the mamillary line. Soulié (1994) locates SP 17 on the lateral thorax: upper edge of the seventh rib (between the sixth and seventh ribs); about two FW (finger width) lateral from the line of the nipple; in a hollow; five FW above SP 16; two FW under SP 18; one FW anterior to LR 14; three FW lateral to ST 19. So (1985) locates SP 17 at 2 divisions lateral to ST 18 and at the same intercostal space.

Sp 18 TIAN XI – HEAVENLY STREAM

⊥ ***0.3 TO 0.5 CUN*** **Δ *5***

Pos: Position of patient: supine.

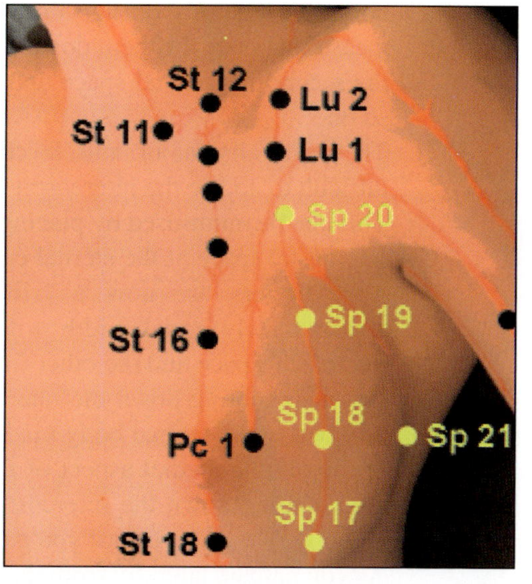

Loc:
a) On the anterior aspect of the torso.
b) On the chest (in the upper jiao).
c) In the fourth intercostal space.
d) 6 cun lateral to the anterior median line.
e) Approximately 1 cun lateral to Pc 1.
f) 2 cun lateral to the nipple.

Cun:
a) The transverse cun measurements for the chest (upper jiao) includes the Kidney, Stomach, Spleen and Lung channels (lateral to the anterior median line). The cun measurements are as follows:
Ki 22 to Ki 27 = 2 cun; St 13 to St 18 = 4 cun; Sp 17 to Sp 20 = 6 cun and Lu 1 to Lu 2 = 6 cun.
b) The transverse measurement for the upper jiao is calculated using the anterior median line and the mid point of the clavicle bone.
c) Identify the mid point of the clavicle by locating the medial end of the clavicle at the sterno-clavicular joint and the lateral end of the acromioclavicular joint, and divide the distance by half.
d) The distance from the anterior median line to the mid point of the clavicle is 4 cun. From here divide again to give 2 cun spaces medial and lateral to 4 cun, therefore giving 2 and 6 cun measurements. The Spleen channel is 6 cun lateral to the anterior median line.
e) The transverse distance between the two nipples (on a man) is 8 cun, thus the distance from the anterior median line to the nipple is 4 cun.

Tip:
a) Locate 6 cun lateral to the anterior median line.
b) The Spleen channel follows the contours of the chest. The flatter the chest the lesser curvature for the Spleen channel.
c) Place your finger in the fourth intercostal space (between the fourth and fifth ribs). The nipple is usually in the fourth intercostal space, therefore a quick and easy reference point. Once you have located the fourth intercostal space, run your finger laterally to 6 cun. Your finger should be in the deepest part of the intercostal space. As you run your finger laterally the intercostal space begins to curve upwards. On women you may need to ask them to lift their breast (left breast, right hand; right breast, left hand) to allow you to access this point at 6 cun lateral to the anterior median line.
d) Palpation at 6 cun lateral to the anterior median line should reveal the accurate location for Sp 18 which is also 1 cun lateral to Pc 1 (also in the fourth intercostal space, but at 1 cun lateral to the centre of the nipple).
e) If there are difficulties feeling for the fourth intercostal space then try feeling for the first and second intercostal spaces which are the easiest to palpate for. Place your index and middle finger in the first and second intercostal spaces on the lateral border of the body of the sternum, then with your two fingers staying at the same measurement move them down one intercostal space so that you have one finger in the second intercostal space and the other finger in the third intercostal space and so on.
f) The pectoralis major muscle covers the surface of the ribs which can make it difficult to locate the intercostal spaces from the third intercostal space downwards. This can be minimised by placing the first and second fingers in the first and second intercostal space at the sternal end of the ribs.
g) Your fingers are now a "rib space" apart. As the intercostal spaces are approximately equal width with each other, placing one finger in the second intercostal space and the other finger should fall into the third intercostal space . As you are counting down the intercostal spaces, the ribs inferior to the sternum are attached to the sternal body via bars of costal or hyaline cartilage. This cartilage opens out the medial aspect of the rib cage more laterally. This means that as you are counting down the intercostal spaces you will need to run your fingers more laterally. The more lateral you palpate the easier the intercostal spaces are to locate. As you palpate laterally from the sternum the intercostal spaces will curve upwards.
h) As a check the fourth intercostal space usually is at the level of the nipple (in a flat chested person).
i) Another way of identifying the intercostal spaces is to count them from the bottom of the rib cage upwards. For the 9th intercostal space (there are 9 intercostal spaces in total) palpate for the inferior border of the rib cage which will be the 10th rib. Place your finger in the intercostal space superior to this rib. You will now be in the 9th intercostal space.
j) When the 9th intercostal space has been established, place the flat of your index or middle finger in the 9th intercostal space and palpate for the 8th intercostal space by feeling for the superior border of the 9th rib. Once you have located the 9th rib, palpate superiorly until you feel a softness, which will be the 8th intercostal space. Use this procedure to palpate and locate the other intercostal spaces.

k) Sp 18 is located in the fourth intercostal space, 6 cun lateral to the anterior median line, or 2 cun lateral to the mamillary line.
l) Palpate laterally from the fourth intercostal space following the contour of the intercostal space until you can feel Sp 18 (at 6 cun lateral to the anterior median line).
m) An easy way to remember which Spleen point lies in which intercostal space is to remember the formula: 22 minus Spleen point X equals intercostal space X. For example, 22 – Sp 18 = 4th intercostal space; 22 – Sp 20 = 2nd intercostal space; etc.

Note: Voisin (1974) locates Sp 18 at the fifth rib, lower border, and at 3 fb (finger breadth) lateral to the mamillary line. Soulié (1994) locates SP 18 on the lateral chest: about mid-distance from the vertical of the npple and the armpit , on the inferior edge of the fifth rib (the third being just under the armpit); in a hollow; two FW (Finger Width) above SP 17; two FW under SP 19; one FW lateral and under PC 1; two FW lateral to ST 17; two FW anterior (medial) to GB 23. So (1985) locates SP 18 at 6 divisions lateral to a point midway between CV 17 and CV 18, between two ribs.

Sp 19 XIONG XIANG – CHEST REGION

⊥ ***0.3 TO 0.5 CUN*** Δ ***5***

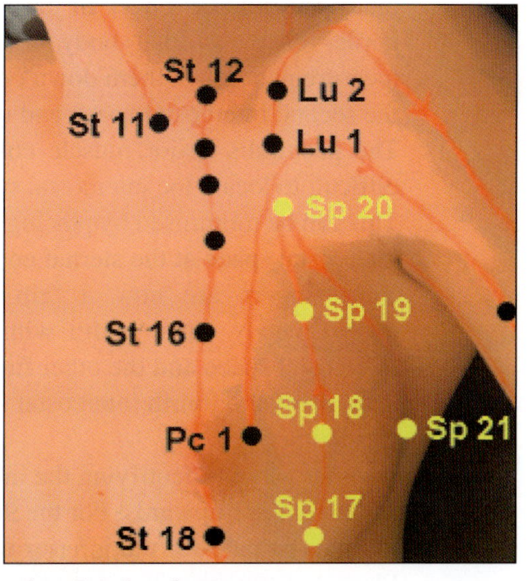

Pos: Position of patient: supine.

Loc: a) On the anterior aspect of the torso.
b) On the chest (in the upper jiao).
c) In the third intercostal space.
d) 6 cun lateral to the anterior median line.
e) 2 cun lateral to the mamillary line.

Cun: a) The transverse cun measurements for the chest (upper jiao) includes the Kidney, Stomach, Spleen and Lung channels (lateral to the anterior median line). The cun measurements are as follows: Ki 22 to Ki 27 = 2 cun; St 13 to St 18 = 4 cun; Sp 17 to Sp 20 = 6 cun and Lu 1 to Lu 2 = 6 cun.
b) The transverse measurement for the upper jiao is calculated using the anterior median line and the mid point of the clavicle bone.
c) Identify the mid point of the clavicle by locating the medial end of the clavicle at the sterno-clavicular joint and the lateral end of the acromioclavicular joint, and divide the distance by half.

d) The distance from the anterior median line to the mid point of the clavicle is 4 cun. From here divide again to give 2 cun spaces medial and lateral to 4 cun, therefore giving 2 and 6 cun measurements. The Spleen channel is 6 cun lateral to the anterior median line.

e) The transverse distance between the two nipples (on a man) is 8 cun, thus the distance from the anterior median line to the nipple is 4 cun.

Tip:

a) Locate 6 cun lateral to the anterior median line.

b) The Spleen channel follows the contours of the chest. The flatter the chest the lesser curvature for the Spleen channel.

c) Place your finger in the third intercostal space (between the third and fourth ribs).The nipple is usually in the fourth intercostal space, therefore a quick and easy reference point. Once you have located the third intercostal space, run your finger laterally to 6 cun. Your finger should be in the deepest part of the intercostal space. As you run your finger laterally the intercostal space begins to curve upwards. On women you may need to ask them to lift their breast (left breast, right hand; right breast, left hand) to allow you to access this point at 6 cun lateral to the anterior median line.

d) Palpation at 6 cun lateral to the anterior median line should reveal the accurate location for Sp 19.

e) If there are difficulties feeling for the third intercostal space then try feeling for the first and second intercostal spaces which are the easiest to palpate for. Place your index and middle finger in the first and second intercostal spaces on the lateral border of the sternal body, then with your two fingers staying at the same measurement move them down one intercostal space so that you have one finger in the second intercostal space and the other finger in the third intercostal space.

f) The pectoralis major muscle covers the surface of the ribs which can make it difficult to locate the intercostal spaces from the third intercostal space downwards. This can be minimised by placing the first and second fingers in the first and second intercostal space at the sternal end of the ribs.

g) Your fingers are now a "rib space" apart. As the intercostal spaces are approximately equal width with each other, placing one finger in the second intercostal space and the other finger should fall into the third intercostal space.

h) As a check the fourth intercostal space usually is at the level of the nipple (in a flat chested person).

i) Another way of identifying the intercostal spaces is to count them from the bottom of the rib cage upwards. For the 9th intercostal space (there are 9 intercostal spaces in total) palpate for the inferior border of the rib cage which will be the 10th rib. Place your finger in the intercostal space superior to this rib. You will now be in the 9th intercostal space.

j) When the 9th intercostal space has been established, place the flat of your index or middle finger in the 9th intercostal space and palpate for the 8th intercostal space by feeling for the superior border of the 9th rib. Once you have located the 9th rib, palpate superiorly until you feel a softness, which will be the 8th intercostal space. Use this procedure to palpate and locate the other intercostal spaces.

k) Sp 19 is located in the third intercostal space, 6 cun lateral to the anterior median line, or 2 cun lateral to the mamillary line.
l) Palpate laterally from the third intercostal space following the contour of the intercostal space until you can feel Sp 19 (at 6 cun lateral to the anterior median line).
m) An easy way to remember which Spleen point lies in which intercostal space is to remember the formula: 22 minus Spleen point X equals intercostal space X.
For example, 22 – Sp 19 = 3rd intercostal space; 22 – Sp 20 = 2nd intercostal space; etc.

Note: Voisin (1974) locates Sp 19 at the 4th rib, lower border, and at 2.5 fb (finger breadth) lateral to the mamillary line. Soulié (1994) locates SP 19 on the lateral thorax: mid-distance from the vertical of the nipple to the vertical of the armpit, on the inferior edge of the fourth rib (the third being just under the armpit); in a hollow; two FW (Finger Width) above SP 18; two FW under SP 20; two FW lateral and slightly under ST 16; two FW medial to GB 23. So (1985) locates SP 19 at 6 divisions lateral to a point midway between CV 18 and CV 19.

Sp 20 ZHOU RONG – ENCIRCLING GLORY

⊥ ***0.3 TO 0.5 CUN*** ***Δ 5***

Pos: Position of patient: supine.

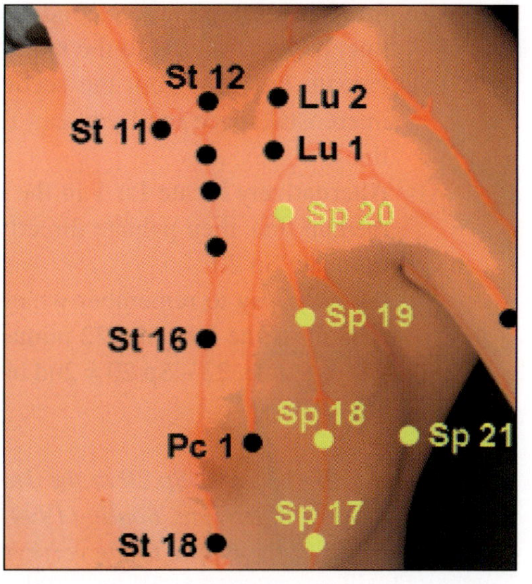

Loc:
a) On the anterior aspect of the torso.
b) On the chest (in the upper jiao).
c) In the second intercostal space.
d) 6 cun lateral to the anterior median line.
e) Inferior to Lu 1.

Cun:
a) The transverse cun measurements for the chest (upper jiao) includes the Kidney, Stomach, Spleen and Lung channels (lateral to the anterior median line). The cun measurements are as follows:
Ki 22 to Ki 27 = 2 cun; St 13 to St 18 = 4 cun; Sp 17 to Sp 20 = 6 cun and Lu 1 to Lu 2 = 6 cun.
b) The transverse measurement for the upper jiao is calculated using the anterior median line and the mid point of the clavicle bone.
c) Identify the mid point of the clavicle by locating the medial end of the clavicle at the sterno-clavicular joint and the lateral end of the acromioclavicular joint, and divide the istance by half.

d) The distance from the anterior median line to the mid point of the clavicle is 4 cun. From here divide again to give 2 cun spaces medial and lateral to 4 cun, therefore giving 2 and 6 cun measurements. The Spleen channel is 6 cun lateral to the anterior median line.

e) The transverse distance between the two nipples (on a man) is 8 cun, thus the distance from the anterior median line to the nipple is 4 cun.

Tip: a) Locate 6 cun lateral to the anterior median line.

b) The Spleen channel follows the contours of the chest. The flatter the chest the lesser curvature for the Spleen channel.

c) Place your finger in the second intercostal space (between the second and third ribs). The nipple is usually in the fourth intercostal space, therefore a quick and easy reference point. Once you have located the second intercostal space, run your finger laterally to 6 cun. Your finger should be in the deepest part of the intercostal space. As you run your finger laterally the intercostal space begins to curve upwards.

d) Palpation at 6 cun lateral to the anterior median line should reveal the accurate location for Sp 20.

e) If there are difficulties feeling for the second intercostal space then place your index and middle finger either side of the second rib on the lateral border of the sternal body, The finger inferior to the second rib is in the second intercostal space.

f) As a check the fourth intercostal space usually is at the level of the nipple (in a flat chested person).

g) Sp 20 is located in the second intercostal space, 6 cun lateral to the anterior median line, or 2 cun lateral to the mamillary line.

h) Palpate laterally from the second intercostal space following the contour of the intercostal space until you can feel Sp 20 (at 6 cun lateral to the anterior median line).

i) Alternatively locate Lu 1 in the first intercostal space, 6 cun lateral to the anterior median line, then palpate directly inferior to Lu 1 into the second intercostal space to locate Sp 20.

j) An easy way to remember which Spleen point lies in which intercostal space is to remember the formula: 22 minus Spleen X point equals intercostal space X.
For example, 22 – Sp 20 = 2nd intercostal space; 22 – Sp 17 = 5th intercostal space; etc.

Note: Voisin (1974) locates Sp 20 at the 3rd rib, slightly above it, and at 2 fb (finger breadth) lateral to the mamillary line. Soulié (1994) locates SP 20 on the lateral chest; mid-distance from the vertical of the nipple to the vertical of the armpit, on the inferior edge of the third rib (which is just under the armpit); in a hollow; two FW (Finger Width) above SP 19; one large FW medial to SP 21 and behind; two FW medial to GB 22; two FW lateral to ST 15; two FW inferior and medial to HT 1; two FW inferior anf lateral to ST 14. So (1985) locates SP 20 at 6 divisions ;ateral to a point midway between CV 19 and CV 20. Legge (1999) locates Sp 20 in the 2nd intercostal space, above Sp 19, directly below Lu 1 and Lu 2, 6 cun lateral to the midline (Ren channel).

The longitudinal distance between the axillary fold to the tip of the 11th rib is measured as 12 cun, when the arm is abducted.

Sp 21 DA BAO – GREAT ENVELOPING

⊥ ***0.3 CUN*** Δ ***3 TO 7***

- EXIT
- GENERAL JUNCTION/Luo/Connecting/Passage/Lo/Lê
- RE-UNION/Crossing/Meeting Point of the Spleen Channel with the Heart Channel – Foot Tai Yin Channel with the Hand Shao Yin Channel

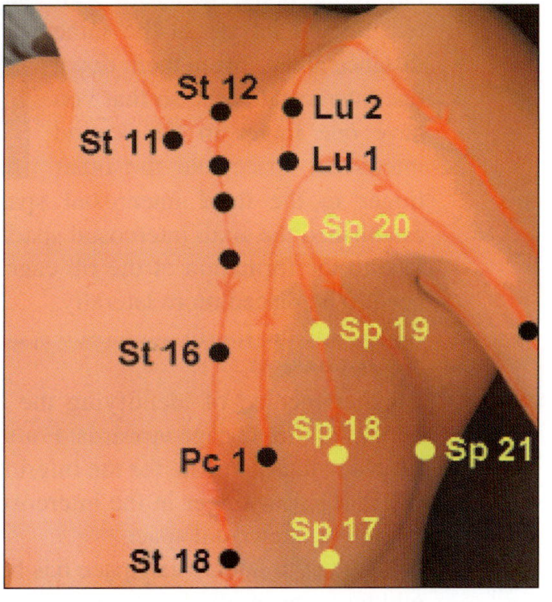

Pos: Position of patient: supine or seated with arm abducted.

Loc: a) On the lateral aspect of the torso.
b) On the lateral chest (in the upper jiao).
c) In the sixth intercostal space (occasionally in the seventh intercostal space).
d) On the mid-axillary line.
e) Inferior and posterior to Sp 17.
f) 2 intercostal spaces inferior or 3 cun inferior to GB 22.

Tip: a) Locate the mid-axillary line which runs from the axilla (armpit) longitudinally along the most lateral aspect of the torso. To establish the mid-axillary line ask the patient to place their hands on their waist and locate the posterior border of the pectoralis major muscle (anterior border of the armpit), and the anterior border of the latissimus dorsi muscle (the posterior border of the armpit). Draw two parallel lines longitudinally along the lateral surface of the torso. and the mid-axillary line is half way between these lines. Alternatively you can visualise where the mid-axillary line should be.
b) Draw a transverse line from the centre of the nipple laterally to the mid axillary line.
c) Sp 21 is used as a reference for GB 22 and GB 23.
d) Sp 21 is located at the intersection of the mid-axillary line and the transverse line in the sixth intercostal space.
e) On a large breasted person you may need to ask them to lift their breast (left breast, right hand; right breast, left hand) to access the point. The nipple is usually in the fourth intercostal space on the anterior aspect of the chest.
f) As Sp 21 may be located in the seventh intercostal space, it is recommended that you use the lines of intersection to locate the sixth intercostal space.

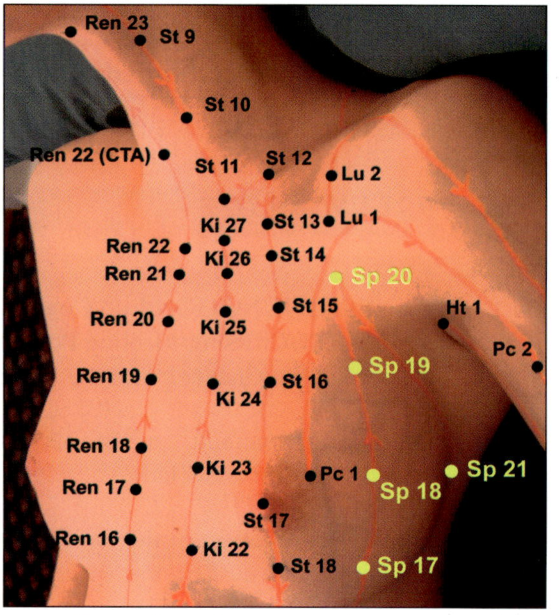

g) The pectoralis major muscle covers the surface of the ribs which can make it difficult to locate the intercostal spaces from the third intercostal space downwards.

h) If it is difficult locate the first and second intercostal spaces which are easier to palpate. Place your index and middle finger in the first and second intercostal spaces on the lateral border of the sternal body, then with your two fingers staying at the same distance apart, place them down one intercostal space so that you have one finger in the second intercostal space and the other finger in the third intercostal space. Repeating this method until you have established the sixth intercostal space.

i) Due to the formation of the rib cage, from the fifth intercostal space your fingers need to be placed more laterally.

j) As a check the fourth intercostal space is usually at the level of the nipple (in a flat chested person).

k) Another method of identifying the intercostal spaces is to count them from the bottom of the rib cage upwards. For the 9th intercostal space (there are 9 intercostal spaces in total) palpate for the inferior border of the rib cage which will be the 10th rib. Place your finger in the intercostal space superior to this rib. You will now be in the 9th intercostal space.

l) When the 9th intercostal space has been established, place the flat of your index or middle finger in the 9th intercostal space and palpate for the 8th intercostal space by feeling for the superior border of the 9th rib. Once you have located the 9th rib, palpate superiorly until you feel a softness, which will be the 8th intercostal space. Use this procedure to palpate and locate the other intercostal spaces. Sp 21 is located in the sixth intercostal space, on the mid axillary line.

m) On some people Sp 21 may be located in the 7th intercostal space. Therefore if you cannot feel a *men* (depression) in 6th intercostal space, palpate in the 7th intercostal space.

n) Palpation will ensure accurate point location.

o) An alternative method is to use cun measurements to locate Sp 21. When the arm is abducted the longitudinal distance between the axillary fold or apex of the axilla to the tip of the 11th rib is measured as 12 cun. Divide 12 cun in half to give 6 cun.

p) Sp 21 is located at approximately 6 cun (halfway) inferior to the axillary fold. This point is located in the 6th (or sometimes 7th) intercostal space so palpation will take overall precedence over the cun measurements.

q) Many people may have more tissue in the area of the tip of the 11th rib. (To locate the tip of the 11th rib, please see Liv 13 tips section).

Note: This point is traditionally located midway between the apex of the axilla and the free end of the 11th rib when the arm is abducted. Voisin (1974) locates Sp 21 at the 6th rib, lower border, on the anterior axillary line. Soulié (1994) locates SP 21 on the lateral chest; sligthly in front of the vertical of the armpit; under the third rib (which is just under the armpit); in the angle of the anterior edge of an intercostal ligament; under the inferior edge of the pectoralis major; in a hollow; one large FW (Finger Width) lateral to SP 20; two FW under HT 1; one large FW inferior and medial to GB 22. Li (1991) locates Sp 21 at 6 cun below the axilla, on the mid-axillary line at the level of the 6th intercostal space.
Shanghai (1993) locates SP 21 at 6 cun below the axilla, on the mid-axillary line, in the 6th intercostal space. Cheng (1987) locates this point on the mid-axillary line, 6 cun below the axilla, midway between the axilla and the free end of the 11th rib. Eachou (1995) locates SP 21 in a supine or lateral position, with the arm raised and on the mid-axillary line, 6 inches below the armpits, or on the mid-axillary line midway between the axilla and the tip of the 11th rib. Yang (1982) locates Sp 21 in the 6th intercostal space, 6 cun directly below the centre of the axilla. Shanghai (1981) locates this point on the mid-axillary line, 6 units below the middle of the axilla in the 7th intercostal space. Legge (1999) locates Sp 21 on the side of the chest, on the mid-axillary line, in the 7th intercostal space. Midway between the axilla and the free end of the 11th rib. Deadman (1998) locates SP 21 on the mid-axillary line, in the 7th intercostal space.

There is a note to this which states that some sources also locate Sp 21 in the 6th intercostal space. Masayoshi (1975) locates SP 21, 6 sun below the axilla on the midaxillar line. Legge (1999) locates Sp 21 on the side of the chest, on the mid-axillary line, in the 7th intercostal space. Midway between the axilla and the free end of the 11th rib. Lotan (2000) locates Sp 21 in the 6th intercostal, inferior to the armpit (axilla) centre; Anterior to the latissimus dorsi muscle; Midpoint between the axilla apex and the 11th rib anterior free end; When the arm is horizontal (abduction), 6 cun inferior to the axilla. Lotan describes an alternative location: in the 7th intercostal, inferior to the armpit centre; anterior to the latissimus dorsi.

REFERENCES FOR THE SPLEEN CHANNEL

Huang-fu Mi. Trans: Yang Shou-zhong and Charles Chace 1993 The Systematic Classic of Acupuncture & Moxibustion – Sp 1: 183

Ellis, Wiseman, Boss 1991 Fundamentals of Chinese Acupuncture – SP 1: 148;

Lotan, Alon 2000 Acupoint Location Guide – Sp 3: 51; Sp 4: 51; Sp 5: 53; Sp 10: 55; Sp 21: 59

Soulié De Morant, George. 1994 Chinese Acupuncture – SP 4: 385/386; SP 5: 386; SP 6: 387; SP 7: 388; SP 8: 388; SP 10: 389; SP 11: 390; SP 12: 390; SP 13: 391; SP 14: 391; SP 15: 392; SP 16: 392; SP 17: 392; SP 18: 393; SP 19: 393; SP 20: 393; SP 21: 394

Voisin, Dr. H 1974 Essentials of Acupuncture – Sp 5: 84; Sp 8: 84; Sp 10: 84; Sp 11: 84 Sp 12: 84; Sp 13: 84; Sp 14: 86; Sp 15: 86; Sp 16: 86; Sp 17: 86; Sp 18: 86; Sp 19: 86; Sp 20: 86; Sp 21: 86

Wu, Wei-P'ing 1973 Chinese Acupuncture – SP 5: 76; SP 6: 76; SP 7: 76; SP 8: 76; SP 10: 77; SP 11: 77; SP 12: 77; SP 13: 77; SP 14: 77; SP 15: 77; SP 16: 78

Lawson – Wood 1973 Acupuncture Handbook – XII 5: 37;

Worsley, J R 1982 Traditional Chinese Acupuncture Volume 1 – Meridians and Points. XII 6: 241; XII 7: 241; XII 8: 241; XII 10: 241; XII 11: 243; XII 12: 243; XII 13: 243; XII 14: 243; XII 16: 245

Lavier, Dr. J 1974 Points of Chinese Acupuncture – SP 6: 39; SP 7: 39; SP 8: 39; SP 10: 39; SP 11: 25; SP 12: 53; SP 13: 53; SP 14: 53; SP 15: 51; SP 16: 51

Legge, David 1999 Acupuncture Points and Meridians – Sp 7: 37; Sp 8: 38; Sp 11: 38; Sp 12: 38; Sp 20: 39; Sp 21: 39

Shanghai College of Traditional Chinese Medicine. 1993 Applied Anatomical Charts of Acupuncture and Moxibustion – SP 7: 46; SP 8: 46; SP 21: 52

Shandong Medical College and Shandong College of Traditional Chinese Medicine 1982 Anatomical Atlas of Chinese Acupuncture Points – Xuehai (Sp 10): 21; Jimen (Sp 11): 21; Chongmen (Sp 12): 21; Fushe (Sp 13): 21

Eachou Chen 1995 Cross-sectional Anatomy of Acupoints – SP 11: 55; SP 21: 194

Masayoshi Hyodo 1975 Ryodoraku Acupuncture – SP 11: 45; SP 12: 45; SP 21: 45

Shanghai College of Traditional Medicine 1981 Acupuncture – A Comprehensive Text – Sp 11: 324; Sp 13: 324 Sp 14: 324; Sp 15: 184; Sp 16: 324; Sp 21: 325

Yang Jiasan (Prof) 1982 The Way to Locate Acu-Points – Sp 13: 54; Sp 21: 55

Qiu Mao-Liang 1996 – Chinese Acupuncture and Moxibustion – SP 14: 89;

So, James Tin Yau (Dr) 1985 The Book of Acupuncture Points: SP 16: 208; SP 17: 208; SP 18: 209; SP 19: 209; SP 20: 210

Li Ding (Prof.). 1991. Acupuncture, Meridian Theory and Acupuncture Points – Sp 21: 305

Cheng Xinnong (Editor) 1987 Chinese Acupuncture and Moxibustion – Sp 21: 154;

Deadman, Peter; Al-Khafaji, Mazin; Baker, Kevin 1998 Manual of Acupuncture, An – SP 21: 204

THE HEART CHANNEL OF THE HAND (SHAO YIN)

Primary Channel

The Heart channel begins at a deep level in the tissues of the heart itself. One deep branch passes down the anterior median line to connect with the small intestine, another travels up from the heart, going alongside the oesophagus, over the pharynx and up to the tongue, around the mouth and up to the optic foramen, where according to Acupuncture theory the eyes are connected with the brain. (Some texts say that this branch continues to connect with the Small Intestine channel in the medial canthus of the eye).

Another deep channel passes from the heart into the aorta and emerges bilaterally through the lungs, passing through the subclavian artery to emerge at a superficial level in the axilla, at Ht 1. The main channel then descends the medial aspect of the anterior surface of the arm and forearm to enter the palm, ending on the radial aspect of the fifth digit, where it links with SI 1.

Divergent Channel

This leaves the primary channel in the axillary fossa, enters the chest and connects with the heart. It then ascends across the throat and emerges on the face, joining the Small Intestine channel at the medial canthus of the eye.

Connecting Channel

This leaves the primary channel at Ht 5 and joins the Small Intestine channel. At about 1.5 cun above the flexure of the wrist it again separates from the Small Intestine channel and follows the Heart primary channel to the heart. It then proceeds to the base of the tongue and connects with the eye.

Muscle Channel

This starts on the medial aspect of the fifth digit, binds with the pisiform bone and again at the medial aspect of the elbow, then proceeds up the arm to enter the chest cavity below the axilla. It crosses the Lung muscle channel in the breast region and binds in the chest. Descending across the diaphragm, it binds at the umbilicus.

THE HEART CHANNEL OF THE HAND

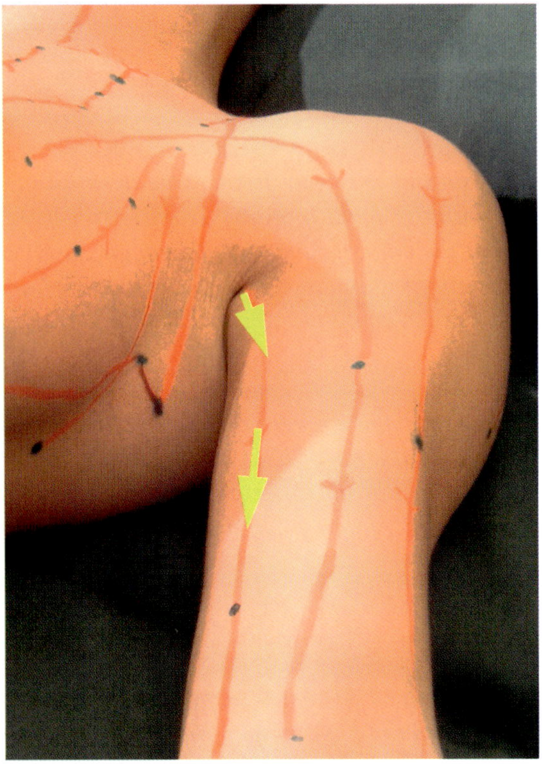

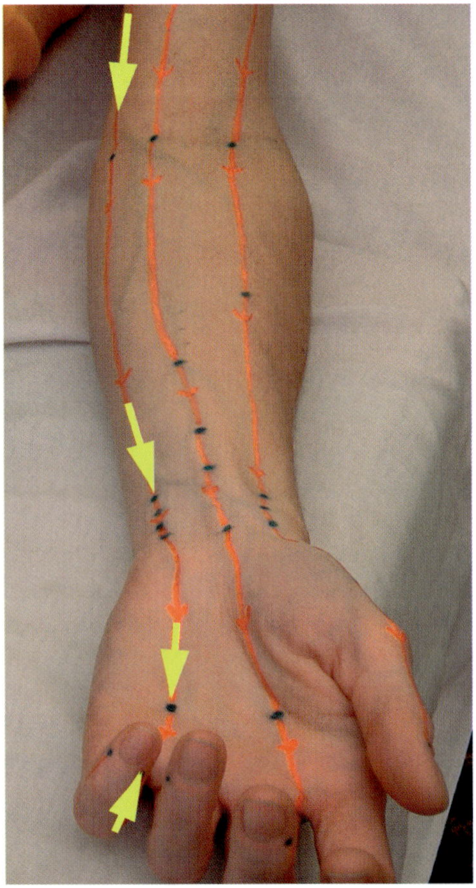

Points of the Heart Channel – Hand Shao Yin (Ht/HT/HE/H/I)

To locate the Heart channel, the arm should be in the anatomical position (with the exception to Ht 1).

Ht 1 is in the axilla, Ht 2 on the medial aspect of the upper arm, Ht 3 on the anterior aspect of the transverse cubital crease of the elbow.

Ht 1 JI QUAN – UTMOST SOURCE

⊥ ***0.3 TO 0.5 CUN*** Δ ***5***

- ENTRY
- RE-UNION/Crossing/Meeting Point of the Heart Channel with the Spleen Channel – Hand Shao Yin Channel with theFoot Tai Yin Channel

Pos: Position of patient: Supine, with hands on the hips so that the arms are flexed at the elbow to expose the axilla (arm pit).

Loc: a) In the axilla.
b) Just posterior to the lower border of the pectoralis major muscle where the arm attaches to the torso.

Tip: a) With the patient's hands on their hips to expose the axilla is exposed (as the arms are not against the torso).
b) The lower border of the pectoralis major muscle forms the anterior wall of the axilla, with the point lying just posterior to it.
c) The point is located by placing your finger in a hook like action just over the lower border of the pectoralis major muscle into the axilla.
d) The point will be too posterior if located in the deepest part of the axilla.

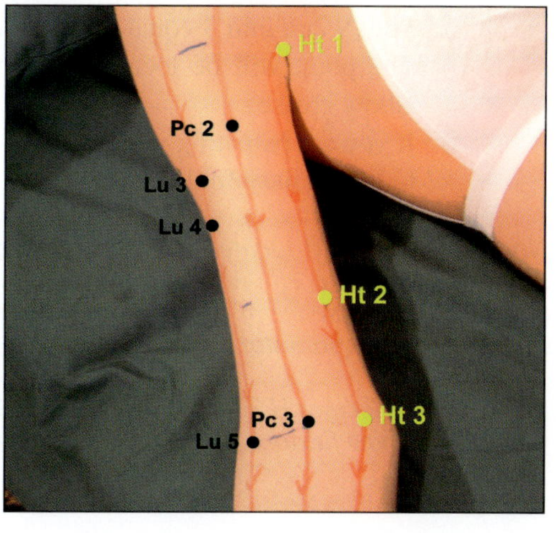

Note: Voisin (1974) locates H 1 on the breast, on the lateral border of the pectoralis major, at the level of the third intercostal space. Worsley (1982) locates I 1 in the axilla, upon the axillary artery. to expose the point, semiabduct the arm and palpate the artery. Shandong (1982) locate Jiquan at the centre of the fossa axillaris on the medial side of the a. axillaris when the arm is abducted. Legge (1999) locates Ht 1 in the centre (the highest point) of the axilla. Lotan (2000) locates H 1, when the arm is raised (abduction), in the centre of the armpit (axilla), medial to the axillary artery.

The distance between the anterior end of the axillary fold to the flexure of the elbow (the transverse cubital crease) is measured as 9 cun.

Ht 2 QING LING – BLUE-GREEN SPIRIT

⊥ *FORBIDDEN TO NEEDLE* Δ ***5 TO 7***
FORBIDDEN TO NEEDLE AND MOXA THIS POINT IN PREGNANCY

Pos: Position of patient: Supine, in the anatomical position (arms at the side and flat on the couch with the palms facing upwards).

Loc: a) On the medial surface of the upper arm.
b) 3 cun proximal to the flexure of the elbow (transverse cubital crease).
c) 6 cun distal to the axillary fold (where the arm joins the torso).
d) In the groove formed by the medial border of the biceps brachii muscle and the humerus.

Tip: a) Flex the elbow against resistance to expose the medial border of the biceps brachii muscle.
b) Once you have identified the muscle, relax the arm and run your finger down from the axilla along the groove formed by the medial border of the biceps brachii muscle towards the elbow. You are running down the Heart channel with the direction of flow.
c) Split 9 cun into 3 equal measurements.
d) The point will be located at approximately 3 cun measurement proximal to the elbow crease.
d) If you are palpating with the flow of the channel, Ht 2 is approximately 6 cun distal to the axillary fold.

Note: Soulié (1994) locates HT 2 on the anteromedial elbow: one FW (Finger Width) lateral to the bone of the elbow (epitrochlea); in the angle between the upper edge of the large transverse prominence of the articulation and the anteior edge of the insertion on an angle on the epitrochlea (pronator teres muscles); in a hollow; two FW above HT 3.

Voisin (1974) locates H 2 on the arm: medial border of the biceps, 3 fb (finger breadth) above the fold of the elbow flexion. Shandong (1982) locate Qingling at 3 cun above Pt. Shaohai (Ht 2).

Ht 3 SHAO HAI – LITTLE SEA

⊥ ***0.3 TO 0.5 CUN*** Δ ***3 TO 7***
FORBIDDEN TO NEEDLE AND MOXA THIS POINT IN PREGNANCY

- WATER
- HE – SEA/Shu – Transporting/Antique

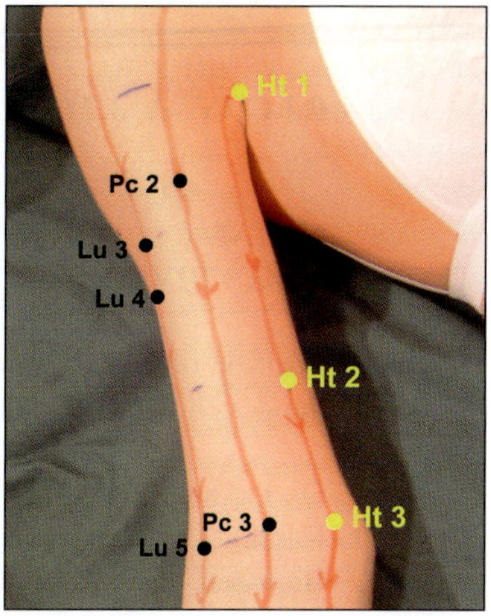

Pos: Position of patient: Supine, in the anatomical position (arms at the side and flat on the couch with the palms facing upwards).

Loc: a) On the anterior surface of the forearm.
b) On the transverse cubital crease (elbow crease).
c) Approximately half-way between the tendon of the biceps brachii muscle and the medial epicondyle of the humerus.

Tip: a) To expose the flexure of the elbow (transverse cubital crease) flex the arm and then draw a line along the formed crease.
b) If more than one crease is exposed, it is usually the most prominent one that is used.
c) To expose the tendon of the biceps brachii muscle, flex the elbow against resistance.
d) If you run your finger with the flow of the channel along the medial border of the biceps brachii, your finger should naturally fall into a hollow at the elbow flexure which is medial to the tendon of the biceps brachii and lateral to the medial epicondyle of the humerus.
e) Where the channel follows with the anatomy this will determine the position of the point relative to the medial aspect of the tendon and the medial epicondyle of the humerus.
f) To reduce patient discomfort when needling this point it is important that you support the arm slightly flexed.

Note: Soulié (1994) locates HT 3 on the medial, anterior elbow: two FW (Finger Width) inferior and lateral to the internal prominence of the bone (epitrochlea); in the angle between the inferior edge of the large transverse rise of the articulation and the upper edge of a large muscle on an angle (pronator teres); in a hollow; medial to the deep brachail artery; two FW under HT 3; one FW medial to PC 3. Voisin (1974) locates H 3 on the elbow: medial extremity of flexion fold.

Shandong (1982) locate Shaohai between the ulnar end of the cubital crease and the epicondylus medialis of the humerus. Legge (1999) locates Ht 3, when the elbow is flexed, the point is 3 cun superior to the medial end of the transverse cubital crease, in the depression anterior to the medial epicondyle of the humerus. Lotan (2000) locates H 3, when the elbow is bent at a right angle, between the medial epicondyle and the cubital crease medial end; When pressing this point, tickling sensation might be felt in the little finger.

The distance between the transverse cubital crease (flexure of the elbow) and the flexure of the wrist is measured as 12 cun. To find the flexure of the wrist, flex and extend the hand and palpate for the articulation at the wrist. The 12 cun measurement is taken between Ht 7 and the flexure of the elbow. Depending on the size of the pisiform bone, Ht 7 may be proximal to the flexure of the wrist.

Ht 4 LING DAO – SPIRIT PATH

⊥ ***0.3 CUN*** Δ ***3 TO 5***
FORBIDDEN TO NEEDLE AND MOXA THIS POINT IN PREGNANCY

- METAL
- JING – RIVER/Shu – Transporting/Antique

Pos: Position of patient: Supine, in the anatomical position (arms at the side and flat on the couch with the palms facing upwards).

Loc:
a) On the anterior surface of the forearm.
b) Radial to the tendon of the flexor carpi ulnaris muscle.
c) Between the tendons of the flexor carpi ulnaris and the flexor digitorum superficialis muscles.
d) 1.5 cun proximal to Ht 7 (wrist flexure).
e) Upon the ulnar artery.

Tip:
a) The point lies in the channel radial to the tendon of the flexor carpi ulnaris muscle which will be prominent and proximal to the pisiform bone when the wrist is flexed against resistance.
b) The point also lies ulnar to the tendon of the flexor digitorum superficialis muscle. This tendon is deep and cannot easily be identified, but if you were to flex and extend the fourth digit you may be able to feel this tendon move under your finger.
c) The distance between Ht 3 and Ht 7 is 12 cun, this point is 1.5 cun proximal to Ht 7.
d) To assist with the location run your finger with the flow of the channel from the flexure of the elbow towards the flexure of the wrist.
e) Upon the ulnar artery – this lies deep and is difficult to palpate.

Note: Soulié (1994) locates HT 4 on the anterior wrist (palm up, in supination); on the line of the little finger; four FW (Finger Width) above the palm; two FW above the head of the ulna; in the angle between the radial (lateral) edge of the ulna and the tendon of the flexor carpi ulnaris muscle, and of the inferior edge of a transverse bulge; on the ulnar edge of the ulnar artery; in a hollow; two FW above HT 5; separated fro PC 5 by the artery and the tendon of the palmaris longus and flexors; separated by the flexor carpi radialis from SI 7; at the level of LU 7. Voisin (1974) locates H 4 on the forearm, anterior aspect: 2.5 fb (finger breadth) proximal to the fold of the wrist flexion. over the ulnar artery.

Ht 5 TONG LI – PENETRATING INSIDE

⊥ ***0.3 CUN*** Δ ***3 TO 5***
FORBIDDEN TO NEEDLE AND MOXA THIS POINT IN PREGNANCY

- JUNCTION/Luo/Connecting/Passage/Lo/Lê
- RE-UNION/Crossing/Meeting Point of theHeart Channel with the Small Intestine Channel – Hand Shao Yin Channel with the Hand Tai Yang Channel
- HOST/GUEST COMBINATION – Source Point with the Junction Point of its Paired Official/Organ Therefore Ht 5 is combined with SI 4
- ONE OF THE HEAVENLY STAR POINTS OF MA DAN-YANG (the others are: Lu 7, LI 4, LI 11, St 36, St 44, Bl 40, Bl 57, Bl 60, GB 34, GB 39 and Liv 3)

Pos: Position of patient: Supine, in the anatomical position (arms at the side and flat on the couch with the palms facing upwards).

Loc:
a) On the anterior surface of the forearm.
b) Radial to the tendon of the flexor carpi ulnaris muscle.
c) Between the tendons of the flexor carpi ulnaris and the flexor digitorum superficialis muscles.
d) Approximately 1 cun proximal to Ht 7 (wrist flexure).
e) In the same channel as Ht 4.
f) Upon the ulnar artery.

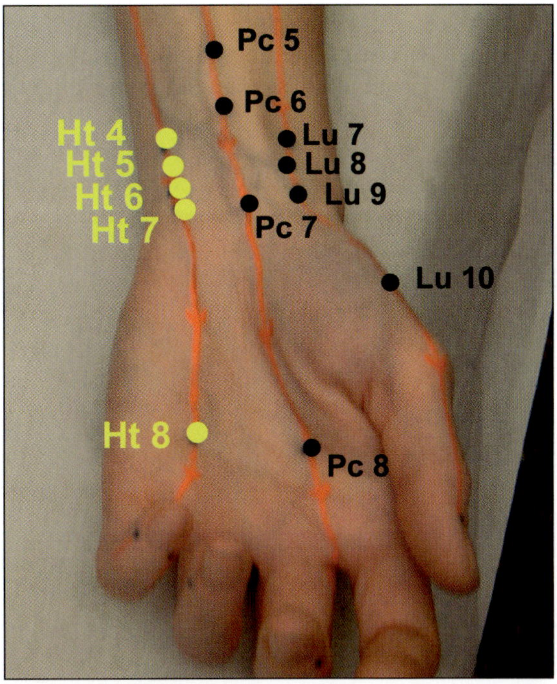

Tip:
a) The point lies in the channel radial to the tendon of the flexor carpi ulnaris muscle which will be prominent and proximal to the pisiform bone when the wrist is flexed against resistance.
b) The point also lies ulnar to the tendon of the flexor digitorum superficialis muscle. This tendon is deep and cannot easily be identified, but if you were to flex and extend the fourth digit you may be able to feel this tendon move under your finger.
c) The distance between Ht 3 and Ht 7 is 12 cun, this point is 1.0 cun proximal to Ht 7.
d) To assist with the location run your finger with the flow of the channel from the flexure of the elbow towards the flexure of the wrist.
e) Upon the ulnar artery – this lies deep and is difficult to palpate.

Note: Soulié (1994) locates HT 5 on the wrist, anterior face (palm up, in supination): on the line of the little finger; in the angle between the superior (posterior) edge of the transverse head of the ulna, and the lateral head of the tendon of the flexor carpi ulnaris muscle, between it and the ulnar artery; in a hollow; two FW (Finger Width) under HT 4; one FW above HT 6; separated from SI 6 by the flexor carpi ulnaris muscle, and from PC 7 by the ulnar artery and the palmaris longus secondus muscle. Voisin (1974) locates H 5 on the forearm, anterior aspect: 1.5 fb (finger breadth) proximal to the fold of the wrist flexion, over the ulnar artery. Shandong (1982) locate Tongli at 1 cun above Pt. Shenmen (Ht 7), on the ulnar side of the tendon of m. flexor Carpi ulnaris.

Ht 6 YIN XI – YIN MOUND

⊥ ***0.3 CUN*** **Δ** ***3 TO 7***
FORBIDDEN TO NEEDLE AND MOXA THIS POINT IN PREGNANCY

- ACCUMULATION/Xi Cleft/Gueki

Pos: Position of patient: Supine, in the anatomical position (arms at the side and flat on the couch with the palms facing upwards).

Loc:
a) On the anterior surface of the forearm.
b) Radial to the tendon of the flexor carpi ulnaris muscle.
c) Between the tendons of the flexor carpi ulnaris and the flexor digitorum superficialis muscles.
d) Approximately 0.5 cun proximal to Ht 7 (wrist flexure).
e) In the same channel as Ht 4 and Ht 5.
f) Upon the ulnar artery.

Tip:
a) The point lies in the channel radial to the tendon of the flexor carpi ulnaris muscle which will be prominent and proximal to the pisiform bone when the wrist is flexed against resistance.
b) The point also lies ulnar to the tendon of the flexor digitorum superficialis muscle. This tendon is deep and cannot easily be identified, but if you were to flex and extend the fourth digit you may be able to feel this tendon move under your finger.
c) The distance between Ht 3 and Ht 7 is 12 cun, this point is 0.5 cun proximal to Ht 7.
d) To assist with the location run your finger with the flow of the channel from the flexure of the elbow towards the flexure of the wrist.
e) Upon the ulnar artery – this lies deep and is difficult to palpate.

Note: Soulié (1994) locates HT 6 on the anterior wrist (palm in supination): on the line of the little finger; in the angle between the inferior edge (towards the palm) of the head of the ulna and of the lateral edge (towards the lateral thumb) of the large tendon of the flexor carpi ulnaris (inserted on the pisiform bone); on the medial (ulnar) edge of the ulnar artery; in a hollow; one FW (Finger Width) below HT 5; one large FW above HT 7; separated by the flexor carpi ulnaris from SI 5. Voisin (1974) locates H 6 on the forearm, anterior aspect: just proximal to the fold of the wrist flexion, over the ulnar artery. Shandong (1982) locate Yinxi at 0.5 cun below Pt. Tongli (Ht 5).

Ht 7 SHEN MEN – SPIRIT GATE

⊥ ***0.3 CUN*** Δ ***3 TO 7***
FORBIDDEN TO NEEDLE AND MOXA THIS POINT IN PREGNANCY

- SOURCE/Yuan/Regulator/Primary
- EARTH
- SEDATION/Reducing/Dispersing
- CHILD
- SHU – STREAM/Shu – Transporting/Antique
- HOST/GUEST COMBINATION – Source Point with the Junction Point of its Paired Official/Organ (Therefore Ht 7 is combined with SI 7)

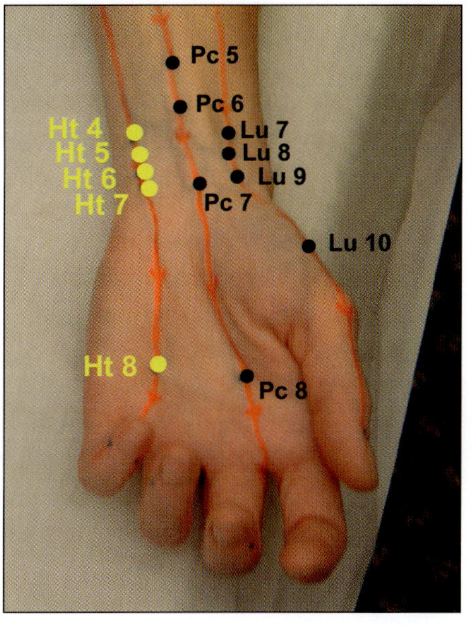

Pos: Position of patient: Supine, in the anatomical position (arms at the side and flat on the couch with the palms facing upwards).

Loc:
a) On the anterior aspect of the wrist, on the wrist flexure.
b) On the proximal radial corner of the pisiform bone.
c) Radial to the tendon of the flexor carpi ulnaris muscle.
d) Upon the ulnar artery.

Tip:
a) The point is described as being on the anterior flexure of the wrist, if however the pisiform bone is large then the point may seem to be more proximal to the wrist articulation.
b) The wrist flexure is not always identified by the wrist crease(s).
c) To help with the location of this point run your finger with the flow of the channel from the flexure of the elbow towards the flexure of the wrist .
d) By flexing and extending the hand a gap may be felt between the pisiform bone and the ulna bone. The point lies in this gap proximal to the radial border of the pisiform bone.
e) Upon the ulnar artery – this lies deep and is difficult to palpate.

Note: Soulié (1994) locates HT 7 on the palm, near the wrist, on the line of the little finger; on the hypothenar eminence; on the inferior and lateral edge (towards the fingers and thumb) of the round bony head (pisiform bone); on the medial edge of the ulnar artery; on the upper edge of the transverse mass (palmar aponeurosis); in the angle between the bone and the lateral edge (towards the thumb) of the insertion of the adductor of the little finger; in a hollow; one large FW (Finger Width) below HT 6; three FW above HT 8; separated by the adductor from SI 4. Wu (1973) locates HE 7 upon the forearm, on the cubital artery at the flexure of the wrist.

Ht 8 on the palmar surface of the hand.

Ht 8 SHAO FU – LESSER PALACE

⊥ *0.2 TO 0.3 CUN* ∆ *3 TO 5*

FORBIDDEN TO NEEDLE AND MOXA THIS POINT IN PREGNANCY EXCEPT FOR HEARTBURN

- FIRE
- HORARY from 11 a m. to 1 p m.
- SEASONAL HORARY – Summer
- YING – SPRING/Shu – Transporting/Antique

Pos: Position of patient: Supine, in the anatomical position (arms at the side and flat on the couch with the palms facing upwards).

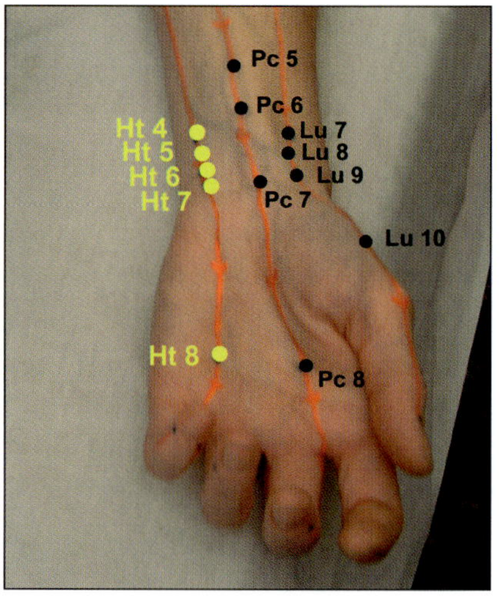

Loc: a) On the palmar surface of the hand.
b) Between the fourth and fifth metacarpal bones.
c) Proximal to the head of the fifth metacarpal.

.

Tip: a) Traditionally the point lies where the tip of the little finger rests when a loose fist is made, however this depends on how loose or how tight the fist is clenched and therefore is not always accurate.
b) This point normally lies just proximal to the distal transverse crease (heart line) of the hand, but the definitive location is in relation to the bone rather than the crease.
c) To locate this point run your finger with the flow of the channel from the flexure of the wrist at Ht 7 towards the radial side of the fifth digit.
d) You can also place one finger on the posterior surface of the hand and feel for the fourth and fifth metacarpo-phalangeal joints (knuckles).
e) Once located feel the metacarpal bones so that you are proximal to the heads of the fourth and fifth metacarpal bones and press in. This will push the bones nearer to the palmar surface of the hand and make the palpation of the anatomy much easier. When you have established this, relax the hand in the anatomical position again so you can palpate for the point.
f) The point lies on the palmar surface of the hand just proximal to the flares formed by the heads of the fourth and fifth metacarpal bones but slightly nearer the fifth metacarpal bone. This is because the Heart channel runs along the radial side of the fifth digit.
g) When you needle this point make sure that the patient's hand is supported and in a relaxed position, this will reduce the sensation felt by the patient on insertion.

Wu (1973) locates Ht 8 upon the palmar surface of the hand, between the fourth and fifth metacarpals, upon the "line of the heart". Lavier (1974) locates Ht 8 exactly on the distal palmar crease. Worsley (1982) locates I 8 on the palmar surface of the hand, between the fourth and the fifth metacarpal bones, on the distal transverse crease, or the 'heart line' of the hand. Soulié (1994) locates HT 8 on the palm, line of the joint of the ring and little fingers, one FW (finger width) above the joint.; just at the superior lateral edge of the prominent angle of the bone at the bottom of the little finger (head of the fifth metacarpal bone). Towards the angle of the head of the fourth metacarpal. Between the bone and the insertion of the small muscle (fourth lumbricalis muscle); in a hollow. On the medial edge of the interosseous artery; on the :heart line."; three FW below HT 7; one FW medial from PC 8, in the angle of the head of the ring finger." Deadman (1998) locates HT 8 generally lying between the two transverse palmar creases.Voisin (1974) locates H 8 on the palm, head of metacarpal 5, radial border. Shandong (1982) locate Shaofu on the ulnar side of Pt. Laogong (Pc 8), between the ossa metacarpale IV and V. Legge (1999) locates Ht 8 between the 4th and 5th metacarpal bones on the palmar surface of the hand. When a fist is made, the point is where the tip of the little finger rests, Lotan (2000) locates H 8 in the depression between the 4th and the 5th metacarpal bones, about 0.3 cun proximal to the bone heads; When fisting the hand, where the tip of the little finger rests; Between the two typical palm transverse creases.

Ht 9 on the posterior aspect of the fifth digit.

Ht 9 SHAO CHONG – LITTLE RUSHING IN

⊥ ***0.1 CUN*** **Δ** ***1 TO 5***

FORBIDDEN TO NEEDLE AND MOXA THIS POINT IN PREGNANCY

- WOOD
- EXIT
- TONIFICATION/Reinforcing
- MOTHER
- JING – WELL/Shu – Transporting/Antique
- RE-UNION/Crossing/Meeting Point of theHeart Channel with the Small Intestine Channel – Hand Shao Yin Channel with the Hand Tai Yang Channel

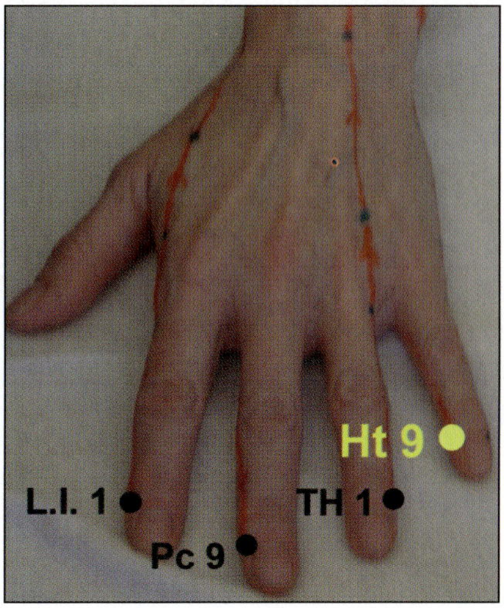

Pos: Position of patient: supine or seated

Loc: a) On the hand.
b) On the posterior aspect of the fifth digit (little finger).
c) The radial nail point of the fifth digit.
d) Approximately 0.1 cun proximal to the corner of the nail.
e) Just distal to the flare of the distal phalanx.

Tip: a) The point is level with the nail bed (where the nail attaches to the skin) rather than the cuticle.
b) Draw a horizontal line across the nail bed.
c) Draw a vertical line from the radial border of the nail towards the nail bed.
d) The lines drawn from b) and c) (vertical and horizontal) form an intersection. This is approximately where the point is located.

Note: Ellis (1991) – the classical location for HT 9 is on the inner side of the little finger, the width of a Chinese leek leaf away from the corner of the nail (The Great Compendium). Huang (1993) locates Ht 9 at the tip of the radial aspect of the small finger, the distance of a leel leaf from the corner of the nail.

REFERENCES FOR THE HEART CHANNEL

Voisin, Dr. H 1974 Essentials of Acupuncture – H 1: 68; H 2: 68; H 3: 68; H 4: 68; H 5: 68; H 6: 68; H 8: 68;
Worsley, J R 1982 Traditional Chinese Acupuncture Volume 1 – Meridians and Points. I 1: 21; I 8: 25
Shandong Medical College and Shandong College of Traditional Chinese Medicine 1982 Anatomical Atlas of Chinese Acupuncture Points – Jiquan (Ht 1): 25; Qingling (Ht 2): 25; Shaohai (Ht 3): 25; Tongli (Ht 5): 25; Yinxi (Ht 6): 25; Shaofu (Ht 8): 25
Legge, David 1999 Acupuncture Points and Meridians – Ht 1: 43; Ht 3: 43; Ht 8: 44
Lotan, Alon 2000 Acupoint Location Guide – H 1: 61; H 3: 61; H 8: 65
Soulié De Morant, George 1994 Chinese Acupuncture (L'Acuponcture Chinoise) – HT 2: 396; HT 3: 396; HT 4: 397; HT 5: 397; HT 6: 398; HT 7: 398; HT 8: 399
Wu, Wei-P'ing 1973 Chinese Acupuncture – HE 7: 80; HE 8: 80
Lavier, Dr. J 1974 Points of Chinese Acupuncture – Upper Arm Pouce Measurement: 8/9; HE 8: 21
Deadman, Peter; Al-Khafaji, Mazin; Baker, Kevin 1998 Manual of Acupuncture, An – HE 8: 221
Huang-fu Mi. Trans: Yang Shou-zhong and Charles Chace 1993 The Systematic Classic of Acupuncture & Moxibustion – Ht 9: 176
Ellis, Wiseman, Boss 1991 Fundamentals of Chinese Acupuncture – HT 9: 171

THE SMALL INTESTINE CHANNEL OF THE HAND (TAI YANG)

Primary channel

The Small Intestine channel starts on the ulnar surface of the little finger (SI 1), and travels up the ulnar aspect of the forearm to the medial aspect of the elbow. After passing between the medial epicondyle of the humerus and the olecranon of the ulna, it runs up the posterior aspect of the arm to the shoulder joint. It crosses the scapula (via Bl 36 and Bl 11) to SI 15 where there is a connection with Du 14, and then comes forward over the shoulder to St 12 in the supraclavicular fossa.

From St 12 a deep branch runs down through the heart and oesophagus, (passing Ren 17), descends through the diaphragm to Ren 13/12 and the stomach, and finally enters the small intestine. The main channel continues to SI 16/17 on the neck, and then up to the cheek. From SI 18 there is one branch passing through GB 1 at the lateral canthus of the eye to SI 19 at the ear (via TH 22), and one passing the lateral side of the nose to link directly with Bl 1 at the medial canthus of the eye.

(Some historical texts also refer to a channel descending to St 39.)

Divergent Channel

This leaves the primary channel at the shoulder, enters the axilla, crosses the heart, and descends to the abdomen to link up with the small intestine.

Connecting Channel

This leaves the primary channel at SI 7 on the forearm and connects with the Heart channel. A second branch continues up the arm, crosses the elbow and meets with the shoulder (LI 15).

Muscle Channel

This starts on the posterior aspect of the fifth digit, binds at the wrist, and travels up the forearm to the elbow, binding with the medial epicondyle of the humerus. It proceeds up the arm and binds below the axilla. One branch passes behind the axilla, spreads out over the scapula, travels in front of the Bladder muscle channel up the neck, and binds behind the ear.

A channel separates behind the pinna to enter the ear, which then reemerges above the pinna, descends the lateral side of the face to bind at the inferior border of the mandible, and ascends again to bind at the lateral canthus of the eye and the temple region. Another branch separates at the mandible, rises up around the teeth and in front of the ear, binds at the lateral canthus of the eye, and rises further to bind at the angle of the natural hairline on the forehead.

THE SMALL INTESTINE CHANNEL OF THE HAND

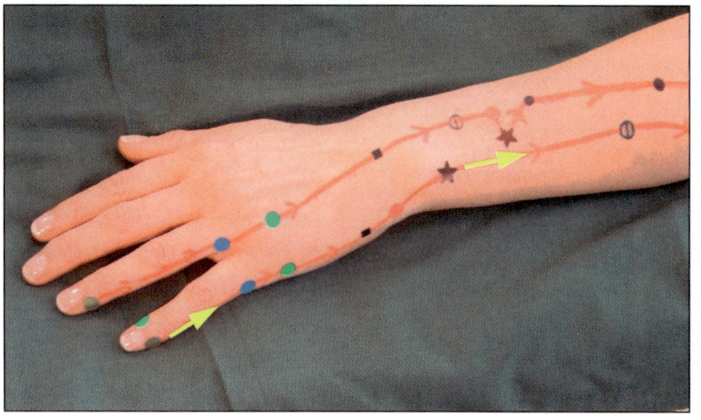

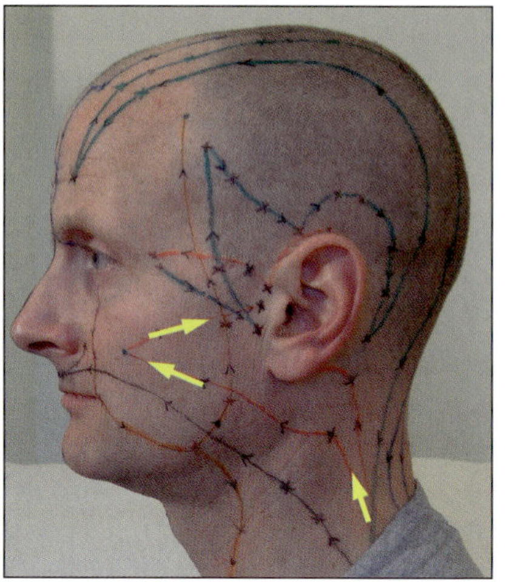

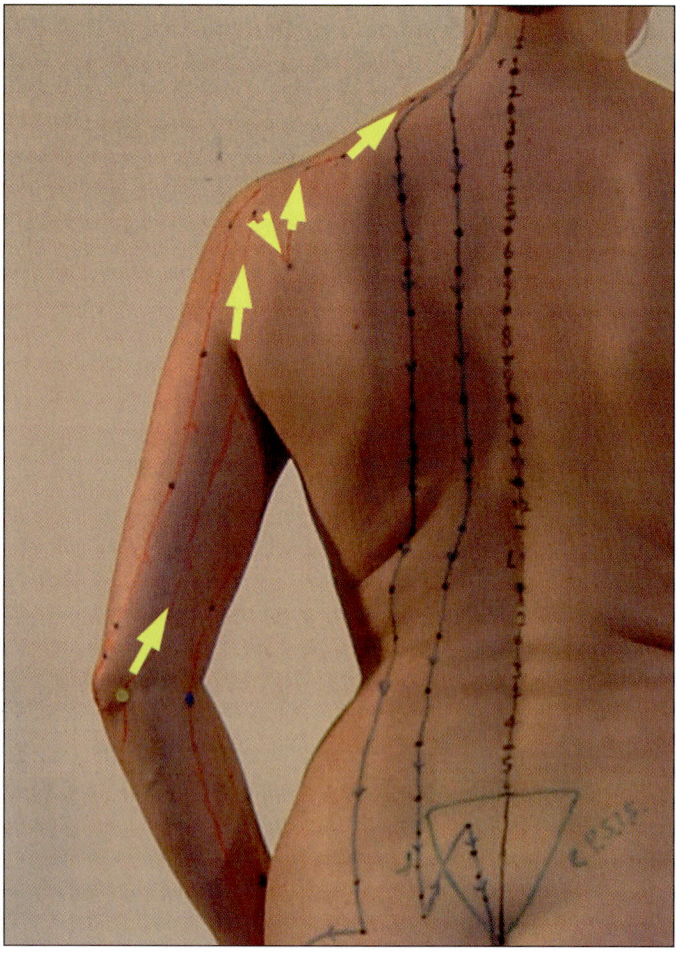

Points of the Small Intestine Channel – Hand Tai Yang (SI/II)

SI points 1-5 are located on the ulnar surface of the fifth digit and hand when the forearm is pronated.

SI 1 SHAO ZE – LITTLE MARSH

⊥ ***0.1 CUN*** ***Δ 3 TO 5***

- METAL
- ENTRY
- JING – WELL/Shu – Transporting/Antique
- RE-UNION/Crossing/Meeting Point of the Small Intestine Channel with the Heart Channel – Hand Tai Yang Channel with the Hand Shao Yin Channel

Pos: Position of patient: supine or seated

Loc: a) On the hand.
b) On the ulnar aspect of the fifth digit (little finger).
c) The ulnar nail point of the fifth digit.
d) Approximately 0.1 cun proximal to the corner of the nail.
e) Just distal to the flare of the distal phalanx.

Tip: a) The point is level with the nail bed (where the nail attaches to the skin) rather than the cuticle.
b) Draw a horizontal line across the nail bed.
c) Draw a vertical line from the ulnar border of the nail towards the nail bed.
d) The lines drawn from b) and c) (vertical and horizontal) form an intersection. This is approximately where the point is located.

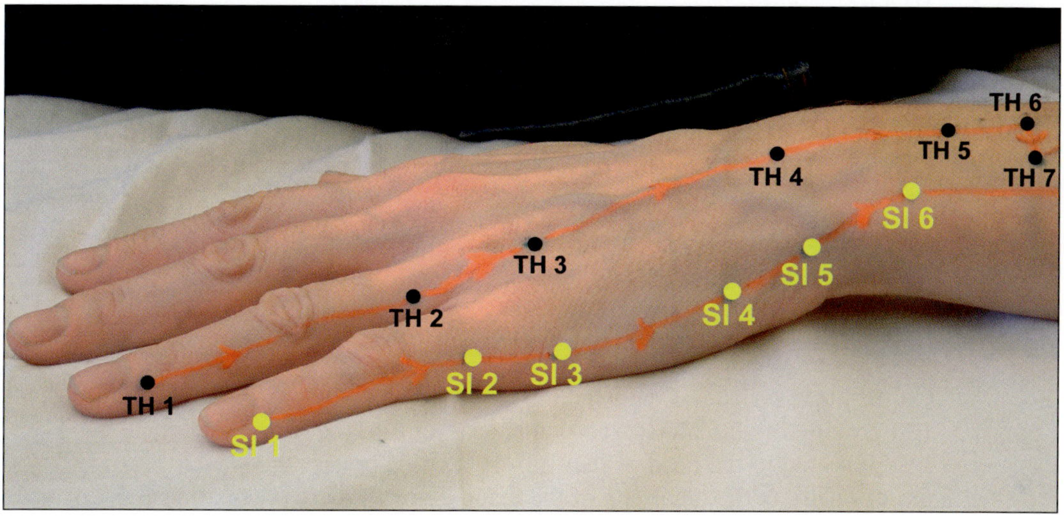

SI 2 QIAN GU – FORWARD VALLEY

⊥ ***0.1 TO 0.3 CUN*** **Δ** ***3 TO 7***

- WATER
- YING – SPRING/Shu – Transporting/Antique

Pos: Position of patient: supine with the forearm pronated.

Loc: a) On the ulnar aspect of the fifth digit (little finger).
b) Just distal to the flare of the base of the proximal phalanx of the fifth digit.
c) Occasionally at the end of the distal metacarpo-phalangeal crease formed when a loose fist is made.

Tip: a) This point may be located with the little finger slightly flexed.
b) Traditionally at the junction of the change in skin colour, where the palmar skin surface meets the posterior skin surface of the hand.
c) To help with the location of this point, run your finger with the flow of the channel from
SI 1 towards the fifth metacarpo-phalangeal joint. As you approach the metacarpophalangeal joint you will feel the base of the proximal phalanx of the fifth digit begin to flare.
d) Just distal to where the base of the proximal phalanx flares is where the point is located.

SI 3 HOU XI – BACK RAVINE

⊥ ***0.2 TO 0.5 CUN*** **Δ** ***3 TO 7***

- WOOD
- TONIFICATION/Reinforcing
- MOTHER
- SHU – STREAM/Shu – Transporting/Antique
- 8 EXTRAORDINARY CHANNELS CONFLUENT/8 Extraordinary Meridians Confluent/8 Extraordinary Vessels Opening/Master Point of Du Mai (Governor Vessel)
- 8 EXTRAORDINARY VESSEL/Coupled Point of the Yang Heel Vessel (Yang Qiao Mai)

Pos: Position of patient: supine with the forearm pronated.

Loc: a) On the ulnar surface of the hand.
b) Just proximal to the metacarpo-phalangeal joint of the fifth digit.
c) Just proximal to the head of the fifth metacarpal bone.
d) Occasionally at the ulnar end of the distal palmar crease when a loose fist is made.

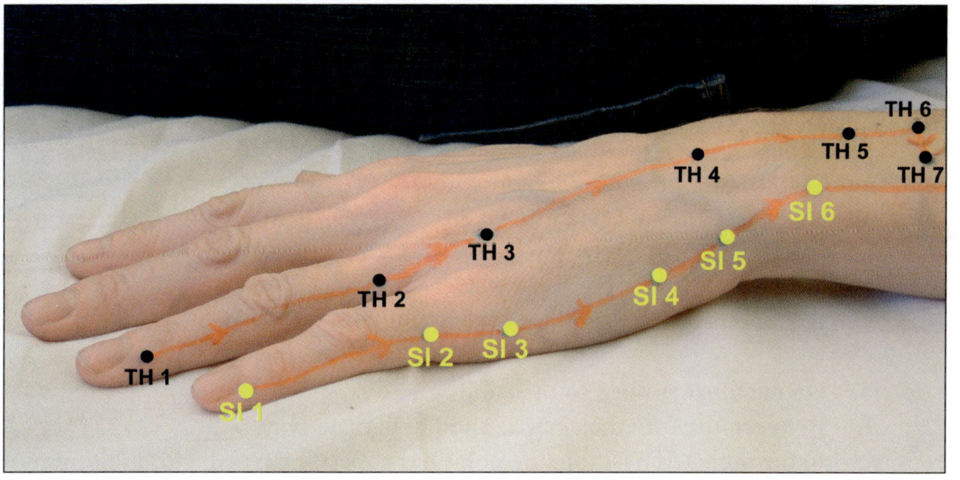

Tip:
a) This point may be located with the little finger slightly flexed.
b) Traditionally at the junction of the change in skin colour, where the palmar skin surface meets the posterior skin surface of the hand.
c) To help with the location of this point, run your finger with the flow of the channel from SI 1 towards the base of the fifth proximal phalanx bone. As you approach the metacarpo-phalangeal joint you will feel the base of the proximal phalanx of the fifth digit begin to flare. Run your finger over the metacarpo-phalangeal joint to where the flare of the head of the fifth metacarpal ends (proximal to the joint), this is proximal to the head of the fifth metacarpal bone where palpation of this area should reveal the location of the point.
d) The heads of the metacarpal bones are the "knuckles" of the hand.

Note: The exact origin of SI 3 half-way along the 5th metacarpal bone is unknown. However Fuye (1956) and Lawson-Wood (1973) locate the point 2cm above the metacarpo-phalangeal articulation of the little finger. Medicine & Health (1980) locates SI 3 the same as our location description but also includes another point named Shang Hou Xi which is located between Hou Xi (SI 3) and Wang Gu (SI 4).

Shanghai College (1981) locates this point, again the same as our explanation but also includes a point (N-UE-4) between SI 3 and SI 4, on the dorsum of the hand, lateral aspect, named Shang Hou Xi (Upper Back Creek or Outer Back Ravine). The reason for including this is that some traditions have this point as SI 3. Worsley (1982) locates II 3 on the ulnar edge of the hand, approximately half-way along the fifth metacarpal bone. (Feel along the bone for the notch.) ("Then palpate for the point directly inferior to the notch on the "fattest" part of the hand.").

SI 4 WAN GU – WRIST BONE

⊥ ***0.2 TO 0.5 CUN*** Δ ***3 TO 7***

- SOURCE/Yuan/Regulator/Primary
- ORIGINAL (for specific symptoms)
- HOST/GUEST COMBINATION – Source Point with the Junction Point of its Paired Official/Organ Therefore SI 4 is combined with Ht 5

Pos: Position of patient: supine with the forearm pronated.

Loc: a) On the ulnar surface of the hand.
b) Between the fifth metacarpal and the hamate bone.
c) In the pronated position, the point lies superior the abductor digiti minimi when the fifth digit is abducted.

Tip: a) Traditionally at the junction of the change in skin colour.
b) To help with the location of this point, run your finger with the flow of the channel from SI 3 towards the flexure of the wrist. As your finger goes over the base of the fifth metacarpal bone you will feel a gap between this bone and the hamate bone.
c) The hamate bone is not very prominent and therefore can easily be mistaken for the triquetral bone which is more prominent and next to the hamate bone.
d) For the height of the point you need to feel for the upper border of the abductor digiti minimi muscle as this point lies just above it. By abducting the little finger this will demonstrate the muscle.
e) Palpation of this area should reveal the location of the point.

Note: Soulié (1994) locates SI 4 on the hand, palm up, in supination; on the medial edge (internal line of the little finger); one large FW (Finger Width) below (distal to) the bony prminence of the ulna; in the angle between the inferior and dorsal edge of the small, round bone to wards the palm (pisiform) and the dorsal edge of the muscle inserted on its inferior face (adductor muscle of the little finger); between it and the unciform bone of the fifth metacarpal, in a hollow; two FW proximal to SI 3; two FW distal and palmar to SI 5; one FW proximal and dorsal to HT 7.

Worsley (1982) locates II 4 on the ulnar edge of the hand, in the hollow between the proximal end of the fifth metacarpal bone and the triquetral bone.

Shandong (1982) locate Hand Wanggu on the ulnar side of the back of the hand, in the depression amid the base of the os metacarpale V the os hamatum and the pisiforme. Legge (1999) locates SI 4 in the depression found distal to the triquetral bone on the ulnar aspect of the wrist. Lotan (2000) locates SI 4 in the depression, at the meeting point of three bones: the triquetral, the pisiform and the base of the 5th metacarpal.

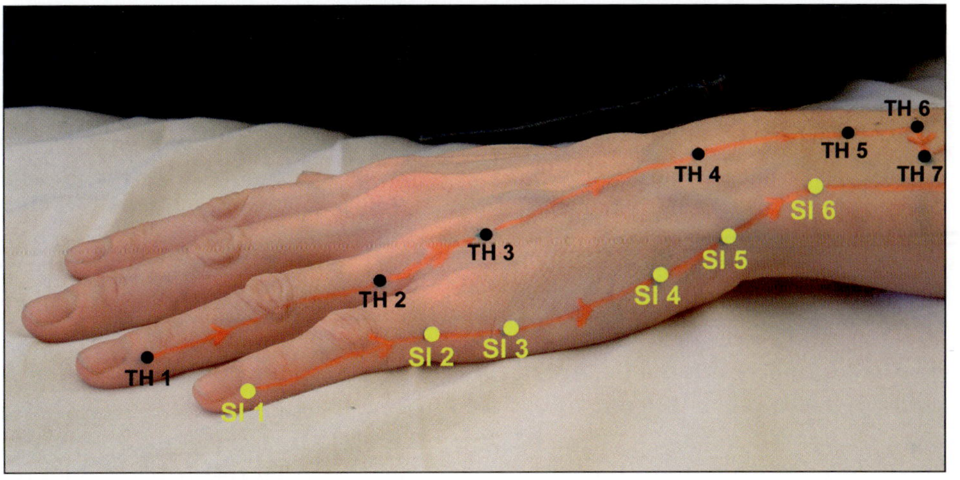

SI 5 YANG GU – YANG VALLEY

⊥ ***0.2 TO 0.3 CUN*** Δ ***3 TO 7***

- FIRE
- HORARY from 1 p m. to 3 p m.
- SEASONAL HORARY – Summer
- JING – RIVER/Shu – Transporting/Antique

Pos: Position of patient: supine with the forearm pronated.

Loc: a) On the ulnar surface of the wrist flexure.
b) Between the triquetral bone and the styloid process of the ulna.

Tip: a) By adducting and abducting the hand (sideways movement) you should be able to feel the gap in between the triquetral bone and the ulna bone. The point lies in a hollow between these two bones.
b) To help with the location of this point, run your finger with the flow of the channel from SI 3 towards the flexure of the wrist. As your finger goes over the base of the fifth metacarpal bone you will feel a gap between this bone and the hamate bone at SI 4.
c) Run your finger from SI 4 towards the gap formed by the triquetral bone and the styloid process of the ulna bone, at the wrist flexure. SI 5 lies in this gap.
d) If you were to draw the channel from SI 1 to the wrist flexure, SI 1, SI 2 and SI 3 are relatively straight, but if you were to draw SI 4 you will see a gradual rise in the channel. SI 5 is higher than SI 4 as the channel has to rise towards SI 6 which is on the upper border of the tendon of the extensor carpi ulnaris muscle.

Soulié (1994) locates SI 5 on the wrist, ulnar edge (on the lateral line of the little finger): in the angle between the inferior edge (towards the fingers) of the dorsal prominence of the ulna and the posterior dorsal edge of the large tendon (flexor carpi ulnaris muscle); in a hollow; separated from SI 6 by the ulnar prominence; two FW (Finger Width) above and dorsal to SI 4. Separated by the tendon of the flexor carpi ulnaris from TW 4. Shandong (1982) locate Yanggu in the depression of the ulnar end of the transverse crease of the back of the wrist, between the processus styloideus of the ulna and the os triquetrum. Lotan (2000) locates SI 5 at the meeting point of three bones: the triquetral, the pisiform and the ulna styloid process; At the ulnar end of the wrist crease.

The distance between the flexure of the wrist (at SI 5) and the humeroulnar joint at the elbow is measured as 12 cun.

In the pronated position, the cun measurements can be taken from the flexure of the wrist (at SI 5) and the medial side of the flexure of the elbow (transverse cubital crease), this is measured as 12 cun.

To locate SI 6 pronate the forearm, abduct and adduct the wrist.

SI 6 YANG LAO – NOURISHING THE OLD

⊥ ***0.3 CUN*** Δ ***3 TO 5***

- ACCUMULATION/Xi Cleft/Gueki

Pos: Position of patient: Supine with the arm pronated. The traditional location has the palmar surface of the hand placed on the chest.

Loc:
a) On the posteromedial surface of the forearm.
b) Just proximal to the flare of the head of the ulna.
c) Between the tendon of the extensor carpi ulnaris muscle and the groove on the medial surface of the head of the ulna. This groove terminates proximal to the head of the ulna as it passes between the head and the styloid process.
d) With the forearm in the pronated position, the tendon of the extensor carpi ulnaris muscle lies in this groove.
e) With the forearm pronated the relative position of the point is between the upper border of the tendon of the extensor carpi ulnaris muscle and the groove in the ulna.
f) Approximately 1 cun proximal to SI 5 (flexure of the wrist), but the anatomy must be prioritised.
g) Traditional location: Just proximal and radial to the prominence of the styloid process of the ulna.

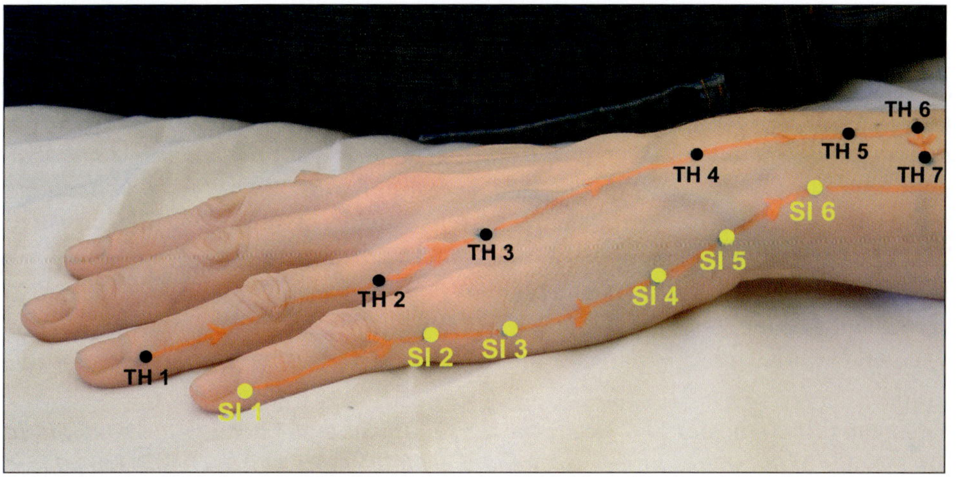

Tip:
a) With the forearm pronated, run your finger with the flow of the channel from SI 3 towards SI 5 (at the wrist flexure) and on to the posteromedial surface of the ulna, this will help you with the location of this point.
b) Moving towards the elbow from the wrist flexure, palpate the head of the ulna, passing over the prominence to where the bone begins to flare (proximal to the head of the ulna), you should be able to feel the groove on the medial surface of the bone.
c) To demonstrate the tendon of the extensor carpi ulnaris muscle, adduct and abduct the hand. You will be able to feel the tendon move as it passes across the surface of the head of the ulna.
d) With the adduction and abduction of the hand you should be able to feel the tendon of the extensor carpi ulnaris muscle within the groove on the medial surface of the ulna.
e) If you place your finger in the groove on the medial surface of the head of the ulna and palpate between the upper and lower margins of the groove, you should be able to feel the tendon of the extensor carpi ulnaris muscle move like a guitar string. This point lies between the upper border of this tendon and the upper margin of the groove in the ulna when the forearm is in the pronated position.
f) The traditional location for SI 6 is best located by feeling for the gap between the styloid process of the ulna bone and the triquetral bone, in the locality of SI 5.
g) Then go towards the median line of the posterior articulation of the wrist, making sure you are still in this gap between the two bones then you should feel a wider gap appear, this is because you have passed the tip of the styloid process of the ulna bone, the point is located in this larger gap.
h) You need to make sure that you do not go far towards the posterior median line, otherwise you may be in the locality of TH 4.

Note: Over many years there have been many locations and confusions as to where this point lies, the traditional location being just proximal and radial to the prominence of the styloid process of the ulna when the hand is facing or the palmar surface of the hand is placed on the chest. In this description when you draw in the channel from SI 5 to SI 6 to SI 7 there is a definite 'kink' in the flow, whereas the above location makes the channel a smoother flow as it does not have to cross any bone or tendon, it follows the seam formed by the ulna bone and the tendon of the extensor carpi ulnaris muscle. Worsley (1982) locates II 6 on the ulna surface of the forearm, 1 ACI (Anatomical Chinese Inch) proximal to II 5, just proximal to the head of the ulna. Lu (1973) in a diagram locates this point proximal to the head of the ulna. Jayasuriya (1982) has two locations for SI 6, the first is on the lateral aspect of the styloid process of the ulna, and the second is on the back of the wrist, proximal to the inferior radio-ulnar joint.

Deadman (1998) locates SI 6 on the the dorsal aspect of the head of the ulna and radial to the prominence of the styloid process of the ulna with the hand on the chest. Eachou (1995) locates SI 6 with the elbow flexed and the palm of the hand facing the chest, on the radial side of the styloid process of the ulna, 1 inch above the dorsal skin crease of the wrist. Voisin (1974) locates SI 6 on the forearm, dorsum, ulnar border, 1.5 fb (finger breadth) proximal to the dorsiflexion fold. Soulié (1994) locates SI 6 on the lower forearm: palm up (in supination); ulnar edge; two FW (Finger Width) above the wrist. A little above the head of the ulna; between the anterior edge of the ulna and the flexor carpi ulnaris muscle. In the angle between the flexor carpi ulnaris and the inferior edge of a transverse mass; in a hollow; separated by the ulnar prominence from SI 5; two large FW below SI 7; one FW superior and medial to TW 6.

Shandong (1982) locate Yangliao with the elbow flexed and the palm against the chest, the point is on the nony cleft on the radial side of the processus styloideus of the ulna. Legge (1999) locates SI 6 with the palm facing the chest, the point is found on the radial side of the styloid process of the ulna. Lotan (2000) locates SI 6, when the palm rests on the breast, in the depression, radial to the ulna styloid tip.

SI 7 lies on the posterior surface of the forearm.
Locate SI 7 with the forearm pronated:

SI 7 ZHI ZHENG – UPRIGHT BRANCH

⊥ ***0.3 TO 0.5 CUN*** **Δ *3***

- JUNCTION/Luo/Connecting/Passage/Lo/Lê
- RE-UNION/Crossing/Meeting Point of the Small Intestine Channel with the Heart Channel – Hand Tai Yang Channel with the Hand Shao Yin Channel
- GREATER INFLUENTIAL /Greater Assembling Point of the Head and Neck
- HOST/GUEST COMBINATION – Source Point with the Junction Point of its Paired Official/Organ Therefore SI 7 is combined with Ht 7

Pos: Position of patient: Supine with the forearm pronated.

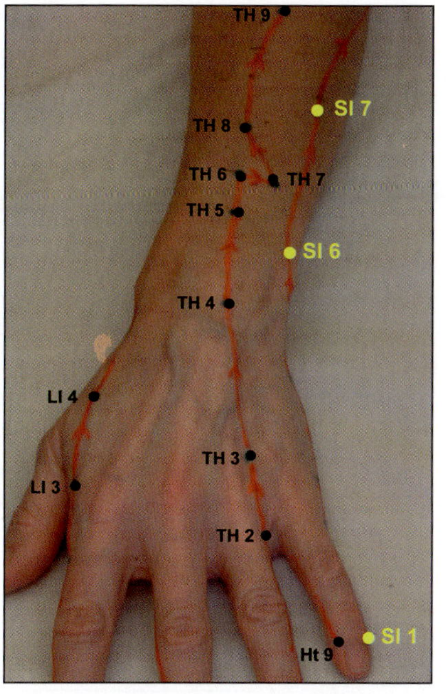

Loc:
a) On the posterior surface of the forearm.
b) On the posterior border of the extensor carpi ulnaris muscle.
c) On the ulna bone.
c) 5 cun proximal to SI 5 (flexure of the wrist).
d) On the line connecting SI 5 with SI 8

Tip:
a) The distance between SI 5 and the lateral side of the flexure of the elbow (transverse cubital crease) is 12 cun, this point is 5 cun proximal to SI 5.
b) With the patients forearm in a pronated position run your finger along from the head of the ulna bone and the posterior border of the extensor carpi ulnaris muscle (SI 6), you should be able to feel a seam as you run your finger along the posterior surface of the forearm towards the elbow, and see that this point is located just on the posterior surface of the forearm, on the ulna bone and at the posterior border of the extensor carpi ulnaris muscle at approximately 5 cun proximal to SI 5 (flexure of the wrist).
c) If you were to rotate the forearm and hand so that the first and second digits were uppermost the point you have located should disappear towards the medial aspect of the forearm when you look at the arm from the fingers to the elbow (end on).
d) To expose the extensor carpi ulnaris muscle, flex and extend the wrist.

Second Common Location:

Pos: Position of patient: Supine or seated with the elbow fully flexed and the forearm rotated so that the fifth digit is in line with the olecranon.

Loc:
a) On the ulnar aspect of the forearm.
b) Between the muscle of the flexor carpi ulnaris and the ulna bone.
c) 5 cun proximal to the flexure of the wrist (at SI 5).
d) On a line between SI 5 and SI 8.

Tip:
a) The distance between SI 5 and the tip of the olecranon of the elbow (transverse cubital crease) is 12 cun, this point is 5 cun proximal to SI 5.
b) With the patients forearm fully flexed and rotated in a position so that the fifth digit is in line with the tip of the olecranon, run your finger along the seam of the border of the flexor carpi ulnaris muscle and the border of the ulna bone.
c) Run your finger from SI 5 towards the elbow in this rotated position and at 5 cun proximal to SI 5 you should be able to palpate for this point as the channel goes towards the humeroulnar joint.

Worsley (1982) locates II 7 on the posterior surface of the forearm, at 5 ACI (Anatomical Chinese Inch) proximal to the flexure of the wrist. With the arm extended and the forearm pronated, it lies in the seam between the ulna and the extensor carpi ulnaris. Deadman (1998) locate SI 7 between the anterior border of the ulna bone and the muscle belly of the flexor carpi ulnaris muscle with the arm either in the supine position or with their arm resting on the chest. Soulié (1994) locates SI 7 on the forearm: palm up, in supination; on the ulnar edge; four FW (Finger Width) above the wrist. Between the anterior edge of the ulna and the flexor carpi ulnaris; in the angle between the flexor carpi ulnaris and the upper edge of a transverse mass; in a hollow; two large FW proximal to SI 6; two FW distal to SI 8; separated by the flat surface of the ulna from TW 8. Many texts simply locate SI 7 on the line joining SI 5 and SI 8, and at 5 cun above SI 5. No reference to anatomy is made. Voisin (1974) locates SI 7 on the forearm, dorsum, ulnar border: midlength of ulna.

Shandong (1982) locate Zhizheng at 5 cun above the ulnar end of the transverse crease of the back of the wrist, on the line between Pt. Yanggu (SI 5) and Pt. Xiaohai (SI 8). Lotan (2000) locates SI 7, when the elbow is flexed and the palm faces the anterior (pronation), on the line connecting SI 5 with SI 8, 5 cun proximal to SI 5. He also describes an alternative location: when the palm rests on the breast, on the line connecting SI 5 with the lateral epicondyle, 5 cun proximal to the wrist crease.

To locate SI 8 on the medial aspect of the flexure of the elbow, flex the elbow with the forearm in an upright position.

SI 8 XIAO HAI – SMALL SEA

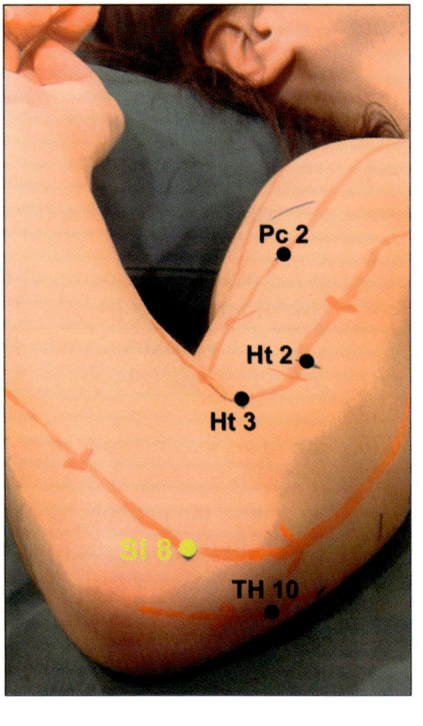

⊥ ***0.2 TO 0.3 CUN*** Δ ***3 TO 7***

- EARTH
- SEDATION/Reducing/Dispersing
- CHILD
- HE – SEA/Shu – Transporting/Antique

Pos: Position of patient: supine with the elbow flexed and the forearm in an upright position, so that the palmar surface of the hand faces anteriorly (the 'stop' position).

Loc: a) On the medial aspect of the flexure of the elbow.
b) Halfway between the olecranon of the ulna bone and the medial epicondyle of the humerus bone.
c) In the humeroulnar joint.

Tip: a) The tip of the elbow is the olecranon of the ulna. Medial to this is a prominence of bone, this is the humerus bone. These two bones form a joint called the humeroulnar joint, and the point is located in this joint.
b) Gentle palpation in the joint will make this point more accessible.
c) When you needle this point make sure that the patients arm is supported, ie. their hand and arm is not in the air. Perhaps place a pillow under the posterior surface of the hand and arm, this will make the arm more relaxed.

Note: The origin of SI 8 at 1 cun distal to the flexure of the elbow is unknown, but is possibly a Japanese location. Worsley (1982) locates II 8 on the posteromedial surface of the forearm, 1 ACI (Anatomical Chinese Inch) distal to the hollow between the medial epicondyle of the humerus and the olecranon when the forearm is semiflexed. Wu (1973) locates SI 8 upon the posterio-internal surface of the elbow, in the hollow of the cubital nerve at one-half pouce below the level of the tip of the elbow.

Soulié (1994) locates SI 8 on the mid-length of the forearm: ulnar edge; palm up, in supination. Between the anterior edge of the ulna and the flexor carpi ulnaris and the superior edge of a transverse mass; ina hollow; two FW (Finger Width) above SI 7; separated from TW 9 by the dorsal width of the bone.

SI 9-13 are found on the posterior torso, with the patient in a seated position. The locations are given relative to the shoulder joint and the scapula.

SI 9 JIAN ZHEN – UPRIGHT SHOULDER

⊥ ***0.5 TO 0.8 CUN*** **Δ *3***

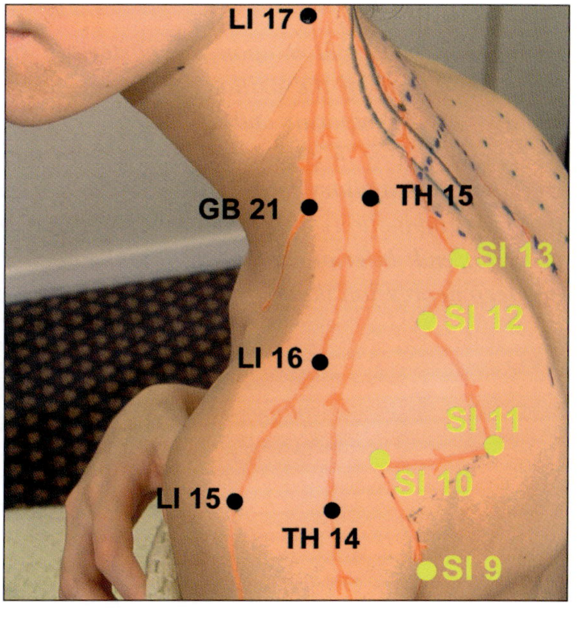

Pos: Position of patient: seated with the forearm adducted against the torso.

Loc: a) On the posterior torso.
b) On the posterior aspect of the shoulder.
c) Inferior to the shoulder joint.
d) Just inferior to the posterior border of the deltoid muscle.
e) Approximately 1 cun directly superior to the meeting point of the upper arm and the torso.

Tip:
a) Run your finger from the meeting point of the upper arm and the torso superiorly while palpating for the point. To locate the meeting point you will need to ask your patient to abduct their arm slightly. When you have located this ask them to adduct their arm again.
b) Feel for the posterior border of the deltoid muscle by asking the person to resist their arm against yours. The point lies just inferior to this border. To locate the point your patient must have their arm relaxed at their side (adducted).
c) Approximately 1 cun superior to this meeting point is where the point is located. Sometimes it maybe 1 cun superior to the posterior axillary crease and sometimes it may not, therefore the 1 cun measurement cannot always be relied upon. Palpation is the most important method of locating this point.
d) If you find there is a discrepancy between the inferior border of the deltoid muscle and the 1 cun superior to the meeting point of the upper arm and torso, palpation is of utmost importance for locating this point.

Note: There are many descriptions for this point, most use the 1 cun superior to the posterior axillary crease. One problem many have found in clinical practice is that the posterior axillary crease can vary in length according to how tight the arm is adducted against the body and also the persons size, and the result of this is that the point may be located too superiorly.

The description does not say which part of the crease the point is superior to, but in a lot of illustrations it seems to be located 1 cun superior to the superior border of the posterior axillary crease. Soulié (1994) locates SI 9 on the posterior shoulder: just under the inferior edge of the scapulohumeral articulation (glenoid fossa); in a hollow; on the superior edge of the teres minor; on the inferor edge of the infraspinatus muscle; arm towards the other side of the body; four FW (Finger Width) lateral and under SI 10; four FW below and posterior to TW 14; at the level of and medial to TW 12.

Wu (1973) locates SI 9 upon the posterior surface of the shoulder, at the height of the posterior flexure of the axilla. Worsley (1982) locates II 9 on the posterior surface of the shoulder, at the superior end of the axillary fold. Shandong (9182) locate Jianzhen with the hands close to the thighs, 1 cun above the posterior axillary fold. Legge (1999) locates SI 9 1 cun above the axillary fold. Lotan (2000) locates SI 9, when the arm lies straight alongside the body (adduction), in the depression, 1 cun superior to the armpit crease (axillary fold) posterior end; Inferior (and medial) to the deltoid; On the latissimus dorsi muscle; Search for the deep depression that can be felt inferior to a meeting of two muscles.

SI 10 NAO SHU – SHOULDER BLADE

⊥ ***0.5 TO 0.7 CUN*** Δ ***3 TO 7***

- 8 EXTRAORDINARY VESSEL/Coalescent Point of the Yang Heel/Yang Motility Vessel (Yang Qiao Mai)
- 8 EXTRAORDINARY VESSEL/Coalescent Point of Yang Linking Vessel (Yang Wei Mai)
- RE-UNION/Crossing/Meeting Point of the Small Intestine Channel with the Bladder Channel, Yang Linking Vessel and Yang Heel/Yang Motility Vessel – Hand Tai Yang Channel with the, Foot Tai Yang Channel, Yang Wei Mai and Yang Qiao Mai

Pos: Position of patient: seated with the forearm adducted against the torso.

Loc: a) On the posterior torso.
b). On the posterior aspect of the shoulder.
c) Superior to the posterior axillary crease.
d) In a depression that is just inferior to the neck of the acromion of the scapular spine.
e) Approximately 1 cun medial to TH 14 (which is at the inferolateral corner of the acromion process at the acromial angle).

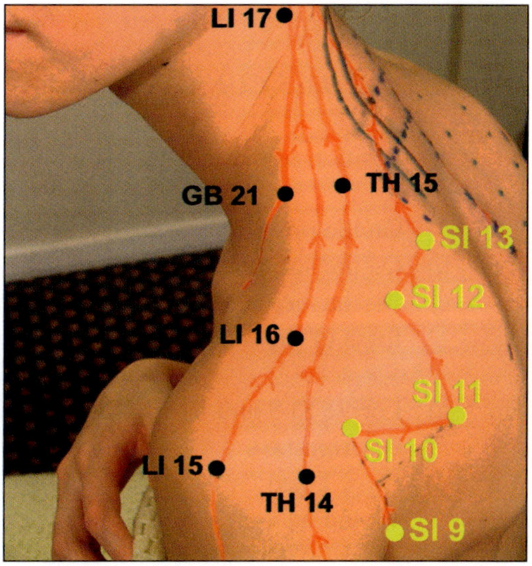

Tip: a) Run your finger from SI 9 superiorly towards the acromion and spine of the scapula. What you have to consider is the structure of the person, are they narrow shouldered or are they broad shouldered? This will determine whether your Small Intestine line is a plumb line, ie. directly superior to SI 9, or whether it goes superior and slightly lateral to SI 9. By running your finger superiorly it will naturally guide you to the neck of the acromion.
b) The neck of the acromion is narrow bone that runs laterally from the spine of the scapula and broadens to form the acromion process. SI 10 is just inferior to the neck of the acromion.
c) SI 10, TH 14 and LI 15 are located in relation to the acromion process of the scapula, SI 10 being inferior to the neck of the acromion, TH 14 is on the inferolateral corner of the the acromion process, at the acromion angle, and LI 15 is inferior to the acromion, between the acromion and the greater tuberosity of the humerus. LI 15 is the most lateral point. 1 cun posterior to this point is TH14 and 1 cun medial to TH 14 is SI 10, so these points are all approximately equidistant from each other. The acromion forms a scallop shape and these three points lie inferior to it.

Note: Soulié (1994) locates SI 10 on the posterior shoulder: just at the upper edge of the articulation of the scapula and humerus (glenoid). On the upper edge of a muscle on an angle (infraspinatus); about one FW (Finger Width) under the spine of the scapula; four FW posterior and above SI 9; two FW lateral to SI 11; two FW below and lateral to TW 15; three FW medial to TW 14.

Wu (1973) locates SI 10 below the acromion, between this and the scapulo-humeral articulation, in the prolongation of the posterior flexure of the axilla. Voisin (1974) locates SI 10 on the scapula: lower border of spine, straight below the tip of the acromion. Shandong (1982) locate Naoshu superior and slightly lateral to the point Jianzhen, at the lower border of the spine scapulae.

SI 11 TIAN ZONG – HEAVENLY ANCESTOR

⊥ ***0.3 TO 0.5 CUN*** Δ ***3 TO 7***

Pos: Position of patient: seated with the forearm relaxed against the torso.

Loc:
a) On the posterior torso.
b) On the scapula bone.
c) At the centre of the infraspinous fossa of the scapula.

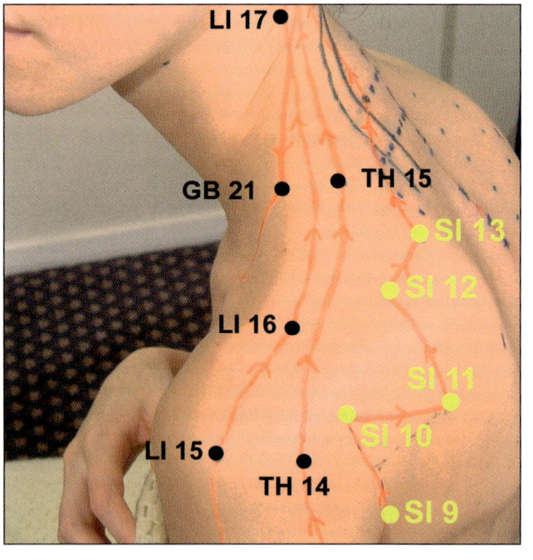

Tip:
a) Locate SI 9 and SI 10 (see separate descriptions).
b) Draw a vertical line from SI 9 to SI 10 and halve it
c) Draw a horizontal line from this half-way mark medially across the scapula, making sure your line is straight (the best way to check this is to stand back from the patient and look at the line from a distance).
e) Next mark in the medial edge of the scapula at the level of your horizontal line.
f) Lateral to the medial edge of the scapula the bone starts to thicken and become prominent to the surface of the posterior torso, you can see this on a lot of people. Where you feel the bone is at its prominence, place a mark on it.
g) So now you should have a vertical line from SI 9 to SI 10, and a horizontal line drawn on the surface of the scapula.
h) The horizontal line needs to be halved. To do this measure half-way from the horizontal line intersecting the vertical line and the mark you made on the prominence of the bone at the medial end of the scapula (not the border/edge) and draw in your mark on the horizontal line.

i) This mark gives you the place where the point can be located most laterally on the horizontal line.
j) Now you need to draw in an equilateral triangle that intersects on your horizontal line.
k) With a pair of dividers or some other means place both tips on SI 9 and SI 10
l) Then as if you were using a compass, lift the end of the dividers off SI 10 and rotate the dividers until the tip passes through the horizontal line, the other tip still being on SI 9, draw in the mark on the horizontal line.
m). Go through l) procedure again but this time lift the end of the dividers off SI 9 and rotate the dividers until the tip passes through the horizontal line, the other tip being on SI 10, draw in the mark on the horizontal line.
n) These two marks l) and m) possibly meet up, but if they do not it does not really matter, as these marks form the place where SI 11 will be located most medially on this horizontal line.
o) On the horizontal line you have marks that tell you how far medial and how far lateral the point can be located. Now you need to palpate for this point along this line with your finger.
p) The reason for this whole procedure is that there are so many places on the scapula that have depressions in them that may be mistaken for the point.

Note: Traditionally SI 11 is said to be at the junction of the upper third and the lower two thirds of a line drawn between the inferior angle of the scapula and the inferior border of the spine of the scapula. It is sometimes described as midway between the medial and lateral borders of the scapula, and occasionally on the level of the 4th thoracic vertebra.

The descriptions and illustrations of SI 11 vary enormously. The idea of SI 11 forming a triangle with SI 9 and 10 still appears in some texts. Academy of Traditional Chinese Medicine (1975), illustrates an equilateral triangle. Some other texts imply an isosceles triangle. Soulié (1994) locates SI 11 on the scapula: one FW (Finger Width) under the inferior medial prominence of the transverse angle of the spine 9of the scapula0; ina hollow; on the infraspinatus; two FW medial and under SI 10; two FW lateral to SI 12; two large FW under TW 15. Wu (1973) locates SI 11 below the thickest part of the spine of the scapula.

Voisin (1974) locates SI 11 on the scapula, infraspinous fossa: posterior border of deltoid. Worsley (1982) locates II 11 on the back, in the middle of the scapula, approximately 1.5 ACI (Anatomical Chinese Inch) inferior to the inferior edge of the middle of the scapular spine. Legge (1999) locates SI 11 at the junction of the upper and middle third of the distance between the midpoint of the scapular spine and the inferior angle of the scapula. Lotan (2000) locates SI 11 level with 1/3 distance between the scapular spine inferior border (e.g. SI 10) and the scapular edge (inferior angle), midway between the scapula's two sides (medial and lateral).

SI 12 BING FENG – GRASPING THE WIND

⊥ ***0.5 CUN*** Δ ***5 TO 7***

- RE-UNION/Crossing/Meeting Point of the Small Intestine Channel with the, Triple Heater, Large Intestines and Gall Bladder Channels – Hand Tai Yang Channel with the Hand Shao Yang, Hand Yang Ming and Foot Shao Yang Channels

Pos: Position of patient: seated with the forearm relaxed against the torso.

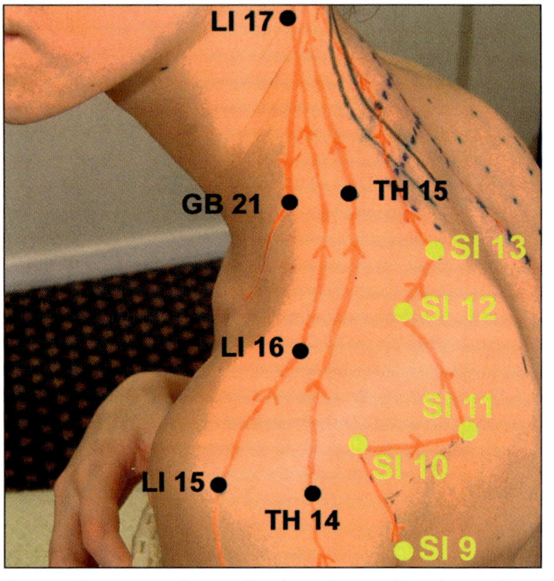

Loc: a) On the posterior torso.
b) Superior to the scapular spine.
c) In the centre of the supraspinous fossa of the scapula.
d) Directly superior to SI 11.
e) In a depression formed when the arm is raised.

Tip: a) Locate SI 11 (see separate description).
b) With your finger on SI 11 (in the infraspinous fossa),run your finger in a straight line superiorly. You should go over the scapular spine and in to the supraspinous fossa.
c) In the supraspinous fossa (hollow above the scapular spine) palpate for the point, making sure that you are not too close to the prominence of the scapular spine.
d) If you make an equilateral triangle using SI 10 and SI 11 as your measurement, this can give you the location for SI 12, or at least the area where you would locate it in the supraspinous fossa, therefore palpation is of utmost importance for this point.

Note: Academy of Traditional Chinese Medicine (1975), illustrates an equilateral triangle. Worsley (1982) locates II 12 on the back, approximately 1 ACI (Anatomical Chinese Inch) superior to the superior edge of the scapular spine ("suggesting that the point should not be too close to the scapular spine, there is no reference to the supraspinous fossa even though the point should be in it."). Soulié (1994) locates SI 12 on the scapula about mid-height: one FW (Finger Width) lateral to the medial edge; one FW medial and inferior to the inferior medial prominence of a transverse rise (spine of the scapula); on the trapezius and infraspiatus; in a hollow; two FW medial to SI 11; two FW below SI 13; at the external level of BL 43. Voisin (1974) locates SI 12 on the scapula, spine, lower border: junction between the medial 1/4 and lateral 3/4. Legge (1999) locates SI 12 in the depression superior to the midpoint of the scapular spine.

SI 13 QU YUAN – CROOKED WALL

⊥ ***0.3 TO 0.5 CUN*** Δ ***3 TO 9***

Pos: Position of patient: seated with the forearm relaxed against the torso.

Loc:
a) On the posterior torso.
b) At the medial end of the supraspinous fossa of the scapula.
c) Approximately midway between SI 10 and the spinous process of the 2nd thoracic vertebra.

Tip:
a) After measuring half-way between SI 10 (please see separate description) and the spinous process of T2 vertebra you need to palpate for the point as the half-way mark is only an approximation.
b) The location of this point should be the same distance superiorly from the scapular spine as SI 12 (please see separate description). This does not mean that the point is in a straight line horizontally but that it is parallel to the superior border of the scapular spine which commonly slopes downwards as you go to the medial border of the scapula towards the location of SI 13.
c) By following the contour of the scapular spine with your finger, you also need to take into account that you should be at the medial end of the supraspinous fossa to locate this point.
d) SI 13 is inferior to and in line with TH 15 and GB 21 (please see separate descriptions). Palpation will accurately locate the point as the description gives you the area in which to palpate.
e) If you cannot locate the spinous process of T2, please follow the following guidelines.
f) First mark out the intervertebral spaces of the thoracic vertebra.
g) To check your C7 and T1 intervertebral space, place your index finger on the prominence of the vertebra you feel may be T1 and your middle finger on the prominence of the vertebra you feel may be C7.
h) Now ask your patient to turn their head to the left and then to the right. Under your middle finger you should feel some slight movement of C7 moving, but under your index finger you should feel no rotation of T1 at all, this is because T1 is attached to a rib whereas C7 is not.
i) A common error is to visualise C7 as being more prominent than T1, Gray's (1978) states it very often can be, but T1 is usually just as prominent and sometimes more so.
j) When you have marked out the intervertebral spaces of the spine, step back and visualise from a short distance the first place that you would be able to attach a first rib to T1 vertebra. The first rib curves anteriorly and inferiorly to the inferior border of the clavicle, so T1 can seem more superior than you may realise. T1 should also be the first vertebra at the base of the neck.
k) Another check you can do is to place your finger in the angle formed on the superior aspect of the shoulder by the acromial extremity of the clavicle and the scapular

spine. From this angle with the patient relaxed run your finger across in a straight line until you meet an intervertebral space – this is the intervertebral space between T2 and T3. In a straight line in this case means following the 3D curvature of the body, not as if you were drawing on a flat piece of paper – 2D image.

l) If you run your finger from the acromial end of the scapular spine along its superior border towards the spine you should meet the intervertebral space of T3 and T4. This is not always as accurate as k) because some scapular spines on people are almost horizontal, therefore they sometimes do not slope downwards as you run your finger to the medial edge of the scapular spine.

m) Once you have located the intervertebral spaces between T1/T2 and T2/T3, palpate for the spinous process of T2 vertebra and draw a mark on the posterior median line.

n) SI 13 is located midway between the mark you made on the spinous process of T2 and SI 10 at the medial end of the supraspinous fossa of the scapula

Note: Worsley (1982) locates II 13 on the back, mid-way between II 12 and the medial border of the scapula, approximately 1 ACI (Anatomical Chinese Inch) superior to the superior edge of the scapular spine, in line with VI 15 (TH 15) and VII 21 (GB 21). Soulié (1994) locates SI 13 on the posterior shoulder: on the superior edge of the scapula; about one-third medial. On the lateral edge of a penetrating angle of the bone (coacoid notch); in the angle of the posterior edge of the muscular insertion; on the trapezius and serratus anterior; on the inferior edge of the infraspinatus; in a hollow; two FW (Finger Width) above SI 12; about four FW inferior and lateral to SI 14; two FW medial to TW 15; two FW lateral to BL 42. Voisin (1974) locates SI 13 on the scapula, upper border: scapular notch.

Wu (1973) locates SI 13 just above the spine of the scapula. Shandong (1982) locate Quyuan on the medial end of the fossa supraspinate of the scapula, at the level of processus spinosus of the 3rd vertebra thoracica. Legge (1999) locates SI 13 in the depression superior to the medial end of the scapular spine. Lotan (2000) locates SI 13 in the depression, in the supraspinous fossa medial side.

SI 14-15 are on the posterior torso.

The distance between the medial border of the scapula and the posterior line is measured as 3 cun, at the level of the 3rd thorac vertebra.

Note: There have been historical differences as to the transverse distance from the scapula to the spine. 3 cun is now the accepted measurement, although some schools use 4 ACI (Anatomical Chinese Inch).

SI 14 JIAN WAI SHU – OUTSIDE THE SHOULDER CORRESPONDNCE

⊥ ***0.3 TO 0.5 CUN*** Δ ***3***

Pos: Position of patient: seated with the forearm relaxed against the torso.

a) On the posterior torso.
b) Level with the intervertebral space between T1 and T2 vertebra.
c) 3 cun lateral to the posterior median line.
d) Level with Du 13 (which is on the posterior median line in the depression formed by the intervertebral space between T1 and T2 vertebra).

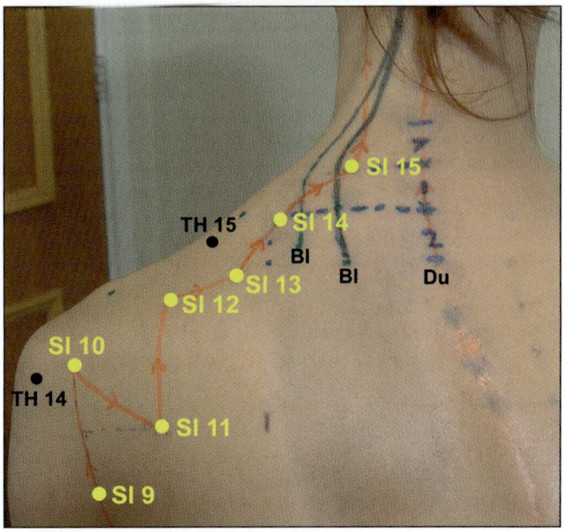

Tip: a) To locate the intervertebral spaces of the upper thoracic vertebra you can use the following landmarks:
b) First mark out the intervertebral spaces of the thoracic vertebra.
c) To check your C7 and T1 intervertebral space, place your index finger on the prominence of the vertebra you feel may be T1 and your middle finger on the prominence of the vertebra you feel may be C7.
d) Now ask your patient to turn their head to the left and then to the right. Under your middle finger you should feel some slight movement of C7 moving, but under your index finger you should feel no rotation of T1 at all, this is because T1 is attached to a rib whereas C7 is not.
e) A common error is to visualise C7 as being more prominent than T1, Gray's (1978) states it very often can be, but is usually just as prominent and sometimes more so.
f) When you have marked out the intervertebral spaces of the spine, step back and visualise from a short distance the first place that you would be able to attach a first rib to T1 vertebra. The first rib curves anteriorly and inferiorly to the inferior border of the clavicle, so T1 can seem more superior than you may realise. T1 should also be the first vertebra at the base of the neck.
g) Another check you can do is to place your finger in the angle formed on the superior aspect of the shoulder by the acromial extremity of the clavicle and the scapular spine. From this angle with the patient relaxed run your finger across in a straight line until you meet an intervertebral space – this is the intervertebral space between T2 and T3. In a straight line in this case means following the 3D curvature of the body, not as if you were drawing on a flat piece of paper – 2D image.

h) If you run your finger from the acromial end of the scapular spine along its superior border towards the spine you should meet the intervertebral space of T3 and T4. This is not always as accurate as f) because some scapula spines on people are almost horizontal, therefore they sometimes do not slope downwards as you run your finger to the medial edge of the scapular spine.
i) The distance between the medial border of the scapula and the posterior median line is measured as 3 cun, at the level of the 3rd thoracic vertebra.
j) Draw a horizontal line from the posterior median line laterally and draw a vertical line from your 3 cun mark. You should palpate for this point where the lines intersect.

Note: Traditionally described as at the level of the lower border of the spinous process of the 1st thoracic vertebra. Wu (1973) locates SI 14 upon the back, at three and one half pouce from the median line at the height of the spinous process of the first thoracic vertebra. Worsley (1982) locates II 14 on the back, 3.5 ACI (Anatomical Chinese Inch) lateral to the tip of the spinous process of the first thoracic vertebra. Soulié (1994) locates SI 14 on the lateral base of the nape: one FW (Finger Width) under the crest of the shoulder; in the angle between the inferior edge of the first rib and the lateral edge of the vertical muscles (iliocostal and levator scapulae muscles); in a hollow; four FW inferior and medial to SI 13; two FW posterior to SI 15; one large FW superior and lateral to BL 41; two FW lateral to GV 14 (Du 14) and slightly above BL 11.

Voisin (1974) locates SI 14 on the trapezius, upper border: at the level of C7 spinous process. Shandong (1982) locate Jianwaishu at 3 cun lateral to the lower border of the processus spinosus of the 1st vertebra thoracic. Legge (1999) locates SI 14 over the bulge of the levator scapula, 3 cun lateral to the tip of the spinous process of the 1st thoracic vertebra.; Lotan (2000) locates SI 14 at 3 cun lateral to T1 spinous process inferior border.

SI 15 JIAN ZHONG SHU – MIDDLE OF THE SHOULDER CORRESPONDENCE

⊥ ***0.3 TO 0.6 CUN*** Δ ***3 TO 10***

Pos: Position of patient: seated with the forearm relaxed against the torso.

Loc: a) On the posterior torso.
b) Level with the intervertebral space between C7 and T1 vertebra.
c) 2 cun lateral to the posterior median line.
d) Level with Du 14 (which is on the posterior median line in the depression formed by the intervertebral space between C7 and T1 vertebra).

Tip: a) To locate the intervertebral spaces of the upper thoracic vertebra you can use the following landmarks:
b) First mark out the intervertebral spaces of the thoracic vertebra.
c) To check your C7 and T1 intervertebral space, place your index finger on the prominence of the vertebra you feel may be T1 and your middle finger on the prominence of the vertebra you feel may be C7.

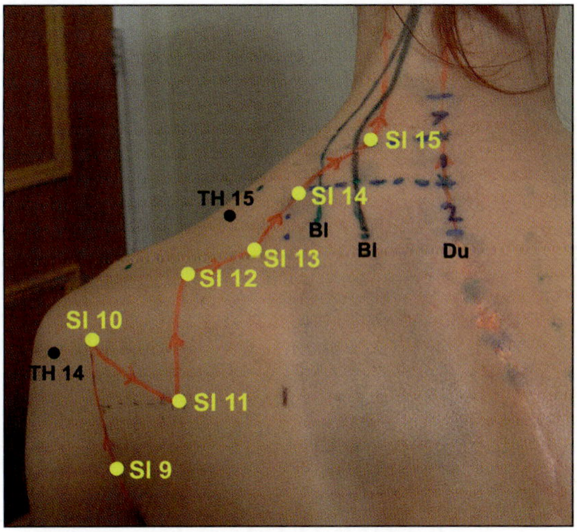

d) Now ask your patient to turn their head to the left and then to the right. Under your middle finger you should feel some slight movement of C7 moving, but under your index finger you should feel no rotation of T1 at all, this is because T1 is attached to a rib whereas C7 is not.

e) A common error is to visualise C7 as being more prominent than T1, Gray's (1978) states it very often can be, but T1 is usually just as prominent and sometimes more so.

f) When you have marked out the intervertebral spaces of the spine, step back and visualise from a short distance the first place that you would be able to attach a first rib to T1 vetrebra. The first rib curves anteriorly and inferiorly to the inferior border of the clavicle, so T1 can seem more superior than you may realise. T1 should also be the first vertebra at the base of the neck.

g) Another check you can do is to place your finger in the angle formed on the superior aspect of the shoulder by the acromial extremity of the clavicle and the scapular spine. From this angle with the patient relaxed run your finger across in a straight line until you meet an intervertebral space – this is the intervertebral space between T2 and T3. In a straight line in this case means following the 3D curvature of the body, not as if you were drawing on a flat piece of paper – 2D image.

h) If you run your finger from the acromial end of the scapular spine along its superior border towards the spine you should meet the intervertebral space of T3 and T4. This is no always as accurate as f) because some scapula spines on people are almost horizontal, therefore they sometimes do not slope downwards as you run your finger to the medial edge of the scapular spine.

i) The distance between the medial border of the scapula and the posterior median line is measured as 3 cun, at the level of the 3rd thoracic vertebra.

j) Split your 3 cun measurement in to 1 cun measurements so you have your 2 cun measurement.

k) Draw a horizontal line from the posterior median line laterally and draw a vertical line from your 2 cun mark. Where the two lines intersect gives you an area to palpate for this point.

Note: Traditionally described at the level of the lower border of the spinous process of the 7th cervical vertebra. Wu (1973) locates SI 15 upon the back, at two and one half pouce from the median line, at the height of the spinous process of the seventh cervical vertebra. Worsley (1982) locates II 15 on the back, 2.5 ACI (Anatomical Chinese Inch) lateral to the tip of the spinous process of the seventh cervical vertebra. Soulié (1994) locates SI 15 on the neck: posterolateral base; between the anterior edge of the trapezius and the posterior edge of the hard vertical muscle (scalenus posterior).

At the level of the sixth cervical vertebra; towards the trapezius and the muscles which it covers (iliocostal and levator scapulae muscles); in a hollow; two FW (Finger Width) ahead of SI 14; mid-height from SI 16; one large FW medial to GB 21. Voisin (1974) locates SI 15 on the trapezius, upper border: at the level of C6 spinous process. Shandong (1982) locate Jianzhongshu 2 cun lateral to the lower border of the 7th vertebra cervicalis. Legge (1999) locates SI 15 at 2 cunlateral to the tip of the spinous process of the 7th cervical vertebra (Du 14). Lotan (2000) locates SI 15 at 2 cun lateral to C 7 spinous process inferior border.

SI 16-17 are found on the lateral aspect of the neck, SI 18-19 are on the face.

SI 16 TIAN CHUANG – HEAVENLY WINDOW

⊥ ***0.3 TO 0.5 CUN*** **Δ 3**

- WINDOW OF THE SKY/Window of Heaven

Pos: Position of patient: supine or seated.

Loc: a) On the lateral surface of the neck.
b). On the posterior border of the sternocleidomastoid muscle.
c) On a contour with the laryngeal prominence, St 9 and LI 18.

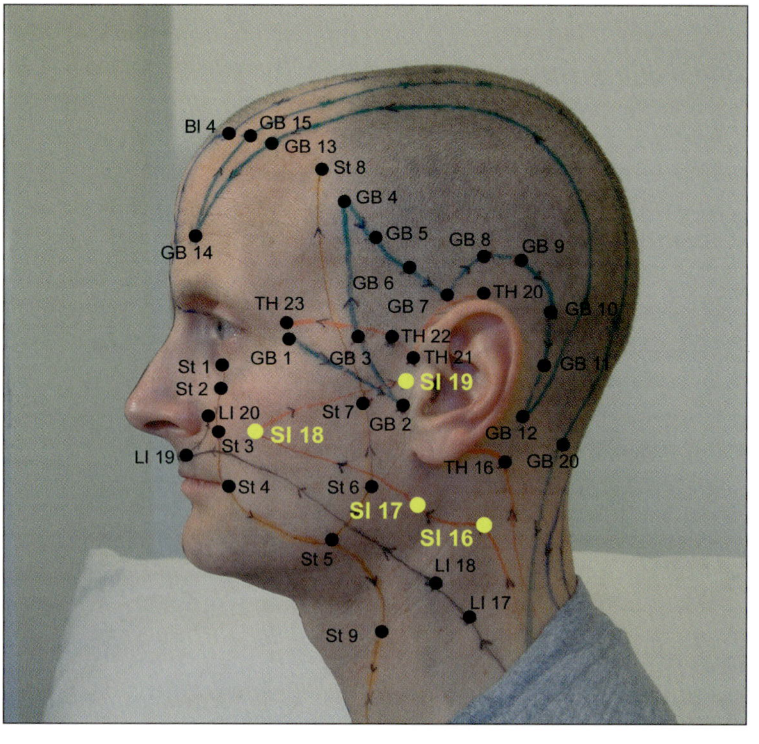

Tip: a) If your patient is supine you may need to ask them to turn their head to one side to locate and therefore to needle the point. If you locate in one position, always needle in the same position otherwise the point may move.

b) To demonstrate the posterior border of the sternocleidomastoid muscle (supine or seated) you need to place your hand on their cheek and to ask them to resist it by getting them to turn their head towards the side your hand is on, the muscle should now be exposed on the opposite side your hand is on.

c) Place your finger on the posterior border of the sternocleidomastoid still under resistance (as in b) and then ask them to relax again. You will feel the muscle relax but you should be able to feel the posterior border. Draw a mark in where you feel the posterior border of the sternocleidomastoid muscle is.

d) Next place your finger on the location of TH 16 (posterior and inferior to the mastoid process of the skull, on the posterior border of the sternocleidomastoid muscle) which is superior to the location of SI 16, then run your finger down from TH 16 along the posterior border of this muscle until your finger starts to feel some resistance. Where you started to feel resistance is where the point is located. The resistance is caused by the thickening or widening of the sternocleidomastoid muscle as it travels towards the clavicle and sternum.

e) Palpation is of utmost importance for the accurate location of this point.

f) Imagine you were to place a choker chain around the persons neck and to let it flop naturally, it would create a natural contour. This would give you a good idea of a contour that exists from the laryngeal prominence through St 9, LI 18 and to SI 16. (Please see separate locations for St 9 and LI 18.)

g) Traditionally level with the laryngeal prominence, but the most common error when locating SI 16, LI 18 and St 9 is that practitioners draw a straight line from the prominence, not taking in to context that the neck is a 3D structure. If a straight line were drawn man of these points would be located too inferior to where they should be.

h) In some cases a line drawn parallel to the contour of the jaw line at the level of the laryngeal prominence has been used but this is not necessarily accurate.

Note: Soulié (1994) locates SI 16 on the lateral side of the neck: three FW (Finger Width) under the prominence behind the ear (mastoid process); in the angle between the posterior edge of the large muscle on an angle towards the front (sternocleidomastoid), and deep, the splenius of the neck, and the inferior and posterior edge of a small round prominence of a deep transverse relief (lateral transverse process of the second cervical vertebra, the axis); in a hollow; two FW inferior and posterior to SI 17; about four FW superior to SI 15; one FW inferior and anterior to TW 16; two FW above LI 17; three FW below TW 17. Wu (1973 locates SI 16 upon the lateral surface of the neck in the hollow below and behind CO 18.

Voisin (1974) locates SI 16 on the sternocleidomastoid, posterior border: behind and below the angle of the mandible. Shandong (1982) locate Tianchuang at 3.5 cun lateral to the laryngeal cartilage, on the posterior border of the m. sterno-cleidomastoideus, 0.5 cun posterior to the Pt. Neck-Futu (LI 18).

SI 17 TIAN RONG – HEAVENLY APPEARANCE

⊥ ***0.3 TO 0.5 CUN*** **Δ** ***3 TO 5***

- WINDOW OF THE SKY/Window of Heaven

Pos: Position of patient: Supine or seated.

Loc: a) On the lateral surface of the neck.
b) On the anterior border of the sternocleidomastoid muscle.
c) Posterior to the angle of the mandible.

Tip: a) To demonstrate the anterior border of the sternocleidomastoid muscle, if the patient is in a seated position, place your palm on the patients forehead and ask them to resist your hand. If in the supine position ask your patient to lift their head slightly off the surface of the pillow. Ask your patient to relax after you have felt for the muscle as you should locate and needle this point with them in a relaxed position. When the patient is relaxed, draw in the anterior border of the sternocleidomastoid muscle.
b) Next with your finger, place it posterior to the angle of the mandible of the jaw near to the ear, then draw the angle in.
c) Then feel for the anterior border of the sternocleidomastoid muscle and draw this in.
d) Between the angle of the mandible (posterior border) and the sternocleidomastoid muscle (anterior border) you will need to palpate for this point.

Note: Wu (1973) locates SI 17 upon the posterior edge of the ramus of the mandible, in a notch in the bone a little above the gonion. Worsley (1982) locates II 17 on the posterior edge of the mandible, in the notch of the bone, slightly superior to the angle of the mandible. Soulié (1994) locates SI 17 on the upper lateral neck; a little behind the posterior, inferior angle of the maxilla; in the angle between the anterior edge of the prominence of the mastoid and the insertion on it of the sternocleidomastoideus; in a hollow; two FW (Finger Width) superior and anterior to SI 16; one FW under TW.17; two FW behind LI 18.

SI 18 QUAN LIAO – CHEEK-BONE

⊥ ***0.3 TO 0.5 CUN*** ***Δ FORBIDDEN TO MOXA***

- RE-UNION/Crossing/Meeting Point of the Small Intestine Channel with the Triple Heater and Gall Bladder Channels – Hand Tai Yang Channel with the Hand Shao Yang and Foot Shao Yang Channels

Pos: Position of patient: supine.

Loc: a) On the face.
b) On the cheek.
c) Directly inferior to the lateral canthus of the eye.
d) In the angle formed by the anterior border of the ramus of the mandible and inferior border of the zygomatic arch of the zygomatic bone.

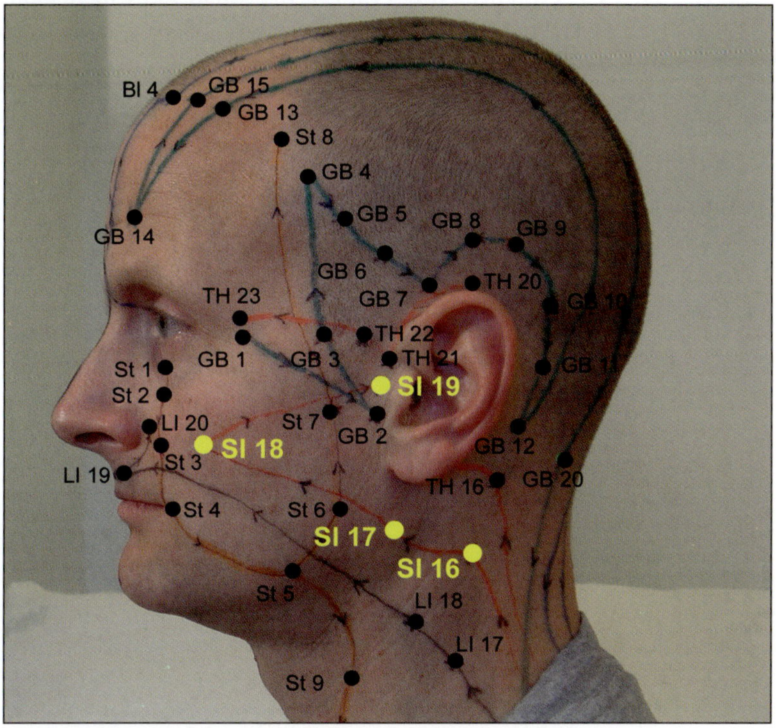

Tip: a) Draw a vertical line down from the lateral canthus of the eye.
b) With your finger running down from the lateral canthus of the eye with you will eventually go over the inferior border of the zygomatic bone. The zygomatic arch is the rounded contour of the zygomatic (cheek) bone.
c) With the mouth partially opening and closing press the hollow of the cheek with your finger and run it superiorly to the inferior border of the zygomatic bone and then go posteriorly until you come to an obstruction, this is the anterior border of the ramus of the of the mandible bone. An angle is formed by these two bones where you cannot go any more superior or posterior with your finger. The point is in this angle.

Note: Soulié (1994) locates SI 18 on the cheek: on the anterior edge of the lobe, at the point where it is attached to the cheek; a bit under the lower bulge of the ear; about two FW (Finger Width) above SI 17; about one FW under TW 21; one FW in front of GB 2. Wu (1973) locates SI 18 upon the face, in the angle formed by the anterior surface of the ramus of the mandible and the inferior edge of the malleus. Shandong (1982) locate Quanliao in the centre of the lower border of the os zygomaticum at the level of Pt. Yingxiang (LI 20), directly below the lateral canthus of the eye. Legge (1999) locates SI 18 directly below the outer corner of the eye, in the depression on the lower border of the zygomatic bone, level with LI 20.

SI 19 TING GONG – LISTENING PALACE

⊥ ***0.2 TO 0.3 CUN*** Δ ***3 TO 5***

- EXIT
- RE-UNION/Crossing/Meeting Point of the Small Intestine Channel with the Triple Heater and Gall Bladder Channels – Hand Tai Yang Channel with the Hand Shao Yang and Foot Shao Yang Channels

Pos: Position of patient: supine.

Loc: a) On the lateral aspect of the face.
b) Anterior to the ear.
c) Anterior to the middle of the tragus of the ear.
d) Posterior to the condyle of the mandible bone.
e) This point lies inferior to TH 21 and superior to GB 2.

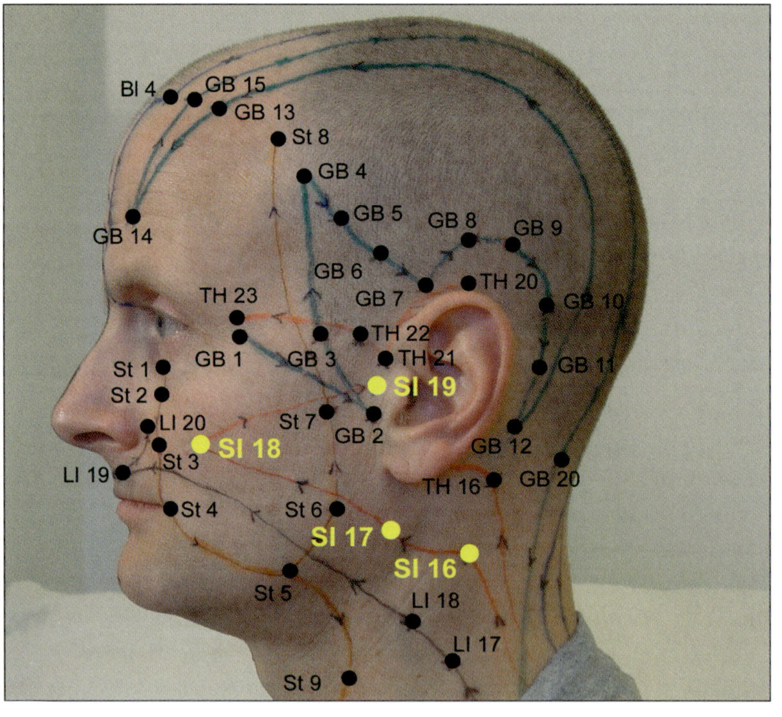

Tip: a) This point is located with the mouth open as the movement of the condyle of the mandible reveals a depression where you would locate SI 19.
b) Make sure you are locating this point level with the middle of the tragus of the ear otherwise you could drift to GB 2 (directly inferior SI 19) or TH 21 (superior to SI 19).
c) If there are two pointed prominences on the tragus you need to use the most superior one as a reference for this point.
d) Perhaps draw a line out from the middle of the tragus of the ear to give you your level, then palpate and needle the point with the mouth open.

Note: Soulié (1994) locates SI 19 on the cheek; in the angle between the anterior edge of the vertical branch of the lower jaw and the superior edge of the large oblique muscle (masseter muscle); about three FW above the inferior edge of the maxilla; preceding point: SI 18, on the lobe; one FW (Finger Width) behind TW 21. Worsley (1982) locates II 19 anterior to the tragus of the ear, on the superficial temporal artery, in the depression formed when the mouth is open. Shandong (1982) locate Tinggong anterior to the helix in the depression posterior to the art. temperomandilaris when opening the mouth. Legge (1999) locates SI 19 in the depression formed between the tragus of the ear and the tepero-mandibular joint when the mouth is slightly open. Lotan (2000) locates SI 19, when the mouth is open, level with the tragus centre, between the tragus and the condylar process.

REFERENCES FOR THE SMALL INTESTINE CHANNEL

Lawson-Wood, D&J 1973 Acupuncture Handbook – II 3: 24

De la Fuye, Dr. Roger 1956 Traiteé d'Acupuncture (le Francois) – SI 3: no page number

Medicine & Health Publishers (No Author) 1980 Explanatory Book of the Newest Illustrations of Acupuncture Points, An – SI 3:15; Shang Hou Xi: 67

Shanghai College of Traditional Medicine 1981 Acupuncture – A Comprehensive Text – SI 3: 240; Shang Hou Xi (N-UE-4) : 352

Worsley, J R 1982 Traditional Chinese Acupuncture Volume 1 -Meridians and Points. II 3: 37; II 4: 37; II 6: 39; II 7: 39; II 8: 39; II 9: 41; II 11: 41; II 12: 43; II 13: 43; II 14: 43; II 15: 43; II 17: 45; II 19: 45

Soulié De Morant, George. 1994 Chinese Acupuncture – SI 4: 403; SI 5: 404; SI 6: 404; SI 7: 405; SI 8: 405; SI 9: 406; SI 10: 406; SI 11: 406; SI 12: 407; SI 13: 407; SI 14: 407; SI 15: 408; SI 16: 408; SI 17: 408; SI 18: 409; SI 19: 409

Shandong Medical College and Shandong College of Traditional Chinese Medicine 1982 Anatomical Atlas of Chinese Acupuncture Points – Hand-Wanggu (SI 4): 28; Yanggu (SI 5): 28; Yangliao (SI 6): 28; Zhizheng (SI 7): 28; Jianzhen (SI 9): 28; Naoshu (SI 10): 28; Quyuan (SI 13): 29; Jianwaishu (SI 14): 29; Jianzhongshu (SI 15): 29; Tianchuang (SI 16): 29; Quanliao (SI 18): 29; Tinggong (SI 19): 29

Legge, David 1999 Acupuncture Points and Meridians – SI 4: 47; SI 6: 47; SI 9: 48; SI 11: 48; SI 12: 48; SI 13: 48; SI 14: 48; SI 15: 48; SI 18: 48; SI 19: 49

Lotan, Alon 2000 Acupoint Location Guide – SI 4: 67: Si 5: 67; SI 7: 69; SI 9: 71; SI 11: 71; SI 13: 73; SI 14: 73; SI 15: 73; SI 19: 75

Lu, Henry C. 1973 Chinese Versions of Modern Acupuncture, The. SI 6: 44

Jayasuriya, Anton 1982 Clinical Acupuncture. SI 6: 6.2

Deadman, Peter; Al-Khafaji, Mazin; Baker, Kevin 1998 Manual of Acupuncture, An – SI 6: 236; SI 7: 238

Eachou Chen 1995 Cross-sectional Anatomy of Acupoints – SI 6: 31

Voisin, Dr. H 1974 Essentials of Acupuncture – SI 6: 82; SI 7: 82; SI 10: 82; SI 11: 82; SI 12: 82; SI 13: 82; SI 14: 82; SI 15: 82; SI 16: 82

Wu, Wei-P'ing 1973 Chinese Acupuncture – SI 8: 82; SI 9: 82; SI 10: 83: SI 11: 83; SI 13: 83; SI 14: 83; SI 15: 83; SI 16: 84; SI 17: 84; SI 18: 84

Academy of Traditional Chinese Medicine, The. 1975 – Outline of Chinese Acupuncture, An. SI 11: 136; SI 12:

Gray, H; Warwick, Roger; Williams, Peter L 1978 Gray's Anatomy 35th Edition. C7/T1 (SI 14): 236; C7/T1 (SI 15): 236

THE BLADDER CHANNEL OF THE FOOT (TAI YANG)

Primary Channel

The Bladder channel starts at the medial corner of the eye at Bl 1. From Bl 2 the channel ascends the median line to Du 24, intersecting the Gallbladder channel at GB 15, then passes through Bl points 3-6. At Bl 7 a deep branch passes to Du 20 at the vertex, then descends the posterior aspect of the head to the ear, connecting with GB 7, 8, 9, 10, 11 and 12. (Japanese tradition has it that from there it is supposed to enter the ear, as well as inside the brain, and reappear again at the top of the head.) A second branch from Bl 7 passes into the brain, links with Du 17, and emerges to meet the main channel at Bl 10.

At Bl 10 the channel splits into two main channels. The medial branch goes down the neck to Du 14/13, runs parallel to the vertebral column from Bl 11 to the sacrum, (via the kidneys and bladder), descends through the gluteal region, and ends in the popliteal fossa at Bl 40 (54). The lateral branch goes straight down along the medial border of the scapula to the buttock, passes through the gluteal region and GB 30, travels down the lateral aspect of the thigh, and rejoins the other branch at the popliteal fossa.

The channel descends the posterior and posterolateral aspects of the lower leg to the lateral malleolus, then runs along the lateral aspect of the foot to the fifth digit, ending at Bl 67. There is a connection between Bl 67 and the origin of the Kidney channel beneath the fifth digit.

At Bl 23 a deep branch enters the body cavity via the paravertebral muscles to connect with the kidney and finally link with the bladder.

Divergent Channel

After separating from the primary channel in the popliteal fossa, the divergent channel travels to a point 5 cun inferior to the sacrum, then detours into the anal region, connects with the bladder and disperses in the kidneys. Then it follows the spine and disperses in the region of the heart before emerging at the neck to rejoin the primary channel.

Connecting Channel

This leaves the primary channel at Bl 58 on the lateral aspect of the lower leg and connects with the Kidney channel.

Muscle Channel

This channel originates at the fifth digit, proceeds to bind at the lateral malleolus and then binds at the knee.

A lower branch extends below the lateral malleolus to the heel, then ascends to bind at the lateral margin of the popliteal fossa. Another branch starts at the joining of the lateral and medial heads of the gastrocnemius muscle, and ascends to bind at the medial margin of the popliteal fossa.

These two branches join in the gluteal region and continue up the side of the spine to the nape of the neck, where a branch passes inwards to the root of the tongue.

Superior to the neck, the channel binds with the occiput and passes over the head to bind at the bridge of the nose. A branch crosses the top of the eye and binds at the inferior border of the nose.

Another branch passes from the lateral margin of the posterior axillary crease to bind with LI 15 on the shoulder. Another channel crosses below the axilla and travels over the chest, emerging at the supraclavicular fossa and ascending to bind at GB 12 posterior to the ear. A further branch emerges from the supraclavicular fossa and crosses the face to a point beside the nose.

THE BLADDER CHANNEL OF THE FOOT

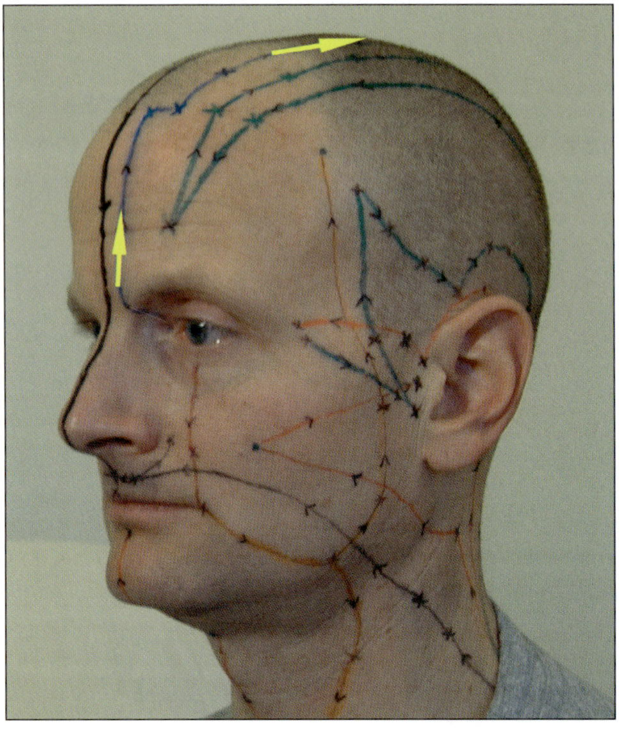

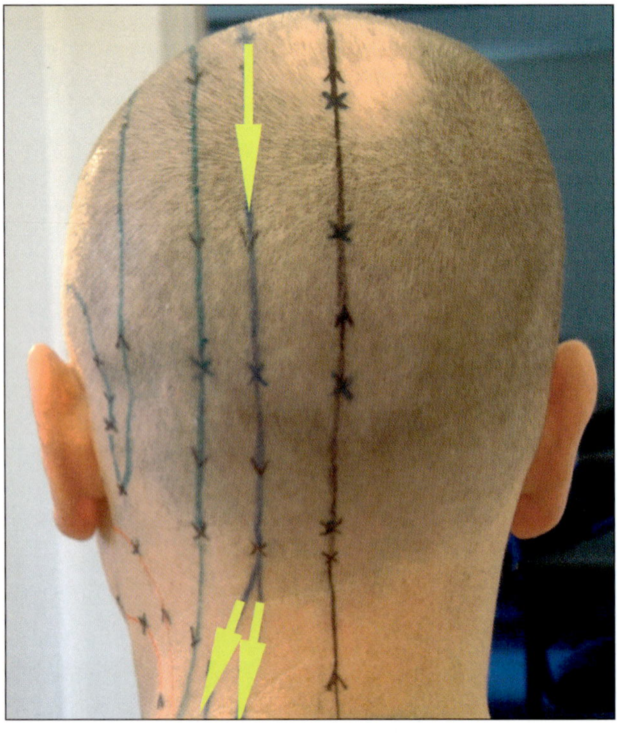

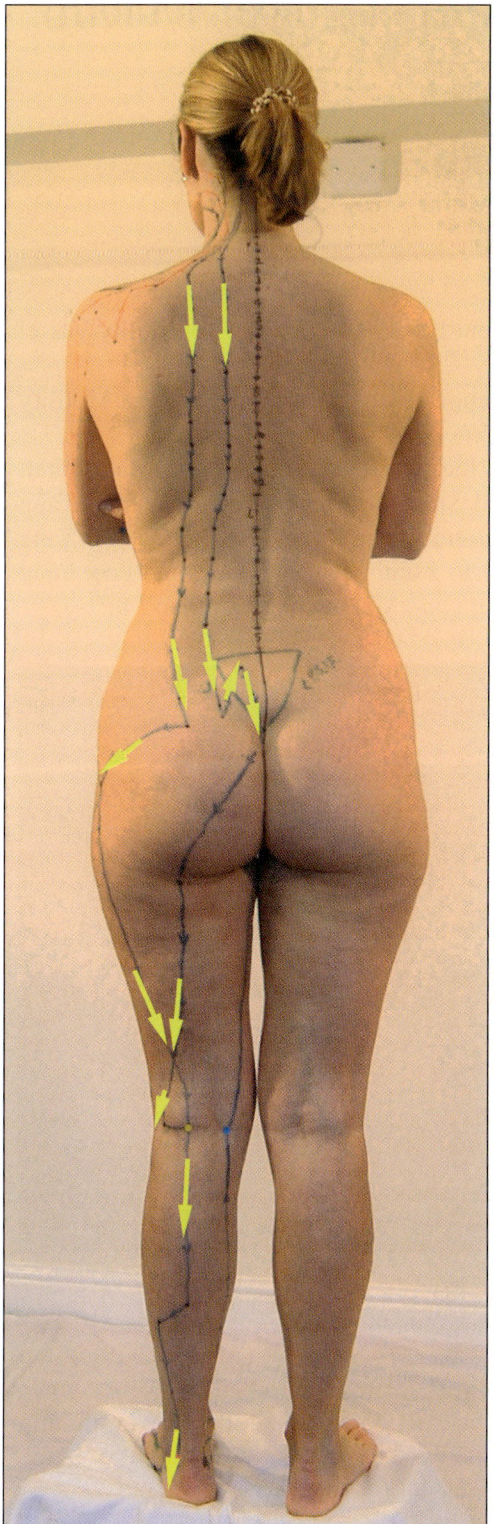

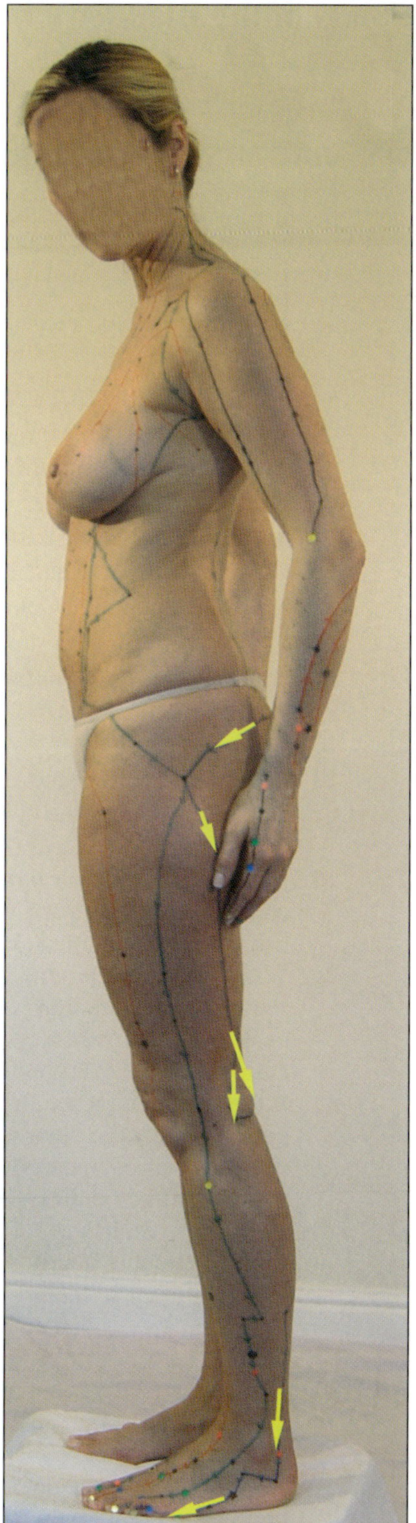

Points of the Bladder Channel – Foot Tai Yang (Bl/BL/B/UB/III)

Bl 1-2 are on the face.

Bl 1 JING MING – EYES BRIGHT

⊥ *0.3 CUN* *Δ FORBIDDEN TO USE MOXA*

- ENTRY
- 8 EXTRAORDINARY VESSEL/Coalescent Point of Yin Heel/Yin Motility Vessel (Yin Qiao Mai)
- 8 EXTRAORDINARY VESSEL/Coalescent Point of the Yang Heel/Yang Motility Vessel (Yang Qiao Mai)
- RE-UNION/Crossing/Meeting Point of the Bladder Channel with the Small Intestine, Triple Heater, Gall Bladder and Stomach Channels, the Du Mai, Yang Motility/Yang Heel Vessel and the Yin Motility/Yin Heel Vessel – Foot Tai Yang Channel with the Hand Tai Yang, Hand Shao Yang, Foot Shao Yang and Foot Yang Ming Channels, the Governor Vessel, Yang Qiao Mai and the Yin Qiao Mai

Pos: Position of patient: supine.

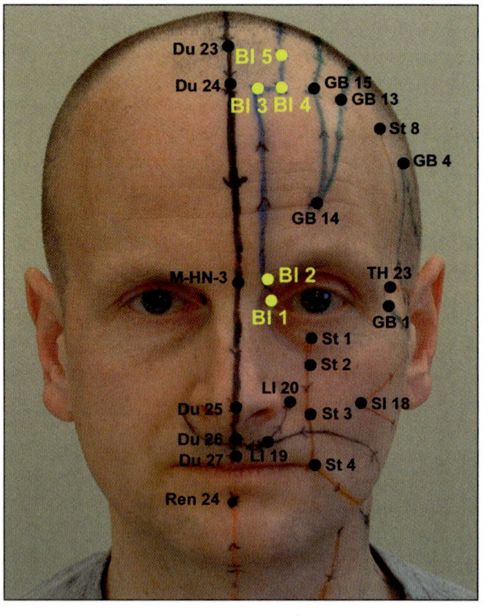

Loc: a) On the face.
b) 0.1 cun superior and medial to the medial canthus of the eye.

Tip: a) As the location of this point has a limited area in which to palpate, you will have to use your observational skills.
b) With some people you will be able to see a clear indentation with the patients eyes open, on others you will find it easier with the eyes gently closed.
c) If you still cannot see the point, ask the patient to gently open and close their eyes. The movement of their eyelids will sometimes show a depression.
d) Another possible way of locating Bl 1 is for the patient to gently close their eyes, and then to close them a little more tightly, but not scrunched up.
e) A visual depression can be revealed by getting the patient to roll their eyes keeping them either open or closed.
f) The human face has two halves, each different from the other, therefore when marking the point on each side of the face Bl 1 could possibly be in slightly different locations, but still using the medial canthus of the eye as a reference.
g) The cun measurement is 0.1 superior and medial to the medial canthus of the eye, but thisis only a guide for accurate location.

h) Some practitioners are reluctant to use this point because of the location. If the needle is angled at 15 degrees towards Bl 2 this will ensure insertion is away from the eyeball.
i) Always needle with the patients eyes closed. If you have located and then needled this point accurately your patients eyes should always water.

Note: Wu (1973) locates BL 1 in the centre of the crease within the medial canthus of the eye. Worsley (1982) locates III 1 at 1 fen superior and medial to the medial canthus of the eye, between two veins. Masayoshi (1975) locates BL 1 2 to 3 mm toward the centre from the medial angle of the eye. Voisin (1974) locates B 1 at the medial commissure of the eyelids, slightly above and medial to it. Legge (1999) locates UB 1 in the depression between the eye and the nose, 0.1 cun superior to the inner corner of the eye. Eachou (1995) locates BL 1 in the fossa 0.1 inch superior to and lateral to the medial angle of the eye. Academy (1975) locates UB 1 0.1 cun lateral and superior to the inner canthus, near the medial orbital border. Soulié (1994) locates BL 1 on the anterior cheek: one small (Finger Width) under the medial corner of the eye; on the inferior edge of the flat bulge of the orbital arch; in the angle of the the medial edge of the insertion of the elevator of the upper lip; in a hollow; lateral and superior to the levator communalis of the upper lip and the wings of the nose; three FW (Finge Width) under BL 2; one FW medial to ST 1; four FW medial to SI 19; one large FW above LI 20.

Bl 2 ZAN ZHU – COLLECT BAMBOO

⊥ ***0.2 TO 0.3 CUN*** *Δ FORBIDDEN TO USE MOXA*

Pos: Position of patient: supine.

Loc: a) On the face.
b) At the medial end of the eyebrow.
c) On the frontal bone of the skull.
d) On the upper orbital margin.
e) Superior to the medial canthus of the eye.
f) In a depression on the superciliary arch of the frontal bone of the skull.
g) In the supraorbital notch.

Tip: a) Depending on hair distribution and cosmetic influences Bl 2 may be located in the eyebrow.
b) At the medial end of the eyebrow you should be able to palpate for a notch on the upper orbital margin of the frontal bone that is superior to Bl 1 (or superior to the medial canthus of the eye).
c) The notch is called the supraorbital notch. This is on the superciliary arch of the frontal bone. The two superciliary arches give rise to the shape of the eyebrows.

Note: Soulié (1994) locates BL 2 on the eyebrows: one half FW (Finger Width) on either side of the medial line; in the angle between the lower edge of the crest of the arch of the eyebrow and the lateral edge of the suture of the nasal bone and frontal bone; one half FW in either side and a bit under M-HN-3/(Du 24.5)/Yintang; three FW above BL 1. Wu (1974) locates BL 2 upon the medial extremity of the eyebrow, at one pouce from the median line. Voisin (1974) locates B 2 on the superciliary arch, 1.5 fb (finger breadth) from the midline of the cranium.

Longitudinal bone proportional measurements of the head:

- **3 cun from between the two eyebrows (M-HN-3, Du 24.5 or Yin Tang) to the natural anterior hairline on the anterior median line.**
- **12 cun from the natural anterior hairline to the posterior hairline on the median line.**
- **3 cun from the posterior hairline to the space between the 7th cervical and 1st thoracic vertebrae (Du 14) on the posterior median line.**
- **15 cun (anterior natural hairline to the space between C7/T1);**
- **18 cun (between the two eyebrows at Du 24.5 or Yin Tang to the space between C7/T1).**

Transverse bone proportional measurements of the head:

- **(Anterior) 9 cun between the two corners of the forehead (St 8).**
- **(Posterior) 9 cun between the bilateral mastoid processes.**

It may be easier to use a length of string so that you can draw on the cun measurements as opposed to drawing the measurements on the scalp itself.

Bl 3-5 are on the anterior aspect of the head, on the frontal bone.

Note: Historically there have been differing opinions concerning the distances between Bl 3-9.

Bl 3 MEI CHONG – EYEBROWS RUSHING

⊥ ***0.3 CUN*** Δ ***3***

Pos: Position of patient: supine or seated.

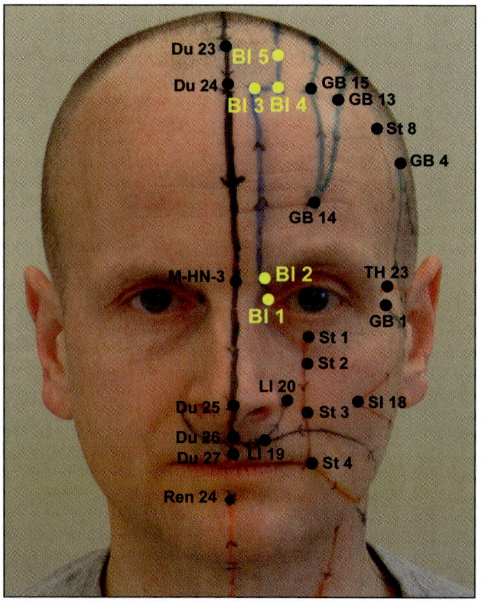

Loc:
a) On the anterior aspect of the head.
b) On the frontal bone.
c) Directly superior to Bl 2 (or the medial end of the eyebrow).
d) 0.75 cun lateral to the anterior median line.
e) 0.5 cun posterior to the natural anterior hairline.
f) Level with Du 24.
g) Between Du 24 and Bl 4.

Cun: a) First mark the median line on the anterior and posterior aspects of the head at the natural anterior and posterior hairline. Many head points are in relation to the natural hairline. The natural hairline may not be apparent due to the hairline receding. Sometimes you can see a definite change in skin texture from the forehead to the scalp, which is usually where the natural hairline was previously.

b) Measure 12 cun from the natural anterior hairline to the natural posterior hairline on the median line. It may be easier to use a length of string or strip of paper so that you can draw on the cun measurements as opposed to drawing the measurements on the scalp itself.

c) Place a mark at 0.5 cun posterior to the natural anterior hairline, Bl 3 should be located on or near to the mark. To assist with the point location palpate with the flow of the channel on the Bladder channel from the medial end of the eyebrow (Bl 2) towards the crown of the head.

d) Transverse bone proportional measurements of the head: (anterior) 9 cun between the two corners of the forehead (St 8) and (posterior) 9 cun between the bilateral mastoid processes.

Tip: a) Mark in the anterior median line and locate St 8 (see St 8 location and tips section), then divide the distance in to 3 equal measurements from the anterior median line to St 8, this will give you 3 equal divisions of 1.5 cun, then divide the 1.5 cun measurement nearest to the anterior median line in to two to give you 0.75 cun lateral to the anterior median line.

b) With your finger on the anterior median line at the natural anterior hairline, palpate laterally (0.75 cun) and posteriorly (0.5 cun) and you should feel a clear depression without having to mark out the cun measurements.

Note: Voisin (1974) locates B 3 on the frontal bone at 4 fb (finger breadth) above Bladder 2 and 1.5 fb from the midline of the cranium. Worsley (1982) locates III 3 on the head, 0.5 ACI (Anatomical Chinese Inch) superior to the natural hair line, 3.5 ACI directly superior to III 2. Wu (1973) locates BL 3 upon the forehead at one and one-half pouce from the median line, at one and one-half pouce above BL 2. Eachou (1995) locates BL 3 at 0.5 inches within the anterior hairline and above the medial border of the eyebrow, or at the midpoint between GV 24 and BL 4.

Soulié (1994) locates BL 3 on top of the forehead, one FW (Finger Width) on either side of the median line, at the posterior edge of the protruberance of the frontal bone at the average hairline (superior edge of the insertion of the frontal muscle); on the lateral edge of the median vertical rise; one FW on either side of GV 24 (Du 24); two FW in front of BL 4; two tightened FW above and medial to GB 15; three FW medial to GB 16. Lavier (1974) in an illustration locates BL 3 superior to the medial end of the eyebrow and almost transversely level with GB 14. Masayoshi (1975) locates BL 3 on the median line, 0.5 sun above the edge of the hairline.

Bl 4 QU CHAI – CROOKED SERVANT

⊥ ***0.2 TO 0.3 CUN*** Δ ***3 TO 5***

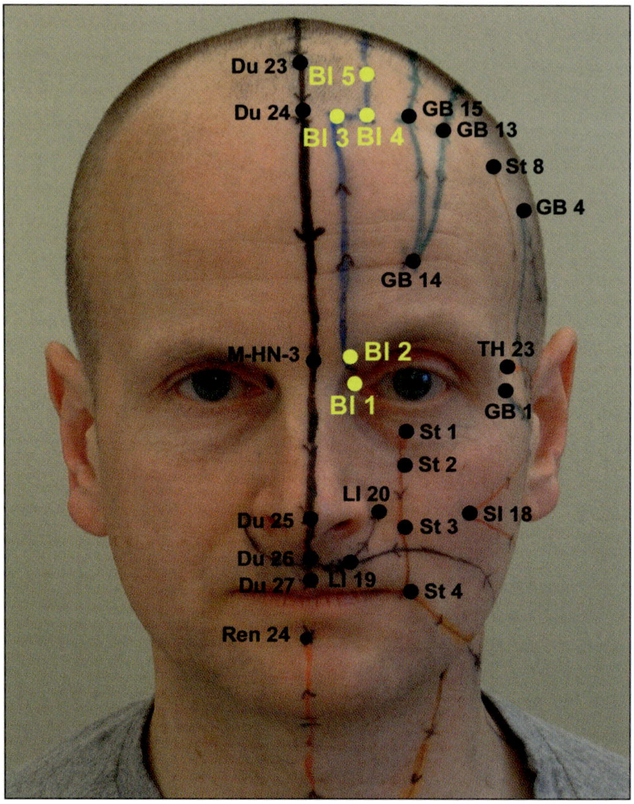

Pos: Position of patient: supine or seated.

Loc:
a) On the anterior aspect of the head.
b) On the frontal bone.
c) 1.5 cun lateral to the anterior median line (at Du 24).
d) 0.5 cun posterior to the natural anterior hairline.
e) One third of the distance lateral from Du 24 to St 8.

Cun:
a) First mark the median line on the anterior and posterior aspects of the head at the natural anterior and posterior hairline. Many head points are in relation to the natural hairline. The natural hairline may not be apparent due to the hairline receding. Sometimes you can see a definite change in skin texture from the forehead to the scalp, which is usually where the natural hairline was previously.
b) Measure 12 cun from the natural anterior hairline to the natural posterior hairline on the median line. It may be easier to use a length of string or strip of paper so that you can draw on the cun measurements as opposed to drawing the measurements on the scalp itself.
c) Transverse bone proportional measurements of the head: (anterior) 9 cun between the two corners of the forehead (St 8) and (posterior) 9 cun between the bilateral mastoid processes.
d) Mark in the anterior median line and locate St 8 (see St 8 location and tips section), then divide the distance in to 3 equal measurements from the anterior median line to St 8, this will give you 3 equal divisions of 1.5 cun.

Tip:
a) Once the cun measurements have been marked palpate for the Bl 4 at 0.5 cun posterior to the natural anterior hairline (1.5 cun lateral to the anterior median line). To assist with the point location palpate with the flow of the channel on the Bladder channel from the front of the head towards the external occipital protruberance.

b) With your finger on the anterior median line at the natural anterior hairline, palpate laterally (1.5 cun) and posteriorly (0.5 cun). You should be able to feel a clear depression without having to mark out the cun measurements. When palpating laterally from the anterior median line you should be able to palpate Bl 3 at approximately 0.75 cun. Palpate laterally the same distance again from Bl 3 (1.5 cun), until you can locate Bl 4 within the groove on the frontal bone.

Note: Wu (1973) locates BL 3 upon the cranium at one and one-half pouce from the median line and three pouce above BL 2. Voisin (1974) locates B 4 on the frontal bone, 4 fb (finger breadth) above Bladder 2 and 1.5 fb from the midline of the cranium. So (1985) locates BL 4 at 1 division lateral to GV 24 (Du 24) in the third cleft from the centre line. Lavier (1974) in an illustration locates BL 4 directly superior to BL 3 which is directly superior to BL 2, and midway between VG 24 (Du) and GB 15.

Soulié (1994) locates BL 4 on the anterior skull, about one FW (Finger Width) on either side of the medial line, two tightened FW (Finger Width) in front of the posterior (superior) edge of the frontal bone.. About mid-distance between the posterior edge of the frontal bone and the transverse rise of the upper insertion of the frontal muscle; in the angle of the lateral edge of the longitudinal rise; in a hollow; on the posterior edge of a slight flat (transverse) rise; two FW posterior to BL 3; two FW anterior to BL 5; two large FW medial and anterior to GB 16; one large FW lateral to GV 23 (Du 23). Masayoshi (1975) locates BL 4 at 1,5 sun lateral to GV 24 (Du 24). Worsley (1982) locates III 4, at 1.3 ACI (Anatomical Chinese Inch) lateral to the median line of the head, 0.5 ACI superior to the natural hairline and 0.5 ACI lateral to III 3.

Bl 5 WU CHU – FIVE PLACES

⊥ ***0.3 CUN*** ***Δ FORBIDDEN TO USE MOXA***

Pos: Position of patient: supine or seated.

Loc:
a) On the anterior aspect of the head.
b) On the frontal bone.
c) 1.5 cun lateral to the anterior median line (at Du 23).
d) 1 cun posterior to the natural anterior hairline.
e) 0.5 cun posterior to Bl 4.

Cun:
a) First mark the median line on the anterior and posterior aspects of the head at the natural anterior and posterior hairline. Many head points are in relation to the natural hairline. The natural hairline may not be apparent due to the hairline receding. Sometimes you can see a definite change in skin texture from the forehead to the scalp, which is usually where the natural hairline was previously.
b) Measure 12 cun from the natural anterior hairline to the natural posterior hairline on the median line. It may be easier to use a length of string or strip of paper so that you can draw on the cun measurements as opposed to drawing the measurements on the scalp itself.

c) Transverse bone proportional measurements of the head: (anterior) 9 cun between the two corners of the forehead (St 8) and (posterior) 9 cun between the bilateral mastoid processes.

d) Mark in the anterior median line and locate St 8 (see St 8 location and tips section), then divide the distance in to 3 equal measurements from the anterior median line to St 8, this will give you 3 equal divisions of 1.5 cun.

Tip: a) Once the cun measurements have been marked palpate for the Bl 5 at 1 cun posterior to the natural anterior hairline (1.5 cun lateral to the anterior median line). To assist with the point location palpate with the flow of the channel on the Bladder channel from Bl 4 towards the external occipital protruberance.

b) Ensure that you palpate posteriorly enough past Bl 4 at 0.5 cun towards Bl 5 at 1 cun posterior to the natural anterior hairline.

c) With your finger on the anterior median line at the natural anterior hairline, palpate laterally (1.5 cun) and posteriorly (1 cun). You should be able to feel a clear depression without having to mark out the cun measurements. When palpating laterally from the anterior median line you should be able to palpate Bl 3 at approximately 0.75 cun. Palpate laterally the same distance again from Bl 3 (0.75 cun), until you can locate Bl 4 (1.5 cun) within the groove on the frontal bone, then palpate 0.5 cun posterior to Bl 4.

Note: Wu (1973) locates BL 5 upon the cranium, at one and one-half pouce from the median line, at three and one-half pouce above BL 2. Lavier (1974) in an illustration locates BL 5 1 pouce posterior to BL 4 and on a level midway between VG 23 and VG 24 (Du). Voisin (1974) locates B 5 on the frontal bone, 5 fb (finger breadth) above Bladder 2, at 1.5 fb from the midline of the cranium. So (1985) locates this point 1 division lateral to GV 23 (Du) in the third cleft from the centre line. Masayoshi (1975) locates BL 5 at 1,5 sun lateral to GV 23 (Du). Worsley (1982) locates III 5 at 1.3 ACI (Anatomical Chinese Inch) lateral to the median line of the head, 0.5 ACI superior to III 4. Soulié (1994) locates BL 5 on the head: in the angle between the posterior edge of the parietal-frontal suture and about one large FW (Finger Width) on either side of the medial line; ina hollow; two FW posterior to BL 4; one large FW anterior to BL 6; one large FW on each side of GV 22 (Du 22); one large FW medial to GB 16,

Bl 6-8 are on the superior aspect of the head, on the parietal bone.

Bl 6 CHENG GUANG – RECEIVE LIGHT

⊥ ***0.3 CUN*** *Δ FORBIDDEN TO USE MOXA*

Pos: Position of patient: supine or seated.

Loc: a) On the top of the head.

b) On the parietal bone.

c) 1.5 cun lateral to the median line.

d) 2.5 cun posterior to the natural anterior hairline.

e) 1.5 cun posterior to Bl 5.

Cun: a) First mark the median line on the anterior and posterior aspects of the head at the natural anterior and posterior hairline. Many head points are in relation to the natural hairline. The natural hairline may not be apparent due to the hairline receding. Sometimes you can see a definite change in skin texture from the forehead to the scalp, which is usually where the natural hairline was previously.

b) Measure 12 cun from the natural anterior hairline to the natural posterior hairline on the median line. It may be easier to use a length of string or strip of paper so that you can draw on the cun measurements as opposed to drawing the measurements on the scalp itself.

c) Transverse bone proportional measurements of the head: (anterior) 9 cun between the two corners of the forehead (St 8) and (posterior) 9 cun between the bilateral mastoid processes.

d) Mark in the anterior median line and locate St 8 (see St 8 location and tips section), then divide the distance in to 3 equal measurements from the anterior median line to St 8, this will give you 3 equal divisions of 1.5 cun.

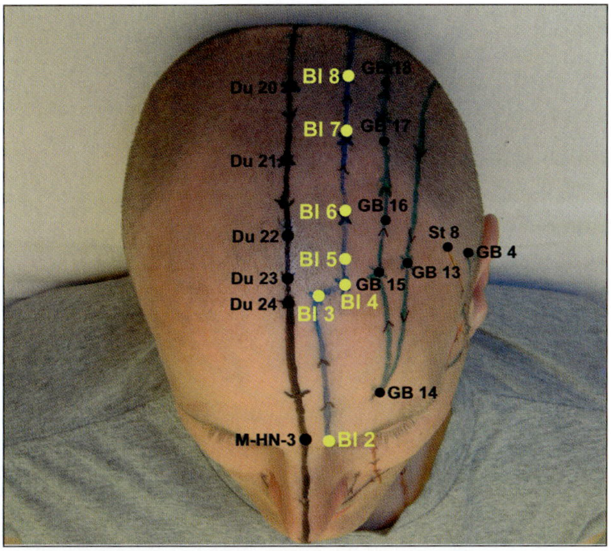

Tip: a) Once the cun measurements have been marked palpate for the Bl 6 at 2.5 cun posterior to the natural anterior hairline (1.5 cun lateral to the anterior median line). To assist with the point location palpate with the flow of the channel on the Bladder channel from Bl 4 towards the external occipital protruberance.

b) Ensure that you palpate posteriorly enough past Bl 4 at 0.5 cun and Bl 5 at 1 cun posterior to the natural anterior hairline to Bl 6 at 2.5 cun.

c) With your finger on the anterior median line at the natural anterior hairline, palpate laterally (1.5 cun) and posteriorly (2.5 cun). You should be able to feel a clear depression without having to mark out the cun measurements. When palpating laterally from the anterior median line you should be able to palpate Bl 3 at approximately 0.75 cun. Palpate laterally the same distance again from Bl 3 (0.75 cun), until you can locate Bl 4 (1.5 cun) within the groove on the frontal bone, then palpate 2 cun posterior to Bl 4.

Note: Soulié (1994) locates BL 6 on top of the head, one large FW (Finger Width) on either side of the medial line, one large FW posterior to the frontal-parietal suture and about two FW in front of the occipital-parietal suture; one large FW posterior to BL 5; one FW in front of BL 7; two FW medial to GB 17; one FW lateral and anterior to GV 21 (Du 21). Voisin (1974) locates B 6 on the parietal bone, 1 fb (finger breadth) behind the coronal suture, 1.5 fb from the midline of the cranium. Wu (1973) locates BL 6 upon the cranium, at one and one-half pouce from the median line, at four pouce above BL 2.

Shanghai (1993) locates BL 6 in the galea aponeurotica, 1.5 cun posterior to BL 5. Worsley (1982) locates III 6 at 1.3 ACI (Anatomical Chinese Inch) lateral to the median line of the head, 1.5 ACI posterior to III 5. Masayoshi (1975) locates BL 6 on the frontal region, 1.5 sun lateral to GV 22 (Du 22).

Bl 7 TONG TIAN – PENETRATE HEAVEN

⊥ ***0.3 CUN*** Δ ***3 TO 5***

Pos: Position of patient: supine or seated.

Loc:
a) On the top of the head.
b) On the parietal bone.
c) 1.5 cun lateral to the median line.
d) 4 cun posterior to the natural anterior hairline.
e) 1.5 cun posterior to Bl 6.

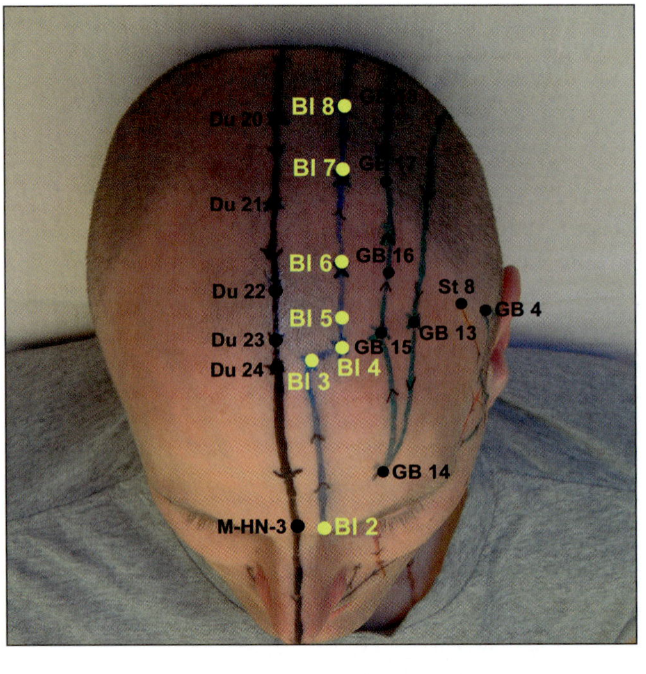

Cun: a) First mark the median line on the anterior and posterior aspects of the head at the natural anterior and posterior hairline. Many head points are in relation to the natural hairline. The natural hairline may not be apparent due to the hairline receding. Sometimes you can see a definite change in skin texture from the forehead to the scalp, which is usually where the natural hairline was previously.

b) Measure 12 cun from the natural anterior hairline to the natural posterior hairline on the median line. It may be easier to use a length of string or strip of paper so that you can draw on the cun measurements as opposed to drawing the measurements on the scalp itself.

c) Transverse bone proportional measurements of the head: (anterior) 9 cun between the two corners of the forehead (St 8) and (posterior) 9 cun between the bilateral mastoid processes.

d) Mark in the anterior median line and locate St 8 (see St 8 location and tips section), then divide the distance in to 3 equal measurements from the anterior median line to St 8, this will give you 3 equal divisions of 1.5 cun.

Tip: a) Once the cun measurements have been marked palpate for the Bl 7 at 4 cun posterior to the natural anterior hairline (1.5 cun lateral to the anterior median line). To assist with the point location palpate with the flow of the channel on the Bladder channel from Bl 4 towards the external occipital protruberance.

b) Ensure that you palpate posteriorly enough past Bl 4 at 0.5 cun, Bl 5 at 1 cun, Bl 6 at 2.5 cun posterior to the natural anterior hairline to Bl 7 at 4 cun.

c) With your finger on the anterior median line at the natural anterior hairline, palpate laterally (1.5 cun) and posteriorly (4 cun).

Note: Wu (1973) locates BL 7 upon the cranium at one and one-half pouce from the median line, at five and one-half pouce above BL 2; Voisin (1974) locates B 7 vertically above the external auditory meatus, 1.5 fb (finger breadth) from the midline of the cranium. So (1985) locates BL 7 1.5 divisions behind BL 6, which is also lateral to a point one division in front of GV 20 (Du), in the third cleft.

Shanghai (1993) locates BL 7 in the galea aponeurotica, 1.5 cun posterior to BL 6. Masayoshi (1975) locates BL 7 1.5 finger widths in front of GV 20 (Du). Soulié (1994) locates BL 7 on top of the head (vertex), one FW (Finger Width) on either side of the median line, one large FW anterior to the occipital-parietal suture, two large FW posterior to the frontal-parietal suture, in a hollow; one FW posterior to BL 6; one large FW anterior to BL 8; one FW lateral and posterior to GV 21 (Du 21); two FW medial to GB 18. Shanghai (1981) locates B 7 1 unit anterior and 1.5 units lateral to Gv 20. Worsley (1982) locates III 7 at 1.3 ACI (Anatomical Chinese Inch) lateral to the median line of the head, 1.5 ACI posterior to III 6. Lavier (1974) in an illustration locates BL 7 lateral to VG 20 (Du) and 1.5 pouce posterior to BL 6.

Bl 8 LUO QUE – LOU END

⊥ ***0.3 CUN*** Δ ***3 TO 5***

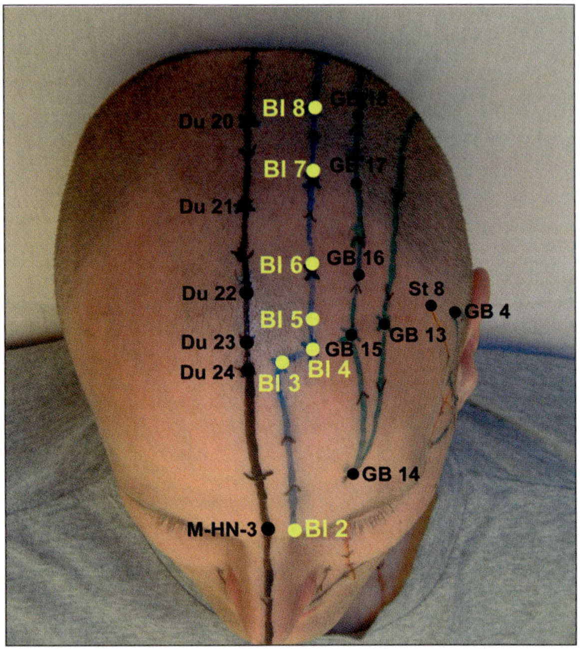

Pos: Position of patient: seated.

Loc:
a) On thetop of the head.
b) On the parietal bone.
c) 1.5 cun lateral to the median line.
d) 5.5 cun posterior to the natural anterior hairline.
e) 1.5 cun posterior to Bl 7.

Cun:
a) First mark the median line on the anterior and posterior aspects of the head at the natural anterior and posterior hairline. Many head points are in relation to the natural hairline. The natural hairline may not be apparent due to the hairline receding. Sometimes you can see a definite change in skin texture from the forehead to the scalp, which is usually where the natural hairline was previously.
b) Measure 12 cun from the natural anterior hairline to the natural posterior hairline on the median line. It may be easier to use a length of string or strip of paper so that you can draw on the cun measurements as opposed to drawing the measurements on the scalp itself.
c) Transverse bone proportional measurements of the head: (anterior) 9 cun between the two corners of the forehead (St 8) and (posterior) 9 cun between the bilateral mastoid processes.
d) Mark in the anterior median line and locate St 8 (see St 8 location and tips section), then divide the distance in to 3 equal measurements from the anterior median line to St 8, this will give you 3 equal divisions of 1.5 cun.

Tip:
a) Once the cun measurements have been marked palpate for the Bl 8 at 5.5 cun posterior to the natural anterior hairline (1.5 cun lateral to the anterior median line). To assist with the point location palpate with the flow of the channel on the Bladder channel from Bl 4 towards the external occipital protruberance.
b) Ensure that you palpate posteriorly enough past Bl 4 at 0.5 cun, Bl 5 at 1 cun, Bl 6 at 2.5 cun, Bl 7 at 4 cun posterior to the natural anterior hairline to 1.5 cun posterior to Bl 7.
c) With your finger on the anterior median line at the natural anterior hairline, palpate laterally (1.5 cun) and posteriorly (5.5 cun).

Note: Lavier (1974) locates BL 8 on a level to and lateral toVG 19 (Du). Wu (1973) locates BL 8 upon the cranium at one and one-half pouce from the median line, at seven pouce above BL 2. Voisin (1974) locates B 8 on the lamboid suture, 1.5 fb (finger breadth) from the midline of the cranium. Worsley (1982) locates III 8 at 1.3 ACI (Anatomical Chinese Inch) lateral to the median line of the head, 1.5 ACI inferior to III 7. Masayoshi (1975) locates BL 8 1.5 finger width lateral to the upper 0.25 median line of the occipital region.

Soulié (1994) locates BL 8 on the summit of the head, posterior and a little lateral, one large FW (Finger Width) to each side of the median line. Just anterior to the occipital-parietal suture, on the parietal bone, on the medial edge of a small bony protruberance; in a hollow; one large FW posterior to BL 7; one large FW on each side of GV 20 (Du 20); two large FW medial to GB 18. So (1985) locates BL 8 1.5 divisions behind BL 7, which is also lateral to a point 0.5 division behind GV 20 (Du), in the third cleft.

Bl 9 is on the posterior aspect of the head, on the occipital bone.

Bl 9 YU ZHEN – JADE PILLOW

⊥ ***0.2 TO 0.3 CUN*** Δ ***3 TO 5***

Pos: Position of patient: seated.

Loc:
a) On the posterior aspect of the head.
b) On the occipital bone.
c) On the level of the superior border of the external occipital protruberance of the occipital bone, Du 17 and GB 19.
d) 1.3 cun lateral to the posterior median line.
e) 9.5 cun posterior to the natural anterior hairline.
f) 2.5 cun superior to the natural posterior hairline

Cun:
a) First mark the median line on the anterior and posterior aspects of the head at the natural anterior and posterior hairline. Many head points are in relation to the natural hairline. The natural hairline may not be apparent due to the hairline receding. Sometimes you can see a definite change in skin texture from the forehead to the scalp, which is usually where the natural hairline was previously.
b) Measure 12 cun from the natural anterior hairline to the natural posterior hairline on the median line. It may be easier to use a length of string or strip of paper so that you can draw on the cun measurements as opposed to drawing the measurements on the scalp itself.
c) Transverse bone proportional measurements of the head: (anterior) 9 cun between the two corners of the forehead (St 8) and (posterior) 9 cun between the bilateral mastoid processes.
d) Mark in the anterior median line and locate St 8 (see St 8 location and tips section), then divide the distance in to 3 equal measurements from the anterior median line to St 8, this will give you 3 equal divisions of 1.5 cun.

Tip: a) First mark the median line on the anterior and posterior aspects of the head at the natural anterior and posterior hairline. Many head points are in relation to the natural hairline. The natural hairline may not be apparent due to the hairline receding. Sometimes you can see a definite change in skin texture from the forehead to the scalp, which is usually where the natural hairline was previously.

b) With your finger on the posterior median line at the natural posterior hairline run your finger superiorly on to the occipital bone. Continue to run your finger superiorly until you come to a bump lnown as the external occipital protruberance.

c) Du 17 is located at the superior border of the external occipital protruberance on the posterior median line. Du 17 can be palpated with relative ease. With your finger on Du 17 palpate laterally until you can a depression which is Bl 9 (just over 1 cun lateral to the posterior median line).

d) Locate Bl 9 by measuring 12 cun from the natural anterior hairline to the natural posterior hairline on the median line. It may be easier to use a length of string or strip of paper so that you can draw on the cun measurements as opposed to drawing the measurements on the scalp.

e) Alternatively place the flat of your finger in between the two muscles of the trapezius on the neck (the muscles eventually partly insert in to the external occipital protruberance of the occipital bone). Half way between the two trapezius muscles on the neck mark the posterior median line.

f) Once you have drawn in the cun measurements you will then be able to palpate for Bl 9 at 2.5 cun superior to the natural posterior hairline (1.3 cun lateral to the posterior median line).

g) Bl 9 is 9.5 cun posterior to the natural anterior hairline or 2.5 cun superior to the natural posterior hairline (1.5 cun lateral to the anterior median line). To assist with the point location palpate with the flow of the channel on the Bladder channel from Bl 4 towards the external occipital protruberance.

h) Ensure that you palpate posteriorly enough past Bl 4 at 0.5 cun, Bl 5 at 1 cun, Bl 6 at 2.5 cun, Bl 7 at 4 cun, Bl 8 at 5.5 posterior to the natural anterior hairline to 4 cun posterior from Bl 8.

i) With your finger on the anterior median line at the natural anterior hairline, palpate laterally with the flow (1.5 cun) and posteriorly (9.5 cun) or laterally (1.5 cun) against the flow and superiorly from the natural posterior hairline (2.5 cun).

Note: Voisin (1974) locates B 9 on the occipital protruberance: upper part, 1.5 fb (finger breadth) from the midline of the cranium. Lavier (1974) in an illustration, locates BL 9 on a level halfway between and lateral to VG 17 and VG 18 (Du). Soulié (1994) locates BL 9 on the lower occiput, two FW (Finger Width) above the inferior edge of the skull, two FW from the median line, in the angle between the inferior edge of a flat, transverse rise and the posterior (medial) edge of a flat rise; in a hollow; two large FW medial to GB 19.

Wu (1973) locates BL 9 upon the cranium at one and one-half pouce from the median line, at eight pouce above BL 2. So (1985) locates BL 9 lateral 1.5 divisions to GV 17 (Du) in the third cleft, also 2 divisions above the back hairline. Deadman (1998) locates BL 9 at 1.3 cun lateral to DU 17 (which is located in the depression superior to the external occipital protruberance), 1.5 cun superior to DU 16.

Eachou (1995) locates this point at 1.5 inches posterior to BL 8, 1.3 inches lateral to GV 17 (Du), and 1.3 inches lateral to the superior nuchal line of the external occipital protruberance, between GV 17 and GB 19. Qiu (1996) locates UB 9 at 2.5 cun directly above the midpoint of the posterior hairline, then 1.3 cun lateral. Shandong (1982) locate Yuzhen on the lateral side of the superior border of the protruberentia occipitalis externa, above Pt. Tianzhu (Bl 10).

Bl 10 is on the posterior aspect of the head, on the nape of the neck.

Bl 10 TIAN ZHU – HEAVENLY PILLAR

⊥ ***0.2 TO 0.5 CUN*** ***Δ 3 TO 5***

- WINDOW OF THE SKY/Window of Heaven
- A POINT OF THE SEA OF QI (or Du 14 and Du 15 – see note) There are two other Sea of Qi Points: Ren 17 and St 9)
- COUSIN in association with St 34

Pos: Position of patient: seated.

Loc: a) On the posterior aspect of the head.
b) On the 'nape' of the neck.
c) On the prominence of the trapezius muscle.
d) 1.3 cun lateral to the posterior median line.
e) 0.5 cun superior to the natural posterior hairline.
f) Level with Du 15.

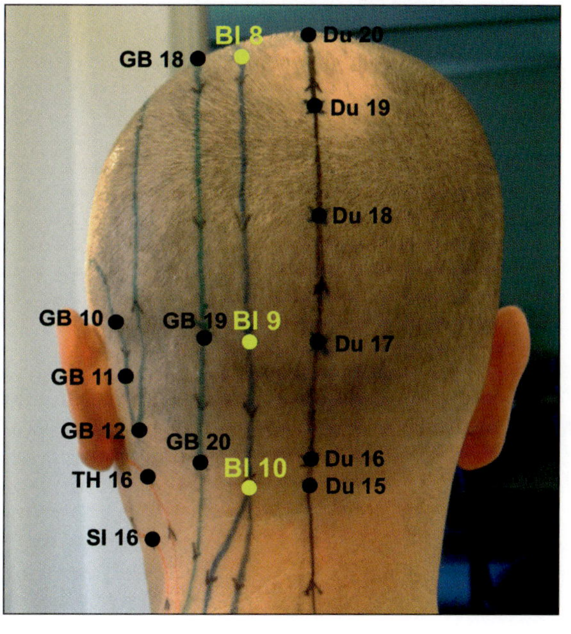

Tip: a) It is advisable not to use the lateral cun measurement to locate this point as the point should be located on the prominence of the trapezius muscle. In the neck the trapezius muscle divides in to two each side of the posterior median line with insertion at the external occipital protruberance. These two narrow bands of muscle can often be seen on the posterior aspect of the neck.

b) Mark the natural posterior hairline, then pinch each side of the left trapezius muscle and palpate for the point on the prominence of the muscle just superior to the natural posterior hairline, then do the same for Bl 10 on the right trapezius muscle.

c) A common error when locating Bl 10 is to mark it medial or lateral to the border of the trapezius muscle Bl 10 is always on the prominence of the muscle.

d) Bl 10 is level with Du 15 which is on the posterior median line in a depression between the first and second cervical vertebrae (the atlas and the axis), 0.5 cun superior to the natural posterior hairline. Locating C1 and C2 is not easy therefore using Du 15 to locate Bl 10 can be difficult.

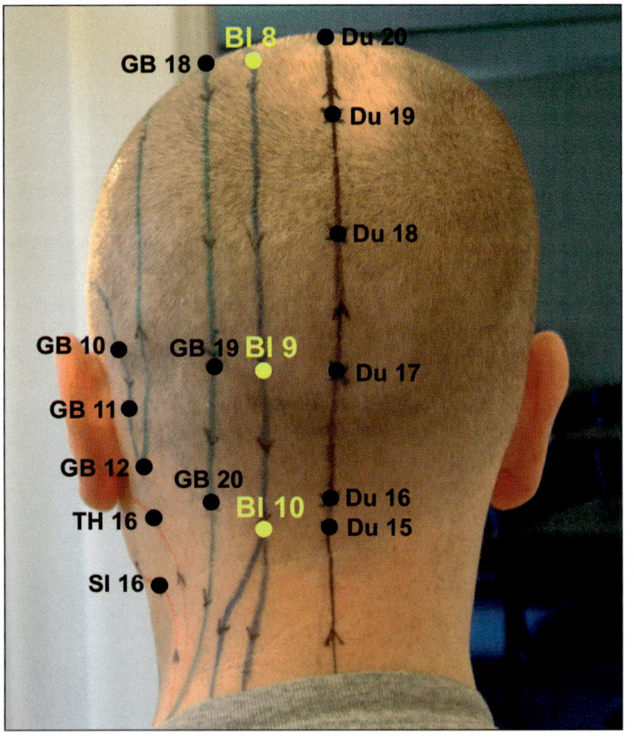

Note: Lavier (1974) illustrates BL 10 level with VG 16 (Du16). Legge (1999) locates UB 10 at 1.3 cun lateral to Du 15, within the posterior hairline, on the lateral side of the upper trapezius. Wu (1973) locates BL 10 upon the posterior surface of the neck, at seven fen (0.7 cun) from the median line and three pouce above the intervertebral depression between the seventh cervical and first thoracic vertebrae. Voisin (1974) locates B 10 on the occipital bone: lower border, 1.5 fb (finger breadth) from the midline of the cranium. Worsley (1982) locates III 10 on the neck, 1.3 ACI (Anatomical Chinese Inch) lateral to the posterior median line, at the base of the occipital bone, on the trapezius, at the level of XIV 16 (Du/GV 16).

Deadman (1998) locates BL 10 on the lateral aspect of the trapezius muscle, 1.3 cun lateral to Du 15. Jayasuriya (1982) locates UB 10 at 0.5 cun above the posterior hairline, between the transverse porcesses of the 1st and 2nd cervical vertebrae, 1.3 cun lateral to Du 17. Shanghai (1993) locates BL 10 on the starting point of the trapezius muscle, in the posterior hairline, in the depression lateral to the tendon, 1.3 cun lateral to Du 15.

Soulié (1994) locates this point on the nape: two FW (Finger Width) from the median line, one FW above the inferior edge of the cranium, in the angle between the posterior (medial) edge of the superimposed insertions of the trapezius and the trachelomastoid muscle and of the deep lower edge of a bony rise.; in a hollow; two FW under BL 9; five FW above BL 11; separated by the trapezius from GB 20; about six FW superior and slightly medial to BL 12; six FW superior and medial to BL 41 So (1985) locates BL 10 0.5 division up from the back hairline in the middle of the trapezius muscle.

Lotan (2000) locates UB 10 level with 0.5 cun inferior to the external occipital protruberance, 1.3 cun lateral to back midline. Li (1991) locates UB 10 at the level of Du 15 on the lateral side of m. trapezius. Academy (1975) locates UB 10 1.3 cun lateral to Du 15, on the lateral side of m. trapezius. Qiu (1996) locates UB 10 0.5 cun directly above the midpoint of the posterior hairline, then 1.3 cun lateral, in the depression on the lateral border of the m.trapezius. Eachou (1995) locates BL 10 1.3 inches lateral to GV 15 (Du 15), at the lateral margin of the trapezius muscle.

Note: The Ling Shu (Spiritual Pivot) Chapter 33 describes areas where the Seas are located rather than point numbers, eg. the middle of the chest is in the region of Ren 17. Ren 17 and St 9 locations seem to have universal agreement as Seas of Qi, but the other Sea of Qi point(s) in the region of the neck, Bl 10 or Du 14/Du 15 seem to have differences of opinion. The College of Traditional Acupuncture favours using Bl 10 instead of Du 14/Du 15. as Du 15 is classified by them as a Sea of Marrow point.

HOW TO MARK OUT AND CHECK THE VERTEBRAE.

The cun measurements of the inner and outer Bladder lines on the posterior torso are constant from the upper to lower posterior torso. They however follow the contours of the posterior torso, and therefore points in the upper lumbar area may lie more lateral, and points in the sacral area may be more medial on a man or equidistant or more lateral on a woman. It is important to follow both the musculature of the torso, and any curvature/tilt of bony structures (scapula, spine, pelvis). You need to recognise any congenital or acquired conditions that can affect the alignment of the vertebrae such as scoliosis, lordosis, spinabifida and ankalosing spondilitis.

Even though the cun measurements do not alter on the posterior torso they are proportional measurements (cun) which means that the inner and outer bladder channels are not on a "plumb" line. Some illustrations show the outer Bladder line between the ribs which can make the points lower than the intervertebral spaces. However the points should be level with the intervertebral spaces regardless of the rib anatomy.

The distance between the medial border of the scapula and the posterior median line is measured as 3 cun at the level of the 3rd thoracic vertebra.
The lateral branch or the outer Bladder line of the Bladder Channel is 3 cun lateral to the posterior median line.

The medial branch or the inner Bladder line of the Bladder Channel is 1.5 cun lateral to the posterior median line.
There are 7 cevical, 12 thoracic and 5 lumbar vertebrae. All of the Bladder points lie in relation to the intervertebral spaces between two vertebrae, eg. T3/4 , which is 1.5 cun lateral to the posterior median line (Bl 13).

Although there are cun measurements for the inner and outer bladder lines of 1.5 cun and 3 cun, it is often much more easy to palpate for the points, especially if you were to place your finger in the intervertebral space and then palpate laterally. Palpating with the flow of the Bladder channel from the top of the back can also help you to locate the points.

The Du points lie in relation to the intervertebral spaces between two vertebrae, eg. T3/4.

Posterior Torso

Normal Spine

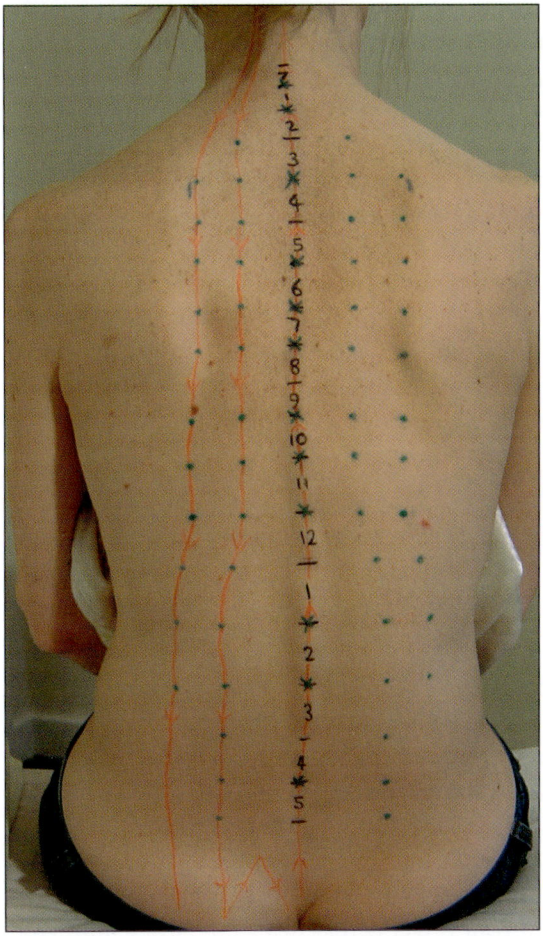

Curvature of the Spine

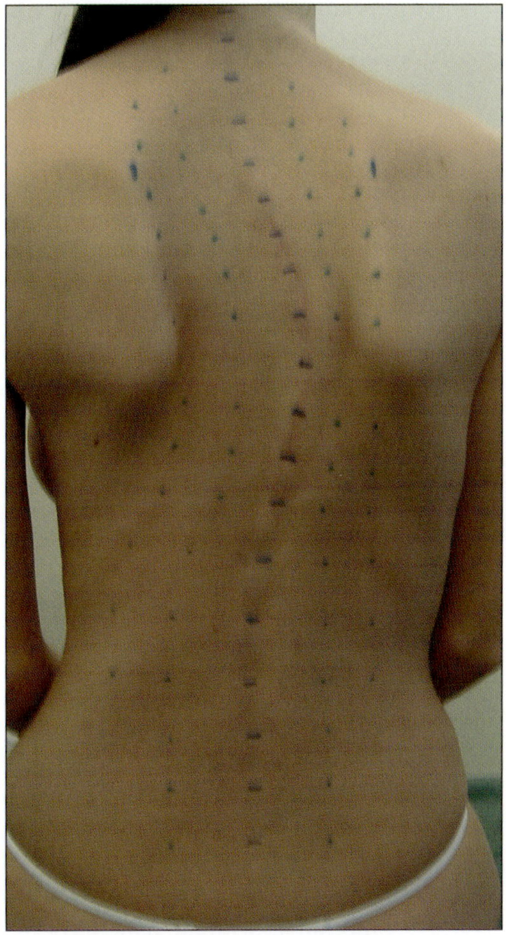

Tip: Using the following landmarks to locate the intervertebral spaces of the upper thoracic vertebrae:

a) First mark out the intervertebral spaces of the thoracic vertebrae.
b) To locate the intervertebral space between C7 and T1, place your index finger on the prominence of the vertebra that may be T1 and your middle finger on the prominence of the vertebra which may be C7.
c) Now ask the patient to turn their head to the left and then to the right. You should feel some slight movement under your middle finger which is C7. You should feel no rotation under your index finger as T1 is attached to a rib whereas C7 is not.
d) A common error is to visualise C7 as being more prominent than T1. Gray's (1978) states it very often can be, but T1 is usually just as prominent and sometimes more so.
e) Place your four fingers from each hand vertically on the each side of the neck so that the radial borders of your fingers are uppermost and the pads are resting lightly against the lateral surface of the neck. Make sure that the ulnar border of the little fingers (5th digit) are resting on the top of the shoulder with the pads of your 5th digits resting on the lateral surface of the neck.
f) Then keeping your left and right 5th digits at this level, bring them together so their tips meet on the posterior median line. They should meet at the level of C7/T1 space or at the spinous process of C7.
g) The illustration below shows how you should have your fingers on the neck and shoulder before the 5th digits meet at the posterior median line:

o (2)	o (2)
o (3)	o (3)
o (4)	o (4)
o (5th digit)	o (5th digit)
(5th digit on top of left shoulder)	(5th digit on top of right shoulder)

h) When you have marked out the intervertebral spaces of the spine, step back and visualise the first place that you would be able to attach the first rib to T1. The first rib curves anteriorly and inferiorly to the inferior border of the clavicle, so T1 can seem more superior than you may realise. T1 should also be the first vertebra at the base of the neck.
i) Another method is to place your finger in the angle formed at the superior aspect of the shoulder by the acromial extremity of the clavicle and the scapular spine. From this angle, with the patient relaxed, run your finger across in a straight line until you meet an intervertebral space – this is the intervertebral space between T2/T3. A straight line means following the 3D curvature of the body, not as if you were drawing on a flat piece of paper – 2D image.
j) To locate the intervertebral space between T3/T4 run your finger from the acromial end of the scapular spine along its superior border towards the spine. You should meet the intervertebral space of T3/T4, however this is not always as accurate as tip i) as some scapula spines are almost horizontal. Therefore they may not slope downwards as you run your finger to the medial edge of the scapular spine.

k) To locate the intervertebral space between L2/L3 place your little finger (5th digit) on top of the iliac crest with your 1st, 2nd and 3rd fingers vertically on top of your little finger. Move your thumb horizontal (at a right angle) to the fingerswhich should bring the thumb in to alignment line with the intervertebral space of L2/L3 as illustrated below:

```
o (2)     o – thumb   L2/L3   thumb – o     o (2)
o (3)                                       o (3)
o (4)                                       o (4)
o (5th digit)                               o (5th digit)
(left iliac crest)                          (right iliac crest)
```

l) To locate the intervertebral space between L3/L4 place your left and right index fingers on the top of the left and right iliac crests with your 1st, 3rd, 4th, and 5th digits at the same level (horizontal). Your thumbs should be at the level of L3/L4 intervertebral space, as illustrated below:

```
o o o o  o – thumb        L3/L4        thumb – o  o o o o
5 4 3 2  1st digit                     1st digit  2 3 4 5
      l                                          l
           index fingers on top of the iliac crest
```

m) To locate the intervertebral space between L4/L5 place your left and right index (2nd) fingers on the top of the left and right iliac crests as above, but this time allowing your thumb to fall away naturally instead of keeping it horizontal with the other digits. The thumb then will be aligned with the intervertebral space of L4/L5, as illustrated below:

```
5 4 3 2 (digits)                 2 3 4 5 (digits)
   o o o o                          o o o o
              o   L4/L5   o
                 thumbs
     index (2nd) fingers on top of the iliac crest
```

On tips g), k), l) and m) "=" is the top of the iliac crest.

n) From the base of L5 the vertebrae are fused and form the sacrum. The size of the sacrum longitudinally is approximately the size of the patient's fist from the knuckle (metacarpo-phalangeal joint) of the thumb to the knuckle (metacarpo-phalangeal joint) of the little finger. If the base of L5 vertebra to the bottom of the sacrum/superior border of the coccyx (sacral body) is longer than the person's fist then you need to re-check the intervertebral spaces again. The sacro-coccygeal articulation may be located at the level of the superior border of the gluteal fold.

Note: The locations of the points on the inner and outer lines of the Bladder Channel on the posterior torso have been unanimous throughout Acupuncture literature, but there are texts that do have different cun measurements for the inner and outer lines of the Bladder Channel. Worsley (1982) uses 2 ACI (Anatomical Chinese Inch) for the inner Bladder line and 4 ACI for the outer Bladder line. Lavier (1974) doesn't use any measurement, the outer Bladder line touches the inner border of the scapula and the inner Bladder line is midway between the border of the scapula and the median line.

Voisin (1974) uses 2 fb (finger breadth) from the midline of the back at the centre of the spinous process for the inner Bladder line and 4 fb from the midline of the back at the centre of the spinous process. Soulié (1994) not only uses various measurements lateral to the vertebra but also uses other anatomy to help locate the points eg, 4 FW (finger width) under the lower angle of the scapula for Bl 19. Wu (1973) uses 2 pouce from the median line for the inner Bladder line measurement and 4 pouce from the median line for the outer Bladder line measurement. Jin Jian uses 2 cun for the medial branch or inner Bladder line.

Points on the posterior torso should be located with the patient in a seated position, with an upright posture.

Bl 11-26 are on the posterior torso, on the medial branch or inner line of the Bladder Channel.

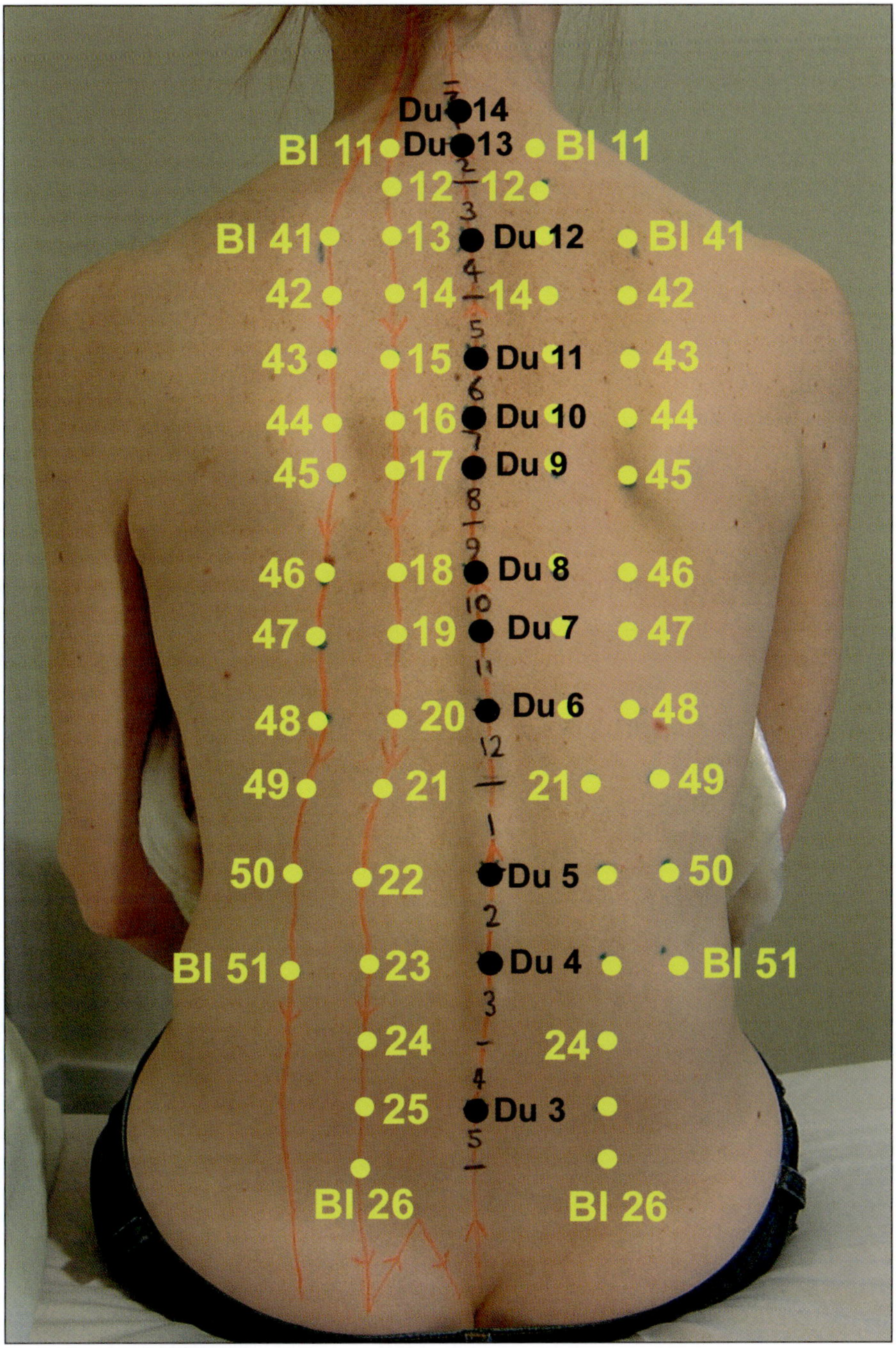

Bl 11 DA ZHU – GREAT SHUTTLE

⊥ ***0.3 CUN*** Δ ***7***

- A Seven External Dragons (E.D's) Point (the other points are Du 20, Bl 23 and Bl 61)
- A POINT OF THE SEA OF BLOOD (for the Upper Body) (There are two other Sea of Blood Points: St 37 and St 39 for the Lower Body)
- INFLUENTIAL/Hui – Meeting/Gathering/Assembling Point of the Bones
- RE-UNION/Crossing/Meeting Point of the Bladder Channel with the Small Intestine, Triple Heater and Gall Bladder Channels, and the Du Mai – Foot Tai Yang Channel with the Hand Tai Yang, Hand Shao Yang, Foot Shao Yang Channels and the Governor Vessel.

Pos: Position of patient: seated and upright.

Loc: a) On the posterior torso.
b) On the inner line or the medial branch of the Bladder channel.
c) 1.5 cun lateral to the posterior median line.
d) Between the 1st and 2nd thoracic vertebrae (level with the base of the spinous process of the 1st thoracic vertebra).
e) Level with Du 13

Tip: a) Please read **"HOW TO MARK OUT AND CHECK THE VERTEBRAE"** for further guidance.
b) The cun measurement from the posterior median line to the inner bladder line is 1.5 cun. Identify the outer Bladder line at 3 cun. This is taken from the posterior median line to the medial border of the scapula at the level of T3.
c) The inner Bladder line is at 1.5 cun (half of 3 cun).
d) Place your finger in the intervertebral space of T1 and T2 and then palpate laterally to 1.5 cun until you feel a *men* (depression).
e) Palpating with the flow of the Bladder channel from the top of the back can assist in locating the point.

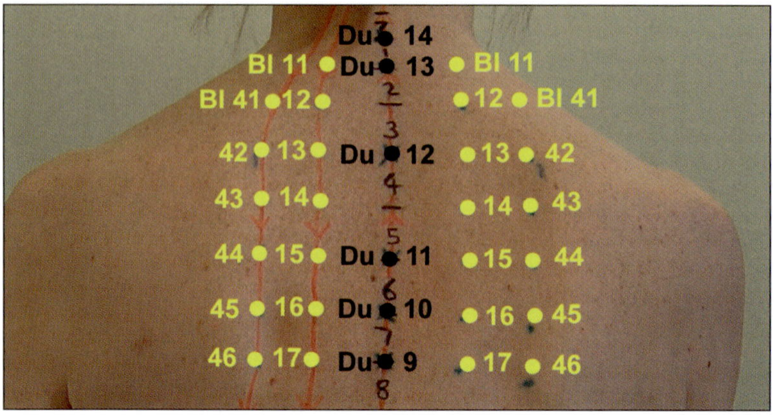

Note: Soulié (1994) locates BL 11 on the upper back, one small FW (Finger Width) from the angle of the inferior lateral edge of the first thoracic vertebra, on the lower edge of the first rib, between two vertical muscles; five FW below BL 10; two FW medial and superior to BL 12; three large FW medial to BL 41; one FW lateral and below GV 14 (Du 14); one large FW medial and above GV 13 (Du 13); two tightened FW below SI 14. Legge (1999) locates UB 11 at 1.5 cun lateral to the tip of the spinous process of the 1st thoracic vertebra. Voisin (1974) locates B 11 at 2 fb (finger breadth) from the midline of the back (centre of spinous process D 1).

Worsley (1982) uses 2 ACI (Anatomical Chinese Inch) for the inner Bladder line and 4 ACI for the outer Bladder line (for the thoracic region of the back). Lavier (1974) doesn't use any measurement, the outer Bladder line touches the inner border of the scapula and the inner Bladder line is midway between the border of the scapula and the median line. Voisin (1974) uses 2 fb (finger breadth) from the midline of the back at the centre of the spinous process for the inner Bladder line and 4 fb from the midline of the back at the centre of the spinous process. Wu (1973) uses 2 pouce from the median line for the inner Bladder line measurement and 4 pouce from the median line for the outer Bladder line measurement. Wu (1973) uses two and four pouce measurements for the inner and outer Bladder lines.

Bl 12 FENG MEN – WIND GATE

⊥ ***0.3 TO 0.5 CUN*** **∆ *5 TO 10***

- 8 EXTRAORDINARY VESSEL/Coalescent Point of Du Mai (Governor Vessel)
- RE-UNION/Crossing/Meeting Point of the Bladder Channel with the Du Mai – Foot Tai Yang Channel with the Governor Vessel.

Pos: Position of patient: seated and upright.

Loc:
a) On the posterior torso.
b) On the inner line or the medial branch of the Bladder channel.
c) 1.5 cun lateral to the posterior median line.
d) Between the 2nd and 3rd thoracic vertebrae (level with the base of the spinous process of the 2nd thoracic vertebra).
e) Level with Bl 41.

Tip:
a) Please read **"HOW TO MARK OUT AND CHECK THE VERTEBRAE"** for further guidance.
b) The cun measurement from the posterior median line to the inner bladder line is 1.5 cun. Identify the outer Bladder line at 3 cun. This is taken from the posterior median line to the medial border of the scapula at the level of T3.
c) The inner Bladder line is at 1.5 cun (half of 3 cun).
d) Place your finger in the intervertebral space of T2 and T3 and then palpate laterally to 1.5 cun until you feel a *men* (depression).
e) Palpating with the flow of the Bladder channel from the top of the back can assist in locating the point.

Note: Soulié (1994) locates BL 12 on the upper back, about two FW (Finger Width) on each side of the first cervical vertebra, in the angle between the inferior edge of the second rib and the medial edge of a vertical muscle (iliocostalis), on the edge of the rhomboids; in a hollow; about two FW lateral and inferior to BL 11; two FW medial and superior to BL 13; two FW inferior and lateral to SI 14.

Legge (1999) locates UB 12 at 1.5 cun lateral to the tip of the spinous process of the 2nd thoracic vertebra. Voisin (1974) locates B 12 2 fb (finger breadth) from the midline of the back (centre of spinous process D 2). Worsley (1982) uses 2 ACI (Anatomical Chinese Inch) for the inner Bladder line and 4 ACI for the outer Bladder line (for the thoracic region of the back).

Lavier (1974) doesn't use any measurement, the outer Bladder line touches the inner border of the scapula and the inner Bladder line is midway between the border of the scapula and the median line. Voisin (1974) uses 2 fb (finger breadth) from the midline of the back at the centre of the spinous process for the inner Bladder line and 4 fb from the midline of the back at the centre of the spinous process. Wu (1973) uses 2 pouce from the median line for the inner Bladder line measurement and 4 pouce from the median line for the outer Bladder line measurement.

Bl 13 FEI SHU – LUNGS CORRESPONDENCE

⊥ ***0.1 TO 0.5 CUN*** **Δ *3 TO 20***

- LUNG BACK SHU/Shu Transporting/AEP (Associated Effect Point)/Approval/ Vesical Reinforcement Point
- A.E (Aggressive Energy) – Needle Depth = 0.1 cun

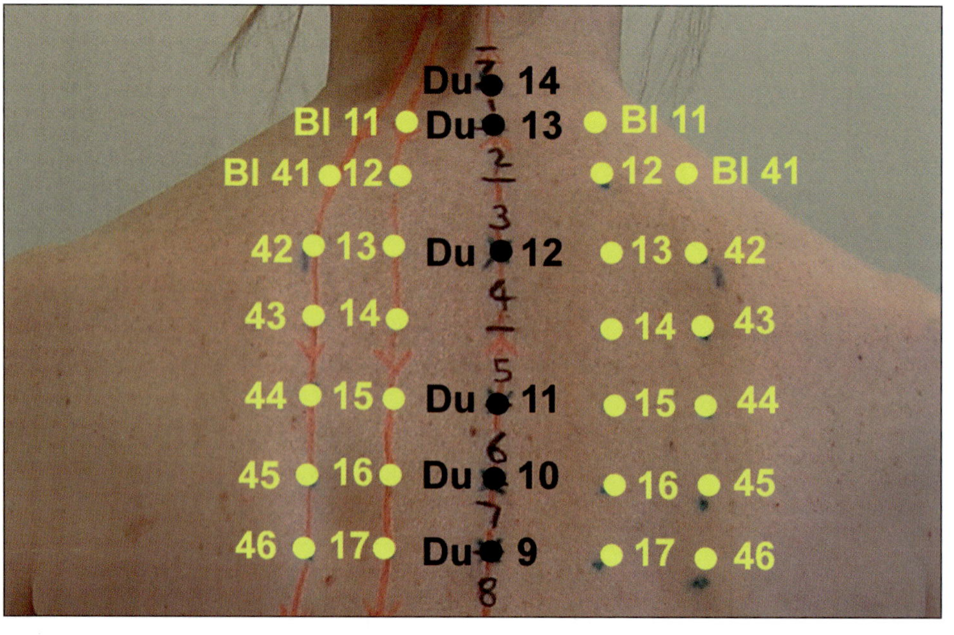

Pos: Position of patient: seated and upright.

Loc: a) On the posterior torso.
b) On the inner line or the medial branch of the Bladder channel.
c) 1.5 cun lateral to the posterior median line.
d) Between the 3rd and 4th thoracic vertebrae (level with the base of the spinous process of the 3rd thoracic vertebra).
e) Level with Du 12 and Bl 42.

Tip: a) Please read **"HOW TO MARK OUT AND CHECK THE VERTEBRAE"** for further guidance.
b) The cun measurement from the posterior median line to the inner bladder line is 1.5 cun. Identify the outer Bladder line at 3 cun. This is taken from the posterior median line to the medial border of the scapula at the level of T3.
c) The inner Bladder line is at 1.5 cun (half of 3 cun).
d) Place your finger in the intervertebral space of T3 and T4 and then palpate laterally to 1.5 cun until you feel a *men* (depression).
e) Palpating with the flow of the Bladder channel from the top of the back can assist in locating the point.

Note: Soulié (1994) locates BL 13 on the upper back, mid-distance from the upper medial point of the scapula to the spinal cord (third thoracic), betwen two vertical muscles (iliocostalis, longissimus dorsi), on the inferior edge of the rhomboid; in a hollow; two FW (Finger Width) under BL 12; two FW above BL 14; two FW lateral to GV 12 (Du 12); two FW medial to BL 42.

Legge (1999) locates UB 13 at 1.5 cun lateral to the tip of the spinous process of the 3rd thoracic vertebra. Voisin (1974) locates B 13 at 2 fb (finger breadth) from the midline of the back (centre of spinous process D 3). Worsley (1982) uses 2 ACI (Anatomical Chinese Inch) for the inner Bladder line and 4 ACI for the outer Bladder line (for the thoracic region of the back).

Lavier (1974) doesn't use any measurement, the outer Bladder line touches the inner border of the scapula and the inner Bladder line is midway between the border of the scapula and the median line. Voisin (1974) uses 2 fb (finger breadth) from the midline of the back at the centre of the spinous process for the inner Bladder line and 4 fb from the midline of the back at the centre of the spinous process. Wu (1973) uses 2 pouce from the median line for the inner Bladder line measurement and 4 pouce from the median line for the outer Bladder line measurement.

Bl 14 JUE YIN SHU – PERICARDIUM CORRESPONDENCE

⊥ ***0.1 TO 0.3 CUN*** Δ *7*

- PERICARDIUM BACK SHU/Shu Transporting/AEP (Associated Effect Point)/ Approval/Vesical Reinforcement Point
- A.E (Aggressive Energy) – Needle Depth = 0.1 cun

Pos: Position of patient: seated and upright.

Loc: a) On the posterior torso.
b) On the inner line or the medial branch of the Bladder channel.
c) 1.5 cun lateral to the posterior median line.
d) Between the 4th and 5th thoracic vertebrae (level with the base of the spinous process of the 4th thoracic vertebra).
e) Level with Bl 43.

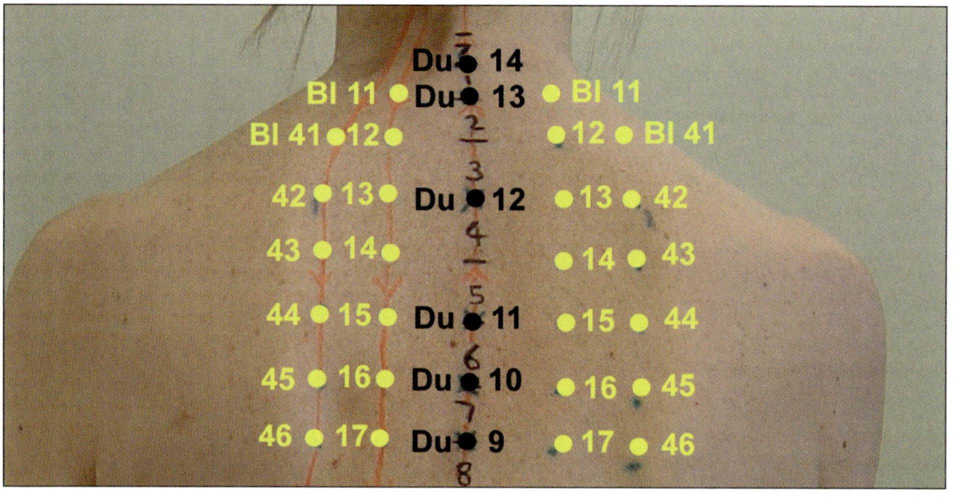

Tip: a) Please read **"HOW TO MARK OUT AND CHECK THE VERTEBRAE"** for further guidance.
b) The cun measurement from the posterior median line to the inner bladder line is 1.5 cun. Ientify the outer Bladder line at 3 cun. This is taken from the posterior median line to the medial border of the scapula at the level of T3.
c) The inner Bladder line is at 1.5 cun (half of 3 cun).
d) Place your finger in the intervertebral space of T4 and T5 and then palpate laterally to 1.5 cun until you feel a *men* (depression).
e) Palpating with the flow of the Bladder channel from the top of the back can assist in locating the point.
f) The posterior torso widens and narrows according to the person's body shape, with the cun measurement being a proportional measurement. Therefore 1.5 cun at the level of T3 may not be the same further down the back, e.g. 1.5 cun at the level of T4/T5 may have a difference of 0.5 cm or more further down the back, especially in the lumbar region.

Note: Soulié (1994) locates BL 14 on the back, mid-distance from the thoracic spine to the scapula at the level of the inferior edge of its crest, between two vertical muscles (iliocostalis and longissimus dorsi), on the inferior edge of the fourth rib, on the trapezius and rhomboid; in a hollow; two FW (Finger Width) under BL 13; two FW above BL 15; two FW medial to BL 43. Legge (1999) locates UB 14 at 1.5 cun lateral to the tip of the spinous process of the 4th thoracic vertebra. Voisin (1974) locates B 14 at 2 fb (finger breadth) from the midline of the back (centre of spinous process D 4).

Worsley (1982) uses 2 ACI (Anatomical Chinese Inch) for the inner Bladder line and 4 ACI for the outer Bladder line (for the thoracic region of the back). Lavier (1974) doesn't use any measurement, the outer Bladder line touches the inner border of the scapula and the inner Bladder line is midway between the border of the scapula and the median line. Voisin (1974) uses 2 fb (finger breadth) from the midline of the back at the centre of the spinous process for the inner Bladder line and 4 fb from the midline of the back at the centre of the spinous process. Wu (1973) uses 2 pouce from the median line for the inner Bladder line measurement and 4 pouce from the median line for the outer Bladder line measurement.

Bl 15 XIN SHU – HEART CORRESPONDENCE

⊥ ***0.1 TO 0.3 CUN*** **Δ *3***

- HEART BACK SHU/Shu Transporting/AEP (Associated Effect Point)/Approval/ Vesical Reinforcement Point
- A.E (Aggressive Energy) – Needle Depth = 0.1 cun

Pos: Position of patient: seated and upright.

Loc: a) On the posterior torso.
b) On the inner line or the medial branch of the Bladder channel.
c) 1.5 cun lateral to the posterior median line.
d) Between the 5th and 6th thoracic vertebrae (level with the base of the spinous process of the 5th thoracic vertebra).
e) Level with Du 11 and Bl 44.

Tip: a) Please read **"HOW TO MARK OUT AND CHECK THE VERTEBRAE"** for further guidance.
b) The cun measurement from the posterior median line to the inner bladder line is 1.5 cun. Identify the outer Bladder line at 3 cun. This is taken from the posterior median line to the medial border of the scapula at the level of T3.
c) The inner Bladder line is at 1.5 cun (half of 3 cun).
d) Place your finger in the intervertebral space of T5 and T6 and then palpate laterally to 1.5 cun until you feel a *men* (depression).
e) Palpating with the flow of the Bladder channel from the top of the back can assist in locating the point.
f) The posterior torso widens and narrows according to the person's body shape, with the cun measurement being a proportional measurement. Therefore 1.5 cun at the level of T3 may not be the same further down the back, e.g. 1.5 cun at the level of T4/T5 may have a difference of 0.5 cm or more further down the back, especially in the lumbar region.

Note: Soulié (1994) locates BL 15 on the back, at the level of the upper third from the spine of the scapula to its lower point, mid-distance from the scapula to the thoracic spine, between two vertical muscles (iliocostalis, longissimus dorsi), just inferior to the edge of the fifth rib; in a hollow; on the trapezius and rhomboid; two FW (Finger Width) under BL 14; two FW above BL 16; at about the level of GV 11 (Du 11); about two FW medial to BL 44. Legge (1999) locates UB 15 at 1.5 cun lateral to the tip of the spinous process of the 5th thoracic vertebra. Voisin (1974) locates B 15 at 2 fb (finger breadth) from the midline of the back (centre of spinous process D 5).

Worsley (1982) uses 2 ACI (Anatomical Chinese Inch) for the inner Bladder line and 4 ACI for the outer Bladder line (for the thoracic region of the back). Lavier (1974) doesn't use any measurement, the outer Bladder line touches the inner border of the scapula and the inner Bladder line is midway between the border of the scapula and the median line. Voisin (1974) uses 2 fb (finger breadth) from the midline of the back at the centre of the spinous process for the inner Bladder line and 4 fb from the midline of the back at the centre of the spinous process. Wu (1973) uses 2 pouce from the median line for the inner Bladder line measurement and 4 pouce from the median line for the outer Bladder line measurement.

Bl 16 DU SHU – GOVERNOR CORRESPONDENCE

⊥ ***0.3 CUN*** Δ ***3***

- GOVERNOR BACK SHU/Shu Transporting/AEP (Associated Effect Point)/ Approval

Pos: Position of patient: seated and upright.

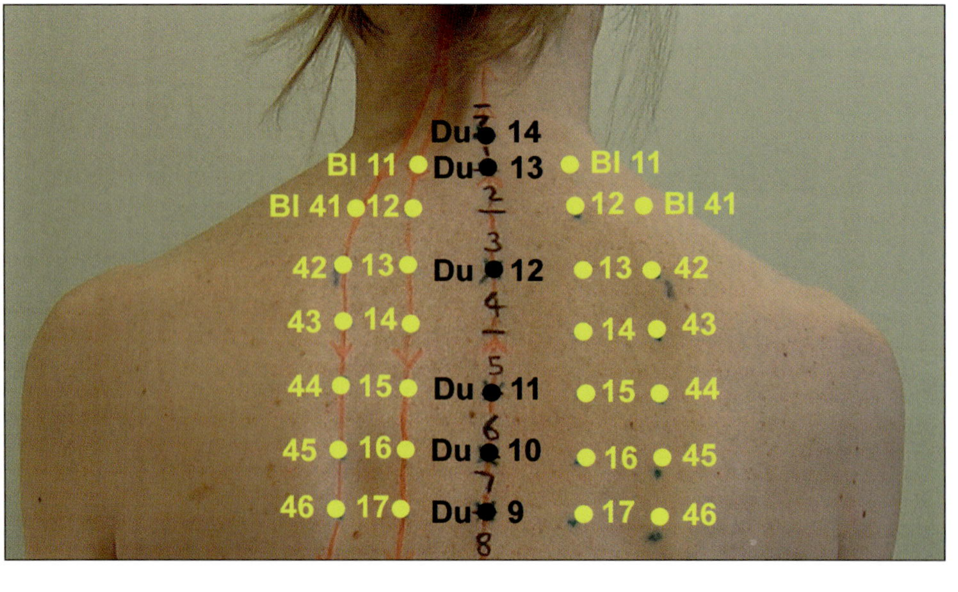

Loc: a) On the posterior torso.
b) On the inner line or the medial branch of the Bladder channel.
c) 1.5 cun lateral to the posterior median line.
d) Between the 6th and 7th thoracic vertebrae (level with the base of the spinous process of the 6th thoracic vertebra).
e) Level with Du 10 and Bl 45.

Tip: a) Please read **"HOW TO MARK OUT AND CHECK THE VERTEBRAE"** for further guidance.
b) The cun measurement from the posterior median line to the inner bladder line is 1.5 cun. Identify the outer Bladder line at 3 cun. This is taken from the posterior median line to the medial border of the scapula at the level of T3.
c) The inner Bladder line is at 1.5 cun (half of 3 cun).
d) Place your finger in the intervertebral space of T6 and T7 and then palpate laterally to 1.5 cun until you feel a *men* (depression).
e) Palpating with the flow of the Bladder channel from the top of the back can assist in locating the point.
f) The posterior torso widens and narrows according to the person's body shape, with the cun measurement being a proportional measurement. Therefore 1.5 cun at the level of T3 may not be the same further down the back, e.g. 1.5 cun at the level of T4/T5 may have a difference of 0.5 cm or more further down the back, especially in the lumbar region.

Note: Soulié (1994) locates BL 16 on the back, three FW (Finger Width) above the inferior point of the scapula, mid-distance from the scapula to the thoracic spine, between two vertical muscles (iliocostalis, longissimus dorsi), on the inferior edge of the sixth rib; in a hollow; two FW under BL 15; two FW above BL 17; about two FW on either side of GV 10 (Du 10); two FW medial to BL 45. Legge (1999) locates UB 16 at 1.5 cun lateral to the tip of the spinous process of the 6th thoracic vertebra. Voisin (1974) locates B 16 at 2 fb (finger breadth) from the midline of the back (centre of spinous process D 6).

Worsley (1982) uses 2 ACI (Anatomical Chinese Inch) for the inner Bladder line and 4 ACI for the outer Bladder line (for the thoracic region of the back). Lavier (1974) doesn't use any measurement, the outer Bladder line touches the inner border of the scapula and the inner Bladder line is midway between the border of the scapula and the median line. Voisin (1974) uses 2 fb (finger breadth) from the midline of the back at the centre of the spinous process for the inner Bladder line and 4 fb from the midline of the back at the centre of the spinous process. Wu (1973) uses 2 pouce from the median line for the inner Bladder line measurement and 4 pouce from the median line for the outer Bladder line measurement.

Bl 17 GE SHU – DIAPHRAGM CORRESPONDENCE

⊥ ***0.3 TO 0.5 CUN*** **Δ *3 TO 5***

- DIAPHRAGM BACK SHU/Shu Transporting/AEP (Associated Effect Point)/ Approval
- INFLUENTIAL/Hui – Meeting/Gathering/Assembling Point of Blood

Pos: Position of patient: seated and upright.

Loc: a) On the posterior torso.
b) On the inner line or the medial branch of the Bladder channel.
c) 1.5 cun lateral to the posterior median line.
d) Between the 7th and 8th thoracic vertebrae (level with the base of the spinous process of the 7th thoracic vertebra).
e) Approximately level with the inferior angle of the scapula.
f) Level with Du 9 and Bl 46.

Tip: a) Please read **"HOW TO MARK OUT AND CHECK THE VERTEBRAE"** for further guidance.
b) The cun measurement from the posterior median line to the inner bladder line is 1.5 cun. Identify the outer Bladder line at 3 cun. This is taken from the posterior median line to the medial border of the scapula at the level of T3.

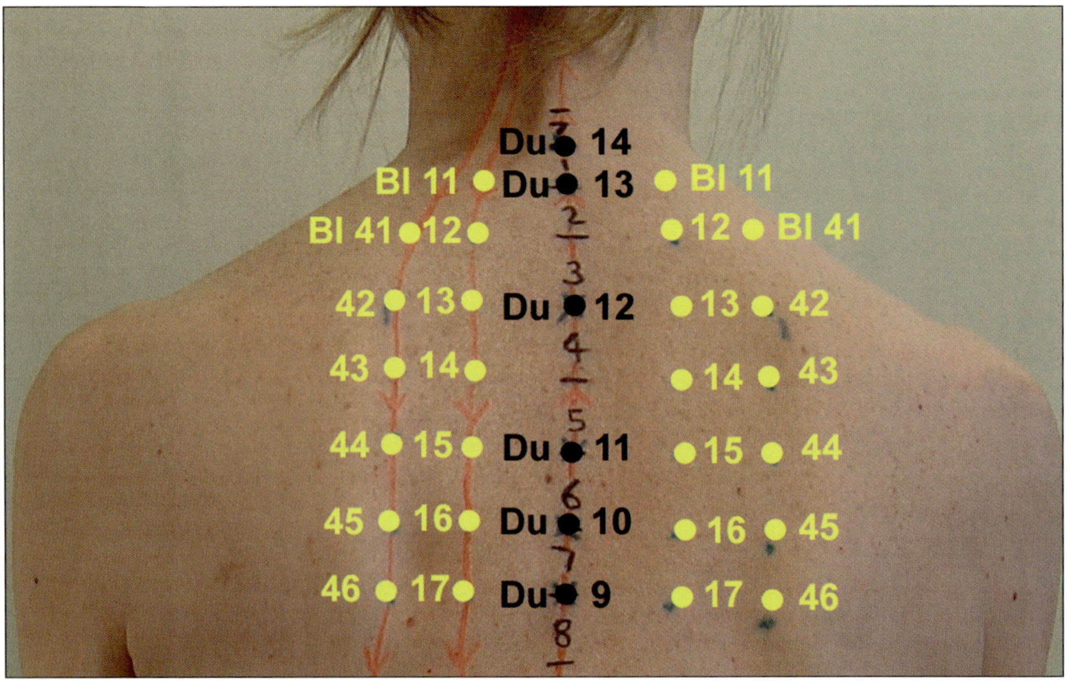

c) The inner Bladder line is at 1.5 cun (half of 3 cun).
d) Place your finger in the intervertebral space of T7 and T8 and then palpate laterally to 1.5 cun until you feel a *men* (depression).
e) Palpating with the flow of the Bladder channel from the top of the back can assist in locating the point.
f) The posterior torso widens and narrows according to the person's body shape, with the cun measurement being a proportional measurement. Therefore 1.5 cun at the level of T3 may not be the same further down the back, e.g. 1.5 cun at the level of T4/T5 may have a difference of 0.5 cm or more further down the back, especially in the lumbar region.

Note: Soulié (1994) locates BL 17 on the back, about two FW (Finger Width) from each side of the thoracic spine (sixth and seventh ribs), at the level of one FW above the inferior point of the scapula, mid-distance from the scapula to the vertebral column, between two vertical muscles (iliocostalis, longissimus dorsi), on the lower edge of the seventh rib; in a hollow; two FW under BL 16; four FW above BL 18; about two FW on either side of GV 9 (Du 9); two FW medial to BL 46. Legge (1999) locates UB 17 at 1.5 cun lateral to the tip of the spinous process of the 7th thoracic vertebra. Voisin (1974) locates B 17 at 2 fb (finger breadth) from the midline of the back (centre of spinous process D 7).

Worsley (1982) uses 2 ACI (Anatomical Chinese Inch) for the inner Bladder line and 4 ACI for the outer Bladder line (for the thoracic region of the back). Lavier (1974) doesn't use any measurement, the outer Bladder line touches the inner border of the scapula and the inner Bladder line is midway between the border of the scapula and the median line. Voisin (1974) uses 2 fb (finger breadth) from the midline of the back at the centre of the spinous process for the inner Bladder line and 4 fb from the midline of the back at the centre of the spinous process. Wu (1973) uses 2 pouce from the median line for the inner Bladder line measurement and 4 pouce from the median line for the outer Bladder line measurement.

Bl 18 GAN SHU – LIVER CORRESPONDENCE

⊥ ***0.1 TO 0.5 CUN*** Δ ***3 TO 20***

- LIVER BACK SHU/Shu Transporting/AEP (Associated Effect Point)/Approval/ Vesical Reinforcement Point
- A.E (Aggressive Energy) – Needle Depth = 0.1 cun

Pos: Position of patient: seated and upright.

Loc: a) On the posterior torso.
b) On the inner line or the medial branch of the Bladder channel.
c) 1.5 cun lateral to the posterior median line.
d) Between the 9th and 10th thoracic vertebrae (level with the base of the spinous process of the 9th thoracic vertebra).
e) Level with Du 8 and Bl 47.

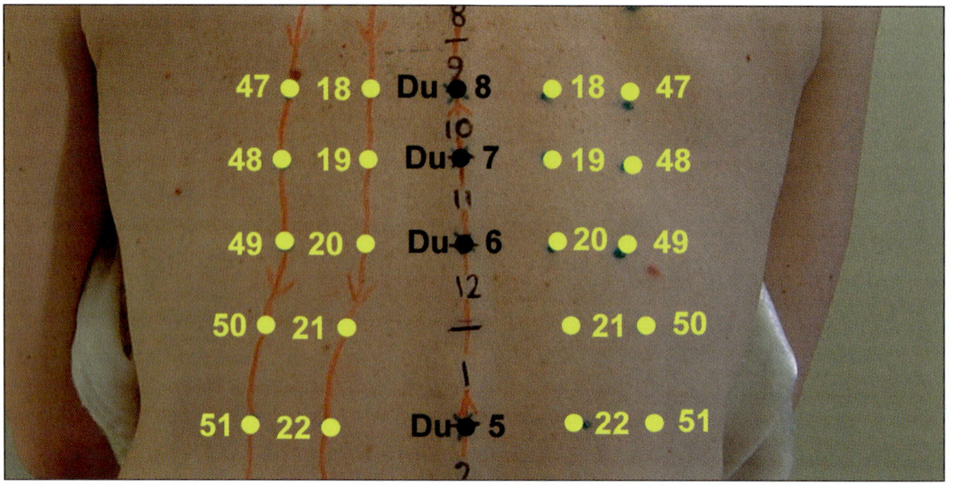

Tip:

a) Please read **"HOW TO MARK OUT AND CHECK THE VERTEBRAE"** for further guidance.

b) The cun measurement from the posterior median line to the inner bladder line is 1.5 cun. Identify the outer Bladder line at 3 cun. This is taken from the posterior median line to the medial border of the scapula at the level of T3.

c) The inner Bladder line is at 1.5 cun (half of 3 cun).

d) Place your finger in the intervertebral space of T9 and T10 and then palpate laterally to 1.5 cun until you feel a *men* (depression).

e) Palpating with the flow of the Bladder channel from the top of the back can assist in locating the point.

f) The posterior torso widens and narrows according to the person's body shape, with the cun measurement being a proportional measurement. Therefore 1.5 cun at the level of T3 may not be the same further down the back, e.g. 1.5 cun at the level of T4/T5 may have a difference of 0.5 cm or more further down the back, especially in the lumbar region.

Note: Soulié (1994) locates BL 18 on the back, one large FW (Finger Width) under the inferior angle of the scapula, about mid-distance from the scapula to the thoracic spine, between two vertical muscles (iliocostalis and longissimus dorsi), on the lower edge of the ninth rib; in a hollow; four FW below BL 17; two FW above BL 19; about two FW lateral to GV 8 (Du 8) on the tenth thoracic vertebra; two FW medial to BL 47. Legge (1999) locates UB 18 at 1.5 cun lateral to the tip of the spinous process of the 9th thoracic vertebra. Voisin (1974) locates B 18 at 2 fb (finger breadth) from the midline of the back (centre of spinous process D 9).

Worsley (1982) uses 2 ACI (Anatomical Chinese Inch) for the inner Bladder line and 4 ACI for the outer Bladder line (for the thoracic region of the back). Lavier (1974) doesn't use any measurement, the outer Bladder line touches the inner border of the scapula and the inner Bladder line is midway between the border of the scapula and the median line.

Voisin (1974) uses 2 fb (finger breadth) from the midline of the back at the centre of the spinous process for the inner Bladder line and 4 fb from the midline of the back at the centre of the spinous process. Wu (1973) uses 2 pouce from the median line for the inner Bladder line measurement and 4 pouce from the median line for the outer Bladder line measurement.

Bl 19 DAN SHU – GALL BLADDER CORRESPONDENCE

⊥ ***0.3 TO 0.5 CUN*** **Δ** ***3 TO 15***

- GALL BLADDER BACK SHU/Shu Transporting/AEP (Associated Effect Point)/ Approval/Vesical Reinforcement Point

Pos: Position of patient: seated and upright.

Loc: a) On the posterior torso.
b) On the inner line or the medial branch of the Bladder channel.
c) 1.5 cun lateral to the posterior median line.
d) Between the 10th and 11th thoracic vertebrae (level with the base of the spinous process of the 10th thoracic vertebra).
e) Level with Du 7 and Bl 48.

Tip: a) Please read **"HOW TO MARK OUT AND CHECK THE VERTEBRAE"** for further guidance.
b) The cun measurement from the posterior median line to the inner bladder line is 1.5 cun. Identify the outer Bladder line at 3 cun. This is taken from the posterior median line to the medial border of the scapula at the level of T3.
c) The inner Bladder line is at 1.5 cun (half of 3 cun).
d) Place your finger in the intervertebral space of T10 and T11 and then palpate laterally to 1.5 cun until you feel a *men* (depression).
e) Palpating with the flow of the Bladder channel from the top of the back can assist in locating the point.
f) The posterior torso widens and narrows according to the person's body shape, with the cun measurement being a proportional measurement. Therefore 1.5 cun at the level of T3 may not be the same further down the back, e.g. 1.5 cun at the level of T4/T5 may have a difference of 0.5 cm or more further down the back, especially in the lumbar region.

Note: Soulié (1994) locates BL 19 on the back, four FW (Finger Width) under the lower angle of the scapula, between two vertical muscles (iliocostalis and longissimus dorsi), at the lower edge of the tenth rib, in a hollow; on the latissimus dorsi; two FW under BL 18; two FW above BL 20; two FW medial to BL 48; two large FW on either side of GV 7 (Du 7). Legge (1999) locates UB 19 at 1.5 cun lateral to the tip of the spinous process of the 10th thoracic vertebra. Voisin (1974) locates B 19 at 2 fb (finger breadth) from the midline of the back (centre of spinous process D 10). Worsley (1982) uses 2 ACI (Anatomical Chinese Inch) for the inner Bladder line and 4 ACI for the outer Bladder line (for the thoracic region of the back).

Lavier (1974) doesn't use any measurement, the outer Bladder line touches the inner border of the scapula and the inner Bladder line is midway between the border of the scapula and the median line. Voisin (1974) uses 2 fb (finger breadth) from the midline of the back at the centre of the spinous process for the inner Bladder line and 4 fb from the midline of the back at the centre of the spinous process. Wu (1973) uses 2 pouce from the median line for the inner Bladder line measurement and 4 pouce from the median line for the outer Bladder line measurement.

Bl 20 PI SHU – SPLEEN CORRESPONDENCE

⊥ ***0.1 TO 0.5 CUN*** Δ ***3 TO 5***

- SPLEEN BACK SHU/Shu Transporting/AEP (Associated Effect Point)/Approval/ Vesical Reinforcement Point
- A.E (Aggressive Energy) – Needle Depth = 0.1 cun

Pos: Position of patient: seated and upright.

Loc: a) On the posterior torso.
b) On the inner line or the medial branch of the Bladder channel.
c) 1.5 cun lateral to the posterior median line.
d) Between the 11th and 12th thoracic vertebrae (level with the base of the spinous process of the 11th thoracic vertebra).
e) Level with Du 6 and Bl 49.

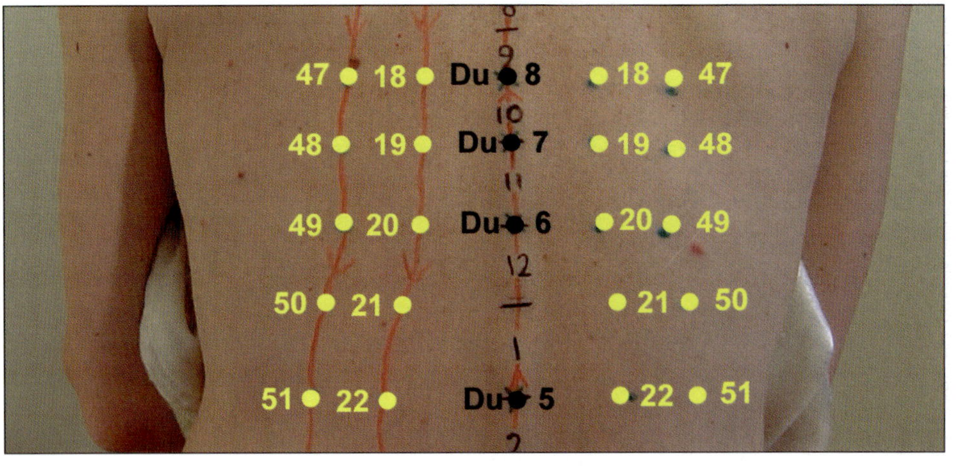

Tip: a) Please read **"HOW TO MARK OUT AND CHECK THE VERTEBRAE"** for further guidance.
b) The cun measurement from the posterior median line to the inner bladder line is 1.5 cun. Identify the outer Bladder line at 3 cun. This is taken from the posterior median line to the medial border of the scapula at the level of T3.
c) The inner Bladder line is at 1.5 cun (half of 3 cun).
d) Place your finger in the intervertebral space of T11 and T12 and then palpate laterally to 1.5 cun until you feel a *men* (depression).
e) Palpating with the flow of the Bladder channel from the top of the back can assist in locating the point.
f) The posterior torso widens and narrows according to the person's body shape, with the cun measurement being a proportional measurement. Therefore 1.5 cun at the level of T3 may not be the same further down the back, e.g. 1.5 cun at the level of T4/T5 may have a difference of 0.5 cm or more further down the back, especially in the lumbar region.

Note: Soulié (1994) locates BL 20 on the back, approximately two FW (Finger Width) on each side of the eleventh thoracic vertebra, between two vertical muscles (iliocostalis and longissimus dorsi), at the lower edge of the eleventh rib, in a hollow; on the latissimus dorsi; two FW below BL 19; two FW superior and slightly lateral to BL 21. In the angle of and under the last rib; two FW on each side of GV 6 (Du 6); two FW medial to BL 49. Legge (1999) locates UB 20 at 1.5 cun lateral to the tip of the spinous process of the 11th thoracic vertebra. Voisin (1974) locates B 20 at 2 fb (finger breadth) from the midline of the back (centre of spinous process D 11).

Worsley (1982) uses 2 ACI (Anatomical Chinese Inch) for the inner Bladder line and 4 ACI for the outer Bladder line (for the thoracic region of the back). Lavier (1974) doesn't use any measurement, the outer Bladder line touches the inner border of the scapula and the inner Bladder line is midway between the border of the scapula and the median line. Voisin (1974) uses 2 fb (finger breadth) from the midline of the back at the centre of the spinous process for the inner Bladder line and 4 fb from the midline of the back at the centre of the spinous process. Wu (1973) uses 2 pouce from the median line for the inner Bladder line measurement and 4 pouce from the median line for the outer Bladder line measurement.

Bl 21 WEI SHU – STOMACH CORRESPONDENCE

⊥ ***0.3 TO 0.5 CUN*** ∆ ***3 TO 21***

- STOMACH BACK SHU/Shu Transporting/AEP (Associated Effect Point)/ Approval/Vesical Reinforcement Point

Pos: Position of patient: seated and upright.

Loc:
a) On the posterior torso.
b) On the inner line or the medial branch of the Bladder channel.
c) 1.5 cun lateral to the posterior median line.
d) Between the 12th thoracic and the 1st lumbar vertebrae (level with the base of the spinous process of the 12th thoracic vertebra).
e) Level with Bl 50.

Tip:
a) Please read **"HOW TO MARK OUT AND CHECK THE VERTEBRAE"** for further guidance.
b) The cun measurement from the posterior median line to the inner bladder line is 1.5 cun. Identify the outer Bladder line at 3 cun. This is taken from the posterior median line to the medial border of the scapula at the level of T3.
c) The inner Bladder line is at 1.5 cun (half of 3 cun).
d) Place your finger in the intervertebral space of T12 and L1 and then palpate laterally to 1.5 cun until you feel a *men* (depression).
e) Palpating with the flow of the Bladder channel from the top of the back can assist in locating the point.
f) The posterior torso widens and narrows according to the person's body shape, with the cun measurement being a proportional measurement. Therefore 1.5 cun at the level of T3 may not be the same further down the back, e.g. 1.5 cun at the level of T4/T5 may have a difference of 0.5 cm or more further down the back, especially in the lumbar region.

Note: Soulié (1994) locates BL 21 on the back, one large FW (Finger Width) on each side of the twelfth thoracic vertebra, on the inferior edge of the last rib, between the muscle along the thoracic spine (longissimus dorsi), and the edge of the twelfth rib, in an angle, on the latissimus dorsi., deep on the lateral superior edge of the transverse process of the first lumbar vertebra; in a hollow; two FW below BL 20; two FW above BL 22; one large FW medial to BL 50. Legge (1999) locates UB 21 at 1.5 cun lateral to the tip of the spinous process of the 12th thoracic vertebra. Voisin (1974) locates B 21 at 2 fb (finger breadth) from the midline of the back (centre of spinous process D 12). Worsley (1982) uses 2 ACI (Anatomical Chinese Inch) for the inner Bladder line and 4 ACI for the outer Bladder line (for the thoracic region of the back).

Lavier (1974) doesn't use any measurement, the outer Bladder line touches the inner border of the scapula and the inner Bladder line is midway between the border of the scapula and the median line. Voisin (1974) uses 2 fb (finger breadth) from the midline of the back at the centre of the spinous process for the inner Bladder line and 4 fb from the midline of the back at the centre of the spinous process. Wu (1973) uses 2 pouce from the median line for the inner Bladder line measurement and 4 pouce from the median line for the outer Bladder line measurement.

Bl 22 SAN JIAO SHU – TRIPLE HEATER CORRESPONDENCE

⊥ ***0.3 TO 0.5 CUN*** **Δ** ***3 TO 20***

- TRIPLE HEATER BACK SHU/Shu Transporting/AEP (Associated Effect Point)/ Approval/Vesical Reinforcement Point

Pos: Position of patient: seated and upright.

Loc: a) On the posterior torso.
b) On the inner line or the medial branch of the Bladder channel.
c) 1.5 cun lateral to the posterior median line.
d) Between the 1st and 2nd lumbar vertebrae (level with the base of the spinous process of the 1st lumbar vertebra).
e) Level with Du 5 and Bl 51.

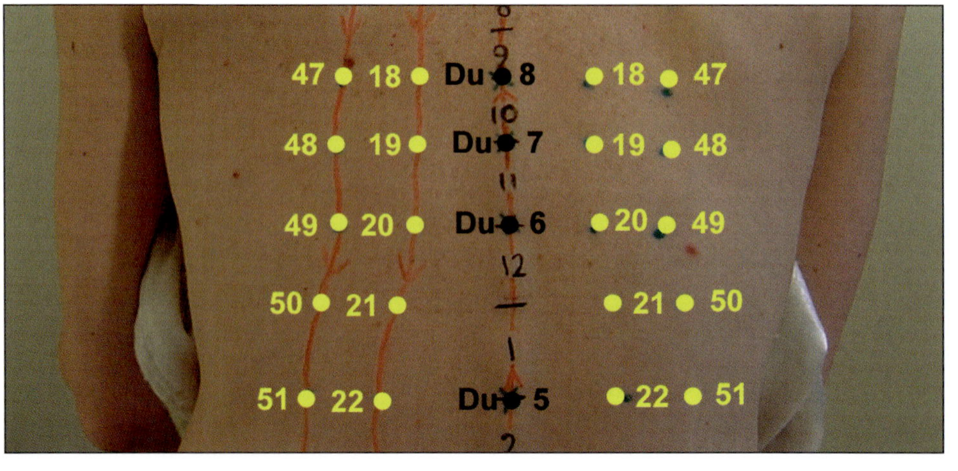

Tip: a) Please read **"HOW TO MARK OUT AND CHECK THE VERTEBRAE"** for further guidance.

b) The cun measurement from the posterior median line to the inner bladder line is 1.5 cun. Identify the outer Bladder line at 3 cun. This is taken from the posterior median line to the medial border of the scapula at the level of T3.

c) The inner Bladder line is at 1.5 cun (half of 3 cun).

d) Place your finger in the intervertebral space of L1 and L2 and then palpate laterally to 1.5 cun until you feel a *men* (depression).

e) Palpating with the flow of the Bladder channel from the top of the back can assist in locating the point.

f) The posterior torso widens and narrows according to the person's body shape, with the cun measurement being a proportional measurement. Therefore 1.5 cun at the level of T3 may not be the same further down the back, e.g. 1.5 cun at the level of T4/T5 may have a difference of 0.5 cm or more further down the back, especially in the lumbar region.

Note: Soulié (1994) locates BL 22 on the lumbar area, one large FW (Finger Width) on each side of the inferior edge of the first lumbar vertebra, two FW under the last rib, between two vertical muscles (iliocostalis, longissimus dorsi), on the superior edge of the transverse process of the second lumbar vertebra, on the latissimus dorsi; in a hollow; two FW below BL 21; two FW above BL 23; two FW medial and slightly above BL 51; two FW on either side of GV 5 (Du 5). Legge (1999) locates UB 22 at 1.5 cun lateral to the tip of the spinous process of the 1st lumbar vertebra. Voisin (1974) locates B 22 at 2 fb (finger breadth) from the midline of the back (centre of spinous process L 1).

Worsley (1982) uses 2.5 ACI (Anatomical Chinese Inch) for the inner Bladder line and 4.5 ACI for the outer Bladder line (for the lumbar region of the back). Lavier (1974) doesn't use any measurement, the outer Bladder line touches the inner border of the scapula and the inner Bladder line is midway between the border of the scapula and the median line. Voisin (1974) uses 2 fb (finger breadth) from the midline of the back at the centre of the spinous process for the inner Bladder line and 4 fb from the midline of the back at the centre of the spinous process. Wu (1973) uses 2 pouce from the median line for the inner Bladder line measurement and 4 pouce from the median line for the outer Bladder line measurement.

Bl 23 SHEN SHU – KIDNEY'S CORRESPONDENCE

⊥ ***0.1 TO 0.8 CUN*** Δ ***3 TO 15***

- KIDNEY BACK SHU/Shu Transporting/AEP (Associated Effect Point)/Approval/ Vesical Reinforcement Point
- A.E (Aggressive Energy) – Needle Depth = 0.1 cun
- A Seven External Dragons (E.D's) Point (the other points are Du 20, Bl 11 and Bl 61)

Pos: Position of patient: seated and upright.

Loc: a) On the posterior torso.
b) On the inner line or the medial branch of the Bladder channel.
c) 1.5 cun lateral to the posterior median line.
d) Between the 2nd and 3rd lumbar vertebrae (level with the base of the spinous process of the 2nd lumbar vertebra).
e) Level with Du 4 and Bl 52.

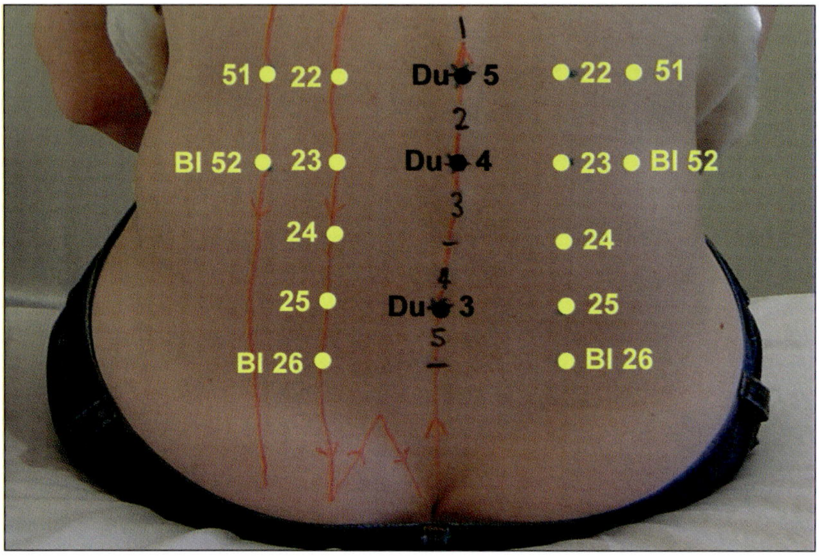

Tip: a) Please read **"HOW TO MARK OUT AND CHECK THE VERTEBRAE"** for further guidance.
b) The cun measurement from the posterior median line to the inner bladder line is 1.5 cun. Identify the outer Bladder line at 3 cun. This is taken from the posterior median line to the medial border of the scapula at the level of T3.
c) The inner Bladder line is at 1.5 cun (half of 3 cun).
d) Place your finger in the intervertebral space of L2 and L3 and then palpate laterally to 1.5 cun until you feel a *men* (depression).
e) Palpating with the flow of the Bladder channel from the top of the back can assist in locating the point.
f) The posterior torso widens and narrows according to the person's body shape, with the cun measurement being a proportional measurement. Therefore 1.5 cun at the level of T3 may not be the same further down the back, e.g. 1.5 cun at the level of T4/T5 may have a difference of 0.5 cm or more further down the back, especially in the lumbar region.

Note: Soulié (1994) locates BL 23 on the lumbar area, approximately one large FW (Finger Width) on each side of the lower edge of the second lumbar vertebra, between the second and third, between two vertical muscles, on the lower edge of the point of the transverse process of the second lumbar vertebra, on the medial edge of the insertion of the greater psoas; in a hollow; two FW below BL 22; two FW above BL 24; two FW medial and slightly inferior to BL 51; two FW on either side of GV 4 (Du 4).

Legge (1999) locates UB 23 at 1.5 cun lateral to the tip of the spinous process of the 2nd lumbar vertebra. Voisin (1974) locates B 23 at 2 fb (finger breadth) from the midline of the back (centre of spinous process L 2). Worsley (1982) uses 2.5 ACI (Anatomical Chinese Inch) for the inner Bladder line and 4.5 ACI for the outer Bladder line (for the lumbar region of the back). Lavier (1974) doesn't use any measurement, the outer Bladder line touches the inner border of the scapula and the inner Bladder line is midway between the border of the scapula and the median line.

Voisin (1974) uses 2 fb (finger breadth) from the midline of the back at the centre of the spinous process for the inner Bladder line and 4 fb from the midline of the back at the centre of the spinous process. Wu (1973) uses 2 pouce from the median line for the inner Bladder line measurement and 4 pouce from the median line for the outer Bladder line measurement.

Bl 24 QI HAI SHU – SEA OF QI CORRESPONDENCE

⊥ ***0.5 TO 0.7 CUN*** ***Δ 3 TO 5***

- SEA OF QI BACK SHU/Shu Transporting/AEP (Associated Effect Point)/ Approval

Pos: Position of patient: seated and upright.

Loc:
a) On the posterior torso.
b) On the inner line or the medial branch of the Bladder channel.
c) 1.5 cun lateral to the posterior median line.
d) Between the 3rd and 4th lumbar vertebrae (level with the base of the spinous process of the 3rd lumbar vertebra).

Tip:
a) Please read **"HOW TO MARK OUT AND CHECK THE VERTEBRAE"** for further guidance.
b) The cun measurement from the posterior median line to the inner bladder line is 1.5 cun. Identify the outer Bladder line at 3 cun. This is taken from the posterior median line to the medial border of the scapula at the level of T3.
c) The inner Bladder line is at 1.5 cun (half of 3 cun).
d) Place your finger in the intervertebral space of L3 and L4 and then palpate laterally to 1.5 cun until you feel a *men* (depression).
e) Palpating with the flow of the Bladder channel from the top of the back can assist in locating the point.
f) The posterior torso widens and narrows according to the person's body shape, with the cun measurement being a proportional measurement. Therefore 1.5 cun at the level of T3 may not be the same further down the back, e.g. 1.5 cun at the level of T4/T5 may have a difference of 0.5 cm or more further down the back, especially in the lumbar region.

Note: Soulié (1994) locates BL 24 on the lumbar area, one large FW (Finger Width) on either side of the interval between the third and fourth lumbar vertebra, on the lateral edge of a vertical muscle, on the inferior edge of the transverse process of the third lumbar vertebra; in a hollow; two FW under BL 23; two FW above BL 25; one FW medial to BL 52. Legge (1999) locates UB 24 at 1.5 cun lateral to the tip of the spinous process of the 3rd lumbar vertebra. Voisin (1974) locates B 24 at 2 fb (finger breadth) from the midline of the back (centre of spinous process L 3). Worsley (1982) uses 2.5 ACI (Anatomical Chinese Inch) for the inner Bladder line and 4.5 ACI for the outer Bladder line (for the lumbar region of the back).

Lavier (1974) doesn't use any measurement, the outer Bladder line touches the inner border of the scapula and the inner Bladder line is midway between the border of the scapula and the median line. Voisin (1974) uses 2 fb (finger breadth) from the midline of the back at the centre of the spinous process for the inner Bladder line and 4 fb from the midline of the back at the centre of the spinous process. Wu (1973) uses 2 pouce from the median line for the inner Bladder line measurement and 4 pouce from the median line for the outer Bladder line measurement.

Bl 25 DA CHANG SHU – LARGE INTESTINES CORRESPONDENCE

⊥ ***0.3 TO 1.0 CUN*** ***Δ 3 TO 20***

- LARGE INTESTINE BACK SHU/Shu Transporting/AEP (Associated Effect Point)/Approval/Vesical Reinforcement Point

Pos: Position of patient: seated and upright.

Loc: a) On the posterior torso.
b) On the inner line or the medial branch of the Bladder channel.
c) 1.5 cun lateral to the posterior median line.
d) Between the 4th and 5th lumbar vertebrae (level with the base of the spinous process of the 4th lumbar vertebra).
e) Level with Du 3.

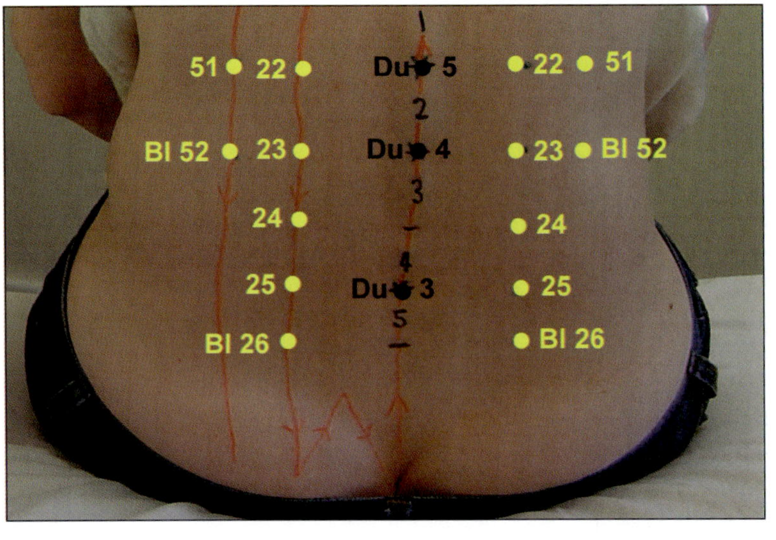

Tip: a) Please read **"HOW TO MARK OUT AND CHECK THE VERTEBRAE"** for further guidance.

b) The cun measurement from the posterior median line to the inner bladder line is 1.5 cun. Identify the outer Bladder line at 3 cun. This is taken from the posterior median line to the medial border of the scapula at the level of T3.

c) The inner Bladder line is at 1.5 cun (half of 3 cun).

d) Place your finger in the intervertebral space of L4 and L5 and then palpate laterally to 1.5 cun until you feel a *men* (depression).

e) Palpating with the flow of the Bladder channel from the top of the back can assist in locating the point.

f) The posterior torso widens and narrows according to the person's body shape, with the cun measurement being a proportional measurement. Therefore 1.5 cun at the level of T3 may not be the same further down the back, e.g. 1.5 cun at the level of T4/T5 may have a difference of 0.5 cm or more further down the back, especially in the lumbar region.

Note: Soulié (1994) locates BL 25 on the lumbar area, one large FW (Finger Width) on either side of the mid-height of the fourth lumbar vertebra, on the upper edge and medial to the prominent angle of the iliac crest, between the muscles (common mass) and the transverse muscles; in a hollow; two FW under BL 24; two FW above BL 26; two FW medial and slightly under BL 52. Legge (1999) locates UB 25 at 1.5 cun lateral to the tip of the spinous process of the 4th lumbar vertebra. Voisin (1974) locates B 25 at 2 fb (finger breadth) from the midline of the back (centre of spinous process L 4).

Worsley (1982) uses 2.5 ACI (Anatomical Chinese Inch) for the inner Bladder line and 4.5 ACI for the outer Bladder line (for the lumbar region of the back). Lavier (1974) doesn't use any measurement, the outer Bladder line touches the inner border of the scapula and the inner Bladder line is midway between the border of the scapula and the median line. Voisin (1974) uses 2 fb (finger breadth) from the midline of the back at the centre of the spinous process for the inner Bladder line and 4 fb from the midline of the back at the centre of the spinous process. Wu (1973) uses 2 pouce from the median line for the inner Bladder line measurement and 4 pouce from the median line for the outer Bladder line measurement.

Bl 26 GUAN YUAN SHU – FIRST GATE CORRESPONDENCE

⊥ ***0.7 TO 1.0 CUN*** **Δ 3**

- FIRST(SOURCE) GATE BACK SHU/Shu Transporting/AEP (Associated Effect Point)/Approval

Pos: Position of patient: seated and upright.

Loc: a) On the posterior torso.

b) On the inner line or the medial branch of the Bladder channel.

c) 1.5 cun lateral to the posterior median line.

d) Between the 5th lumbar and the 1st sacral vertebrae (level with the base of the spinous process of the 5th lumbar vertebra).

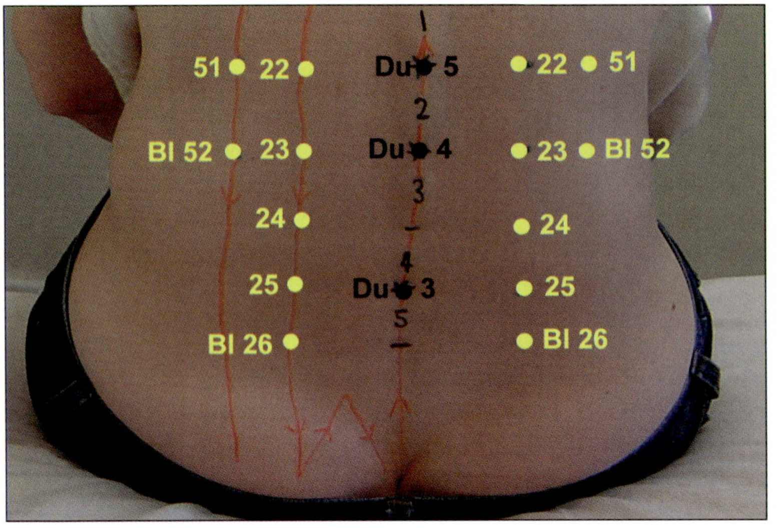

Tip:
- a) Please read **"HOW TO MARK OUT AND CHECK THE VERTEBRAE"** for further guidance.
- b) The cun measurement from the posterior median line to the inner bladder line is 1.5 cun. Identify the outer Bladder line at 3 cun. This is taken from the posterior median line to the medial border of the scapula at the level of T3.
- c) The inner Bladder line is at 1.5 cun (half of 3 cun).
- d) Place your finger in the intervertebral space of L5 and S1 and then palpate laterally to 1.5 cun until you feel a *men* (depression).
- e) Palpating with the flow of the Bladder channel from the top of the back can assist in locating the point.
- f) The posterior torso widens and narrows according to the person's body shape, with the cun measurement being a proportional measurement. Therefore 1.5 cun at the level of T3 may not be the same further down the back, e.g. 1.5 cun at the level of T4/T5 may have a difference of 0.5 cm or more further down the back, especially in the lumbar region.

Note: Soulié (1994) locates BL 26 on the lumbar area, in the deep angle of the upper edge of the sacrum and the medial edge of the hip bone, at the upper opening of the sacroiliac articulation, on the lower edge of the transverse process of the fifth lumbar vertebra. One FW (Finger Width) on either side of the lumbosacral articulation; in a hollow; on the common mass of lumbar and vertebral muscles; two FW under BL 25; two FW superior and medial to BL 27; above BL 31; one FW either side of GV 3 (Du 3). Legge (1999) locates UB 26 at 1.5 cun lateral to the tip of the spinous process of the 5th lumbar vertebra. Voisin (1974) locates B 26 at 2 fb (finger breadth) from the midline of the back (centre of spinous process L 5).

Worsley (1982) uses 2.5 ACI (Anatomical Chinese Inch) for the inner Bladder line and 4.5 ACI for the outer Bladder line (for the lumbar region of the back). Lavier (1974) doesn't use any measurement, the outer Bladder line touches the inner border of the scapula and the inner Bladder line is midway between the border of the scapula and the median line. Voisin (1974) uses 2 fb (finger breadth) from the midline of the back at the centre of the spinous process for the inner Bladder line and 4 fb from the midline of the back at the centre of the spinous process. Wu (1973) uses 2 pouce from the median line for the inner Bladder line measurement and 4 pouce from the median line for the outer Bladder line measurement.

THE SACRUM.

The sacrum is triangular in shape and is formed by five fused vertebrae. At its superior border it articulates with the base of the fifth lumbar vertebra, and at its inferior border it articulates with the coccyx (sacrococcygeal articluation or sacral hiatus which is a semi moveable joint). On each side of the posterior median line there are four pelvic sacral foramina where acupuncture points are located. These foramina run longitudinally on the body of the sacrum. The foramina are located more medially as the sacrum begins to narrow downwards.
The sacroiliac joint is located between the lateral border of the body of the sacrum and the medial border of the iliac crest towards the posterior superior iliac spine (PSIS) of the ilium. The ilium is part of the hip bone or the innominate bone. Longitudinally the sacroiliac joint tends to run in a straight line. Acupuncture points are located level with the four sacral foramina.

Tip a) From the base of L5 there are fused vertebrae that form the sacrum. The longitudinal size of the sacrum is approximately the size of the patient's fist from the knuckle (metacarpo-phalangeal joint) of the thumb to the knuckle (metacarpo-phalangeal joint) of the little finger. If the measurement from the base of L5 to the bottom of the sacrum/superior border of the coccyx (sacrococcygeal articulation) is longer than the person's fist the sacrum appears too long. Likewise if the measurement is less than the size of the patient's fist, then the sacrum appears to be too small. Therefore re-check the intervertebral spaces of the whole back. The sacrococcygeal articulation is located approximately at the superior border of the gluteal fold.

b) Marking the lumbar this will ensure you have the correct location of the base of L5 and the superior border of the sacrum body. Please see tips c) to e) for guidance.

c) To check the vertebrae place your little fingers (5th digit) on top of the iliac crest with your 1st, 2nd and 3rd fingers vertically on top of the little finger. By placing your thumbs horizontally and parallel to the spaces of the vertebrae, they should line up with the intervertebral space of L2/L3 as illustrated below:

```
o (2)        o – thumb   L2/L3   thumb – o        o (2)
o (3)                                             o (3)
o (4)                                             o (4)
o (5th digit)                                     o (5th digit)
             (left iliac crest)(right iliac crest)
```

d) By placing your left and right index fingers on the top of the left and right iliac crests and with your 1st, 3rd, 4th, and 5th digits at the same level (transverse), your thumbs should be at the level of L3/L4 intervertebral space, as illustrated below:

```
o o o o  o – thumb         L3/L4        thumb – o  o o o o
 5 4 3 2  1st digit                       1st digit  2 3 4 5
          l                                        l
          index (2nd) fingers on top of the iliac crest
```

e) Another check is to place your left and right index (2nd) fingers on the top of the left and right iliac crests as above, but this time allowing your thumb to fall away naturally instead of keeping it transverse with the other digits. By allowing your thumb to drop away they should line up with L4/L5 intervertebral space, as illustrated below:

5 4 3 2 (digits)   2 3 4 5 (digits)

o o o o̲   o̲ o o o

o   L4/L5   o

thumbs

index (2nd) fingers on top of the iliac crest

Tips c), d) and e) "=" indicates the top of the iliac crest.

f) Further tips for Bladder sacral points located are included with the individual points.

Bl 27-34 are on the posterior torso, on the sacrum, Bl 35 is lateral to the coccyx. These points can be located with the patient in a seated position, or prone (in which case place a pillow under the pelvis to emphasise the sacral structures).

Bl 27 XIAO CHANG SHU – SMALL INTESTINES CORRESPONDENCE

⊥ ***0.3 TO 1.0 CUN***   Δ ***3 TO 20***

Palpation and treatment of sacral points in pregnancy is forbidden as they may induce labour.

- SMALL INTESTINE BACK SHU/Shu Transporting/AEP (Associated Effect Point)/ Approval/Vesical Reinforcement Point

Pos: Position of patient: seated and upright, or prone with a pillow under the pelvis.

Loc: a) On the posterior torso.
b) On the sacrum.
c) At the medial border of the sacroiliac joint.
d) Approximately half way between Bl 26 and Bl 28.
e) Level with the 1st sacral foramen (Bl 31).
f) 1.5 cun lateral to the posterior median line.

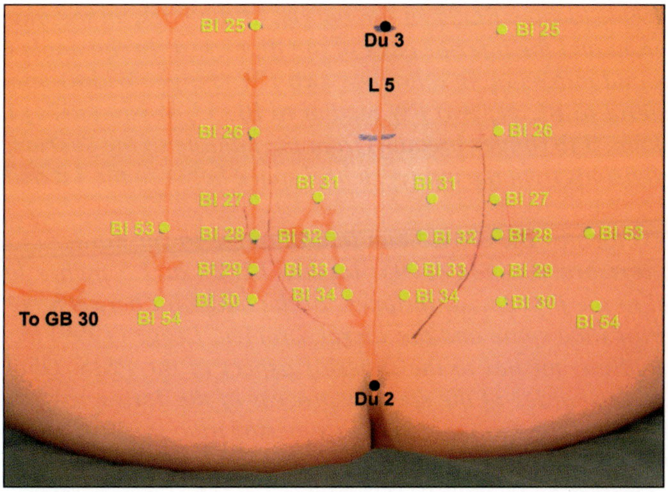

Tip:
a) Please read "THE SACRUM" for guidance. Mark out the superior and inferior borders of the sacrum body.
b) Locate the sacroiliac joint of the ilium, the Bladder channel flows through the joint and is more or less a 'plumb' line. Palpate laterally firmly and sensitively from the posterior median line of the body of the sacrum until you locate the sacroiliac joint.
c) If you cannot feel the joint, locate Bl 26 first (see separate location) and then palpate with your finger inferiorly. If you still cannot feel the joint draw a longitudinal line directly below Bl 26, then palpate for Bl 27 as you will be in the area laterally from the posterior median line to the sacroiliac joint.
d) The posterior superior iliac spine of the ilium (PSIS) is a bony protruberence that may be palpated on people with a light to medium covering of tissue. Alternatively locate the top of the iliac crest and follow the contour of the bone towards the sacrum where you should feel a bony protruberence.
e) The inferior and medial borders of the posterior superior iliac spine form an 'L' shape on the right side of the body and a reversed 'L' on the left side of the body. On the corner of the 'L' in the sacroiliac joint is Bl 28. Approximately half way between Bl 26 and Bl 28 is Bl 27.
f) Palpation will accurately locate the point in the sacroiliac joint.
g) If you cannot locate the posterior superior iliac spine of the ilium you need to locate the second sacral foramen. This is usually the easiest one to locate as it has a large *men* (depression) to palpate, and the curvature of the sacrum bulges out more than the location of the first sacral foramen.
h) The second sacral foramen is usually level with the inferior border of the posterior superior iliac spine of the ilium, on the sacrum body. The inferior border is a bony protruberence that may be palpated on people that have a light to medium covering of tissue.
i) When you have located the second sacral foramen, palpate superiorly and very slightly laterally until you feel the depression of the first sacral foramen. Level with the first sacral foramen palpate laterally to the sacroiliac joint where Bl 27 is located.

Note: Soulié (1994) locates BL 27 at the bottom of the back, in the angle between the lateral edge of the sacrum and the inferior edge of the iliac crest. In the angle of the insertions of the gluteus medius and maximus; in a hollow; two FW (Finger Width) inferior and lateral to BL 26; one FW lateral to BL 31; two FW medial to BL 53. Voisin (1974) locates B 27 at S 1, in the sacroiliac joint, 3 fb (finger breadth) from the midline of the sacrum. So (1985) locates BL 27 lateral 1.5 divisions from the intervertebral space between the 1st and 2nd sacral vertebrae.

Shanghai (1993) locates BL 27, 1.5 cun lateral to the lower border of the spinous process of the 1st sacral vertebra. Eachou (1995) locates BL 27 at 1.5 inches lateral to the posterior midline, lateral to the first sacral foramen, at the midpoint between the medial margin of the posterior superior iliac spine and the sacral foramen. Legge (1999) locates UB 27 at 1.5 cun lateral to the midline, medial to the superior aspect of the PSIS. Qiu (1996) locates UB 27 level with the lower border of the spinous process of the 1st sacral vertebra, 1.5 cun lateral. Lawson-Wood locates III 27 on the postero-superior iliac spine, 4 cm lateral to the first sacral foramen. Shandong (1982) locate Xiaochangshu at 1.5 cun lateral to the lower border of the 1st vertebra sacrales. Academy (1975) locates UB 27, 1.5 cun lateral to the midline of the back, level to the 1st posterior sacral foramen, in the depression between the medial border of the posterior superior iliac spine and the sacrum..

Worsley (1982) uses 2.5 ACI (Anatomical Chinese Inch) for the inner Bladder line and 4.5 ACI for the outer Bladder line (for the sacral region of the back). Lavier (1974) doesn't use any measurement, the outer Bladder line touches the inner border of the scapula and the inner Bladder line is midway between the border of the scapula and the median line. Voisin (1974) uses 2 fb (finger breadth) from the midline of the back at the centre of the spinous process for the inner Bladder line and 4 fb from the midline of the back at the centre of the spinous process. Wu (1973) uses 2 pouce from the median line for the inner Bladder line measurement and 4 pouce from the median line for the outer Bladder line measurement.

Bl 28 PANG GUANG SHU – BLADDER CORRESPONDENCE

⊥ ***0.3 TO 1.0 CUN*** **Δ *3 TO 15***

Palpation and treatment of sacral points in pregnancy is forbidden as they may induce labour.

- BLADDER BACK SHU/Shu Transporting/AEP (Associated Effect Point)/ Approval/Vesical Reinforcement Point

Pos: Position of patient: seated and upright, or prone with a pillow under the pelvis.

Loc: a) On the posterior torso.
b) On the sacrum.
c) At the medial border of the sacroiliac joint.
d) At the level of the inferior and medial borders of the posterior superior iliac spine (PSIS).
e) Level with the 2nd sacral foramen (Bl 32).
f) 1.5 cun lateral to the posterior median line.

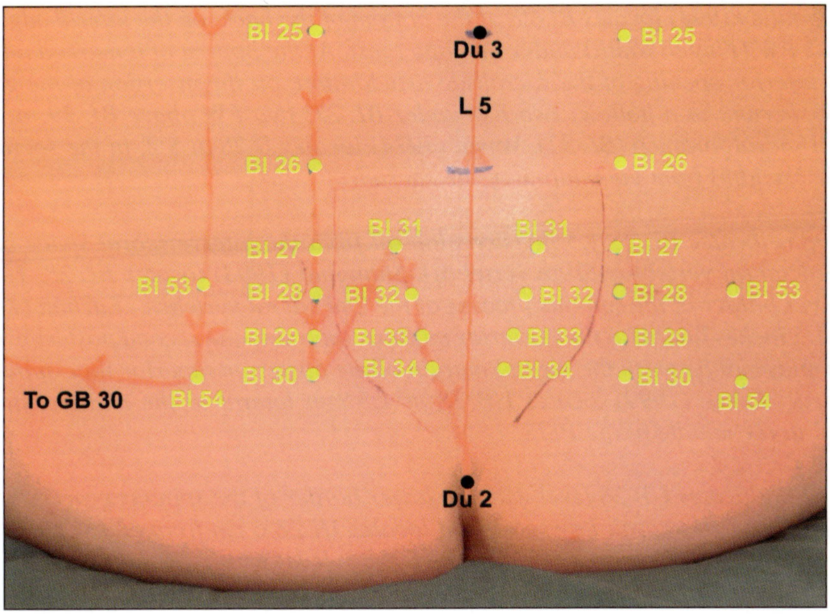

Tip:

a) Please read "THE SACRUM" for guidance. Mark out the superior and inferior borders of the sacrum body.

b) Locate the sacroiliac joint of the ilium, the Bladder channel flows through the joint and is more or less a 'plumb' line. Palpate laterally firmly and sensitively from the posterior median line of the body of the sacrum until you locate the sacroiliac joint.

c) If you cannot feel the joint, locate Bl 26 first (see separate location) and then palpate with your finger inferiorly. If you still cannot feel the joint draw a longitudinal line directly below Bl 26, then palpate for Bl 27 as you will be in the area laterally from the posterior median line to the sacroiliac joint. Bl 28 is located approximately the same distance as between Bl 26 and Bl 27 and inferior to Bl 27.

d) The posterior superior iliac spine of the ilium (PSIS) is a bony protruberence that may be palpated on people with a light to medium covering of tissue. Alternatively locate the top of the iliac crest and follow the contour of the bone towards the sacrum where you should feel a bony protruberence.

e) The inferior and medial borders of the posterior superior iliac spine form an 'L' shape on the right side of the body and a reversed 'L' on the left side of the body. On the corner of the 'L' in the sacroiliac joint is Bl 28.

f) Palpation will accurately locate the point in the sacroiliac joint.

g) If you cannot locate the posterior superior iliac spine of the ilium you need to locate the second sacral foramen. This is usually the easiest one to locate as it has a large *men* (depression) to palpate, and the curvature of the sacrum bulges out more than the location of the first sacral foramen. On a level with the second sacral foramen palpate laterally to the sacroiliac joint to locate Bl 28.

h) The second sacral foramen is usually level with the inferior border of the posterior superior iliac spine of the ilium, on the sacrum body.

Note: Soulié (1994) locates BL 28 at the bottom of the back, on the lateral edge of the sacrum, about 2 FW (Finger Width) under the iliac crest. At the bottom of a marked notch of the bone, at the inferior opening of the sacroiliac articulation, on the insertion of the gluteus maximus on the sacrum; in a hollow; two FW under BL 27; two FW above BL 29; at the level of the second sacral foramen (BL 32). Voisin (1974) locates B 28 at S 2, in the sacroiliac joint, 3 fb (finger breadth) from the midline of the sacrum.

So (1985) locates BL 28 1.5 divisions lateral from the intervertebral space between the 2nd and 3rd sacral vertebrae (19th vertebra). Shanghai (1993) locates BL 28, 1.5 cun lateral to the lower border of the spinous process of the 2nd sacral vertebra. Eachou (1995) locates BL 28 at 1.5 inches lateral to the posterior midline, lateral to the second posterior sacral foramen, at the midpoint between the medial margin of the posterior superior iliac spine and the sacral foramen. Legge (1999) locates UB 28 at 1.5 cun lateral to the midline, in the depression medial to the middle of the PSIS.

Qiu (1996) locates UB 28 level with the lower border of the spinous process of the 2nd sacral vertebra, 1.5 cun lateral. Lawson-Wood locates III 28 6 cm from and slightly below the third sacral foramen. Academy (1975) locates UB 28, level with the 2nd posterior sacral foramen, 1.5 cun lateral to Du Mai, in the depression between the lower medial border of the posterior superior iliac spine and the sacrum. Ellis (1991) locates BL 28 at the level of the 2nd sacral foramen, 1.5 inches lateral to the governing vessel, in the depression between the medial border of the posterior superior iliac spine and the sacrum.

Worsley (1982) uses 2.5 ACI (Anatomical Chinese Inch) for the inner Bladder line and 4.5 ACI for the outer Bladder line (for the sacral region of the back). Lavier (1974) doesn't use any measurement, the outer Bladder line touches the inner border of the scapula and the inner Bladder line is midway between the border of the scapula and the median line. Voisin (1974) uses 2 fb (finger breadth) from the midline of the back at the centre of the spinous process for the inner Bladder line and 4 fb from the midline of the back at the centre of the spinous process.

Soulié (1994) not only uses various measurements lateral to the vertebra but also uses other anatomy to help locate the points. Wu (1973) uses 2 pouce from the median line for the inner Bladder line measurement and 4 pouce from the median line for the outer Bladder line measurement. Shandong (1982) locates Pangguanshu at 1.5 cun lateral to the lower border of the 2nd vertebra sacrales.

Bl 29 ZHONG LU SHU – MIDDLE OF THE BACKBONE CORRESPONDENCE

⊥ ***0.3 TO 0.5 CUN*** Δ ***3 TO 15***

Palpation and treatment of sacral points in pregnancy is forbidden as they may induce labour.

- MIDDLE OF THE SPINE BACK SHU/Shu Transporting/AEP (Associated Effect Point)/Approval

Pos: Position of patient: seated and upright, or prone with a pillow under the pelvis.

Loc: a) On the posterior torso.
b) On the sacrum.
c) On the lateral edge of the body of the sacrum.
d) Inferior to Bl 28.
e) Approximately half way between Bl 28 and Bl 30 (see separate locations).
f) Level with the 3rd sacral foramen (Bl 33).
g) 1.5 cun lateral to the posterior median line.

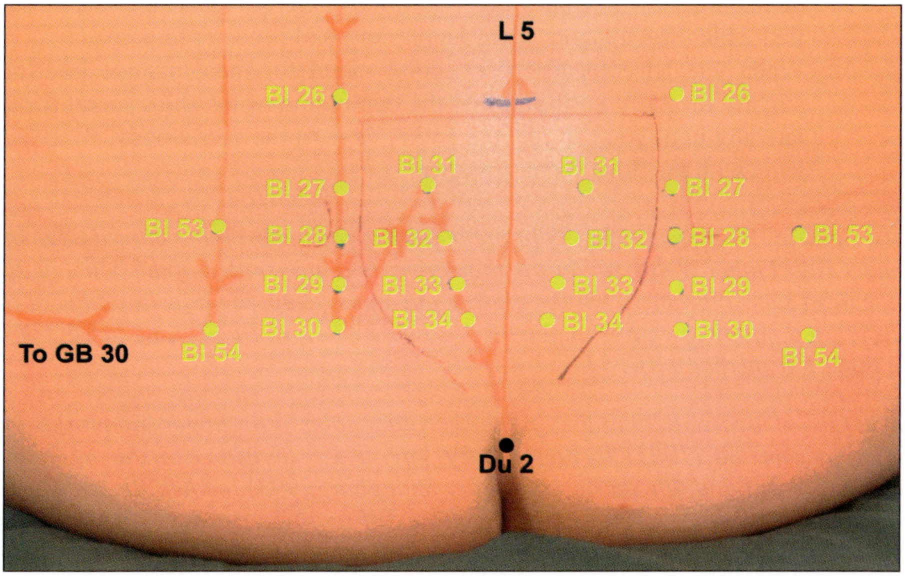

Tip: a) Please read "THE SACRUM" for guidance. Mark out the superior and inferior borders of the sacrum body.
b) Locate the sacroiliac joint of the ilium, the Bladder channel flows through the joint and is more or less a 'plumb' line. Palpate laterally firmly and sensitively from the posterior median line of the body of the sacrum until you locate the sacroiliac joint.
c) If you cannot feel the joint, locate Bl 26 (see separate location) and palpate inferiorly. If you still cannot feel the joint draw a longitudinal line directly below Bl 26 and then palpate for Bl 27 which is located lateral to the edge of the body of the sacrum in the sacroiliac joint. Bl 28 is located approximately the same distance as between Bl 26 and Bl 27 and inferior to Bl 27.

d) If Bl 28 is difficult to locate please refer to Bl 28 location.
e) The posterior superior iliac spine of the ilium (PSIS) is a bony protruberence that may be palpated on people with a light to medium covering of tissue. Alternatively locate the top of the iliac crest and follow the contour of the bone towards the sacrum where you should feel a bony protruberence.
f) The inferior and medial borders of the posterior superior iliac spine form an 'L' shape on the right side of the body and a reversed 'L' on the left side of the body. On the corner of the 'L' in the sacroiliac joint is Bl 28.
g) Palpation will accurately locate the point in the sacroiliac joint.
h) If you cannot locate the posterior superior iliac spine of the ilium you need to locate the second sacral foramen. This is usually the easiest one to locate as it has a large *men* (depression) to palpate, and the curvature of the sacrum bulges out more than the location of the first sacral foramen. On a level with the second sacral foramen palpate laterally to the sacroiliac joint to locate Bl 28.
i) Locate and mark Bl 30 (see separate location). Bl 29 is located approximately half way between Bl 28 and Bl 30.
j) Bl 29 is level with the third sacral foramen (Bl 33) which can be difficult to locate as it is one of the smaller sacral foramen. The area of the third sacral foramen is often covered with a thick layer of tissue, therefore locate the second sacral foramen first which has a larger *men* (depression) and is easier to palpate.
k) When you have located the second sacral foramen, palpate inferiorly and very slightly medially until you feel the depression of the third sacral foramen. Palpate laterally until you can feel the lateral edge of the sacral body. Bl 29 is located on a level with the third sacral foramen.

Note: Soulié (1994) locates BL 29 at the bottom of the back, on the lateral edge of the sacrum, about 4 FW (Finger Width) under the iliac crest. In a large notch of the bone, at about the level of the third sacral foramen. On the gluteus maximus; deep, the inferiior edge of the piriformis muscle; in a hollow; two FW under BL 28; two FW above BL 30; one large FW lateral to BL 33; three FW medial to BL 54.

Voisin (1974) locates B 29 at S 3, in the sacroiliac joint, 3 fb (finger breadth) from the midline of the sacrum. So (1985) locates BL 29 lateral 1.5 divisions to the intervertebral space between the 3rd and 4th sacral vertebrae. Shanghai (1993) locates BL 29, 1.5 cun lateral to the lower border of the spinous process of the 3rd sacral vertebra. Qiu (1996) locates UB 29 level with the lower border of the spinous process of the 3rd sacral vertebra, 1.5 cun lateral.

Worsley (1982) uses 2.5 ACI (Anatomical Chinese Inch) for the inner Bladder line and 4.5 ACI for the outer Bladder line (for the sacral region of the back). Lavier (1974) doesn't use any measurement, the outer Bladder line touches the inner border of the scapula and the inner Bladder line is midway between the border of the scapula and the median line.

Voisin (1974) uses 2 fb (finger breadth) from the midline of the back at the centre of the spinous process for the inner Bladder line and 4 fb from the midline of the back at the centre of the spinous process. Wu (1973) uses 2 pouce from the median line for the inner Bladder line measurement and 4 pouce from the median line for the outer Bladder line measurement.

Bl 30 BAI HUAN SHU – WHITE RING CORRESPONDENCE

⊥ ***0.3 TO 0.8 CUN*** Δ ***FORBIDDEN TO MOXA***

Palpation and treatment of sacral points in pregnancy is forbidden as they may induce labour.

- WHITE RING BACK SHU/Shu Transporting/AEP (Associated Effect Point)/ Approval

Pos: Position of patient: seated and upright, or prone with a pillow under the pelvis.

Loc: a) On the posterior torso.
b) On the sacrum.
c) On the lateral edge of the body of the sacrum.
d) Level with the 4th sacral foramen (Bl 34).
e) Inferior to Bl 29.
f) 1.5 cun lateral to the posterior median line.

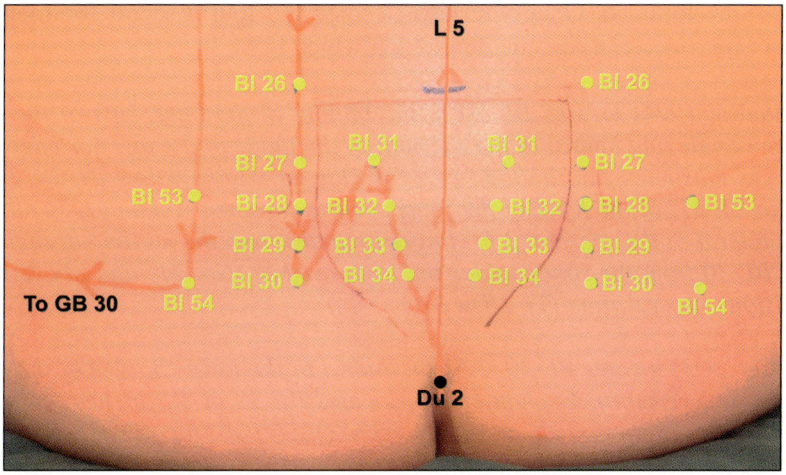

Tip: a) Please read "THE SACRUM" for guidance. Mark out the superior and inferior borders of the sacrum body.
b) Locate the sacroiliac joint of the ilium, the Bladder channel flows through the joint and is more or less a 'plumb' line. Palpate laterally firmly and sensitively from the posterior median line of the body of the sacrum until you locate the sacroiliac joint.
c) If you cannot feel the joint , locate Bl 26 (see separate location) and palpate with inferiorly. If you still cannot feel the joint draw a longitudinal line directly below Bl 26. Continue drawing your line towards the gluteus maximus muscle. The line will give you an approximation of the lateral edge of the sacrum body.
d) Bl 30 is located from the lateral edge of the sacral and the longitudinal line drawn from Bl 26. The lateral edge of the sacral body begins to narrow from the level of the third or fourth sacral foramen to the sacrococcygeal articulation (base of the sacrum). Bl 30 is usually on a line directly inferior to Bl 26, Bl 27, Bl 28 and Bl 29 but may appear to be located a little more medially to these points.

e) Another method of locating Bl 30 is to palpate for the sacrococcygeal articulation, which is a small gap between the base of the sacral body and the transverse process of the coccyx. The sacrococcygeal articulation is approximately at the superior border of the gluteal fold.

f) Once the sacrococcygeal articulation has been located, palpate superiorly and slightly lateral from the posterior median line and feel for the fourth sacral foramen (Bl 34). The depression of the fourth sacral foramen is relatively small. Palpate laterally until you feel a depression which is softer than the surrounding tissue, which is the location of Bl 30.

g) Another method of locating Bl 30 is to feel for the second sacral foramen. This is usually the easiest one to locate as it has a large *men* (depression) to palpate, and the curvature of the sacrum bulges out more than the location of the first sacral foramen.

h) Palpate from the second sacral foramen towards the sacrococcygeal articulation where should be able to palpate two smaller depressions of the third and fourth sacral foramen. You will need to palpate firmly but sensitively to be able to feel for the foramen. Once you have located the fourth sacral foramen, palpate laterally until you can feel the depression which is Bl 30.

Note: Soulié (1994) locates BL 30 at the bottom of the back, just at the edge of the lower prominent angle and lateral to the sacrum; in the angle of the inferior edge of the insertion of the gluteus maximus; in a hollow; two FW (Finger Width) below BL 29; two FW above and lateral to BL 35; at the level of the fourth sacral foramen. Voisin (1974) locates B 30 at S 4, slightly lateral to the sacrum, 3 fb (finger breadth) from the midline of the sacrum. So (1985) locates BL 30 from the space under the last vertebra (No. 21) and above the coccyx, lateral 1.5 divisions (lateral from GV 2/Du 2).

Shanghai (1993) locates BL 30, 1.5 cun lateral to the lower border of the spinous process of the 4th sacral vertebra. Eachou (1995) locates BL 30 at 1.5 inches lateral to the posterior midline, lateral to the fourth sacral foramen. Qiu (1996) locates UB 30 level with the lower border of the spinous process of the 4th sacral vertebra, 1.5 cun lateral.

Worsley (1982) uses 2.5 ACI (Anatomical Chinese Inch) for the inner Bladder line and 4.5 ACI for the outer Bladder line (for the sacral region of the back). Lavier (1974) doesn't use any measurement, the outer Bladder line touches the inner border of the scapula and the inner Bladder line is midway between the border of the scapula and the median line.

Voisin (1974) uses 2 fb (finger breadth) from the midline of the back at the centre of the spinous process for the inner Bladder line and 4 fb from the midline of the back at the centre of the spinous process.

Wu (1973) uses 2 pouce from the median line for the inner Bladder line measurement and 4 pouce from the median line for the outer Bladder line measurement. Shandong (1982) locate Baihuanshu on the lower border of the processus spinosus of the 4th vertebra sacrales, 1.5 cun lateral to Pt. Yaoshu (Du 2).

Bl 31 SHANG LIAO – UPPER SACRAL BONE

⊥ ***0.7 TO 1.0 CUN*** Δ ***3 TO 15***

FORBIDDEN TO NEEDLE AND MOXA THIS POINT IN PREGNANCY – ONLY TO BE USED FOR INDUCTION

- RE-UNION/Crossing/Meeting Point of the Bladder Channel with the Gall Bladder Channel – Foot Tai Yang Channel with the Foot Shao Yang Channel.

Pos: Position of patient: seated and upright, or prone with a pillow under the pelvis.

Loc: a) On the posterior torso.
b) On the sacrum.
c) In the 1st sacral foramen.
d) Approximately at the midpoint of the posterior superior iliac spine and the posterior median line (Du Mai).
e) Level with Bl 27.

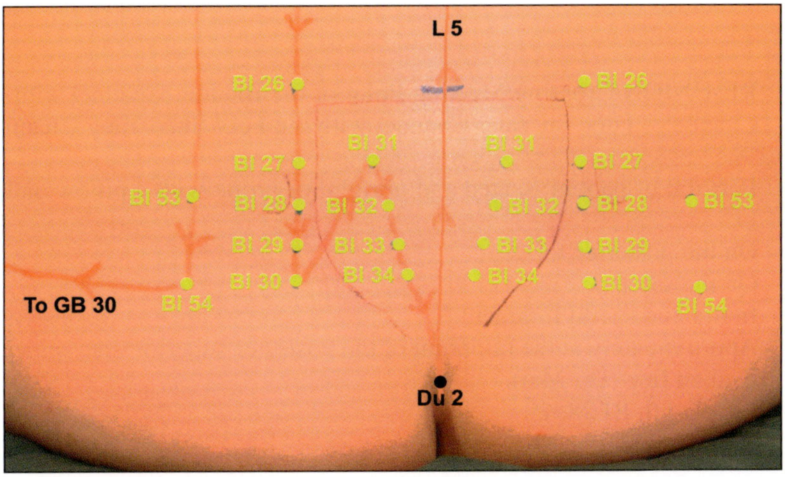

Tip: a) Please read "THE SACRUM" for guidance. Mark out the superior and inferior borders of the sacrum body.
b) Locate the second sacral foramen first as this is usually the easiest one to locate as it quite a large hole to palpate, it is often in the area of the sacrum where the sacrum body is most prominent.
c) The second sacral foramen is usually on a level with the inferior border of the posterior superior iliac spine of the ilium, on the sacrum body. The inferior border is a bony protruberence that may be palpated on people that have a light to medium covering of tissue.
d) The posterior superior iliac spine of the ilium (PSIS) is a bony protruberence that may be palpated on people with a light to medium covering of tissue. Alternatively locate the top of the iliac crest and follow the contour of the bone towards the sacrum where you should feel a bony protruberence.

e) The inferior and medial borders of the posterior superior iliac spine form an 'L' shape on the right side of the body and a reversed 'L' on the left side of the body. Bl 28 is on the corner of the 'L' in the sacroiliac joint. The second sacral foramen (Bl 32) is level with the bottom of the 'L' and on the sacral body.

f) From the second sacral foramen, palpate superiorly and very slightly laterally until you feel the *men* (depression) of the first sacral foramen (Bl 31).

Note: So (1985) locates BL 31 under the 1st sacral vertebra (No. 18 vertebra), lateral 1.25 divisions. Voisin (1974) locates B 31 in S 1, 0.5 fb (finger breadth) from the midline of the sacrum. Shandong (1982) locate Shangliao opposite to the posterior 8 sacralia foramena. Pt. Shangliao (Bl 31), Pt. Ciliao (Bl 32), Pt. Zongliao (Bl 33), Pt. Xialiao (Bl 34) are located at the 1st, 2nd, 3rd, 4th posterior sacral foramen respectively.

Bl 32 CI LIAO – SECOND SACRAL BONE

⊥ ***0.7 TO 1.0 CUN*** Δ ***7 TO 15***
FORBIDDEN TO NEEDLE AND MOXA THIS POINT IN PREGNANCY – ONLY TO BE USED FOR INDUCTION

- RE-UNION/Crossing/Meeting Point of the Bladder Channel with the Gall Bladder Channel – Foot Tai Yang Channel with the Foot Shao Yang Channel.

Pos: Position of patient: seated and upright, or prone with a pillow under the pelvis.

Loc: a) On the posterior torso.
b) On the sacrum.
c) In the 2nd sacral foramen.
d) Approximately at the midpoint of the posterior superior iliac spine and the posterior median line (Du Mai).
e) Level with Bl 28.

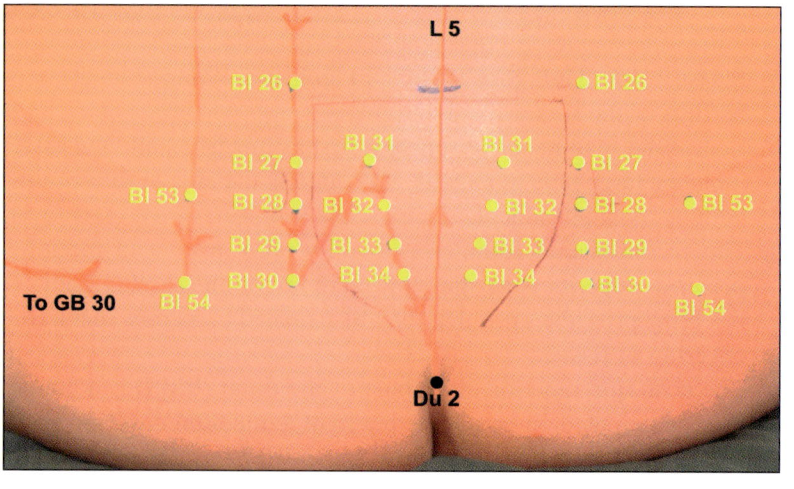

Tip:
a) Please read "THE SACRUM" for guidance. Mark out the superior and inferior borders of the sacrum body.
b) Locate the second sacral foramen first as this is usually the easiest one to locate as it quite a large hole to palpate, it is often in the area of the sacrum where the sacrum body is most prominent.
c) The second sacral foramen is usually on a level with the inferior border of the posterior superior iliac spine of the ilium, on the sacrum body. The inferior border is a bony protruberence that may be palpated on people that have a light to medium covering of tissue.
d) The posterior superior iliac spine of the ilium (PSIS) is a bony protruberence that may be palpated on people with a light to medium covering of tissue. Alternatively locate the top of the iliac crest and follow the contour of the bone towards the sacrum where you should feel a bony protruberence.
e) The inferior and medial borders of the posterior superior iliac spine form an 'L' shape on the right side of the body and a reversed 'L' on the left side of the body. Bl 28 is on the corner of the 'L' in the sacroiliac joint. The second sacral foramen (Bl 32) is level with the bottom corner of the 'L' (Bl 28) and on the sacral body.

Note: So (1985) locates BL 32 under the 2nd sacral vertebra (No. 19 vertebra), lateral 1.25 divisions. Voisin (1974) locates B 32 in S 2, 0.5 fb (finger breadth) from the midline of the sacrum. Shandong (1982) locate Ciliao opposite to the posterior 8 sacralia foramena. Pt. Shangliao (Bl 31), Pt. Ciliao (Bl 32), Pt. Zongliao (Bl 33), Pt. Xialiao (Bl 34) are located at the 1st, 2nd, 3rd, 4th posterior sacral foramen respectively.

Bl 33 ZHONG LIAO – MIDDLE SACRAL BONE

⊥ ***0.7 TO 1.0 CUN*** Δ ***3 TO 15***

FORBIDDEN TO NEEDLE AND MOXA THIS POINT IN PREGNANCY – ONLY TO BE USED FOR INDUCTION

- RE-UNION/Crossing/Meeting Point of the Bladder Channel with the Gall Bladder Channel – Foot Tai Yang Channel with the Foot Shao Yang Channel.

Pos: Position of patient: seated and upright, or prone with a pillow under the pelvis.

Loc:
a) On the posterior torso.
b) On the sacrum.
c) In the 3rd sacral foramen.
d) Approximately midway between Bl 29 and the posterior median line (Du Mai).
e) Level with Bl 29.

Tip:
a) Please read "THE SACRUM" for guidance. Mark out the superior and inferior borders of the sacrum body.
b) Locate the second sacral foramen first as this is usually the easiest one to locate as it quite a large hole to palpate, it is often in the area of the sacrum where the sacrum body is most prominent.

c) The second sacral foramen is usually on a level with the inferior border of the posterior superior iliac spine of the ilium, on the sacrum body. The inferior border is a bony protruberence that may be palpated on people that have a light to medium covering of tissue.
d) The posterior superior iliac spine of the ilium (PSIS) is a bony protruberence that may be palpated on people with a light to medium covering of tissue. Alternatively locate the top of the iliac crest and follow the contour of the bone towards the sacrum where you should feel a bony protruberence.
e) The inferior and medial borders of the posterior superior iliac spine form an 'L' shape on the right side of the body and a reversed 'L' on the left side of the body. Bl 28 is on the corner of the 'L' in the sacroiliac joint. The second sacral foramen (Bl 32) is level with the bottom corner of the 'L' (Bl 28) and on the sacral body.
f) When you have located the second sacral foramen, palpate inferiorly and very slightly medially from it until you feel the depression of the third sacral foramen (Bl 33).

Note: So (1985) locates BL 33 under the 3rd sacral vertebra (No. 20 vertebra), lateral 1 division. Voisin (1974) locates B 33 in S 3, 0.5 fb (finger breadth) from the midline of the sacrum. Shandong (1982) locate Zongliao opposite to the posterior 8 sacralia foramena. Pt. Shangliao (Bl 31), Pt. Ciliao (Bl 32), Pt. Zongliao (Bl 33), Pt. Xialiao (Bl 34) are located at the 1st, 2nd, 3rd, 4th posterior sacral foramen respectively.

Bl 34 XIA LIAO – LOWER SACRAL BONE

⊥ ***0.6 TO 0.8 CUN*** Δ ***3 TO 15***

FORBIDDEN TO NEEDLE AND MOXA THIS POINT IN PREGNANCY – ONLY TO BE USED FOR INDUCTION

- RE-UNION/Crossing/Meeting Point of the Bladder Channel with the Gall Bladder Channel – Foot Tai Yang Channel with the Foot Shao Yang Channel.

Pos: Position of patient: seated and upright, or prone with a pillow under the pelvis.

Loc:
a) On the posterior torso.
b) On the sacrum.
c) In the 4th sacral foramen.
d) Approximately midway between Bl 30 and the posterior median line (Du Mai).
e) Level with Bl 30.

Tip:
a) Please read "THE SACRUM" for guidance. Mark out the superior and inferior borders of the sacrum body..
b) Locate the second sacral foramen first as this is usually the easiest one to locate as it quite a large hole to palpate, it is often in the area of the sacrum where the sacrum body is most prominent.

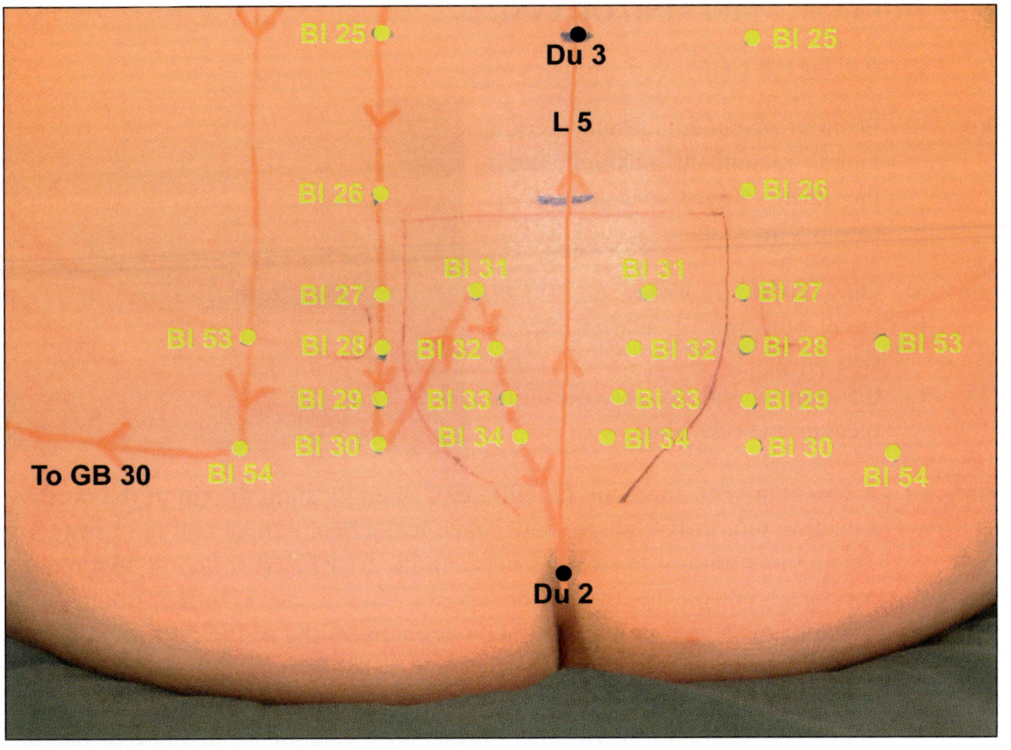

c) The second sacral foramen is usually on a level with the inferior border of the posterior superior iliac spine of the ilium, on the sacrum body. The inferior border is a bony protruberence that may be palpated on people that have a light to medium covering of tissue.

d) The posterior superior iliac spine of the ilium (PSIS) is a bony protruberence that may be palpated on people with a light to medium covering of tissue. Alternatively locate the top of the iliac crest and follow the contour of the bone towards the sacrum where you should feel a bony protruberence.

e) The inferior and medial borders of the posterior superior iliac spine form an 'L' shape on the right side of the body and a reversed 'L' on the left side of the body. Bl 28 is on the corner of the 'L' in the sacroiliac joint. The second sacral foramen (Bl 32) is level with the bottom corner of the 'L' (Bl 28) and on the sacral body.

f) When you have located the second sacral foramen, palpate inferiorly and very slightly medially from it until you feel the depression of the third sacral foramen (Bl 33). From the third sacral foramen palpate inferiorly and slightly medially until you feel the relatively small depression of Bl 34 in the fourth sacral foramen.

Note: So (1985) locates BL 34 under the 4th sacral vertebra (No. 21 vertebra), lateral 1 division. Voisin (1974) locates B 34 in S 4, 0.5 fb (finger breadth) from the midline of the sacrum. Shandong (1982) locate Xialiao opposite to the posterior 8 sacralia foramena. Pt. Shangliao (Bl 31), Pt. Ciliao (Bl 32), Pt. Zongliao (Bl 33), Pt. Xialiao (Bl 34) are located at the 1st, 2nd, 3rd, 4th posterior sacral foramen respectively.

Bl 35 HUI YANG – MEETING OF YANG

⊥ ***0.4 TO 0.8 CUN*** Δ ***5***

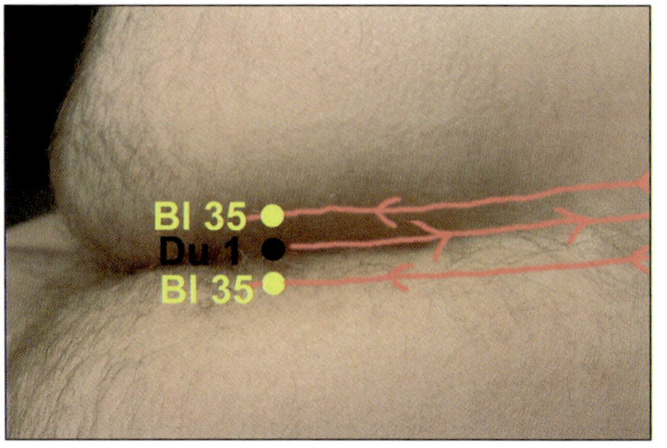

Pos: Position of patient: prone or in a lateral recumbant position, with the knees flexed and pulled up towards the chin.

Loc: a) On the posterior torso.
b) Level with the tip of the coccyx (Du 1).
c) 0.5 cun lateral to the posterior median line (Du Mai).

Tip: a) A common error made by practitioners when locating the tip of the coccyx is not palpating inferiorly enough, hence they feel a boney ridge that falls away to tissue. This is often one of the spaces between the four fused vertebrae that make up the coccygeal body. The tip of the coccyx should curve further round under the posterior torso so that you can feel a definate ending of the coccygeal body.
b) Once you have located the tip of the coccyx (Du 1), palpate laterally approximately 0.5 cun to locate Bl 35.
c) Some Five Element practitioners prefer to locate Bl 35 at 0.5 cun lateral to the sacro-coccygeal articulation. If so the patient should be in a seated position bending forward a little. Palpate down the posterior median line of the sacrum until you feel a gap at the base of the sacrum, which is the sacrococcygeal articulation (Du 2). Palpate approximately 0.5 cun laterally to this point to locate Bl 35.

Note: Wu (1973) locates Bl 35 in the gluteal furrow, upon the external edge of the coccyx, at the height of the sacro-coccygeal articulation. Soulie (1994) locates BL 35 in the coccygeal region: at the level and one large FW (Finger Width) on either side of the interval between the first and second coccygeal vertebrae, one large FW under the lower edge of the sacrum; in a hollow; about two FW inferior and medial to BL 30; two FW under BL 34; four FW above BL 36. Lavier (1974) illustrates the point on a level with GV 2 (Du). Worsley (1982) locates III 35 on the buttock, lateral to the sacrococcygeal articulation, 0.5 ACI (Anatomical Chinese Inch) lateral to the median line. Voisin (1974) locates B 35 at the sacrococcygeal joint, lateral border, 0.5 fb (finger breadth) from the midline of the sacrum.

Cun Measurements of the Upper Leg

The distance from a line drawn transversely between the gluteal groove and the level of the lower border of the symphysis pubis (where the medial side of the upper leg joins the torso) to the medial popliteal crease (flexure of the knee) is measured as 14 cun.

The distance between the popliteal crease to the superior border of the greater trochanter of the femur (when the leg is abducted), is measured as 19 cun. There are discrepancies with other descriptions of the anatomy which use the 19 cun measurement, i.e. 19 cun from the popliteal crease to the superior and inferior borders of the pubic symphysis.

The bone proportional measurement of the thigh is accepted as being 14 cun.

Note: The points Bl 36-55 on the Bladder channel are listed using the current adopted Chinese numbering system:

The points are numbered on the medial branch from the upper back down to the knee crease, i.e. points 11-40, then the points on the lateral branch from the upper to lower back, i.e.points 41-54.

The numbers in brackets have been adopted predominantly by some schools of Five Element acupuncture and also feature in the following books: Shanghai College of Traditional Medicine 1984 Acupuncture – A Comprehensive Text; Worsley, J R 1982 Traditional Chinese Acupuncture Volume 1 – Meridians and Points; Wu, Wei-P'ing 1973 Chinese Acupuncture; Voisin, Dr. H 1974 Essentials of Acupuncture; Lavier, Dr. J 1974 Points of Chinese Acupuncture; Soulié De Morant, George. 1994 Chinese Acupuncture; So, James TinYao 1985 Book of Acupuncture Points, The; Yoshiaki Omura 1982 Acupuncture Medicine.

These differences arise after Bl 35 as the channel flows on down from the sacrum to the popliteal crease. The numbering system in brackets runs from Bl 35 to Bl 54 from the top of outer (lateral) Bladder channel to the popliteal crease (e.g. Bl 43 in this text would be Bl 38 in the sources referenced above).

Bl 36-38 are on the posterior aspect of the thigh

Bl 36 (50) CHENG FU – RECEIVE AND SUPPORT

⊥ *0.8 TO 1.5 CUN* Δ *FORBIDDEN TO MOXA*

Pos: Position of patient: prone with the feet hanging over the end of the couch.

Loc:
a) On the posterior surface of the upper thigh.
b) On the inferior border of the gluteus maximus muscle.
c) At the mid-point of the gluteal groove.
d) Between the muscles of the semitendinosus and the biceps femoris.

Cun:
a) The distance from a line drawn transversely between the gluteal groove and the level of the lower border of the symphysis pubis (where the medial side of the upper leg joins the torso) to the medial popliteal crease (flexure of the knee) is measured as 14 cun.
b) The distance between the popliteal crease to the superior border of the greater trochanter of the femur (when the leg is abducted), is measured as 19 cun. There are discrepancies with other descriptions of the anatomy which use the 19 cun measurement, i.e. 19 cun from the popliteal crease to the superior and inferior borders of the pubic symphysis.
c) The bone proportional measurement of the thigh is accepted as being 14 cun.

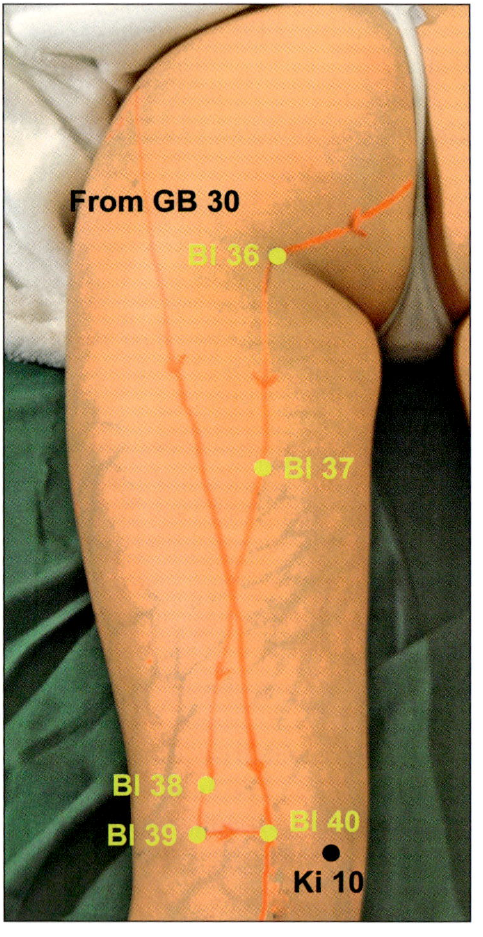

Tip:
a) To locate the posterior median line of the upper leg place the palms of your hands either side of the thigh and visualise the mid line between the two hands.
b) Palpate for the point on the mid-point of the gluteal groove at the inferior border of the gluteus maximus muscle.
c) The point can be palpated at the level of the gluteal groove between the two hamstring muscles, the semitendinosus and the biceps femoris.

Bl 37 (51) YIN MEN – PROSPEROUS GATE

⊥ *0.7 TO 1.5 CUN* Δ *FORBIDDEN TO MOXA*

Pos: Position of patient: prone with the feet hanging over the end of the couch.

Loc:
a) On the posterior surface of the upper thigh.
b) On the line connecting Bl 36 and Bl 40 (see separate descriptions).
c) 6 cun inferior to Bl 36.
d) 8 cun proximal to the posterior aspect of the popliteal crease (flexure) of the knee.
e) Between the muscles of the semitendinosus and the biceps femoris.

Cun:
a) The distance from a line drawn transversely between the gluteal groove and the level of the lower border of the symphysis pubis (where the medial side of the upper leg joins the torso) to the medial popliteal crease (flexure of the knee) is measured as 14 cun.
b) The distance between the popliteal crease to the superior border of the greater trochanter of the femur (when the leg is abducted), is measured as 19 cun. There are discrepancies with other descriptions of the anatomy which use the 19 cun measurement, i.e. 19 cun from the popliteal crease to the superior and inferior borders of the pubic symphysis.
c) The bone proportional measurement of the thigh is accepted as being 14 cun.

Tip:
a) Mark out 14 cun then run the flat of your finger with the flow of the Bladder channel, 6 cun inferior to the gluteal groove at Bl 36 (51). Bl 37 is located in this area between the muscles of the semitendinosus and the biceps femoris.
c) Palpate for accurate point location.
d) If you are having difficulty locating the posterior aspect of the popliteal crease ask the patient to flex their leg, and then mark the crease.

Note: Wu (1973) locates BL 51 (Bl 37) at 7 pouce proximal to the knee flexure. There is no reference in Wu's book for the measurement of the thigh (knee crease to gluteal region). Worsley (1982) uses 13 ACI (Anatomical Chinese Inch) from the medial extremity of the knee crease to the medial extremity of the groin. III 51 (Bl 37) is located on the posterior surface of the thigh, at the midpoint between the biceps femoris and the semitendinosus, 7 ACI (Anatomical Chinese Inch) proximal to the knee crease. So (1985) uses 18 divisions from the tip of the prominence of the femur at the hip to the knee crease. BL 51 (Bl 37) is located 6 divisions directly below BL 50 (Bl 36), in the centre of the back of the thigh. Voisin (1974) locates B 51 (Bl 37) midway between the subgluteal and popliteal folds, on the midwidth of the thigh.

There is no reference in Voisin's book for the measurement of the thigh (knee crease to gluteal region) Lavier (1974) uses 13 pouce as the measurement from the popliteal crease to the great trochanter. In an illustration BL 51 (Bl 37) is located on the posterior thigh, 7 pouce proximal to the popliteal crease, between the semitendinosus and the biceps femoris muscles. Shanghai (1981) uses 19 units between the greater trochanter of the femur and the middle of the popliteal crease. B 51 (Bl 37) is located on the back of the thigh, 6 units directly below B 50 (Bl 36).

Soulié (1994) uses 13 cun from the middle eminence of the greater trochanter to the superior border of the patella. He locates BL 51 (Bl 37) on the posterior thigh, around the median line, a little lateral; five FW (Finger Width) under the point of the ischium. In the angle between two large muscles (biceps femoris and semitendinosis); in a hollow; five FW below BL 50 (Bl 36). Masayoshi (1975) locates BL 37 in the center of the posterior thigh, midway between BL 36 and BL 40. There is no reference for the measurements of the thigh.

Bl 38 (52) FU XI – FLOATING RESERVE

⊥ ***0.5 TO 0.7 CUN*** Δ ***3 TO 7***

Pos: Position of patient: prone with the leg slightly flexed.

Loc:
a) On the posterior surface of the lower thigh.
b) Just medial to the tendon of the biceps femoris muscle.
c) On the line connecting Bl 36 and Bl 40 (see separate descriptions).
d) 1 cun proximal to the lateral end of the posterior aspect of the popliteal crease (flexure) of the knee.

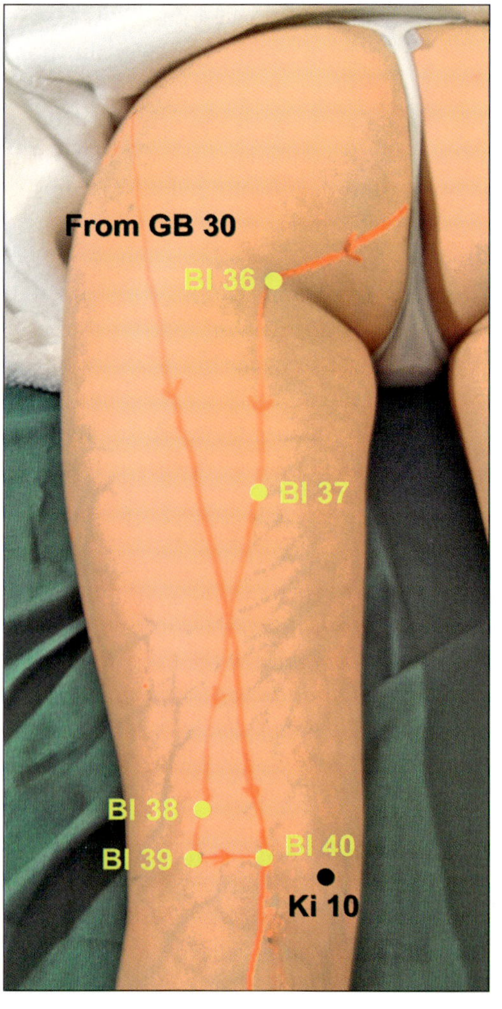

Cun:
a) The distance from a line drawn transversely between the gluteal groove and the level of the lower border of the symphysis pubis (where the medial side of the upper leg joins the torso) to the medial popliteal crease (flexure of the knee) is measured as 14 cun.
b) The distance between the popliteal crease to the superior border of the greater trochanter of the femur (when the leg is abducted), is measured as 19 cun. There are discrepancies with other descriptions of the anatomy which use the 19 cun measurement, i.e. 19 cun from the popliteal crease to the superior and inferior borders of the pubic symphysis.
c) The bone proportional measurement of the thigh is accepted as being 14 cun.

Tip: a) With the patient prone, feel for the medial border of the biceps femoris muscle on the posterior aspect of the popliteal crease and palpate and mark the border of the muscle running superiorly along the thigh for approximately three inches. Usually you should see a dimple at the lateral end of the posterior aspect of the popliteal crease, which is formed by the medial border of the biceps femoris muscle.

b) Once you have located this dimple palpate with the flow of the Bladder channel down the thigh until you are approximately 1 cun proximal to the posterior aspect of the popliteal crease. Point location is usually accurate enough by palpation without the need to mark the cun measurements.

c) If you prefer to use the cun measurements then mark out 14 cun, then run the flat of your finger with the flow of the Bladder channel to 1 cun proximal to the posterior aspect of the popliteal crease.

d) Palpate for the point 1 cun proximal to the posterior aspect of thepopliteal crease.

e) If you are having difficulty locating the posterior aspect of the popliteal crease ask the patient to flex their leg, and then mark in the crease.

Note: Wu (1973) locates BL 52 (Bl 38) upon the posterior surface of the thigh, at one pouce above the popliteal flexure, within the tendon of the longum of the femoral biceps. There is no reference in Wu's book for the measurement of the thigh (knee crease to gluteal region).

Worsley (1982) uses 13 ACI (Anatomical Chinese Inch) from the medial extremity of the knee crease to the medial extremity of the groin. III 52 (Bl 38) is located on the posterior surface of the thigh, 1 ACI (Anatomical Chinese Inch) proximal to the lateral end of the knee crease, medial to the tendon of the biceps femoris.

So (1985) uses 18 divisions from the tip of the prominence of the femur at the hip to the knee crease. BL 52 (Bl 38) is located one division above BL 53 (Bl 39).

Voisin (1974) locates B 52 (Bl 38) in the popliteal cavity, 3 fb (finger breadth) above and lateral to its center, against the medial border of the biceps tendon (lateral hamstring). There is no reference in Voisin's book for the measurement of the thigh (knee crease to gluteal region)

Lavier (1975) locates BL 52 (Bl 38) on the posterior thigh, 1 pouce proximal to the popliteal crease, medial to the tendon of the biceps femoris muscle.

Shanghai (1981) uses 19 units between the greater trochanter of the femur and the middle of the popliteal crease. B 52 (B 38) is located 1 unit above B 53 (Bl 39).

Soulié (1994) uses 13 cun from the middle eminence of the greater trochanter to the superior border of the patella. He locates BL 52 (Bl 38) on the lateral posterior knee; in the angle between the superior edge of the large projection (lateral condyle of the femur) and the medial edge of the tendons on an angle (plantaris muscle, lateral gastrocnemius muscle); in a hollow; on the edge of the plantaris, five FW (Finger Width) below the ischium; three FW above BL 53 (Bl 39), Shandong (1982) locate Fuxi lateral to the popliteal fossa, 1 cun above Pt. Weiyang (Bl 39).

Bl 39 (53) WEI YANG – EQUILIBRIUM YANG

⊥ ***0.5 TO 0.7 CUN*** Δ ***3 TO 5***

- ACCUMULATION/Xi Cleft/Gueki of the Yang Heel/Yang Motility Vessel (Yang Qiao Mai)
- LOWER HE-SEA point of the Triple Heater

Pos: Position of patient: prone with the feet hanging over the end of the couch.

Loc: a) On the posterior surface of the leg.
b) On the posterior aspect of the popliteal crease (flexure) of the knee.
c) Just medial to the tendon of the biceps femoris muscle (in a dimple).
d) On the line connecting Bl 36 and Bl 40 (see separate descriptions).

Tip: a) With the patient prone, feel for the medial border of the biceps femoris muscle on the posterior aspect of the popliteal crease and palpate for the point. Usually you can see a dimple at the lateral end of the posterior aspect of the popliteal crease, which is formed by the medial border of the biceps femoris muscle.
b) Run the flat of your finger with the flow of the Bladder channel to the posterior aspect of the popliteal crease . This will take you to a dimple where the point is located.
c) If you are having difficulty locating the posterior aspect of the popliteal crease ask the patient to flex their leg, and then mark in the crease.

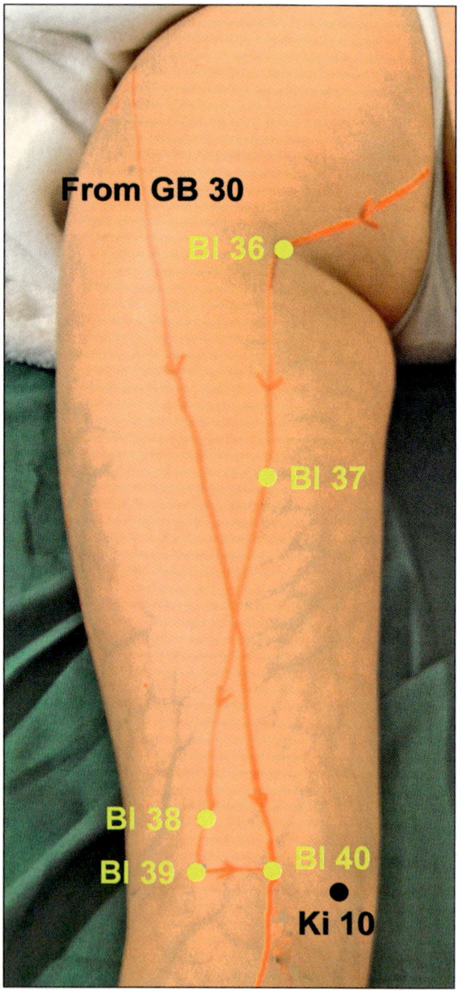

Note: Wu (1973) locates BL 53 (Bl 39) in the popliteal fold, upon the crease of the flexure, at two pouce external to the median line of the member. Voisin (1974) locates B 53 (Bl 39) in the popliteal cavitity 1.5 fb (finger breadth) from the lateral border. Shanghai (1981) B 53 (Bl 39) is located on the back of the knee, 1 unit lateral to B 54 (Bl 40). Eachou (1995) locates BL 39 on the lateral side of the skin crease of the popliteal fossa, 1 inch lateral to BL 40, and medial to the tendon of the biceps femoris muscle, Shandong (1982) locate Weiyang above the popliteal crease, 1 cun lateral to Weizhong (Bl 40).

Soulié (1994) locates BL 53 (Bl 39) on the posterolateral knee. At the lateral extremity of the crease of the flexion: between the medial edge of the great tendon of the biceps femoris and the lateral edge of the lateral gastrocnemius; in a hollow; three FW (Finger Width) below BL 52 (Bl 38); three FW superior and lateral to BL 55; one FW lateral to BL 54 (Bl 40).

Bl 40 is on the posterior aspect of the popliteal crease, (on the median branch of the Bladder channel).

Bl 40 (54) WEI ZHONG – EQUILIBRIUM MIDDLE

⊥ ***0.5 CUN*** Δ ***FORBIDDEN TO MOXA***

- EARTH
- HE – SEA/Shu – Transporting/Antique
- LOWER HE-SEA point of the Bladder
- GREATER INFLUENTIAL /Greater Assembling Point of the Back and Vertebrae.
- ONE OF THE HEAVENLY STAR POINTS OF MA DAN-YANG (the others are: Lu 7, LI 4, LI 11, St 36, St 44, Bl 57, Bl 60, Ht 5, GB 34, GB 39 and Liv 3)

Pos: Position of patient: prone with the feet hanging over the end of the couch.

Loc: a) On the posterior surface of the leg.
b) On the posterior aspect of the popliteal crease (flexure) of the knee.
c) Mid-way between the tendons of the biceps femoris muscle and the semitendinosus muscle.
d) On the line connecting Bl 36 and Bl 40 (see separate descriptions).

Tip: a) With the patient prone, on the posterior aspect of the popliteal crease, locate the medial border of the biceps femoris muscle and the lateral border of the semitendinosus muscle. These borders are often visible as dimples on the medial and lateral aspects of the popliteal crease.
b) Bl 40 is located mid way between the borders of the tendons or dimples on the popliteal crease.
c) Palpate for accurate point location which can be in quite a large depression.
d) Bl 40 is located where the inner and outer bladder channels from the posterior torso and the upper leg meet.
e) If you are having difficulty locating the posterior aspect of the popliteal crease ask the patient to flex their leg, and then mark in the crease.

Note: Soulié (1994) locates BL 54 (Bl 40) on the knee, posterior face (popliteal crease); lateral third of the crease of the flexion; one FW (Finger Width) medial to the lateral ropy tendon (biceps femoris); in the angle between the lower edge of the crease of the flexion and the medial edge of the lateral gastrocnemius; in a hollow; one FW medial to BL 53 (Bl 39); two FW above BL 55. Shandong (1982) locate Weizhong at the midpoint of the popliteal transverse crease.

HOW TO MARK OUT AND CHECK THE VERTEBRAE.

The cun measurements of the inner and outer Bladder lines on the posterior torso are constant from the upper to lower posterior torso. They however follow the contours of the posterior torso, and therefore points in the upper lumbar area may lie more lateral, and points in the sacral area may be more medial on a man or equidistant or more lateral on a woman. It is important to follow both the musculature of the torso, and any curvature/tilt of bony structures (scapula, spine, pelvis). Even though the cun measurements do not alter as you go down the posterior torso they are proportional measurements (cun) which means that the inner and outer bladder channels are not therefore on a "plumb" line.

In some illustrations the outer Bladder line appears to be in between the ribs which can sometimes make the points lower than the spaces between the vertebrae, this is incorrect as the points should stay level with the intervertebral spaces of the vertebra and not in between the ribs.

The distance between the medial border of the scapula and the posterior median line is measured as 3 cun at the level of the 3rd thoracic vertebra.

The lateral branch or the outer Bladder line of the Bladder Channel is 3 cun lateral to the posterior median line.

The medial branch or the inner Bladder line of the Bladder Channel is 1.5 cun lateral to the posterior median line.

There are 7 cevical, 12 thoracic and 5 lumbar vertebrae. All of the Bladder points lie in relation to the intervertebral spaces between two vertebrae, eg. T3/4 , which is 3 cun lateral to the posterior median line (Bl 42).

Although there are cun measurements for the inner and outer bladder lines of 1.5 cun and 3 cun, it is often much more easy to palpate for the points, especially if you were to place your finger in the intervertebral space and then palpate laterally. Palpating with the flow of the Bladder channel from the top of the back can assist with point location.

Tip: Using the following landmarks to locate the intervertebral spaces of the upper thoracic vertebrae:

a) First mark out the intervertebral spaces of the thoracic vertebrae.
b) To locate the intervertebral space between C7 and T1, place your index finger on the prominence of the vertebra that may be T1 and your middle finger on the prominence of the vertebra which may be C7.
c) Now ask the patient to turn their head to the left and then to the right. You should feel some slight movement under your middle finger which is C7. You should feel no rotation under your index finger as T1 is attached to a rib whereas C7 is not.
d) A common error is to visualise C7 as being more prominent than T1. Gray's (1978) states it very often can be, but T1 is usually just as prominent and sometimes more so.

e) Place your four fingers from each hand vertically on the each side of the neck so that the radial borders of your fingers are uppermost and the pads are resting lightly against the lateral surface of the neck. Make sure that the ulnar border of the little fingers (5th digit) are resting on the top of the shoulder with the pads of your 5th digits resting on the lateral surface of the neck.

f) Then keeping your left and right 5th digits at this level, bring them together so their tips meet on the posterior median line. They should meet at the level of C7/T1 space or at the spinous process of C7.

g) The illustration below shows how you should have your fingers on the neck and shoulder before the 5th digits meet at the posterior median line:

o (2)	o (2)
o (3)	o (3)
o (4)	o (4)
o (5th digit)	o (5th digit)
(5th digit on top of left shoulder)	(5th digit on top of right shoulder)

h) When you have marked out the intervertebral spaces of the spine, step back and visualise the first place that you would be able to attach the first rib to T1. The first rib curves anteriorly and inferiorly to the inferior border of the clavicle, so T1 can seem more superior than you may realise. T1 should also be the first vertebra at the base of the neck.

i) Another method is to place your finger in the angle formed at the superior aspect of the shoulder by the acromial extremity of the clavicle and the scapular spine. From this angle, with the patient relaxed, run your finger across in a straight line until you meet an intervertebral space – this is the intervertebral space between T2/T3. A straight line means following the 3D curvature of the body, not as if you were drawing on a flat piece of paper – 2D image.

j) To locate the intervertebral space between T3/T4 run your finger from the acromial end of the scapular spine along its superior border towards the spine. You should meet the intervertebral space of T3/T4, however this is not always as accurate as tip i) as some scapula spines are almost horizontal. Therefore they may not slope downwards as you run your finger to the medial edge of the scapular spine.

k) To locate the intervertebral space between L2/L3 place your little finger (5th digit) on top of the iliac crest with your 1st, 2nd and 3rd fingers vertically on top of your little finger. Move your thumb horizontal (at a right angle) to the fingerswhich should bring the thumb in to alignment line with the intervertebral space of L2/L3 as illustrated below:

o (2)	o – thumb	L2/L3	thumb – o	o (2)
o (3)				o (3)
o (4)				o (4)
o (5th digit)				o (5th digit)
(left iliac crest)				(right iliac crest)

l) To locate the intervertebral space between L3/L4 place your left and right index fingers on the top of the left and right iliac crests with your 1st, 3rd, 4th, and 5th digits at the same level (horizontal). Your thumbs should be at the level of L3/L4 intervertebral space, as illustrated below:

```
o o o o  o – thumb        L3/L4        thumb – o  o o o o
 5 4 3 2  1st digit                      1st digit  2 3 4 5
            1                                     1
               index fingers on top of the iliac crest
```

m) To locate the intervertebral space between L4/L5 place your left and right index (2nd) fingers on the top of the left and right iliac crests as above, but this time allowing your thumb to fall away naturally instead of keeping it horizontal with the other digits. The thumb then will be aligned with the intervertebral space of L4/L5, as illustrated below:

```
 5 4 3 2 (digits)                       2 3 4 5 (digits)
    o o o o                                o o o o
                    o   L4/L5   o
                        thumbs
        index (2nd) fingers on top of the iliac crest
```

On tips g), k), l) and m) "=" is the top of the iliac crest.

n) From the base of L5 the vertebrae are fused and form the sacrum. The size of the sacrum longitudinally is approximately the size of the patient's fist from the knuckle (metacarpo-phalangeal joint) of the thumb to the knuckle (metacarpo-phalangeal joint) of the little finger. If the base of L5 vertebra to the bottom of the sacrum/superior border of the coccyx (sacral body) is longer than the person's fist then you need to re-check the intervertebral spaces again. The sacro-coccygeal articulation may be located at the level of the superior border of the gluteal fold.

Note: The locations of the points on the inner and outer lines of the Bladder Channel on the posterior torso have been unanimous throughout Acupuncture literature, but there are texts that do have different cun measurements for the inner and outer lines of the Bladder Channel. Worsley (1982) uses 2 ACI (Anatomical Chinese Inch) for the inner Bladder line and 4 ACI for the outer Bladder line. Lavier (1974) doesn't use any measurement, the outer Bladder line touches the inner border of the scapula and the inner Bladder line is midway between the border of the scapula and the median line.

Voisin (1974) uses 2 fb (finger breadth) from the midline of the back at the centre of the spinous process for the inner Bladder line and 4 fb from the midline of the back at the centre of the spinous process. Soulié (1994) not only uses various measurements lateral to the vertebra but also uses other anatomy to help locate the points eg, 4 FW (finger width) under the lower angle of the scapula for Bl 19. Wu (1973) uses 2 pouce from the median line for the inner Bladder line measurement and 4 pouce from the median line for the outer Bladder line measurement. Jin Jian uses 2 cun for the medial branch or inner Bladder line.

The numbers in brackets have been adopted predominantly by some schools of Five Element acupuncture and also feature in the following books: Shanghai College of Traditional Medicine 1984 Acupuncture – A Comprehensive Text; Worsley, J R 1982 Traditional Chinese Acupuncture Volume 1 – Meridians and Points; Wu, Wei-P'ing 1973 Chinese Acupuncture; Voisin, Dr. H 1974 Essentials of Acupuncture; Lavier, Dr. J 1974 Points of Chinese Acupuncture; Soulié De Morant, George. 1994 Chinese Acupuncture; So, James TinYao 1985 Book of Acupuncture Points, The; Yoshiaki Omura 1982 Acupuncture Medicine.

These differences arise after Bl 35 as the channel flows on down from the sacrum to the popliteal crease. The numbering system in brackets runs from Bl 35 to Bl 54 from the top of outer (lateral) Bladder channel to the popliteal crease (e.g. Bl 43 in this text would be Bl 38 in the sources referenced above).

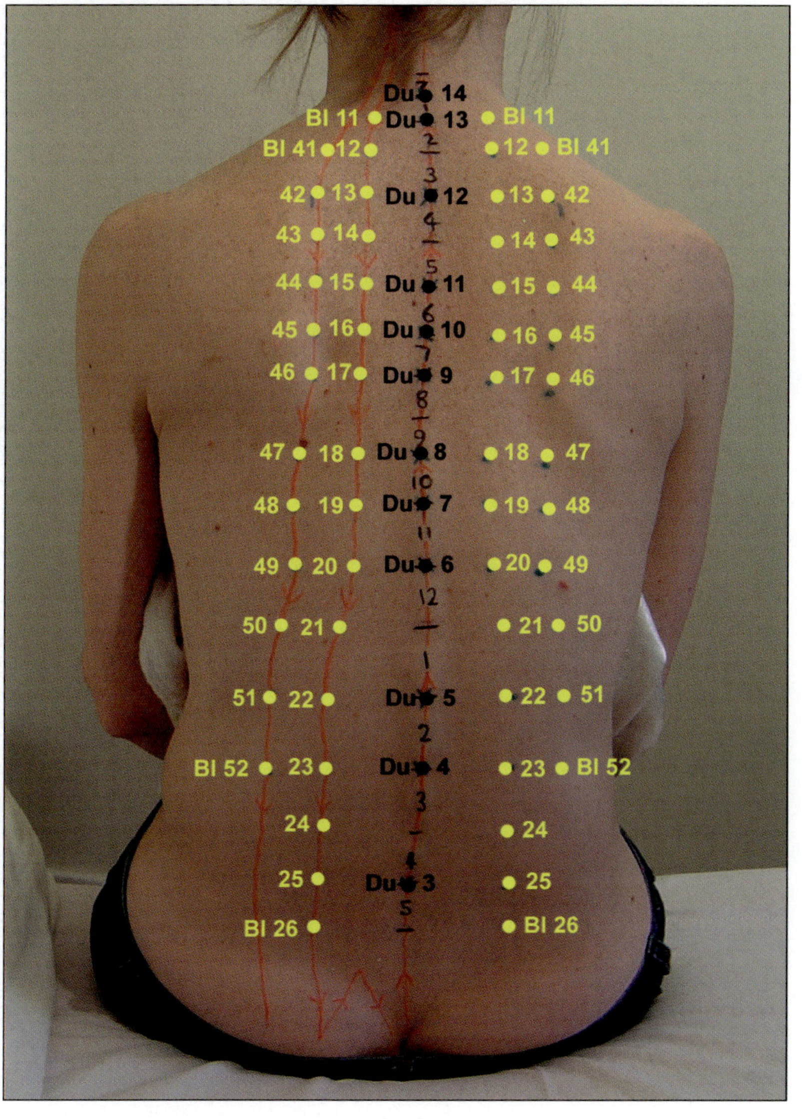

Bl 41-52 are on the posterior torso, (on the lateral branch of the Bladder channel).

Bl 41 (36) FU FEN – NEAR DIVISION

⊥ ***0.3 TO 0.5 CUN*** **Δ** ***5 TO 7***

- RE-UNION/Crossing/Meeting Point of the Bladder Channel with the Small Intestine Channel – Foot Tai Yang Channel with the Hand Tai Yang Channel.

Pos: Position of patient: seated and upright.

Loc: a) On the posterior torso.
b) On the outer line or the lateral branch of the Bladder channel.
c) 3 cun lateral to the posterior median line.
d) Between the 2nd and 3rd thoracic vertebrae (level with the base of the spinous process of the 2nd thoracic vertebra).
e) Level with Bl 12.

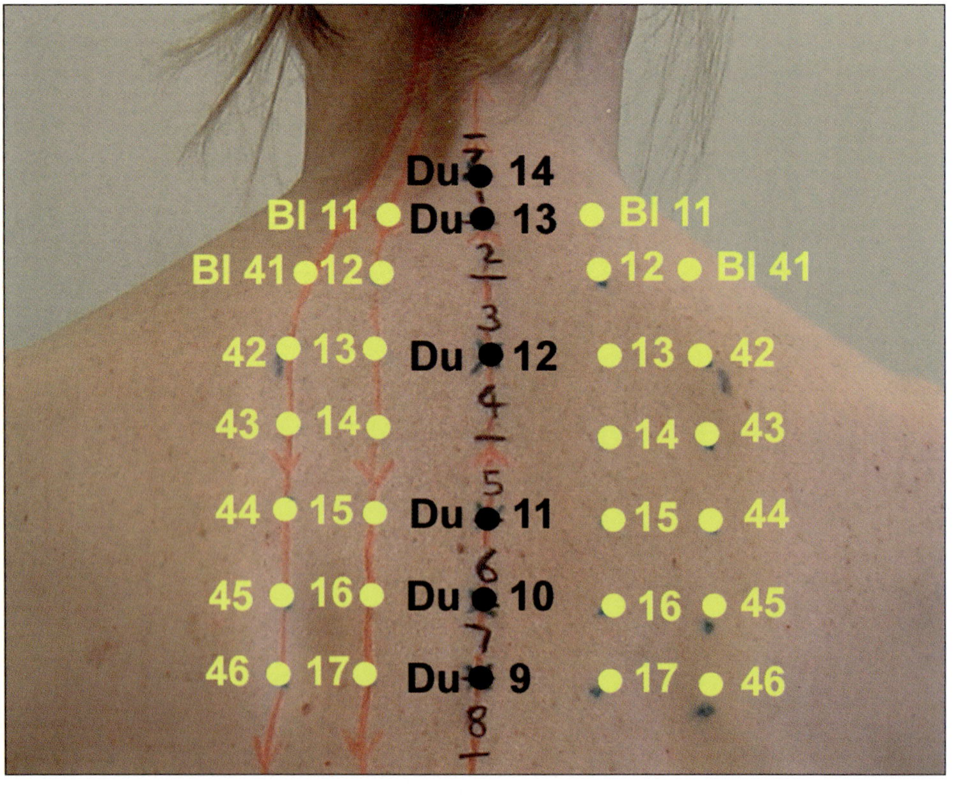

Tip: a) Please read **"HOW TO MARK OUT AND CHECK THE VERTEBRAE"** for further guidance.

b) The cun measurement from the posterior median line to the outer bladder line is 3 cun. This is taken from the posterior median line to the medial border of the scapula at the level of T3.

c) Place your finger in the intervertebral space of T2 and T3 and then palpate laterally to 3 cun until you feel a *men* (depression).

d) Palpating with the flow of the Bladder channel from the top of the back may also help you to locate the points.

e) The point is transversely level with the base of the spinous process of the 2nd thoracic vertebra. This may mean that you are not between the 2nd and 3rd ribs but on the 2nd rib. The ribs do not play any part in the location of the point.

f) As the cun measurement is a proportional measurement, 3 cun at the level of T3 may not be the same further down the back, as the posterior torso widens and narrows according to the persons own body shape, e.g. 3 cun at the level of T4/T5 may have a difference of approximately 1 cm further down the back, especially in the lumbar region.

Note: Soulié (1994) locates BL 36 (Bl 41) on the upper back: one FW (Finger Width) above the medial superior angle of the scapula; on the superior edge of the second rib; on the lateral edge of the superimposed vertical muscles (iliocostalis under the levator scapulae); in a hollow; one very large FW lateral to BL 11; one very large FW above BL 37 (Bl 42); one large FW under and a bit lateral to SI 14.

Legge (1999) locates UB 41 at 3 cun lateral to the tip of the spinous process of the 2nd thoracic vertebra. Voisin (1974) locates B 36 (Bl 41) 4 fb (finger breadth) from the midline of the back (centre of spinous process D 2).

Eachou (1995) locates BL 41 3 inches lateral to the posterior midline, on the medial margin of the scapula between the second and third ribs. Worsley (1982) uses 4 ACI (Anatomical Chinese Inch) for the outer Bladder line (for the thoracic region of the back). Lavier (1974) doesn't use any measurement, the outer Bladder line touches the inner border of the scapula. In an illustration he shows the direction of the flow comes from below, possibly from the inner Bladder line, rather than from Bl 10.

Voisin (1974) uses 4 fb (finger breadth) lateral from the midline of the back at the centre of the spinous process for the outer Bladder line. Wu (1973) uses 4 pouce from the median line for the outer Bladder line measurement.

Bl 42 (37) PO HU – SOUL DOOR

⊥ ***0.3 TO 0.5 CUN*** Δ ***5 TO 15***

Pos: Position of patient: seated and upright.

Loc: a) On the posterior torso.
b) On the outer line or the lateral branch of the Bladder channel.
c) 3 cun lateral to the posterior median line.
d) Between the 3rd and 4th thoracic vertebrae (level with the base of the spinous process of the 3rd thoracic vertebra).
e) Level with Du 12 and Bl 13.

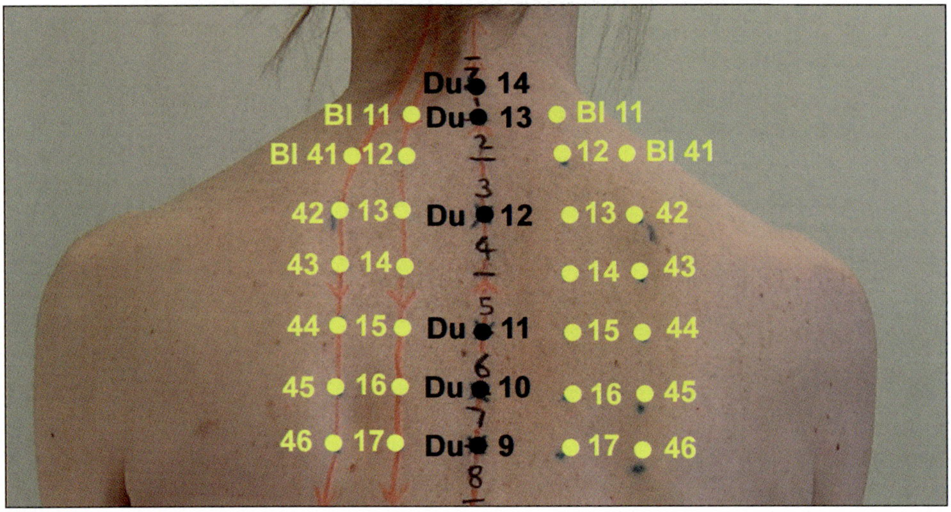

Tip: a) Please read **"HOW TO MARK OUT AND CHECK THE VERTEBRAE"** for further guidance.
b) The cun measurement from the posterior median line to the outer bladder line is 3 cun. This is taken from the posterior median line to the medial border of the scapula at the level of T3.
c) Place your finger in the intervertebral space of T3 and T4 and then palpate laterally to 3 cun until you feel a *men* (depression).
d) Palpating with the flow of the Bladder channel from the top of the back may also help you to locate the points.
e) The point is transversely level with the base of the spinous process of the 3rd thoracic vertebra. This may mean that you are not between the 3rd and 4th ribs but on the 3rd rib. The ribs do not play any part in the location of the point.
f) As the cun measurement is a proportional measurement, 3 cun at the level of T3 may not be the same further down the back, as the posterior torso widens and narrows according to the persons own body shape, e.g. 3 cun at the level of T4/T5 may have a difference of approximately 1 cm further down the back, especially in the lumbar region.

Note: Soulié (1994) locates BL 37 (Bl 42) on the upper back: On the medial edge of the scapula, at the angle between its superior and medial thirds. and the inferior edge of the second rib. On the medial inferior edge of the insertion of the levator scapulae. On the lateral edge of the iliocostalis muscle; in a hollow; on the rhomboid; one very large FW (Finger Width) below BL 36 (Bl 41); one very large FW above BL 38 (Bl 43); two FW lateral to BL 13; two FW medial to SI 13. Legge (1999) locates UB 42 at 3 cun lateral to the tip of the spinous process of the 3rd thoracic vertebra. Voisin (1974) locates B 37 (Bl 42) 4 fb (finger breadth) from the midline of the back (centre of spinous process D 3). Eachou (1995) locates BL 42 3 inches lateral to the posterior midline, on the medial margin of the scapula between the third and fourth ribs. Worsley (1982) uses 4 ACI (Anatomical Chinese Inch) for the outer Bladder line (for the thoracic region of the back). Lavier (1974) doesn't use any measurement, the outer Bladder line touches the inner border of the scapula. In an illustration he shows the direction of the flow comes from below, possibly from the inner Bladder line, rather than from Bl 10. Voisin (1974) uses 4 fb (finger breadth) lateral from the midline of the back at the centre of the spinous process for the outer Bladder line. Wu (1973) uses 4 pouce from the median line for the outer Bladder line measurement.

Bl 43 (38) GAO HUANG SHU – RICH FOR THE VITALS CORRESPONDENCE

⊥ ***0.3 TO 0.5 CUN*** Δ ***7 TO 50***

Pos: Position of patient: seated and upright.

Loc:
a) On the posterior torso.
b) On the outer line or the lateral branch of the Bladder channel.
c) 3 cun lateral to the posterior median line.
d) Between the 4th and 5th thoracic vertebrae (level with the base of the spinous process of the 4th thoracic vertebra).
e) Level with Bl 14.

Tip:
a) Please read **"HOW TO MARK OUT AND CHECK THE VERTEBRAE"** for further guidance.
b) The cun measurement from the posterior median line to the outer bladder line is 3 cun. This is taken from the posterior median line to the medial border of the scapula at the level of T3.
c) Place your finger in the intervertebral space of T4 and T5 and then palpate laterally to 3 cun until you feel a *men* (depression).
d) Palpating with the flow of the Bladder channel from the top of the back may also help you to locate the points.
e) The point is transversely level with the base of the spinous process of the 4th thoracic vertebra. This may mean that you are not between the 4th and 5th ribs but on the 4th rib. The ribs do not play any part in the location of the point.
f) As the cun measurement is a proportional measurement, 3 cun at the level of T3 may not be the same further down the back, as the posterior torso widens and narrows according to the persons own body shape, e.g. 3 cun at the level of T4/T5 may have a difference of approximately 1 cm further down the back, especially in the lumbar region.

Note: Soulié (1994) locates BL 38 (Bl 43) on the upper back: elbows held in front in order to separate the scapulae, which cover the point when they are in the normal position. By following the inferior edge, towards the back, of the relief on an angle to the spine of the scapula, the finger falls between the third and fourth ribs, in a triangular hollow. The point is in the lateral inferior angle of the hollow, on the superior edge of the fourth rib and of a tendon (serratus anterior), in a groove on an angle between rhomboids major and minor, on the trapezius; one very large FW (Finger Width) below BL 37 (Bl 42); one very large FW above BL 39 (Bl 44); two FW lateral to BL 14; two FW lateral and slightly above SI 12.

Legge (1999) locates UB 43 at 3 cun lateral to the tip of the spinous process of the 4th thoracic vertebra. Voisin (1974) locates B 38 (Bl 43) 4 fb (finger breadth) from the midline of the back (centre of spinous process D 4). Eachou (1995) locates BL 43 at 3 inches lateral to the posterior midline, on the medial margin of the scapula between the fourth and fifth ribs. Worsley (1982) uses 4 ACI (Anatomical Chinese Inch) for the outer Bladder line (for the thoracic region of the back). Lavier (1974) doesn't use any measurement, the outer Bladder line touches the inner border of the scapula. In an illustration he shows the direction of the flow comes from below, possibly from the inner Bladder line, rather than from Bl 10. Voisin (1974) uses 4 fb (finger breadth) lateral from the midline of the back at the centre of the spinous process for the outer Bladder line. Wu (1973) uses 4 pouce from the median line for the outer Bladder line measurement.

Bl 44 (39) SHEN TANG – SPIRIT HALL

⊥ ***0.3 TO 0.5 CUN*** Δ *5*

Pos: Position of patient: seated and upright.

Loc: a) On the posterior torso.
b) On the outer line or the lateral branch of the Bladder channel.
c) 3 cun lateral to the posterior median line.
d) Between the 5th and 6th thoracic vertebrae (level with the base of the spinous process of the 5th thoracic vertebra).
e) Level with Du 11 and Bl 15.

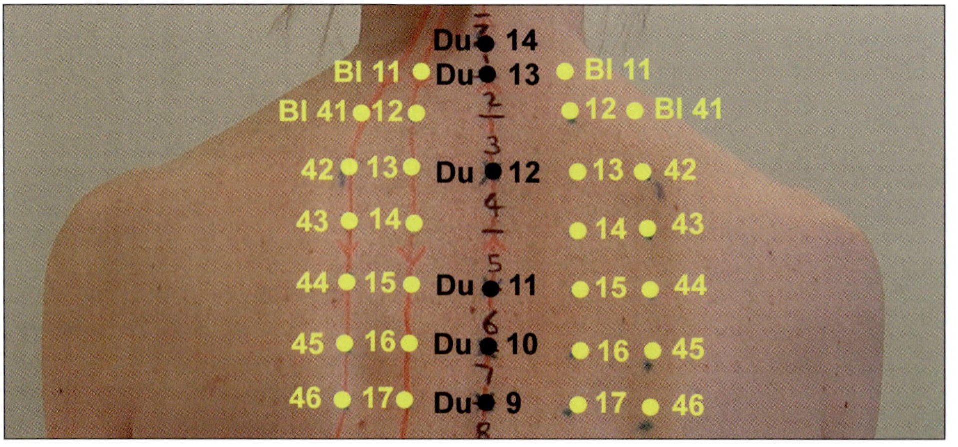

Tip: a) Please read **"HOW TO MARK OUT AND CHECK THE VERTEBRAE"** for further guidance.

b) The cun measurement from the posterior median line to the outer bladder line is 3 cun. This is taken from the posterior median line to the medial border of the scapula at the level of T3.

c) Place your finger in the intervertebral space of T5 and T6 and then palpate laterally to 3 cun until you feel a *men* (depression).

d) Palpating with the flow of the Bladder channel from the top of the back may also help you to locate the points.

e) The point is transversely level with the base of the spinous process of the 5th thoracic vertebra. This may mean that you are not between the 5th and 6th ribs but on the 5th rib. The ribs do not play any part in the location of the point.

f) As the cun measurement is a proportional measurement, 3 cun at the level of T3 may not be the same further down the back, as the posterior torso widens and narrows according to the persons own body shape, e.g. 3 cun at the level of T4/T5 may have a difference of approximately 1 cm further down the back, especially in the lumbar region.

Note: Soulié (1994) locates BL 39 (Bl 44) on the back: at the level of one third from the spine of the scapula to the lower angle; in the angle between the medial edge of the scapula and the inferior edge of the fifth rib in a hollow; between the bone and the iliocostalis muscle; on the rhomboid; one very large FW (Finger Width) below BL 38 (Bl 43); one very large FW above BL 40 (Bl 45); two FW lateral to BL 15; at the level of GV 11 (Du 11). Legge (1999) locates UB 44 at 3 cun lateral to the tip of the spinous process of the 5th thoracic vertebra.

Voisin (1974) locates B 39 (Bl 44) at 4 fb (finger breadth) from the midline of the back (centre of spinous process D 5). Eachou (1995) locates BL 44, 3 inches lateral to the posterior midline, on the medial margin of the scapula between the fifth and sixth ribs. Worsley (1982) uses 4 ACI (Anatomical Chinese Inch) for the outer Bladder line (for the thoracic region of the back). Lavier (1974) doesn't use any measurement, the outer Bladder line touches the inner border of the scapula. In an illustration he shows the direction of the flow comes from below, possibly from the inner Bladder line, rather than from Bl 10.

Voisin (1974) uses 4 fb (finger breadth) lateral from the midline of the back at the centre of the spinous process for the outer Bladder line. Wu (1973) uses 4 pouce from the median line for the outer Bladder line measurement.

Bl 45 (40) YI XI – WAIL OF GRIEF

⊥ ***0.3 TO 0.5 CUN*** Δ ***5 TO 15***

Pos: Position of patient: seated and upright.

Loc: a) On the posterior torso.
b) On the outer line or the lateral branch of the Bladder channel.
c) 3 cun lateral to the posterior median line.
d) Between the 6th and 7th thoracic vertebrae (level with the base of the spinous process of the 6th thoracic vertebra).
e) Level with Du 10 and Bl 16.

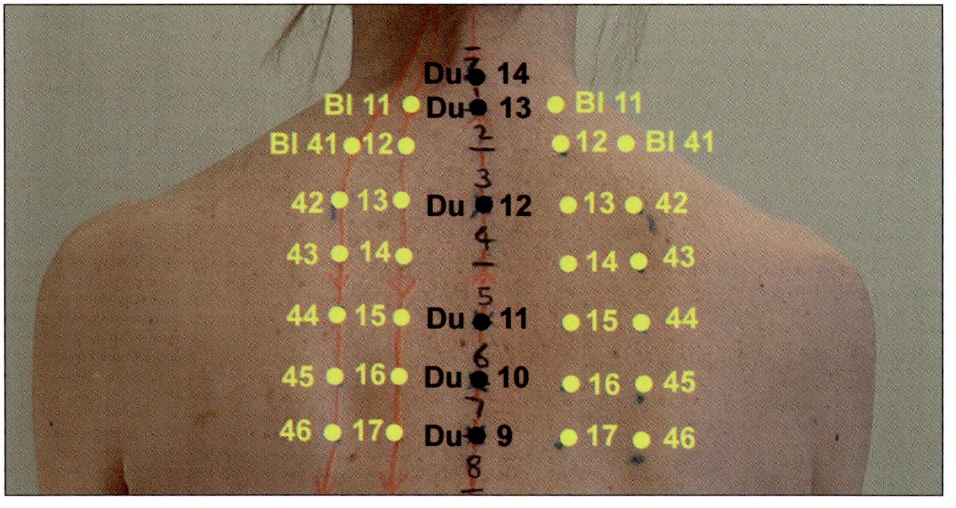

Tip: a) Please read **"HOW TO MARK OUT AND CHECK THE VERTEBRAE"** for further guidance.
b) The cun measurement from the posterior median line to the outer bladder line is 3 cun. This is taken from the posterior median line to the medial border of the scapula at the level of T3.
c) Place your finger in the intervertebral space of T6 and T7 and then palpate laterally to 3 cun until you feel a *men* (depression).
d) Palpating with the flow of the Bladder channel from the top of the back may also help you to locate the points.
e) The point is transversely level with the base of the spinous process of the 6th thoracic vertebra. This may mean that you are not between the 6th and 7th ribs but on the 6th rib. The ribs do not play any part in the location of the point.
f) As the cun measurement is a proportional measurement, 3 cun at the level of T3 may not be the same further down the back, as the posterior torso widens and narrows according to the persons own body shape, e.g. 3 cun at the level of T4/T5 may have a difference of approximately 1 cm further down the back, especially in the lumbar region.

Note: Soulié (1994) locates BL 40 (Bl 45) on the back: at the level of two thirds from the spine of the scapula to its lower angle; at the medial edge of the scapula, and at the lower edge of the sixth rib; in a hollow; on the rhomboid; one very large FW below BL 39 (Bl 44); one very large FW above BL 41 (Bl 46); two FW lateral to BL 16; four FW on either side of GV 10 (Du 10). Legge (1999) locates UB 45 at 3 cun lateral to the tip of the spinous process of the 6th thoracic vertebra. Voisin (1974) locates B 40 (Bl 45) 4 fb (finger breadth) from the midline of the back (centre of spinous process D 6).

Eachou (1995) locates BL 45 at 3 inches lateral to the posterior midline, on the medial margin of the scapula between the sixth and seventh ribs. Worsley (1982) uses 4 ACI (Anatomical Chinese Inch) for the outer Bladder line (for the thoracic region of the back). Lavier (1974) doesn't use any measurement, the outer Bladder line touches the inner border of the scapula. In an illustration he shows the direction of the flow comes from below, possibly from the inner Bladder line, rather than from Bl 10. Voisin (1974) uses 4 fb (finger breadth) lateral from the midline of the back at the centre of the spinous process for the outer Bladder line. Wu (1973) uses 4 pouce from the median line for the outer Bladder line measurement.

Bl 46 (41) GE GUAN – DIAPHRAGM BORDER

⊥ ***0.3 TO 0.5 CUN*** ∆ ***3 TO 15***

Pos: Position of patient: seated and upright.

Loc:
- a) On the posterior torso.
- b) On the outer line or the lateral branch of the Bladder channel.
- c) 3 cun lateral to the posterior median line.
- d) Between the 7th and 8th thoracic vertebrae (level with the base of the spinous process of the 7th thoracic vertebra).
- e) Approximately level with the inferior angle of the scapula.
- f) Level with Du 9 and Bl 17.

Tip:
- a) Please read **"HOW TO MARK OUT AND CHECK THE VERTEBRAE"** for further guidance.
- b) The cun measurement from the posterior median line to the outer bladder line is 3 cun. This is taken from the posterior median line to the medial border of the scapula at the level of T3.
- c) Place your finger in the intervertebral space of T7 and T8 and then palpate laterally to 3 cun until you feel a *men* (depression).
- d) Palpating with the flow of the Bladder channel from the top of the back may also help you to locate the points.
- e) The point is transversely level with the base of the spinous process of the 7th thoracic vertebra. This may mean that you are not between the 7th and 8th ribs but on the 7th rib. The ribs do not play any part in the location of the point.
- f) As a guide the point lies approximately level with the inferior angle of the scapula.
- g) As the cun measurement is a proportional measurement, 3 cun at the level of T3 may not be the same further down the back, as the posterior torso widens and narrows according to the persons own body shape, e.g. 3 cun at the level of T4/T5 may have a difference of approximately 1 cm further down the back, especially in the lumbar region.

Note: Soulié (1994) locates BL 41 (Bl 46) on the back: at the level of one FW (Finger Width) above the inferior angle of the scapula; in the angle between the scapula and the lower edge of the seventh rib; in a hollow on the latissimus dorsi, rhomboid; one very large FW below BL 40 (Bl 45); four FW above BL 42 (Bl 47); two FW lateral to BL 17; four FW on either side of GV 9 (Du 9), superior edge of T7. Legge (1999) locates UB 46 at 3 cun lateral to the tip of the spinous process of the 7th thoracic vertebra. Voisin (1974) locates B 41 (Bl 46) 4 fb (finger breadth) from the midline of the back (centre of spinous process D 7).

Eachou (1995) locates BL 46 at 3 inches lateral to the posterior midline, on the medial margin of the scapula between the seventh and eighth ribs. Worsley (1982) uses 4 ACI (Anatomical Chinese Inch) for the outer Bladder line (for the thoracic region of the back). Lavier (1974) doesn't use any measurement, the outer Bladder line touches the inner border of the scapula. In an illustration he shows the direction of the flow comes from below, possibly from the inner Bladder line, rather than from Bl 10.

Voisin (1974) uses 4 fb (finger breadth) lateral from the midline of the back at the centre of the spinous process for the outer Bladder line. Wu (1973) uses 4 pouce from the median line for the outer Bladder line measurement.

Bl 47 (42) HUN MEN – SPIRITUAL SOUL GATE

⊥ ***0.3 TO 0.5 CUN*** ***Δ 3 TO 15***

Pos: Position of patient: seated and upright.

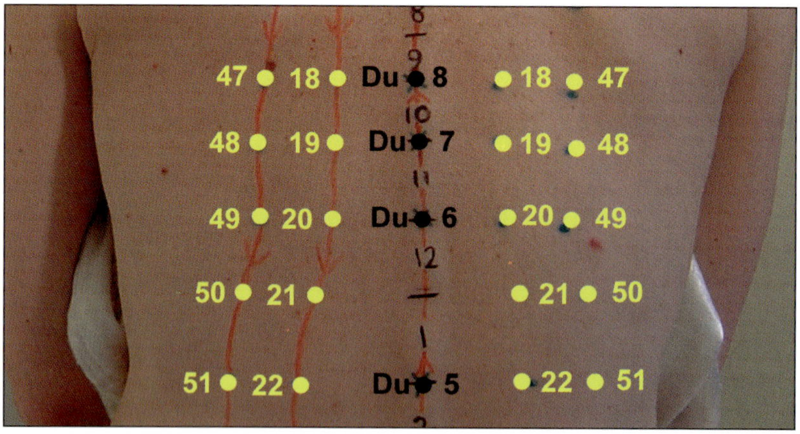

Loc: a) On the posterior torso.

b) On the outer line or the lateral branch of the Bladder channel.

c) 3 cun lateral to the posterior median line.

d) Between the 9th and 10th thoracic vertebrae (level with the base of the spinous process of the 9th thoracic vertebra).

e) Level with Du 8 and Bl 18.

Tip:
a) Please read **"HOW TO MARK OUT AND CHECK THE VERTEBRAE"** for further guidance.
b) The cun measurement from the posterior median line to the outer bladder line is 3 cun. This is taken from the posterior median line to the medial border of the scapula at the level of T3.
c) Place your finger in the intervertebral space of T9 and T10 and then palpate laterally to 3 cun until you feel a *men* (depression).
d) Palpating with the flow of the Bladder channel from the top of the back may also help you to locate the points.
e) The point is transversely level with the base of the spinous process of the 9th thoracic vertebra. This may mean that you are not between the 9th and 10th ribs but on the 9th rib. The ribs do not play any part in the location of the point.
f) As the cun measurement is a proportional measurement, 3 cun at the level of T3 may not be the same further down the back, as the posterior torso widens and narrows according to the persons own body shape, e.g. 3 cun at the level of T4/T5 may have a difference of approximately 1 cm further down the back, especially in the lumbar region.

Note: Soulié (1994) locates BL 42 (Bl 47) on the back: at the level of three FW (Finger Width) below the lower angle of the scapula; four FW on either side of the upper edge of the tenth thoracic vertebra; on the inferior edge of the ninth rib; on the vertical of the medial edge of the scapula; in a hollow; four FW below BL 41 (Bl 46); two FW above BL43 (Bl 48); two FW lateral to BL 18. Legge (1999) locates UB 47 at 3 cun lateral to the tip of the spinous process of the 9th thoracic vertebra. Voisin (1974) locates B 42 (Bl 47) 4 fb (finger breadth) from the midline of the back (centre of spinous process D 9).

Eachou (1995) locates BL 47 at 3 inches lateral to the posterior midline, between the ninth and tenth ribs. Worsley (1982) uses 4 ACI (Anatomical Chinese Inch) for the outer Bladder line (for the thoracic region of the back). Lavier (1974) doesn't use any measurement, the outer Bladder line touches the inner border of the scapula. In an illustration he shows the direction of the flow comes from below, possibly from the inner Bladder line, rather than from Bl 10.

Voisin (1974) uses 4 fb (finger breadth) lateral from the midline of the back at the centre of the spinous process for the outer Bladder line. Wu (1973) uses 4 pouce from the median line for the outer Bladder line measurement.

Bl 48 (43) YANG GANG – YANG NET

⊥ *0.3 TO 0.5 CUN* Δ *3 TO 5*

Pos: Position of patient: seated and upright.

Loc: a) On the posterior torso.
b) On the outer line or the lateral branch of the Bladder channel.
c) 3 cun lateral to the posterior median line.
d) Between the 10th and 11th thoracic vertebrae (level with the base of the spinous process of the 10th thoracic vertebra).
e) Level with Du 7 and Bl 19.

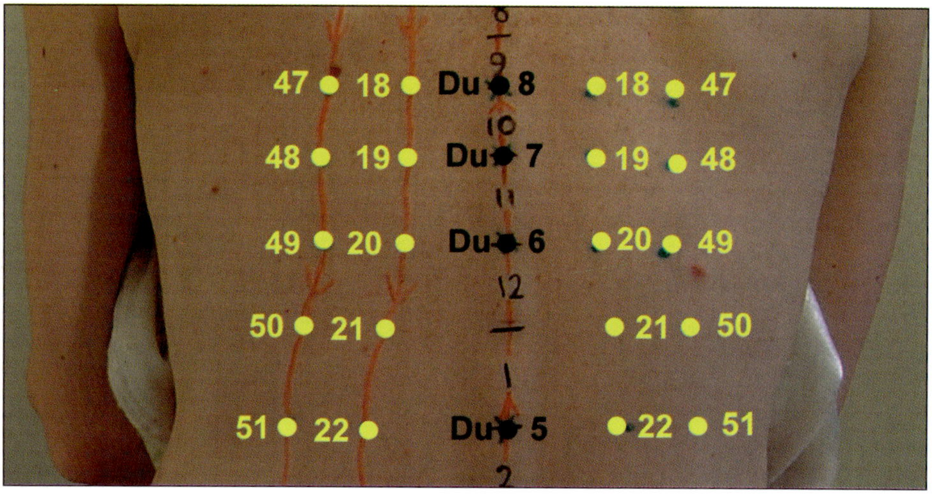

Tip: a) Please read **"HOW TO MARK OUT AND CHECK THE VERTEBRAE"** for further guidance.
b) The cun measurement from the posterior median line to the outer bladder line is 3 cun. This is taken from the posterior median line to the medial border of the scapula at the level of T3.
c) Place your finger in the intervertebral space of T10 and T11 and then palpate laterally to 3 cun until you feel a *men* (depression).
d) Palpating with the flow of the Bladder channel from the top of the back may also help you to locate the points.
e) The point is transversely level with the base of the spinous process of the 10th thoracic vertebra. This may mean that you are not between the 10th and 11th ribs but on the 10th rib. The ribs do not play any part in the location of the point.
f) As the cun measurement is a proportional measurement, 3 cun at the level of T3 may not be the same further down the back, as the posterior torso widens and narrows according to the persons own body shape, e.g. 3 cun at the level of T4/T5 may have a difference of approximately 1 cm further down the back, especially in the lumbar region.

Note: Soulié (1994) locates BL 43 (Bl 48) on the back: approximately four FW (Finger Width) under the inferior edge of the last rib; approximately four FW on either side of the superior edge of the eleventh thoracic vertebra; in a hollow on the inferior edge of the tenth rib; two FW below BL 42 (Bl 47); one large FW above BL 44 (Bl 49); two FW lateral to BL 19; four FW on either side of GV 6 (Du 6). Legge (1999) locates UB 48 at 3 cun lateral to the tip of the spinous process of the 10th thoracic vertebra. Voisin (1974) locates B 43 (Bl 48) 4 fb (finger breadth) from the midline of the back (centre of spinous process D 10).

Eachou (1995) locates BL 48 at 3 inches lateral to the posterior midline, between the tenth and eleventh ribs. Worsley (1982) uses 4 ACI (Anatomical Chinese Inch) for the outer Bladder line (for the thoracic region of the back). Lavier (1974) doesn't use any measurement, the outer Bladder line touches the inner border of the scapula. In an illustration he shows the direction of the flow comes from below, possibly from the inner Bladder line, rather than from Bl 10. Voisin (1974) uses 4 fb (finger breadth) lateral from the midline of the back at the centre of the spinous process for the outer Bladder line. Wu (1973) uses 4 pouce from the median line for the outer Bladder line measurement.

Bl 49 (44) YI SHE – THOUGHT DWELLING

⊥ ***0.3 TO 0.5 CUN*** Δ ***3 TO 15***

Pos: Position of patient: seated and upright.

Loc:
- a) On the posterior torso.
- b) On the outer line or the lateral branch of the Bladder channel.
- c) 3 cun lateral to the posterior median line.
- d) Between the 11th and 12th thoracic vertebrae (level with the base of the spinous process of the 11th thoracic vertebra).
- e) Level with Du 6 and Bl 20

Tip:
- a) Please read **"HOW TO MARK OUT AND CHECK THE VERTEBRAE"** for further guidance.
- b) The cun measurement from the posterior median line to the outer bladder line is 3 cun. This is taken from the posterior median line to the medial border of the scapula at the level of T3.
- c) Place your finger in the intervertebral space of T11 and T12 and then palpate laterally to 3 cun until you feel a *men* (depression).
- d) Palpating with the flow of the Bladder channel from the top of the back may also help you to locate the points.
- e) The point is transversely level with the base of the spinous process of the 11th thoracic vertebra. This may mean that you are not between the 11th and 12th ribs but on the 11th rib. The ribs do not play any part in the location of the point.
- f) As the cun measurement is a proportional measurement, 3 cun at the level of T3 may not be the same further down the back, as the posterior torso widens and narrows according to the persons own body shape, e.g. 3 cun at the level of T4/T5 may have a difference of approximately 1 cm further down the back, especially in the lumbar region.

Note: Soulié (1994) locates BL 44 (Bl 49) on the inferior lateral back: about four FW (Finger Width) on either side of the twelfth thoracic vertebra; approximately two FW above the lower edge of the twelfth rib; on the lower edge of the eleventh rib; nearly above the end of the twelfth rib; in a hollow; one very large FW below BL 43 (Bl 48); two FW above BL 45 (Bl 50), lateral to BL 20; four FW on either side of GV 5 (Du 5). Legge (1999) locates UB 49 at 3 cun lateral to the tip of the spinous process of the 11th thoracic vertebra. Voisin (1974) locates B 44 (Bl 49) 4 fb (finger breadth) from the midline of the back (centre of spinous process D 11).

Eachou (1995) locates BL 49 at 3 inches lateral to the posterior midline, between the eleventh and twelfth ribs. Worsley (1982) uses 4 ACI (Anatomical Chinese Inch) for the outer Bladder line (for the thoracic region of the back). Lavier (1974) doesn't use any measurement, the outer Bladder line touches the inner border of the scapula. In an illustration he shows the direction of the flow comes from below, possibly from the inner Bladder line, rather than from Bl 10.

Voisin (1974) uses 4 fb (finger breadth) lateral from the midline of the back at the centre of the spinous process for the outer Bladder line. Wu (1973) uses 4 pouce from the median line for the outer Bladder line measurement.

Bl 50 (45) WEI CANG – STOMACH GRANARY

⊥ ***0.3 TO 0.5 CUN*** ∆ ***3 TO 10***

Pos: Position of patient: seated and upright.

Loc: a) On the posterior torso.
b) On the outer line or the lateral branch of the Bladder channel.
c) 3 cun lateral to the posterior median line.
d) Between the 12th thoracic and 1st lumbar vertebrae (level with the base of the spinous process of the 12th thoracic vertebra).
e) Level with Bl 21.

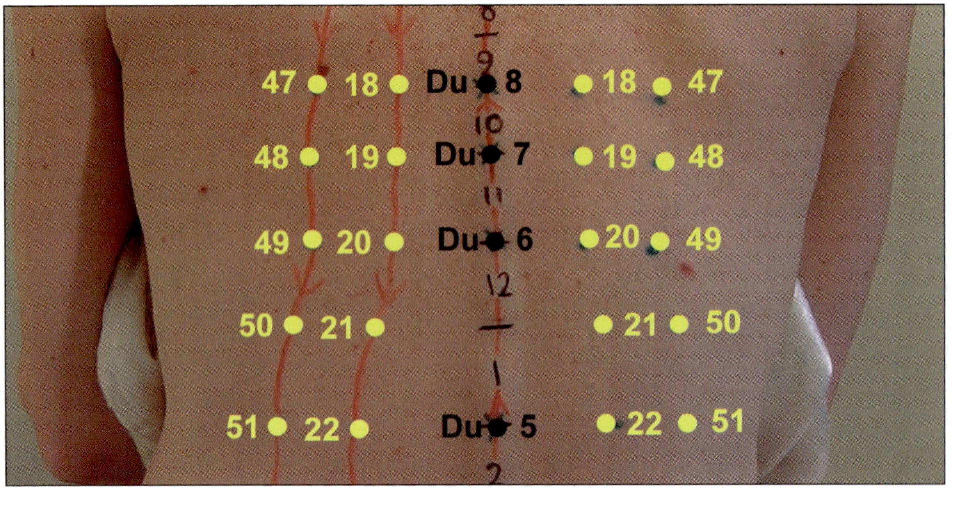

Tip:
- a) Please read **"HOW TO MARK OUT AND CHECK THE VERTEBRAE"** for further guidance.
- b) The cun measurement from the posterior median line to the outer bladder line is 3 cun. This is taken from the posterior median line to the medial border of the scapula at the level of T3.
- c) Place your finger in the intervertebral space of T12 and L1 and then palpate laterally to 3 cun until you feel a *men* (depression).
- d) Palpating with the flow of the Bladder channel from the top of the back may also help you to locate the points.
- e) The point is transversely level with the base of the spinous process of the 12th thoracic vertebra. The ribs do not play any part in the location of the point.
- f) As the cun measurement is a proportional measurement, 3 cun at the level of T3 may not be the same further down the back, as the posterior torso widens and narrows according to the persons own body shape, e.g. 3 cun at the level of T4/T5 may have a difference of approximately 1 cm further down the back, especially in the lumbar region.

Note: Soulié (1994) locates BL 45 (Bl 50) in the lumbar area: on the lower edge of the last rib (twelfth rib); about three. FW (Finger Width) on either side of the twelfth thoracic vertebra; in a hollow; on the lateral edge of the mass of lumbar muscles; two FW below and slightly medial to BL 44 (Bl 49); slightly above BL 46 (Bl 51); three FW on either side of GV 6 (Du 6); one large FW lateral to BL 32. Legge (1999) locates UB 50 at 3 cun lateral to the tip of the spinous process of the 12th thoracic vertebra. Voisin (1974) locates B 45 (Bl 50) at 4 fb (finger breadth) from the midline of the back (centre of spinous process of Rib 12: lower border). Eachou (1995) locates BL 50 at 3 inches lateral to the posterior midline, inferior to the twelfth rib.

Worsley (1982) uses 4 ACI (Anatomical Chinese Inch) for the outer Bladder line (for the thoracic region of the back). Lavier (1974) doesn't use any measurement, the outer Bladder line touches the inner border of the scapula. In an illustration he shows the direction of the flow comes from below, possibly from the inner Bladder line, rather than from Bl 10.

Voisin (1974) uses 4 fb (finger breadth) lateral from the midline of the back at the centre of the spinous process for the outer Bladder line. Wu (1973) uses 4 pouce from the median line for the outer Bladder line measurement.

Bl 51 (46) HUANG MEN – DIAPHRAGM GATE OF VITALITY

⊥ *0.3 TO 0.5 CUN* Δ *3 TO 15*

Pos: Position of patient: seated and upright.

Loc:
a) On the posterior torso.
b) On the outer line or the lateral branch of the Bladder channel.
c) 3 cun lateral to the posterior median line.
d) Between the 1st and 2nd lumbar vertebrae (level with the base of the spinous process of the 1st lumbar vertebra).
e) Level with Du 5 and Bl 22

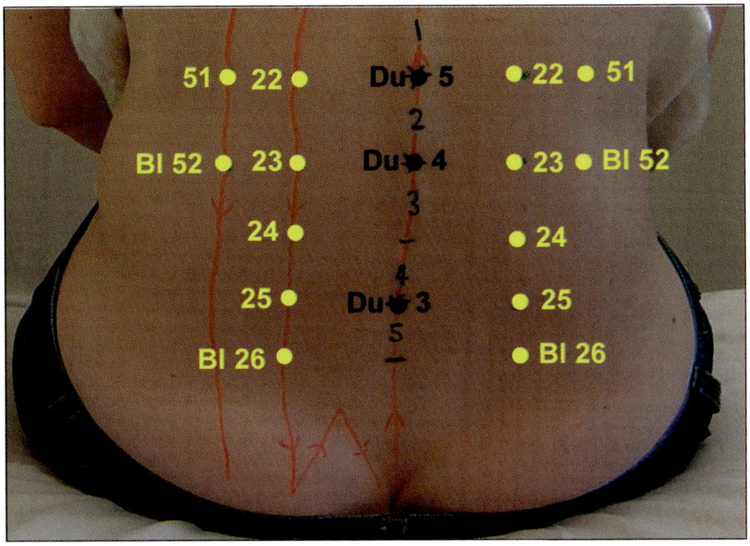

Tip:
a) Please read **"HOW TO MARK OUT AND CHECK THE VERTEBRAE"** for further guidance.
b) The cun measurement from the posterior median line to the outer bladder line is 3 cun. This is taken from the posterior median line to the medial border of the scapula at the level of T3.
c) Place your finger in the intervertebral space of L1 and L2 and then palpate laterally to 3 cun until you feel a *men* (depression).
d) Palpating with the flow of the Bladder channel from the top of the back may also help you to locate the points.
e) The point is transversely level with the base of the spinous process of the 1st lumbar vertebra.
f) As the cun measurement is a proportional measurement, 3 cun at the level of T3 may not be the same further down the back, as the posterior torso widens and narrows according to the persons own body shape, e.g. 3 cun at the level of T4/T5 may have a difference of approximately 1 cm further down the back, especially in the lumbar region.

Note: Soulié (1994) locates BL 46 (Bl 51) in the lumbar area: about one FW (Finger Width) below the last rib; about three FW on either side of the thoracic spine (second lumbar vertebra); on the lateral edge of the lumbar muscles; deep, at the level of the lower edge of the extremity of the transverse process of the first lumbar vertebra.; in a hollow; one FW below BL 45 (Bl 50); two FW above BL 47 (Bl 52); one large FW lateral to BL 22; three FW lateral to GV 5 (Du 5). Legge (1999) locates UB 51 at 3 cun lateral to the tip of the spinous process of the 1st lumbar vertebra;.

Voisin (1974) locates B 46 (Bl 51) at 4 fb (finger breadth) from the midline of the back (centre of spinous process of L 1). Worsley (1982) uses 4.5 ACI (Anatomical Chinese Inch) for the outer Bladder line (for the lumbar and sacral regions of the back). Lavier (1974) doesn't use any measurement, the outer Bladder line touches the inner border of the scapula. In an illustration he shows the direction of the flow comes from below, possibly from the inner Bladder line, rather than from Bl 10.

Voisin (1974) uses 4 fb (finger breadth) lateral from the midline of the back at the centre of the spinous process for the outer Bladder line. Wu (1973) uses 4 pouce from the median line for the outer Bladder line measurement.

Bl 52 (47) ZHI SHI – AMBITION ROOM

⊥ ***0.5 TO 0.8 CUN*** **Δ *3 TO 15***

Pos: Position of patient: seated and upright.

Loc:
a) On the posterior torso.
b) On the outer line or the lateral branch of the Bladder channel.
c) 3 cun lateral to the posterior median line.
d) Between the 2nd and 3rd lumbar vertebrae (level with the base of the spinous process of the 2nd lumbar vertebra).
e) Level with Du 4 and Bl 23.

Tip:
a) Please read **"HOW TO MARK OUT AND CHECK THE VERTEBRAE"** for further guidance.
b) The cun measurement from the posterior median line to the outer bladder line is 3 cun. This is taken from the posterior median line to the medial border of the scapula at the level of T3.
c) Place your finger in the intervertebral space of L2 and L3 and then palpate laterally to 3 cun until you feel a *men* (depression).
d) Palpating with the flow of the Bladder channel from the top of the back may also help you to locate the points.
e) The point is transversely level with the base of the spinous process of the 2nd lumbar vertebra.
f) As the cun measurement is a proportional measurement, 3 cun at the level of T3 may not be the same further down the back, as the posterior torso widens and narrows according to the persons own body shape, e.g. 3 cun at the level of T4/T5 may have a difference of approximately 1 cm further down the back, especially in the lumbar region.

Note: Soulié (1994) locates BL 47 (Bl 52) in the lumbar area; a little above the iliac crest; about three large FW (Finger Width) on either side of the upper edge of the fourth lumbar vertebra; on the latissimus dorsi and lumbar muscles; in a hollow; two FW below BL 46 (Bl 51); three FW above and medial to BL 48 (Bl 53); two FW lateral to BL 25; about two FW medial to BL 26. Legge (1999) locates UB 52 at 3 cun lateral to the tip of the spinous process of the 2nd lumbar vertebra. Voisin (1974) locates B 47 (Bl 52) 4 fb (finger breadth) from the midline of the back (centre of spinous process of L 2).

Worsley (1982) uses 4.5 ACI (Anatomical Chinese Inch) for the outer Bladder line (for the lumbar and sacral regions of the back). Lavier (1974) doesn't use any measurement, the outer Bladder line touches the inner border of the scapula. In an illustration he shows the direction of the flow comes from below, possibly from the inner Bladder line, rather than from Bl 10. Voisin (1974) uses 4 fb (finger breadth) lateral from the midline of the back at the centre of the spinous process for the outer Bladder line. Wu (1973) uses 4 pouce from the median line for the outer Bladder line measurement.

Bl 53 and 54 are on the buttock, (on the lateral branch of the Bladder channel).

Bl 53 (48) BAO HUANG – WOMB AND HEART DIAPHRAGM

⊥ ***0.5 TO 0.8 CUN*** △ ***3 TO 10***

Pos: Position of patient: seated and upright, or prone with a pillow under the pelvis.

Loc: a) On the posterior torso.
b) On the buttock.
c) Level with the sacrum.
d) On the outer line or the lateral branch of the Bladder channel.
e) 3 cun lateral to the posterior median line.
f) Level with the 2nd sacral foramen.
g) Level with Bl 28 and Bl 32.

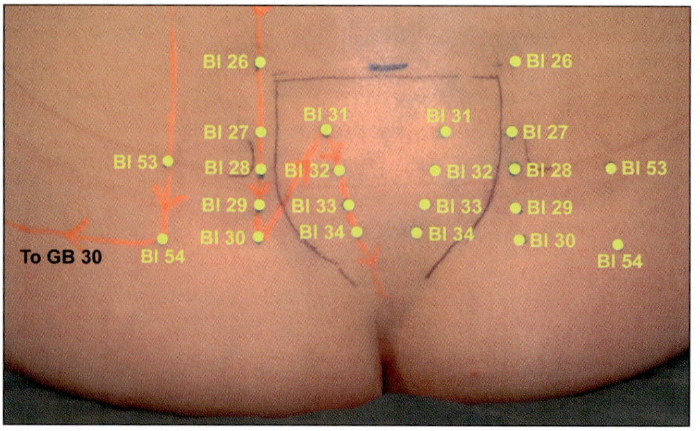

Tip: a) Mark out the superior and inferior edges of the sacrum body. Please read "THE SACRUM" for guidance.

b) The second sacral foramen is the easiest of the four sacral foramina to locate as it is often the most prominent area of the sacrum.

c) The posterior superior iliac spine of the ilium (PSIS) is a bony protruberence that may be palpated on people with a light to medium covering of tissue. Alternatively locate the top of the iliac crest and follow the contour of the bone towards the sacrum where you should feel a bony protruberence.

d) The inferior and medial borders of the posterior superior iliac spine form an 'L' shape on the right side of the body and a reversed 'L' on the left side of the body. On the corner of the 'L' in the sacroiliac joint is Bl 28. Level with the bottom of the 'L' and on the sacrum body is the second sacral foramen (Bl 32).

e) Run your finger laterally level with the second sacral foramen to 3 cun lateral to the posterior median line, but remember that the 3 cun mark made at the level of the 3rd thoracic vertebra (between the medial border of the scapula and the posterior median line) is not necessarily a 'plumb' line. You need to look at the contour of the persons body – the 3 cun measurement is a proportional measurement so it can look wider or narrower depending on the persons' body shape.

f) For accurate location of Bl 53, palpate with your finger at approximately 3 cun lateral to the posterior median line.

Note: Soulié (1994) locates BL 48 (Bl 53) on the upper buttock: two FW (Finger Width) lateral to the top of the sacrum; in the angle of the inferior edge, very deep to the edge of the iliac crest; on the medial edge of a muscular bundle (gluteus medius); deep, the insertion of the gluteus minimus; in a hollow; three FW inferior and lateral to BL 47 (Bl 52); four FW above BL 49 (Bl 54); two FW lateral to BL 27; about four FW medial to GB 27.

Legge (1999) locates UB 53 at 3 cun lateral to the tip of the spinous process of the 2nd sacral vertebra (S 2), 1.5 cun lateral to UB 28. Voisin (1974) locates B 48 (Bl 53) 4 fb (finger breadth) from the midline of the back (centre of spinous process of S 2). Worsley (1982) uses 4.5 ACI (Anatomical Chinese Inch) for the outer Bladder line (for the lumbar and sacral regions of the back). Lavier (1974) doesn't use any measurement, the outer Bladder line touches the inner border of the scapula. In an illustration he shows the direction of the flow comes from below, possibly from the inner Bladder line, rather than from Bl 10.

Voisin (1974) uses 4 fb (finger breadth) lateral from the midline of the back at the centre of the spinous process for the outer Bladder line. Wu (1973) uses 4 pouce from the median line for the outer Bladder line measurement. Shandong (1982) locate Baohuang at 3 cun lateral to the midline of the back, between the processus spinosus of the 2nd and 3rd vertebrae sacrales.

Bl 54 (49) ZHI BIAN – ORDERLY FRONTIER

⊥ ***0.5 TO 1.0 CUN*** ***Δ 3 TO 7***

Pos: Position of patient: seated and upright, or prone with a pillow under the pelvis.

Loc:
a) On the posterior torso.
b) On the buttock.
c) Level with the sacrum.
d) On the outer line or the lateral branch of the Bladder channel.
e) 3 cun lateral to the posterior median line.
f) Level with the 4th sacral foramen.
g) Lateral to the sacral hiatus of the sacrum.
h) Level with Bl 30 and Bl 34.

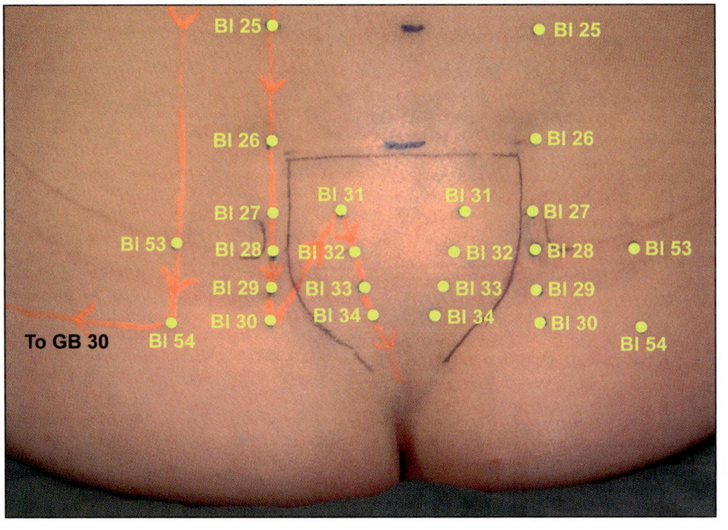

Tip:
a) Mark out the superior and inferior edges of the sacrum body. Please read "THE SACRUM" for guidance.
b) The second sacral foramen is the easiest of the four sacral foramina to locate as it is often the most prominent area of the sacrum.
c) The posterior superior iliac spine of the ilium (PSIS) is a bony protruberence that may be palpated on people with a light to medium covering of tissue. Alternatively locate the top of the iliac crest and follow the contour of the bone towards the sacrum where you should feel a bony protruberence.
d) The inferior and medial borders of the posterior superior iliac spine form an 'L' shape on the right side of the body and a reversed 'L' on the left side of the body. On the corner of the 'L' in the sacroiliac joint is Bl 28. Level with the bottom of the 'L' and on the sacrum body is the second sacral foramen (Bl 32).
e) Run your finger laterally level with the second sacral foramen to 3 cun lateral to the posterior median line.

f) When you have located the second sacral foramen, palpate inferiorly and very slightly medially from it until you feel the depression of the third sacral foramen (Bl 33). Palpate inferiorly and slightly medially again from the third sacral foramen and you should be able to feel a relatively small depression which is the fourth sacral foramen where Bl 34 is located.

g) Run your finger laterally level with the fourth sacral foramen to 3 cun lateral to the posterior median line. Remember that the 3 cun mark made at the level of the 3rd thoracic vertebra (between the medial border of the scapula and the posterior median line) is not necessarily a 'plumb' line. You have to look at the contour of the persons body – the 3 cun measurement is a proportional measurement so it can look wider or narrower depending on the persons' body shape.

h) For accurate location of Bl 54, palpate with your finger at approximately 3 cun lateral to the posterior median line.

Note: Soulié (1994) locates BL 49 (Bl 54) on the buttock:s: mid-width and mid-height; deep, the superior edge of the neck of the femur, articulating in the hip, also a transverse muscle (piriformis muscle); on the inferior edge of the gluteus medius; on the gluteus maximus; in a hollow; four FW below BL 48 (Bl 53); six FW below BL 50 (Bl 36); three large FW lateral to BL 29; four FW medial to GB 30. Legge (1999) locates UB 54 at 3 cun lateral to S 4 or the hiatus of the sacrum. Voisin (1974) locates B 49 (Bl 54) 4 fb (finger breadth) from the midline of the back (centre of spinous process of S 3).

Worsley (1982) uses 4.5 ACI (Anatomical Chinese Inch) for the outer Bladder line (for the lumbar and sacral regions of the back). Lavier (1974) doesn't use any measurement, the outer Bladder line touches the inner border of the scapula. In an illustration he shows the direction of the flow comes from below, possibly from the inner Bladder line, rather than from Bl 10. Voisin (1974) uses 4 fb (finger breadth) lateral from the midline of the back at the centre of the spinous process for the outer Bladder line. Wu (1973) uses 4 pouce from the median line for the outer Bladder line measurement. Shandong (1982) locate Zhibian at 3 cun lateral to the midline of the back, on the lower border of the 4th vertebrae sacrales.

Bl 55-59 are on the posterior and posterolateral aspects of the lower leg. The distance between the flexure of the knee and the prominence of the lateral malleolus of the fibula is 16 cun.

Bl 55 HE YANG – UNITING YANG

⊥ ***0.5 TO 0.7 CUN*** **Δ** ***3 TO 7***

- 8 EXTRAORDINARY VESSEL/ Coalescent Point of Yang Heel/Yang Motility Vessel (Yang Qiao Mai) – see note below

Pos: Position of patient: prone with the feet hanging over the end of the couch.

Loc:
a) On the posterior aspect of the lower leg.
b) On the posterior median line of leg
c) Between the medial and lateral heads of the gastrocnemius muscle.
d) On the line connecting Bl 40 and Bl 57.
e) 2 cun inferior to Bl 40 (with the flow of the channel).
f) 14 cun proximal to the prominence of the lateral malleolus.

Tip:
a) Locate the posterior aspect of the popliteal (knee) crease by flexing the patient's leg.
b) The measurement from the popliteal crease on the posterior and lateral sides of the knee flexure to the prominence of the lateral malleolus (ankle) is 16 cun.
c) At 2 cun inferior to Bl 40 the channel flows part of the way down the posterior median line of the lower leg. Palpating from Bl 40 you should be able to feel a seam formed by the medial and lateral heads of the gastrocnemius muscle. The Bladder channel flows down the leg along the seam.
d) The cun measurements are not always accurate, therefore should only be used as a guide for palpation of the point.
e) Run your finger from the crease at Bl 40 (mid-way between two dimples formed by the tendons of the biceps femoris muscle and the semitendinosus muscle) with the flow of the Bladder channel down the leg to locate the point. Bl 55 is 2 cun inferior to Bl 40 or 14 cun proximal to the prominence of the lateral malleolus (ankle bone).

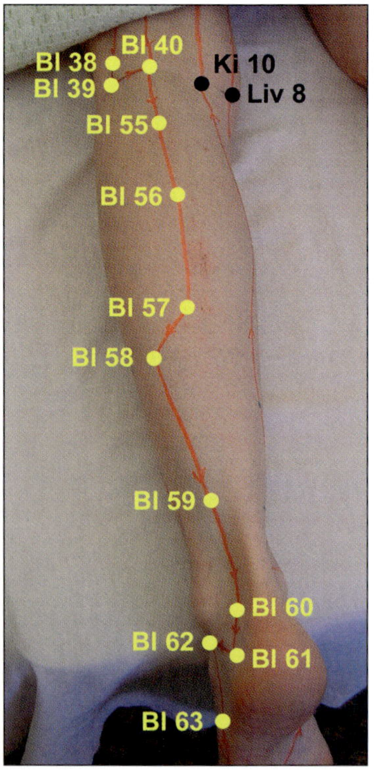

Note: In some texts Bl 55 is listed as an 8 EXTRAORDINARY VESSEL/Coalescent Point of Yang Qiao Mai (Yang Heel/Yang Motility Vessel), whereas in others it is omitted. Wu (1973) locates BL 55 on the posterior surface of the leg, at two and a half pouce below the popliteal crease, between the gastrocnemius muscles.

Bl 56 CHENG JIN – SUPPORTING MUSCLES

⊥ ***FORBIDDEN TO NEEDLE*** **Δ *3 TO 7***

Pos: Position of patient: prone with the feet hanging over the end of the couch.

Loc:
a) On the posterior aspect of the lower leg.
b) On the posterior median line of leg
c) In the centre of the belly of the gastrocnemius muscle.
d) On the line connecting Bl 40 and Bl 57.
e) 5 cun inferior to Bl 40 (with the flow of the channel).
f) 11 cun proximal to the prominence of the lateral malleolus bone.
g) Midway between Bl 55 and Bl 57.

Tip:
a) Locate the posterior aspect of the popliteal (knee) crease by flexing the patient's leg.
b) The measurement from the popliteal crease on the posterior and lateral sides of the knee flexure to the prominence of the lateral malleolus (ankle) is 16 cun.
c) The Bladder channel usually flows part of the way down the posterior median line to approximately 8 cun. As you palpate from the knee crease at Bl 40 you should be able to feel a seam formed by the medial and lateral heads of the gastrocnemius muscle. From here the Bladder channel runs down the centre of the belly of the gastrocnemius muscle.
d) Some people have well developed leg muscles and the Bladder channel may not be on the median line of the leg, therefore the belly of the gastrocnemius muscle takes precedence.
e) Occasionally the cun measurements are not always accurate, but should be used as a guide for palpation and location of the point.
f) Bl 56 is 5 cun inferior to Bl 40 or 11 cun proximal to the prominence of the lateral malleolus (ankle bone).

Note: Historically the cun measurements of Bl 56/57/58 have varied, but the bone proportional cun measurements are not as reliable as the muscular landmarks.

Note: Worsley (1982) locates III 56 on the posterior surface of the leg, 12 ACI (Anatomical Chinese Inch) proximal to the level of the prominence of the lateral malleolus, between the lateral and medial heads of the gastrocnemius. Wu (1973) locates BL 56 upon the posterior surface of the leg, at four pouce below the popliteal crease, between the gastrocnemius muscles.

Lavier (1974) locates BL 56 at 12 pouce proximal to the prominence of the external malleolus and in the centre of the belly of the gastrocnemius muscle. Soulié (1994) locates BL 56 on the calf: mid-height, mid-width, between the two sides of the gastrocnemius; in the angle letween the gastrol (BL 55); two FW (Finger Width) below BL 55; two FW above BL 57. Vosin (1974) locates B 56 on the gastrocnemius: between the two heads, centre of its muscle mass.

Bl 57 CHENG SHAN – SUPPORTING MOUNTAIN

⊥ ***0.7 CUN*** **Δ** ***3 TO 15***

- ONE OF THE HEAVENLY STAR POINTS OF MA DAN-YANG (the others are: Lu 7, LI 4, LI 11, St 36, St 44, Bl 40, Bl 60, Ht 5, GB 34, GB 39 and Liv 3)

Pos: Position of patient: prone with the feet hanging over the end of the couch.

Loc:
a) On the posterior aspect of the lower leg.
b) On the posterior median line of leg.
c) On the line connecting Bl 40 and Bl 57.
d) At the point where the junction of the two halves of the belly of the gastrocnemius muscle meets with the tendocalcaneus (achilles tendon).
e) Approximately 8 cun inferior to Bl 40 (with the flow of the channel).
f) Approximately 8 cun proximal to the prominence of the lateral malleolus bone.
g) Midway between Bl 40 and Bl 60.

Tip:
a) Locate the posterior aspect of the popliteal crease (knee) by flexing the patient's leg.
b) At approximately 8 cun inferior to Bl 40 the channel flows part of the way down the posterior median line of the lower leg. As you palpate from Bl 40 you should be able to feel a seam formed by the medial and lateral heads of the gastrocnemius muscle. The Bladder channel runs in the seam in the centre of the belly of the gastrocnemius muscle.
c) With well developed leg muscles the Bladder channel may not be on the median line of the leg, therefore the belly of the gastrocnemius muscle takes precedence.
d) Occasionally the cun measurements are not accurate, but should be used as a guide for palpation and point location.
e) Approximately 8 cun (halfway between the popliteal crease and the prominence of the lateral malleolus) you should be able to feel a *men* (depression) where the gastrocnemius muscle and the achilles tendon changes from muscle to tendon.
f) The measurement from the popliteal crease on the posterior and lateral sides of the knee flexure to the prominence of the lateral malleolus (ankle) is 16 cun.
g) Bl 57 is 8 cun inferior to Bl 40 or 8 cun proximal to the prominence of the lateral malleolus or halfway between Bl 40 and Bl 60.
h) To assist in palpation and point location run your finger from the crease at Bl 40 (midway between two dimples formed by the tendons of the biceps femoris muscle and the semitendinosus muscle) with the flow of the Bladder channel.
i) To locate Bl 57 ask the patient to push against your thigh with the ball of their foot so their heel is raised. Place your finger in the depression formed by the junction at the inferior border of the two halves of the belly of the gastrocnemius muscle. Ask the patient to relax their foot so you will feel the depression slightly inferior to your finger when the heel was raised.
j) The patient is always in the same position for point location and needling.

Note: Historically the cun measurements of Bl 56/57/58 have varied, but the bone proportional cun measurements are not as reliable as the muscular landmarks.

Note: Wu (1973) locates BL 57 upon the posterior surface of the leg, between the gastrocnemius muscles, where the tendon emerges, at seven pouce below the popliteal crease. Lavier (1974) in an illustration locates BL 57 at 9 pouce proximal to the prominence of the lateral malleolus. The illustration also locates the point just inferior to the junction of the two halves of the belly of the gastrocnemius muscle. Worsley (1982) locates III 57 on the posterior surface of the leg, 9 ACI (Anatomical Chinese Inch) proximal to the level of the prominence of the lateral malleolus, between the lateral and medial heads of the gastrocnemius. Voisin (1974) locates B 57 on the Gastrocnemius: lower part of muscle mass, upper part of hollow visible upon rising of toes.

Bl 58 FEI YANG – FLY AND SCATTER

⊥ ***0.3 TO 0.7 CUN*** Δ ***3 TO 7***

- JUNCTION/Luo/Connecting/Passage/Lo/Lê
- RE-UNION/Crossing/Meeting Point of the Bladder Channel with the Kidney Channel – Foot Tai Yang Channel with the Foot Shao Yin Channel
- HOST/GUEST COMBINATION – Source Point with the Junction Point of its Paired Official/Organ Therefore Bl 58 is combined with Ki 3

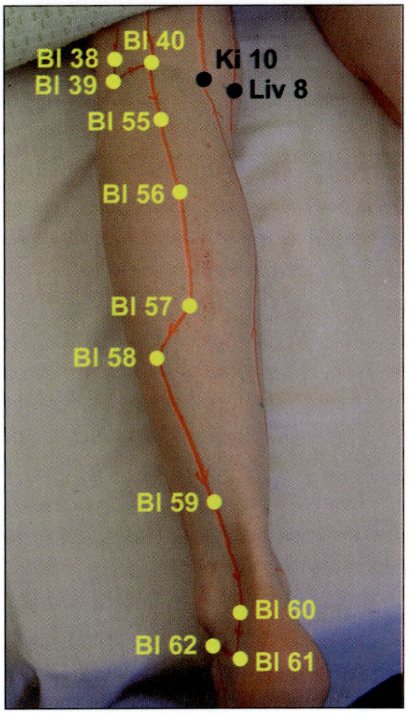

Pos: Position of patient: prone with the feet hanging over the end of the couch.

Loc: a) On the posterolateral aspect of the lower leg.
b) Between the fibula bone and the tendocalcaneus (achilles tendon).
c) On the lateral border of the tendocalcaneus (sometimes the lateral border of the gastrocnemius muscle) – see tip c).
d) Approximately 1 cun lateral to Bl 57 – see tip d).
e) Approximately 1 cun inferior to Bl 57.
f) Approximately 9 cun inferior to Bl 40 (with the flow of the channel).
g) Approximately 7 cun proximal to the prominence of the lateral malleolus (ankle).
h) Directly superior to Bl 59 and Bl 60.

Tip: a) Run your finger in the groove formed by the posterior border of the prominence of the lateral malleolus bone and the lateral border of the tendocalcaneus (achilles tendon) towards the knee.

b) The groove formed by the posterior border of the fibula and the tendocalcaneus will narrow as you run your finger up the leg (against the flow of the channel).

c) The point is located approximately 7 cun proximal to the prominence of the lateral malleolus in the groove which is formed by the posterior border of the fibula lateral border of the tendocalcaneus or the lateral border of the gastrocnemius muscle (depending on the area where the tissue alters from muscle to tendon).

d) The point should be located on the lateral border of the tendon or muscle and not on it, therefore the point may not appear to be at 1 cun lateral to Bl 57 as the anatomy takes precedence.

e) Occasionally Bl 58 may not be located at the cun measurement, therefore palpation is important to accurately locate the point.

f) There are 16 cun from the popliteal crease on the posterior and lateral sides of the knee flexure to the prominence of the lateral malleolus. Bl 58 is 9 cun inferior to Bl 40 or 7 cun proximal to the prominence of the lateral malleolus.

Note: Historically the cun measurements of Bl 56/57/58 have varied, but the bone proportional cun measurements are not as reliable as the muscular landmarks.

Note: Lawson-Wood (1973) locates III 58 on the postero-extern of the leg, half-way between the external malleolus and the tibio-femoral articulation, on the external gastrocnemius. Voisin (1974) locates B 58 at the gastrocnemius: musculotendinous junction, vertically above the posterior border of the lateral malleolus. Lavier (1974) in an illustration locates BL 58 at 8 pouce proximal to the prominence of the external malleolus, on the lateral border of the tendocalcaneus or soleus muscle. Shandong (1982) locate Feiyang at 7 cun above Pt. Kunlun (Bl 60), latero-inferior to Pt. Chengshan (Bl 57).

Worsley (1982) locates III 58 on the posterolateral surface of the leg, 8 ACI (Anatomical Chinese Inch) proximal to the level of the prominence of the lateral malleolus, between the gastrocnemius and soleus. So (1985) locates BL 58 one division below BL 57, one-half a division lateral to the outside of the calf between two muscles. Wu (1973) locates BL 58 on the posterio-external surface of the leg, between the peroneus longus and the soleus, at eight pouce above the centre of the external malleus.

Soulié (1994) locates BL 58 on the posterolateral lower leg, about mid-height: seven FW (Finger Width) above the lateral malleolus. One large FW posterior to the peroneus muscle; one small FW under the lateral union of the lateral gastrocnemius muscle on the Achilles tendon; on the lateral edge of the tendon, in a transverse groove; on the soleus muscle; two FW below and lateral to BL 57; three FW above and posterior to BL 59; one small FW lateral and slightly below GB 36

To locate Bl 59-62 the foot should be dorsiflexed.

Bl 59 FU YANG – FOOT BONE YANG

⊥ ***0.5 TO 0.7 CUN*** Δ ***3 TO 7***

- ACCUMULATION/Xi Cleft/Gueki Point of the Yang Linking/Yang Heel Vessel (Yang Qiao Mai)
- 8 EXTRAORDINARY VESSEL/Coalescent Point of the Yang Linking/Yang Heel Vessel (Yang Qiao Mai)

Pos: Position of patient: prone with the feet hanging over the end of the couch.

Loc:
a) On the lateral aspect of the lower leg.
b) In a seam between the tendocalcaneus (achilles tendon) and the posterior border of the fibula bone.
c) Directly superior to Bl 60.
d) Approximately 13 cun inferior to Bl 40 (with the flow of the channel).
e) Approximately 3 cun proximal to the prominence of the lateral malleolus bone (ankle).

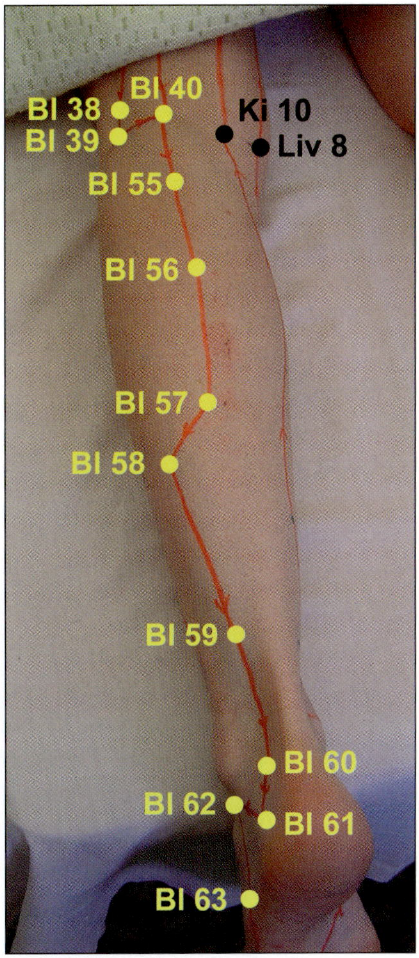

Tip:
a) Run your finger from the ankle towards the knee in the groove formed by the posterior border of the prominence of the lateral malleolus and the lateral border of the tendocalcaneus towards the knee.
b) The groove formed by the posterior border of the fibula and the tendocalcaneus will narrow as you run your finger up the leg (against the flow of the channel).
c) The point is located in the groove approximately 3 cun proximal to the prominence of the lateral malleolus.
d) Occasionally Bl 59 may not be located at the cun measurement, therefore palpation is important to accurately locate the point.
e) There are 16 cun from the popliteal crease on the posterior and lateral sides of the knee flexure to the prominence of the lateral malleolus. Bl 59 is 13 cun inferior to Bl 40 or 3 cun proximal to the prominence of the lateral malleolus.

Note: Voisin (1974) locates B 59 between the Achilles tendon and the fibula, 3 fb (finger breadth) above the lateral malleolus. Wu (1973) locates BL 59 upon the posterio-external surface of the leg, behind the peroneus, at three pouce above the centre of the external malleus. Worsley (1982) locates III 59 on the posterolateral surface of the leg, 3 ACI (Anatomical Chinese Inch) proximal to the level of the prominence of the lateral malleolus, posterior to the peroneus longus, directly proximal to III 60 (Bl 60).

Soulié (1994) locates BL 59 on the lateral leg: four FW (Finger Width) above the lateral malleolus, just at the posterior edge of the peroneus; on the upper edge of a transverse mass; on the anterior edge of the soleus muscle; in a hollow; three FW below and slightly anterior to BL 58; four FW above BL 60; one very large FW posterior to GB 37. Shanghai (1981) locates B 59 at 3 units above B 60, at the lateral aspect of the gastrocnemius muscle. Shandong (1982) locate Fuyang at 3 cun above Pt. Kunlun, posterior to the malleolus lateralis.

Bl 60 is on the lateral aspect of the leg, level with the prominence of the lateral malleolus of the fibula. The distance from the prominence of the lateral malleolus to the inferior edge of the heel is measured as 3 cun.

Bl 60 KUN LUN – KUN LUN MOUNTAIN

⊥ ***0.3 TO 0.5 CUN*** **Δ** ***3 TO 7***

- FIRE
- JING – RIVER/Shu – Transporting/Antique
- ONE OF THE HEAVENLY STAR POINTS OF MA DAN-YANG (the others are: Lu 7, LI 4, LI 11, St 36, St 44, Bl 40, Bl 57, Ht 5, GB 34, GB 39 and Liv 3)

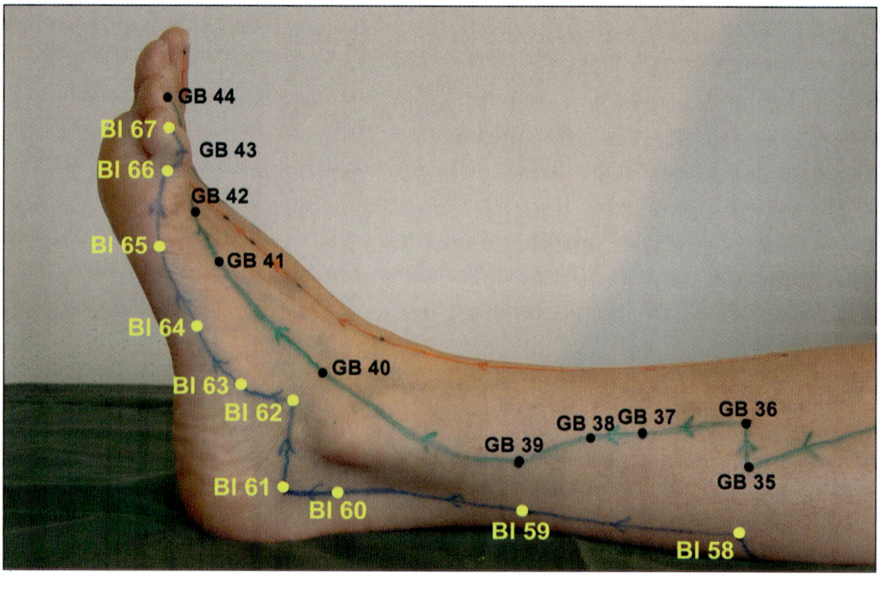

Pos: Position of patient: prone with the feet hanging over the end of the couch or supine.

Loc: a) On the lateral aspect of the lower leg.
b) Posterior to the prominence of the lateral malleolus (ankle).
c) In a groove between the tendocalcaneus (achilles tendon) and the prominence of the lateral malleolus.

Tip: a) To accurately locate the prominence of the lateral malleolus, stand at the opposite side of the patient, i.e. stand on the left side for the prominence of the right lateral malleolus and vice versa. Look directly over the anterior surface of the leg for the contour of the lateral malleolus. From the prominence of the lateral malleolus draw a line towards the tendo-calcaneus. Palpate for the prominence if it is not visible due to localised swelling.
b) Place your finger on the lateral surface of the lower leg approximately a quarter of the way up the leg from the lateral malleolus in the groove formed by the posterior border of the fibula and the lateral border of the tendocalcaneus.
c) Palpate for Bl 60 with your finger in the deepest part of the groove level with the posterior border of the prominence of the lateral malleolus and the anterior border of the tendo-calcaneus.
d) The level of the prominence of the lateral malleolus is an important reference mark when locating 16 cun from the popliteal crease on the posterior and lateral sides of the knee flexure to the prominence of the lateral malleolus.
e) The distance from the prominence of the lateral malleolus to the inferior edge of the heel is 3 cun.

Note: Wu (1973), Worsley (1982), and Soulié (1994) also locate this point in relation to the peroneal artery, upon the artery, Wu (1973 locates BL 60 upon the external surface of the ankle, between the external malleus and the Achilles tendon, above the superior edge of the calcaneum, upon the peroneal artery. Worsley (1982) locates III 60 mid-way between the prominence of the lateral malleolus and the achilles tendon, on the peroneal artery.

Soulié (1994) locates BL 60 on the posterolateral ankle; in the angle between the posterolateral edge of the lateral malleolus and the upper edge of the calcaneus and the anterior edge of the posterior peroneal tendons. Anterior to the poterior peroneal artery, external saphenus nerve and vein; in a hollow; four FW (Finger Width) below BL 59; two tightened FW above BL 61. So (1985) locates BL 60 posterior to the lateral maleolus 1/2 division; between the edge of the ankle and the tendon. Voisin (1974) locates B 60 between the Achilles tendon and lateral malleolus, upper border of calcaneus.

Bl 61-66 are on the lateral aspect of the foot.

Bl 61 PU SHEN – SERVANT'S AIDE

⊥ ***0.3 CUN*** Δ ***3 TO 7***

- A Seven External Dragons (E.D's) Point (the other points are Du 20, Bl 11 and Bl 23)
- 8 EXTRAORDINARY VESSEL/Coalescent Point of Yang Heel/Yang Motility Vessel (Yang Qiao Mai)
- RE-UNION/Crossing/Meeting Point of the Bladder Channel with the Yang Motility/Yang Heel Vessel – Foot Tai Yang Channel with the Yang Qiao Mai.

Pos: Position of patient: supine or prone with the feet hanging over the end of the couch.

Loc: a) On the lateral aspect of the foot.
b) On the calcaneus.
c) Approximately 1.5 cun directly inferior to Bl 60 (at the level of the prominence of the lateral malleolus)
d) At the junction of the change in skin colour.

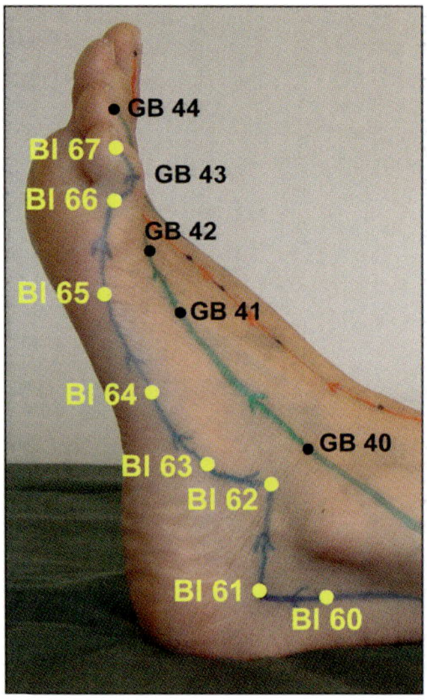

Tip: a) To accurately locate the prominence of the lateral malleolus, stand at the opposite side of the patient, i.e. stand on the left side for the prominence of the right lateral malleolus and vice versa. Look directly over the anterior surface of the leg for the contour of the lateral malleolus. From the prominence of the lateral malleolus draw a line towards the tendo-calcaneus. Palpate for the prominence if it is not visible due to localised swelling.
b) Measure 3 cun from the prominence of the lateral malleolus to the inferior edge of the heel and mark 1.5 cun.
c) At the level of the prominence of the lateral malleolus, palpate in the groove until you are on the calcaneus approximately 1.5 cun inferior to Bl 60. The groove is formed by the tendocalcaneus and the posterior border of the fibula.)
d) Bl 61 is located approximately 1.5 cun directly inferior to Bl 60 at the change of skin colour. You will need to palpate for the point especially if there is no change in skin colour.

Note: Yang (1982) locates UB 61 at 2 cun directly below Kunlun (UB 60). Soulié (1994) locates BL 61 on the lateral heel: below the angle between the anterior edge of the vertical long tendon and the posterior edge of the ankle (lateral malleolus) and the eminence of the bone; one FW (Finger Width) below BL 60, and two FW above BL 62. Worsley (1982) locates III 61 on the superior edge of the lateral surface of the calcaneus, directly inferior to III 60 (Bl 60). So (1985) locates BL 61 at 2 divisions below BL 60, 1/4 of a division towards the back of the heel in the cleft on the heel bone. Legge (1999) locates UB 61 at 1 cun directly below Kunlun (UB 60), at the junction of the red and white skin. Voisin (1974) locates B 61 at 1 fb (finger breadth) below B 60. Wu (1973) locates BL 61 upon the foot, at the centre of the external surface of the calcaneum, below BL 60. Shandong (1982) locate Pushen below Pt. Kunlun (Bl 60), in the depression of the calcaneus.

Bl 62 SHEN MAI – EXTENDED MERIDIAN

⊥ ***0.3 CUN*** **Δ *FORBIDDEN TO MOXA***

- 8 EXTRAORDINARY VESSEL/Coalescent Point of Yang Heel/Yang Motility Vessel (Yang Qiao Mai)
- 8 EXTRAORDINARY CHANNELS CONFLUENT/8 Extraordinary Meridians Confluent/8 Extraordinary Vessels Opening/Master Point of the Yang Heel/Yang Motility Vessel (Yang Qiao Mai)
- 8 EXTRAORDINARY VESSEL/Coupled Point of the Du Mai (Governor Vessel)
- SUN SI-MIAO GHOST (Gui) – Ghost Point Name: Gui Lu – Ghost Path

Pos: Position of patient: supine.

Loc: a) On the lateral aspect of the foot.
b) Directly inferior to the prominence of the lateral malleolus.
c) Approximately 0.5 cun inferior to the inferior border of the lateral malleolus.

Tip: a) To accurately locate the prominence of the lateral malleolus, stand at the opposite side of the patient, i.e. stand on the left side for the prominence of the right lateral malleolus and vice versa. Look directly over the anterior surface of the leg for the contour of the lateral malleolus. From the prominence of the lateral malleolus draw a line towards the tendo-calcaneus. Palpate for the prominence if it is not visible due to localised swelling.
b) Locate the inferior border of the lateral malleolus by palpation.
c) Measure 3 cun from the prominence of the lateral malleolus to the inferior edge of the heel and mark 1.5 cun. Divide the upper 1.5 cun into 3 to give you three 0.5 cun measurements.
d) From the inferior border of the lateral malleolus, use one of the 0.5 cun measurements and mark 0.5 cun inferior to the inferior border of the lateral malleolus.
e) Draw two longitudinal marks at the 0.5 cun measurement of the anterior and posterior borders of the lateral malleolus, then divide these two marks in half to give an approximate area to accurately palpate for the point.
f) The fibularis longus (peroneus longus) and fibularis brevis (peroneus brevis) muscles are frequently used to locate Bl 62. However in clinical reality these two tendons can often be in different locations at 0.5 cun inferior to the lateral malleolus. They can vary so much that the location of the point can be either anterior, posterior, superior or even in between them. As long as you palpate directly below the middle of the inferior border of the lateral malleolus at 0.5 cun, you should be able to accurately palpate for Bl 62.
g) Actively evert and plantar flex the foot to expose the tendons of the fibularis longus and fibularis brevis.

Note: Voisin (1974) locates B 62 at 1.5 fb (finger breadth) below and slightly in front of the lateral malleolus. Wu (1973) locates BL 62 upon the foot, at one-half pouce below the point of the external malleus, between the two tendons. Legge (1999) locates UB 62 in the depression directly below the external malleolus and anterior and superior to the peroneal tendond as they wrap around the posterior aspect of the lateral malleolus.

Worsley (1982) locates III 62 one half ACI (Anatomical Chinese Inch) distal to the tip of the lateral malleolus, between the tendons of the peroneus longus and the peroneus brevis. So (1985) locates BL 62 1/2 division below the centre of the lateral malleolus, between two small tendons.

Lotan (2000) locates UB 62 inferior to the lateral malleolus, vertically inferior to the malleolus peak, between the peroneal tendons and the malleolus. Deadman (1998) locates BL 62 on the lateral side of the foot, approximately 0.5 cun inferior to the inferior border of the lateral malleolus, in a depression posterior to the peroneal tendons. Masayoshi (1975) locates BL 62 dorectly below the lateral malleolus, at the lower edge of the tendon, sheath of short fibular muscle. Shanghai (1993) locates BL 62 on the lateral aspect of the foot, directly below the lateral malleolus, in the depression below the trochlear process of the calcaneum.

Soulié (1994) locates BL 62 on the lateral foot: just under the lateral malleolus, below the lower edge of the calcaneus bone; in the angle between the posterior edge of the tendons turning towards the front (peroneus longus muscle, and under it, the posterior peroneus brevis), and the superior edge of a horizontal muscle (abductor digiti minimi muscle); about two FW (Finger Width) below BL 61 and one large FW posterior to BL 63. Shandong (1982) locate Shenmai in the depression at the lower border of the malleolus lateralis.

Bl 63 JIN MEN – GOLDEN GATE

⊥ ***0.3 CUN*** Δ ***3 TO 5***

- ACCUMULATION/Xi Cleft/Gueki
- 8 EXTRAORDINARY VESSEL/Coalescent Point of Yang Linking Vessel (Yang Wei Mai)
- RE-UNION/Crossing/Meeting Point of the Bladder Channel with the Yang Linking Vessel – Foot Tai Yang Channel with the Yang Wei Mai.

Pos: Position of patient: supine.

Loc: a) On the lateral aspect of the foot.
b) Proximal to the tuberosity of the fifth metatarsal bone.
c) Just inferior to the inferior border of the cuboid bone.
d) Anterior (distal) and inferior to Bl 62.

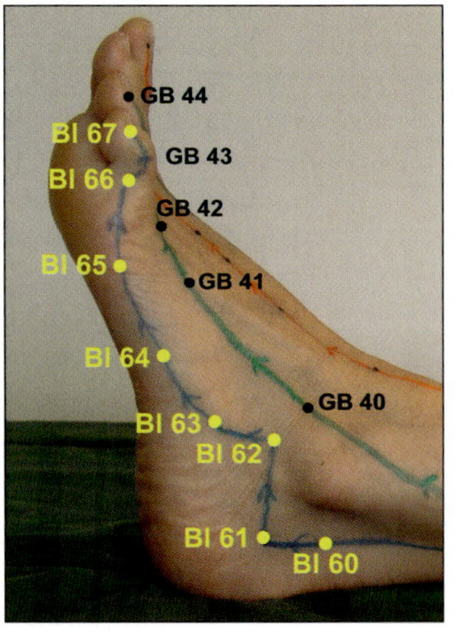

Tip: a) Visualise the lateral aspect of the foot before you palpate for Bl 63. Usually you can see a bony prominence inferior and slightly distal to the lateral malleolus, this is the tuberosity of the fifth metatarsal bone.

b) Run your finger with the direction of flow of the Bladder channel from the inferior border of the lateral malleolus (near to Bl 62) both inferiorly and anteriorly (distally) towards the tuberosity of the the fifth metatarsal.

c) Palpate for the proximal border of the tuberosity of the fifth metatarsal and draw the border of the tuberosity (circular shape).

d) Visualise the circle as a clock face, the point can be palpated between 9 and 10 on the right foot and between 2 and 3 on the left foot (12 is towards the plantar surface of the foot). Therefore the point is more inferior than the widest aspect of the foot. Bl 63 is inferior to the inferior border of the cuboid bone (which is the bone more proximal and slightly superior to the fifth metatarsal bone).

Note: There appears to be great confusion about this point in various texts. The location has been given as "directly inferior to the anterior border of the lateral malleolus, on the inferior border of the cuboid bone", and also "at the mid-point of the line joining Bl 62 and Bl 64, in the depression lateral to the cuboid bone", as well as "anterior and inferior to Bl 62, in the depression posterior to the tuberosity of the fifth metatarsal bone".

Wu (1973) locates BL 63 upon the foot, at one pouce in front of the external malleus. Voisin (1974) locates B 63 on the dorsum of the foot: at the junction of the calcaneus, talus and cuboid bones. Lotan (2000) locates UB 63 vertically inferior to the lateral malleolus anterior border, posterior to the cuboid, about 1 cun inferior and anterior to UB 62. Legge (1999) locates UB 63 anterior and inferior to UB 62, on the lateral and inferior aspect of the cuboid bone, posterior to the proximal head of the 5th metatarsal bone. Lavier (1974) in an illustration locates BL 63 on the lateral aspect of the foot, anterior to the prominence of the lateral malleolus, in the joint between the talus and cuboid bones. So (1985) locates BL 63 one division below BL 62, and 1/2 division distal. Just inder the apex of the triangular bone.

Soulié (1994) locates BL 63 on the lateral edge of the foot: about two FW (Finger Width) below and a little in front of the lateral malleolus. In the angle between the upper edge of a horizontal muscle at the edge of the sole (abductor digiti minimi muscle), and the posterior edge of the inferior point of the cuboid bone; in front of the calcaneus; one large FW in front of BL 62; two FW posterior to BL 64. Qiu (1996) locates UB 63 at the midpoint of the line joining UB 62 and UB 64 in the depression lateral to the cuboid bone. Masayoshi (1974) locates BL 63 on the outer side of the cuboid joit of the heel, joint of the calcaneous and cuboid bone.

Cheng (1987) locates B 63 anterior and inferior to B 62, in the depression lateral to the cuboid bone. Ellis (1991) locates BL 63 anterior and inferior to BL 62, in the depression inferior to the cuboid bone. Shanghai (1993) locates BL 63 on the lateral aspect of the foot, anterior and inferior to the lateral maleolus, between BL 64 and BL 62, on the lateral and inferior border of the cuboid bone. Shandong (1982) locate Jinmen antero-inferior to Pt. Shenmai (Bl 62), in the lateral depression of the os cuboideum.

Bl 64 JING GU – CAPITAL BONE

⊥ ***0.3 TO 0.5 CUN*** Δ ***3 TO 7***

- SOURCE/Yuan/Regulator/Primary
- ORIGINAL (for specific symptoms)
- HOST/GUEST COMBINATION – Source Point with the Junction Point of its Paired Official/Organ Therefore Bl 64 is combined with Ki 4

Pos: Position of patient: supine.

Loc: a) On the lateral aspect of the foot.
b) Just inferior and distal to the tuberosity of the fifth metatarsal bone.
c) Distal to the flare of the base of the fifth metatarsal bone.
d) Traditionally at the junction of the change in skin colour.

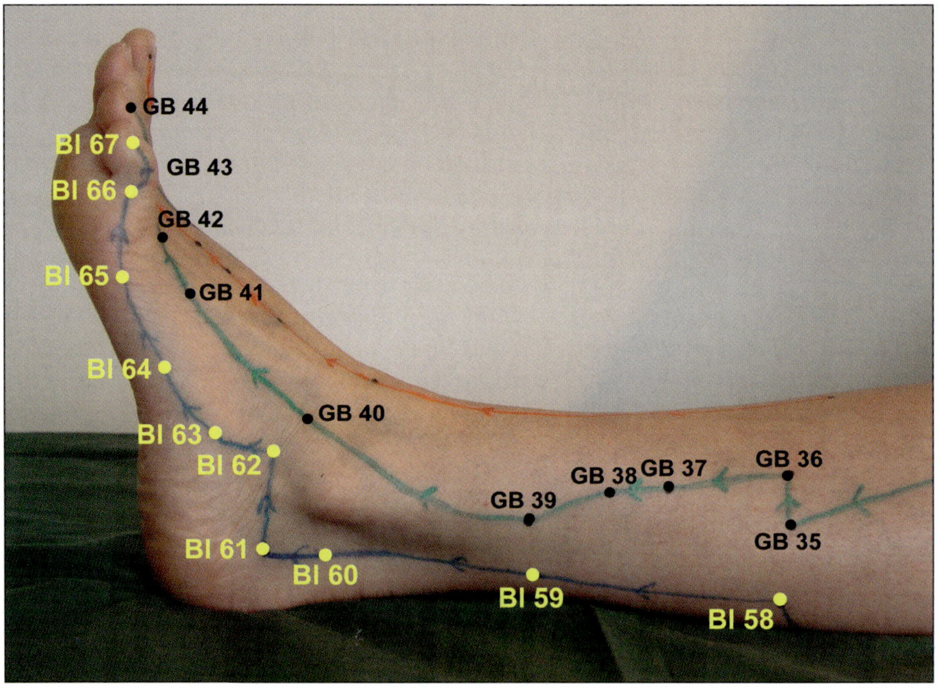

Tip: a) Visualise the lateral aspect of the foot before you palpate for Bl 63. Usually you can see a bony prominence inferior and slightly distal to the lateral malleolus, this is the tuberosity of the fifth metatarsal bone.
b) Run your finger with the direction of flow of the Bladder channel from the inferior border of the lateral malleolus (near to Bl 62) both inferiorly and anteriorly (distally) towards the tuberosity of the the fifth metatarsal.
c) Palpate for the proximal border of the tuberosity of the fifth metatarsal and draw the border of the tuberosity (circular shape).

d) Visualise the circle as a clock face, the point can be palpated between 4 and 5 on the right foot and between 7 and 8 on the left foot (12 is towards the plantar surface of the foot). Therefore the point is more inferior than the widest aspect of the foot. Bl 64 is inferior and distal to the tuberosity of the fifth metatarsal bone.
e) Palpation is important as Bl 64 may not be at the junction of the change in skin colour.
f) A common error when locating Bl 64 is locating it too high and the point is needled on the metatarsal bone. The point is always inferior to the bone.
g) Think of the lateral aspect of the foot as a filling to a sandwich and you are pressing the sandwich down to 'bulge' the filling out. The line of the Bladder channel flows towards the fifth digit on the widest or most prominent aspect of the bulge which may not be at the change in skin colour.

Note: Many texts locate Bl 64 inferior to the tuberosity of the base of the 5th metatarsal bone, whereas many others locate it distal/anterior to the tuberosity. So (1985) locates BL 64 at 2 divisions proximal to the head of the 5th metatarsal bone on the outer side of the foot where the yin and yang skin meet. Lavier (1974) in an illustration locates BL 64 on the lateral aspect of the foot, proximal to the tuberosity of the fifth metatarsal bone, directly inferior to GB 40. Wu (1973) locates BL 64 on the external edge of the foot, behind the tubercle of the fifth metatarsal.

Qiu (1996) locates UB 64 below the tuberosity of the 5th metatarsal bone, at the junction of the red and white skin, Eachou (1995) locates BL 64 proximal to the tuberosity of the fifth metatarsal bone, on the lateral part of the foot. Lawson-Wood (1973) locates III 64 on the external border of the foot, under the tubercle of the fifth metatarsal. Voisin (1974) locates B 64 at the metatarsal 5, lateral border, in a hollow just behind its tuberosity.

Soulié (1994) locates BL 64 on the lateral edge of the foot: one half FW (Finger Width) in front of the big bony eminence at mid-length (tubercle of the fifth metatarsal); in the angle between the upper edge of the metatarsal and the anterior edge of the insertion of the peroneus brevis; on the upper edge of the muscle froming the edge of the sole (abductor digiti minimi muscle), in a hollow; two FW anterior to BL 63; two FW posterior to BL 65.

Legge (1999) locates UB 64 inferior to the proximal head of the 5th metatarsal bone, at the junction of the red and white skin. Ellis (1991) locates BL 64 on the lateral side of the dorsum of the foot, proximal to the tuberosity of the 5th metatarsal bone, at the border of the red and white skin. Shanghai (1993) locates BL 64 on the lateral aspect of the foot, in the depression below the tuberosity of the 5th metatarsal bone, at the junction of the red and white skin.

Cheng (1987) locates B 64 below the tuberosity of the fifth metatarsal bone, at the junction of the red and white skin. Academy (1975) locates UB 64 below the tuberosity of the 5th metatarsal bone at the junction of the red and white skin.

Masayoshi (1975) locates BL 64 on the posterior outer side of the near end of the 5th metatarsas. Jayasuriya (1982) locates UB 64 in the depression inferior to the tuberosity of the 5th metatarsal bone, at the border of the two colours of the skin. Huang (1993) locates Bl 64 on the lateral aspect of the foot below the major bone in a depression on the border of the red and white flesh. Shandong (1982) locate Jinggu postero-inferior to the tuberosity of the 5th os metatarsale.

Bl 65 SHU GU – BONE BINDER

⊥ ***0.3 CUN*** **∆ *3 TO 5***

- WOOD
- SEDATION/Reducing/Dispersing
- CHILD
- SHU – STREAM/Shu – Transporting/Antique

Pos: Position of patient: supine.

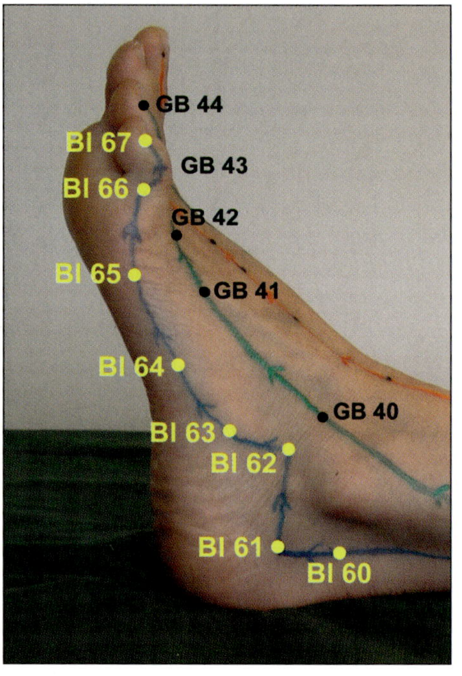

Loc:
a) On the lateral aspect of the foot.
b) Proximal and inferior to the flare of the head of the fifth metatarsal bone.
c) Proximal and inferior to the fifth metatarsophalangeal joint.
d) Traditionally at the junction of the change in skin colour.

Tip:
a) Look at the lateral aspect of the foot before you palpate for the point. Usually you can see a bony prominence at the base of the fifth digit which is the fifth metatarsophalangeal joint or the 'knuckle' of the fifth digit.
b) Palpate for the flare just proximal to the fifth metatarsophalangeal joint. The flare forms part of the head of the fifth metatarsal.
c) Palpation is important as Bl 65 may not be at the junction of the change in skin colour.
d) A common error when locating Bl 65 is locating it too high and the point is needled on the metatarsal bone. The point is always inferior to the bone.
e) Think of the lateral aspect of the foot as a filling to a sandwich and you are pressing the sandwich down to 'bulge' the filling out. The line of the Bladder channel flows towards the fifth digit on the widest or most prominent aspect of the bulge which may not be at the change in skin colour.
f) Palpate with the flow of the Bladder channel from the tuberosity of the fifth metatarsal bone along the widest aspect of the foot towards the metatarsophalangeal joint. You will feel a resistance where the joint begins to prominate. Palpate for Bl 65 just proximal and inferior to the joint.

Bl 66 ZU TONG GU – PENETRATING VALLEY

⊥ ***0.2 CUN*** Δ ***3 TO 5***

- WATER
- HORARY from 3 p.m. to 5 p.m.
- SEASONAL HORARY – Winter
- YING – SPRING/Shu – Transporting/Antique

Pos: Position of patient: supine.

Loc:
a) On the lateral aspect of the foot.
b) Just distal and inferior to the flare of the base of the fifth proximal phalanx.
c) Just distal and inferior to the fifth metatarsophalangeal joint.
d) Traditionally at the junction of the change in skin colour.

Tip:
a) Look at the lateral aspect of the foot before you palpate for the point. Usually you can see a bony prominence at the base of the fifth digit (little toe) which is the fifth metatarsophalangeal joint or the 'knuckle' of the fifth digit.
b) Palpate for the flare just distal and inferior to the fifth metatarsophalangeal joint. The flare forms part of the base of the fifth proximal phalanx.
c) The point is usually at the junction of the change in skin colour.
d) A common error when locating Bl 64 is locating it too high and the point is needled on the metatarsal bone. The point is always inferior to the bone. Bl 66 is just inferior to the metatarsophalangeal joint or just inferior to the flare of the base of the proximal phalanx of the fifth digit.
e) Palpate with the flow of the Bladder channel from the tuberosity of the fifth metatarsal bone along the widest aspect of the foot to the metatarsophalangeal joint. Run your finger distal to the joint until you are just distal to the flare. You should be able to palpate for the point just distal and inferior to the metatarsophalangeal joint or just distal and inferior to the base of the fifth proximal phalanx.
f) When you are palpating for Bl 66 think about the location of Bl 67 as the Bladder channel rises superiorly towards the lateral nail point of the fifth digit The channel begins to rise very slightly at Bl 66 as the channel flows towards the exit point of the Bladder channel (Bl 67).

Note: Eachou (1995) also locates as above, he also locates it in the lateral skin crease of the 5th toe. So (1985) locates BL 66 justdistal to the head of the 5th metatarsal bone in front of the joint, on the side of the foot, on top of the bone.

Bl 67 on the lateral aspect of the fifth digit.

Bl 67 ZHI YIN – EXTREMITY OF YIN

⊥ ***0.1 CUN*** ***Δ 3***
FORBIDDEN TO NEEDLE OR MOXA DURING PREGNANCY EXCEPTION BEING MOXA ROLL WHICH MAY BE USED TO TURN A BREECH BABY

- METAL
- EXIT
- TONIFICATION/Reinforcing
- MOTHER
- JING – WELL/Shu – Transporting/Antique
- RE-UNION/Crossing/Meeting Point of the Bladder Channel with the Kidney Channel – Foot Tai Yang Channel with the Foot Shao Yin Channel.

Pos: Position of patient: supine.

Loc: a) On the foot.
b) On the lateral aspect of the fifth digit (little toe).
c) The lateral nail point of the fifth digit.
d) Approximately 0.1 cun proximal to the corner of the nail.
e) Just distal to the flare of the distal phalanx.

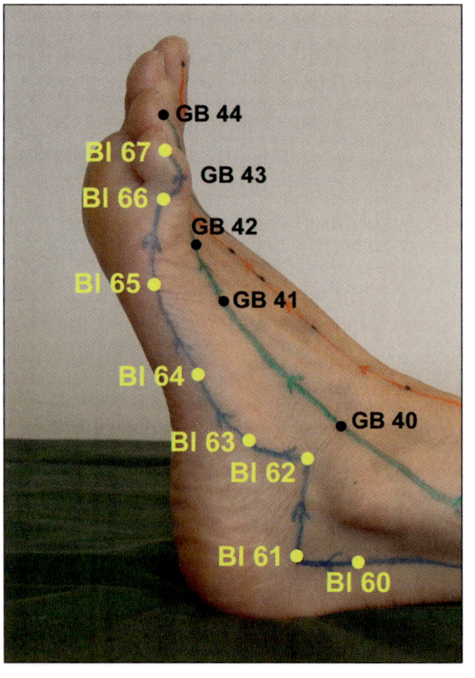

Tip: a) The point is level with the nail bed (where the nail attaches to the skin) rather than the cuticle.
b) Draw a horizontal line across the nail bed.
c) Draw a vertical line from the lateral border of the nail towards the nail bed.
d) The lines drawn from b) and c) (vertical and horizontal) form an intersection. This is approximately where the point is located.

Note: Ellis (1991) in a classical description locates BL 67 on the outer side of the small toe, the width of a Chinese leek leaf away from the corner of the nail (The Great Compendium). Huang (1993) locates Bl 67 at the lateral aspect of the small toe, the distance of a leek leaf from the corner of the nail.

REFERENCES FOR THE BLADDER CHANNEL

Wu, Wei-P'ing 1973 Chinese Acupuncture – BL 1: 85; BL 2: 85; BL 3: 85; BL 4: 85; BL 5: 86; BL 6: 86; BL 7: 86; BL 8: 86; BL 9: 86; BL 10: 86; Inner Bladder Line: 87/88/89/90/91; Outer Bladder Line: 92/93/94; BL 35: 91; Bl 37 (BL 51): 94; Bl 38 (BL 52): 95; Bl 39 (BL 53): 95; BL 55: 95; BL 56: 95; BL 57: 96; BL 58: 96; BL 59: 96; BL 60: 96; BL 61: 96; BL 62: 96; BL 63: 97; BL 64: 97;

Worsley, J R 1982 Traditional Chinese Acupuncture Volume 1 – Meridians and Points. III 1: 61; III 3: 61; III 4: 61; III 5: 61; III 6: 63; III 7: 63; III 8: 63; III 10: 63; Inner Bladder Line: 65/67/69/71/73; Outer Bladder Line: 12/75/77/79; III 35: 73; Thigh Measurement: 12; Bl 37 (III 51): 81; Bl 38 (III 52): 81; III 56: 83; III 57: 83; III 58: 83; III 59: 83; III 60: 85; III 61: 85; III 62: 85

Masayoshi Hyodo 1975 Ryodoraku Acupuncture – BL 1: 54; BL 3: 54; BL 4: 54; BL 5: 54; BL 6: 54; BL 7: 54; BL 8: 54; BL 37: 56; BL 62: 57; BL 63: 57; BL 64: 57

Voisin, Dr. H 1974 Essentials of Acupuncture – B 1: 52: B 3: 52; B 4: 52; B 5: 52; B 6: 52; B 7: 52; B 8: 52; B 9: 52; B 10: 52; Inner Bladder Line: 52; Outer Bladder Line: 54; B 11: 52; B 12: 52; B 13: 52; B 14: 52; B 15: 52; B 16: 52; B 17: 52; B 18: 52; B 19: 52; B 20: 52; B 21: 52; B 22: 52; B 23: 52; B 24: 52; B 25: 52; B 26: 52; B 27: 52; B 28: 52; B 29: 52; B 30: 52; B 31: 52; B 32: 52; B 33: 52; B 34: 52; B 35: 52; Bl 37 (B 51): 56; Bl 38 (B 52): 56; Bl 41 (B 36): 54; Bl 42: (B 37): 54; Bl 43 (B 38): 54; Bl 44 (B 39): 54; Bl 45 (B 40): 54; Bl 46 (B 41): 54; Bl 47 (B 42): 54; Bl 48 (B 43): 54; Bl 49 (B 44): 54; Bl 50 (B 45): 54; Bl 51 (B 46): 54; Bl 52 (B 47): 54; Bl 53 (B 48): 54; Bl 54 (B 49): 54; B 56: 56; B 57: 56; B 58: 56; B 59: 56; B 60: 56; B 61: 56; B 62: 56; B 63: 56; B 64: 56

Legge, David 1999 Acupuncture Points and Meridians – UB 1: 53; UB 10: 53; UB 11: 54; UB 12: 54; UB 13: 54; UB 14: 54; UB 15: 54; UB 16: 54; UB 17: 55; UB 18: 55; UB 19: 55; UB 20: 55; UB 21: 55; UB 22: 55; UB 23: 55; UB 24: 55; UB 25: 55; UB 26: 55; UB 27: 55; UB 28: 56; UB 41: 57; UB 42: 57; UB 43: 57; UB 44: 57; UB 45: 57; UB 46: 57; UB 47: 57; UB 48: 57; UB 49: 57; UB 50: 57; UB 51: 57; UB 52: 58; UB 53: 58; UB 54: 58; UB 61: 58; UB 62: 58; UB 63: 59; UB 64: 59

Eachou Chen 1995 Cross-sectional Anatomy of Acupoints – BL 1: 209; BL 3: 104; BL 9: 112; BL 10: 136; BL 27: 183; BL 28: 184; BL 30: 184; BL 39: 64; BL 41: 187; BL 42: 188; BL 43: 188; BL 44: 189; BL 45: 189; BL 46: 189; BL 47: 190; BL 48: 190; BL 49: 191; BL 50: 191; BL 64: 93; BL 66: 97

Academy of Traditional Chinese Medicine, The. 1975 – Outline of Chinese Acupuncture, An. UB 1: 138; UB 10: 142; UB 27: 146;; UB 64: 154

Soulié De Morant, George. 1994 Chinese Acupuncture – BL 1: 410; BL 2: 411; BL 3: 411; BL 4: 411/412; BL 5: 412; BL 6: 412; BL 7: 413; BL 8: 413; BL 9: 413; BL 10: 414; BL 11: 415; BL 12: 415; BL 13: 416; BL 14: 416; BL 15: 417; BL 16: 417; BL 17: 418; BL 18: 418; BL 19: 419; BL 20: 419; BL 21: 420; BL 22: 420; BL 23: 421; BL 24: 421; BL 25: 422; BL 26: 422; BL 27: 423; BL 28: 423; BL 29: 424; BL 30: 424; BL 35: 426; Thigh Measurements: 69; Bl 37 (BL 51): 432; Bl 38 (BL 52): 433; Bl 39 (BL 53): 433; Bl 40: (BL 54): 434; Bl 41(BL 36): 426; Bl 42 (BL 37): 427; Bl 43 (BL 38): 427; Bl 44 (BL 39): 428; Bl 45 (BL 40): 428; Bl 46 (BL 41): 429; Bl 47 (BL 42): 429; Bl 48 (BL 43): 429; Bl 49 (BL 44): 430; Bl 50 (BL 45): 430; Bl 51 (BL 46): 430; Bl 52 (BL 47): 431; Bl 53 (BL 48): 431; Bl 54 (BL 49): 432; BL 56: 435; BL 58: 436; BL 60: 437; BL 61: 437; BL 62: 438; BL 63: 439; BL 64: 439

Lavier, Dr. J 1974 Points of Chinese Acupuncture – BL 3: 79; BL 4: 79; BL 5: 81; BL 7: 81; BL 8: 83; BL 9: 83; BL 10: 83; Inner/Outer Bladder Line: 58; BL 35: 61; Thigh Measurements: 27; Bl 37 (BL 51): 27; Bl 38 (BL 52): 27; BL 56: 35; BL 57: 35; BL 58: 35; BL 63: 45; BL 64: 45

So, James Tin Yau (Dr) 1985 The Book of Acupuncture Points: BL 4: 236; BL 5: 236; BL 7: 237; BL 8: 238; BL 9: 238; BL 10: 18; BL 27: 89; BL 28: 90; BL 29: 240; BL 30: 90; BL 31: 91; BL 32: 91; BL 33: 92; BL 34: 92; Thigh Measurements: 1; Bl 37 (BL 51): 244; Bl 38 (BL 52): 245; BL 58: 246; BL 60: 158; BL 61: 247; BL 62: 158; BL 63: 159; BL 64: 248; BL 66: 249

Shanghai College of Traditional Chinese Medicine. 1993 Applied Anatomical Charts of Acupuncture and Moxibustion – BL 6: 70; BL 7: 70; BL 10: 72; BL 27: 80; BL 28: 80; BL 29: 82; BL 30: 82; BL 62: 98; BL 63: 98; BL 64: 98/100;

Shanghai College of Traditional Medicine 1981 Acupuncture – A Comprehensive Text – B 7: 143; Thigh Measurements: 125; Bl 37 (B 51): 265; Bl 38 (B 52): 318; Bl 39 (B 53): 279; B 59: 318;

Deadman, Peter; Al-Khafaji, Mazin; Baker, Kevin 1998 Manual of Acupuncture, An – BL 9: 262; BL 10: 263; BL 62: 320

Qiu Mao-Liang 1996 – Chinese Acupuncture and Moxibustion – UB 9: 104; UB 10: 104; UB 27: 108; UB 28: 108; UB 29: 108; UB 30: 108; UB 63: 114; UB 64: 114

Shandong Medical College and Shandong College of Traditional Chinese Medicine 1982 Anatomical Atlas of Chinese Acupuncture Points – Yuzhen (Bl 9): 32; Xiaochangshu (Bl 27): 34; Pangguanshu (Bl 28): 34; Baihuanshu (Bl 30): 34; Shangliao (Bl 31): 34; Ciliao (Bl 32): 34; Zongliao (Bl 33): 34; Xialiao (Bl 34): 34; Fuxi (Bl 38): 34; Weiyang (Bl 39): 34; Weizhong (Bl 40): 34; Baohuang (Bl 53): 35; Zhibian (Bl 54): 35; Feiyang (Bl 58): 36; Fuyang (Bl 59): 36; Pushen (Bl 61): 36; Shenmai (Bl 62): 36; Jinmen (Bl 63): 36; Jinggu (Bl 64): 36

Jayasuriya, Anton 1982 Clinical Acupuncture – UB 10: 395; UB 64: 398

Lotan, Alon 2000 Acupoint Location Guide – UB 10: 79; UB 62: 97; UB 63: 99

Li Ding (Prof.). 1991. Acupuncture, Meridian Theory and Acupuncture Points – UB 10: 248

Lawson – Wood 1973 Acupuncture Handbook – III 27: 56; III 28: 57; III 58: 50; III 64: 42

Ellis, Wiseman and Boss. 1991 Fundamentals of Chinese Acupuncture – BL 28: 213; BL 63: 233; BL 64: 233; BL 67: 236

Gray, H; Warwick, Roger; Williams, Peter L 1978 Gray's Anatomy 35th Edition. C7/T1: 236; Ilium: 344/345; Sacrum: 242/243; Coccyx: 244/245

Yang Jiasan (Prof) 1982 The Way to Locate Acu-Points – UB 61: 42

Yoshiaki Omura. 1982 Acupuncture Medicine – Numbering of Bladder points: Various Page Numbers

Cheng Xinnong (Editor) 1987 Chinese Acupuncture and Moxibustion – B 63: 180; B 64: 180

Huang-fu Mi. Trans: Yang Shou-zhong and Charles Chace 1993 The Systematic Classic of Acupuncture & Moxibustion – Bl 64: 195; Bl 67: 195

THE KIDNEY CHANNEL OF THE FOOT (SHAO YIN)

Primary Channel

The Kidney channel begins on the plantar surface of the fifth digit, goes towards the sole, and emerges at Ki 1. It travels along the medial aspect of the foot from the inferior border of the navicular bone, goes to the medial malleolus, and then travels upwards to the medial aspect of the knee, linking with Sp 6 between Ki 8 and Ki 9. From Ki 10 at the medial aspect of the flexure of the knee the channel travels superficially as far as the groin.

Here it passes deep to join with Du 1 at the tip of the coccyx, travels up the spinal column to Du 4, then passes forward to Ren 4, down to Ren 3 and emerges again at Ki 11. The channel travels through the lower jiao, (from Ki 16 entering the kidney and connecting with the bladder), and middle and upper jiao to end at Ki 27 inferior to the clavicle. (Some texts say there is a link with the kidney and bladder direct from Du 1.)

A deep channel from the kidney rises up through the abdomen, passing through the liver, diaphragm and lungs, and up through the trachea and larynx to finish at the root of the tongue. Another short branch travels from Ki 25 to the lungs and the heart, and on to Ren 17 where it joins the Pericardium channel and disperses in the chest.

Divergent Channel

After separating from the primary channel in the popliteal fossa, the divergent channel intersects the divergent channel of the Bladder on the thigh, then proceeds upwards and connects with the kidney before crossing the Dai Mai at about the level of the 7th thoracic vertebra. From here it ascends to the base of the tongue and continues up to emerge at the nape of the neck, joining the Bladder primary channel.

Connecting Channel

After leaving the primary channel at Ki 4 on the medial aspect of the ankle, it crosses the heel and connects with the Bladder channel. A branch follows the Kidney channel upwards to a point inferior to the pericardium, then passes into the lumbar vertebrae.

Muscle Channel

This originates beneath the fifth digit, and together with the Spleen muscle channel crosses inferior to the medial malleolus and binds at the heel, where it joins the Bladder muscle channel. It then passes up the leg, binding at the inferomedial aspect of the knee, joins with the Spleen muscle channel, and travels up the medial aspect of the thigh to bind at the genital region. A branch ascends the side of the spine to the nape of the neck, binding with the occiput and linking up with the Bladder muscle channel.

THE KIDNEY CHANNEL OF THE FOOT

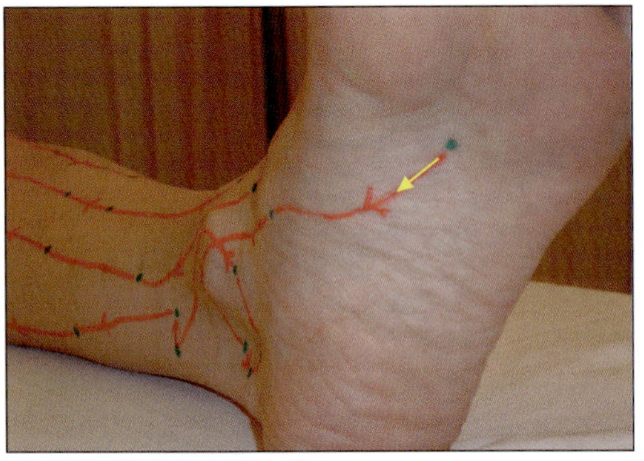

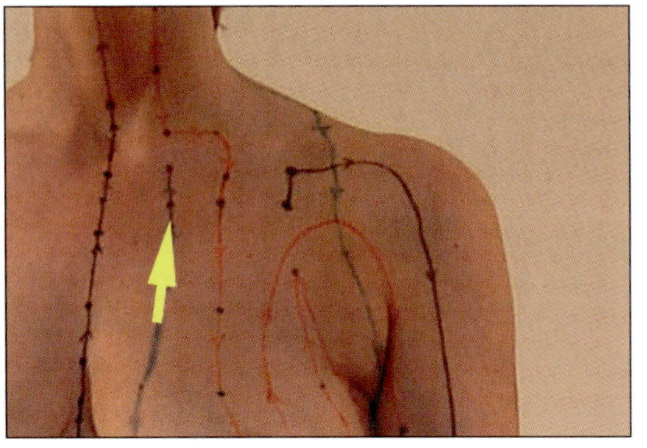

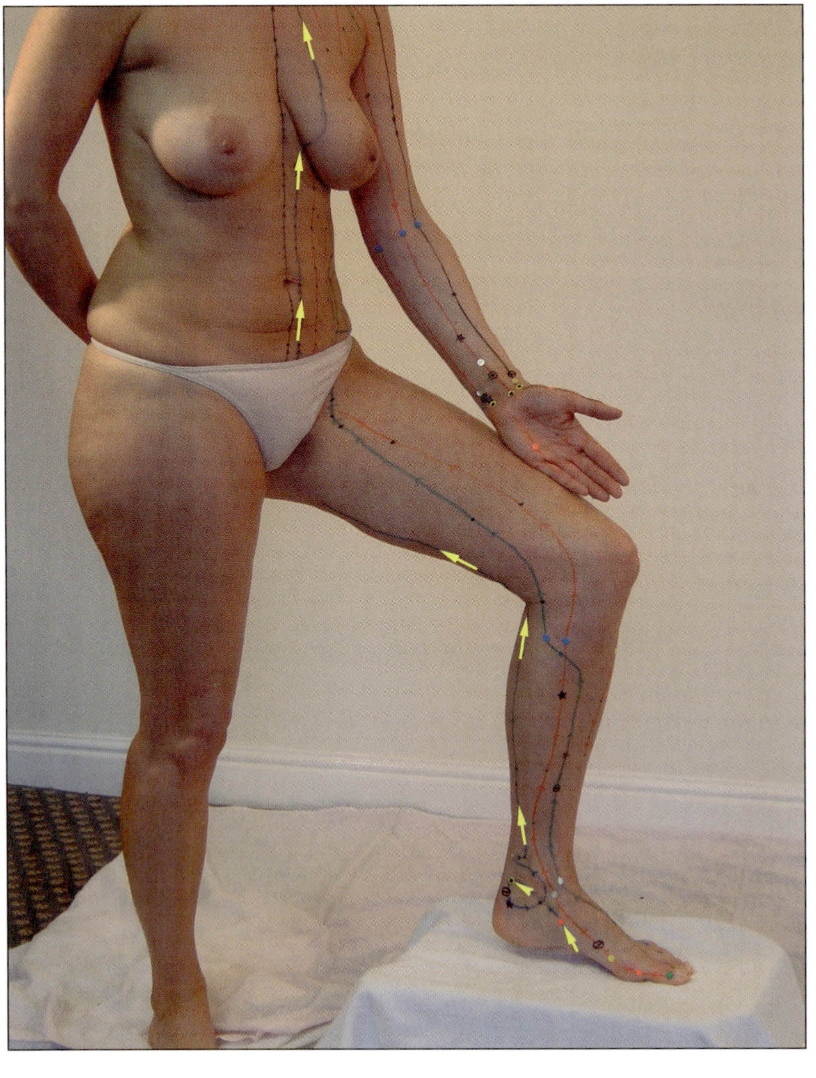

Points of the Kidney Channel – Foot Shao Yin (Ki/KI/K/KID/IV)

Ki 1 is on the sole of the foot, Ki 2 on the medial aspect of the foot, Ki 3-6 at the medial aspect of the ankle.

Ki 1 YONG QUAN – BUBBLING SPRING

⊥ ***0.3 TO 0.5 CUN*** Δ ***3 TO 7***

- WOOD
- ENTRY
- SEDATION/Reducing/Dispersing
- CHILD
- JING – WELL/Shu – Transporting/Antique
- RE-UNION/Crossing/Meeting Point of the Kidney Channel with the Bladder Channel – Foot Shao Yin Channel with the Foot Tai Yang Channel.

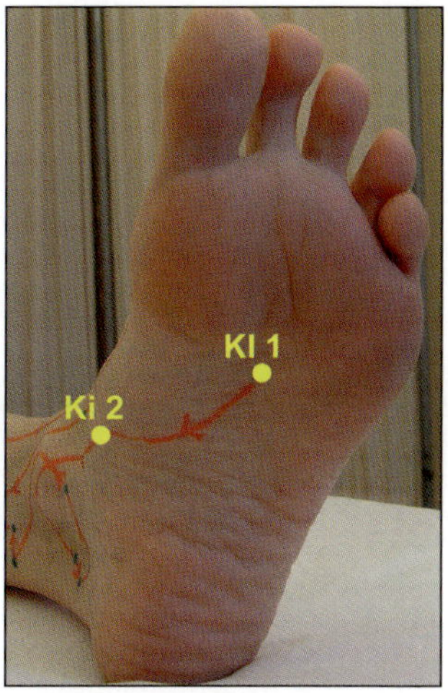

Pos: Position of patient: supine.

Loc:
a) On the foot.
b) On the plantar surface or the sole of the foot.
c) In between the second and third metatarsal bones.
d) Proximal to the heads of the second and third metatarsal bones.
e) Distal to the bases of the second and third metatarsal bones.
f) Approximately one third the distance from the base of the second proximal phalanges (base of toe) to the posterior aspect of the heel.
g) Approximately at the anterior one third and posterior two thirds of the plantar surface of the foot.
h) Traditionally in the depression formed when the foot is plantar flexed.

Tip:
a) The plantar surface of the foot has two main points of contact with the ground which are the heel and the head of the five metatarsals. The majority of people will have a natural arch between these two areas on the medial side of the foot.
b) Gently press the area of the heads of the second and third metatarsals (nearest the toes). If in the correct area the second and third digits should move, if not you may be between the first and second or third and fourth metatarsals.
c) To measure the anterior one third and posterior two thirds of the plantar surface of the foot draw a horizontal line across the base of the second phalanx (where it joins the main body of the foot) and visualise the posterior edge of the heel.
d) Divide the foot in to three from the horizontal line to the posterior edge of the heel. The point is located approximately at the anterior one third of the foot just proximal to the metatarsophalangeal joint on the plantar surface of the foot, just on the arch of the foot.
e) Plantar flex the foot (a claw shape) to form a depression or stand back and visualise the area. The point is slightly more proximal to the edge of the metatarsophalangeal joint towards the heel.
f) The location can vary in people, therefore palpation will ensure accuracy as the description does not indicate how close the point is to the base or head of the second and third metatarsal.

Note: Voisin (1974) locates K 1 on the sole of the foot, in the centre of the hollow formed upon flexing the toes. Wu (1973) locates KI 1 upon the sole of the foot within the crease formed when the toes are flexed. Worsley (1982) locates IV 1 on the plantar surface of the foot, between the second and third metatarsal bones, in the crease formed when the toes are flexed.

Soulié (1994) locates KI 1on the sole of the foot: about one-third lateral, approximately mid-length: at the level of and at two FW (Finger Width) medial to the anterior edge of the lateral eminence of the foot (tubercle of the fifth metatarsal); in the angle between the medial edge of the abductor digiti minimi and the anterior edge of a transverse mass; in a hollow. Slightly lateral to the flexor digitorum brevis muscle.; two FW lateral and in front of KI 2 Yang (1982) locates K 1 on the sole, in the depression which is at the junction of the anterior and middle third of the sole.

Huang (1993) locates Ki 1 in the centre of the sole where a hole appears when the foot is arched and the toes bent downwards. Li (1991) locates K 1 in the depression appearing on the sole when the foot is in plantar flexion. Legge (1999) locates Ki 1 in the deepest depression on the sole of the foot, where the longitudinal and transverse arches of the foot intersect. Approximately two thirds the distance between the heel and the base of the second toe.

So (1985) locates KI 1 on the distal half of the sole of the foot where the midline of the sole intersects a line level to the bottom edge of the big toe metatarsophalangeal joint. Or, you can find the point by pressing with the fingernail down the midline of the sole of the foot, from the top of the foot. The first depression is the point. Lawson-Wood (1973) locates IV 1 on the sole of the foot, between the two pads at the base of the first and other toes. Masayoshi (1975) locates KI 1 at the depression slightly forward from the centre of the sole of the foot.

Ki 2 RAN GU – BLAZING VALLEY

⊥ ***0.3 TO 0.5 CUN*** Δ ***3 TO 5***

- FIRE
- YING – SPRING/Shu – Transporting/Antique

Pos: Position of patient: supine.

Loc:
a) On the foot.
b) On the medial aspect of the foot.
c) Just inferior to the tuberosity of the navicular bone.
d) Traditionally at the junction of the change in skin colour.

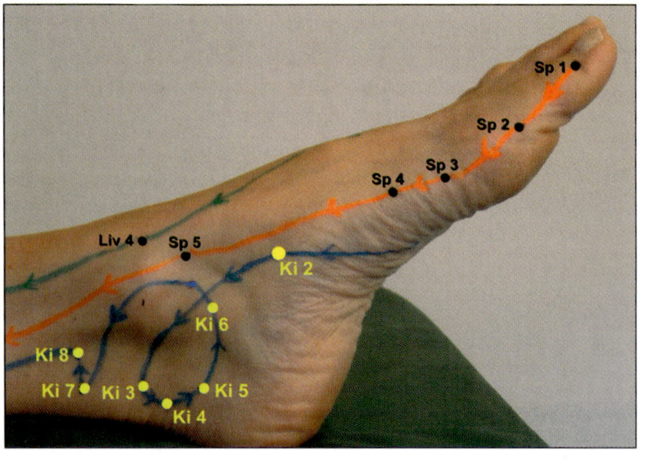

Tip: a) To locate the navicular bone, place the pad of your finger on Ki 1 (see seperate description) or the highest point of the arch of the foot. Follow the Kidney channel as it flows towards the navicular bone.

b) Imagine water being poured on to the plantar surface of the foot, the water will flow medially towards the navicular bone. A common error when locating Ki 2 is to locate the medial cuneiform bone which is distal to the navicular bone.

c) Although the traditional description states this point is at the junction of the change in skin colour, this can often be innacurate as the junction can vary considerably.

d) Palpation is important as this point is usually located just inferior to the tuberosity of the navicular bone. It can often be located just inferior and slightly distal to the tuberosity.

Wu (1973) locates KI 2 upon the internal side of the foot, one and one-half pouce before the internal malleus, below the navicular eminence. Voisin (1974) locates K 2 on the medial aspect of the foot, 2 fb (finger breadth) in front and below the medial malleolus, just below the navicular tuberosity. Masayoshi (1975) locates KI 2 at the inner side of the centre of the sole at the lower end of the joint of the first cuneiform and navicular bone. Deadman (1998) locates KID 2 on the medial side of the foot, distal and inferior to the medial malleolus, in the depression distal and inferior to the navicular tuberosity.

Eachou (1995) locates KI 2 anterior to the medial malleolus, anterior and inferior to the tuberosity of the navicular bone, approximately 1 inch posterior to SP 4. Shanghai (1993) locates KI 2 on the medial aspect of the foot, anterior and inferior to the medial malleolus, in the depression anterior and inferior to the tuberosity of the navicular bone. Yang (1982) locates K 2 in the depression on anterior and inferior to the tuberosity of the navicular bone.

Soulié (1994) locates KI 2 on the sole of the foot; one-fourth of the width; one large FW (Finger Width) in front of the heel bone (calcaneus); in the angle between the anterior edge of a transverse mass and the lateral edge of the muscle forming the medial edge (abductor, and deeper, the flexor of the great toe); in a hollow; on the medial edge of the flexor digitorum brevis muscle; three FW in front of and lateral to KI 6; two FW posterior and medial to KI 1. At the level of and lateral to SP 5 and the scaphoid eminence. Academy (1975) locates K 2 anterior and inferior to the medial malleolus, in a depression at the anterior and inferior border of the navicular bone.

To locate KI 3-6, the foot should be fully dorsiflexed, and held in this position to needle by the practitioner (so the patient's foot can be relaxed).

Ki 3 TAI XI – GREATER MOUNTAIN STREAM

⊥ ***0.3 TO 0.5 CUN*** **Δ *3 TO 5***

- SOURCE/Yuan/Regulator/Primary
- EARTH
- SHU – STREAM/Shu – Transporting/Antique
- HOST/GUEST COMBINATION – Source Point with the Junction Point of its Paired Official/Organ Therefore Ki 3 is combined with Bl 58

Pos: Position of patient: supine or seated.

Loc: a) On the ankle.
b) On the medial aspect of the ankle.
c) Level with the prominence of the medial malleolus of the tibia.
d) In a groove midway between the borders of the medial malleolus and the tendocalcaneus (achilles tendon)

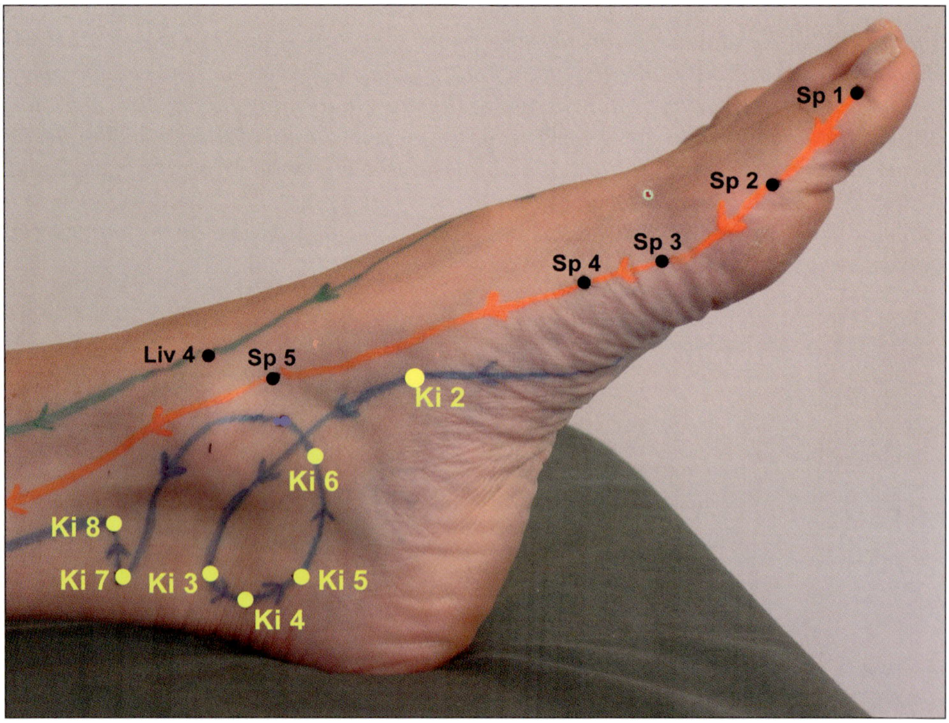

Tip:
a) The easiest way of marking and hence needling this point is to have the patients' foot at the end of the couch so they can rest it against your body.
b) To accurately locate the prominence of the medial malleolus, stand at the opposite side of the patient, i.e. stand on the left side for the prominence of the right medial malleolus and vice versa. Look directly over the anterior surface of the leg for the contour of the medial malleolus. From the prominence of the medial malleolus draw a line towards the tendo-calcaneus. Palpate for the prominence if it is not visible due to localised swelling.
c) Place the flat of your finger in the groove between the prominence of the medial malleolus and the tendocalcaneus and palpate for the point on the drawn line. The point is located in the deepest part of the groove, not necessarily halfway between the malleolus and the tendocalcaneus.
d) The groove may not be apparent if the person has swollen ankles but the point is often easier to palpate.
e) The point is easier to locate and needle with the patient supine rather than seated.
f) If the patient is in a supine position, the proximity of the couch to the tendocalcaneus can make this point difficult to locate. Therefore ask the patient to rotate their leg slightly outwards, so you can reach the area for accurate point location. You will also need to needle the point in this position.

Note: Worsley (1982) locates IV 3 on the medial surface of the leg. 1 ACI (Anatomical Chinese Inch) proximal to the prominence of the medial malleolus, upon the posterior tibial artery. (He Locates IV 4 (Ki 4) where we locate Ki 3). Wu (1973) locates KI 3 upon the internal side of the foot, at one-half pouce behind the internal malleus, above the superior edge of the calcaneum upon the tibial posterior artery.

Lavier (1974) in an illustration locates KI 3 level with the inferior border of the medial malleolus, in a groove between the posterior border of the medial malleolus and the anterior border of the achilles tendon. Voisin (1974) numbers Ki 3 as K 5 and locates the point on the medial aspect of the foot: 1 fb (finger breadth) behind the medial malleolus. slightly above the calcaneum. Voisin modified the pathway of the Kidney meridian between K 3 and K 7, in accordance with observations made by Dr. Ferreyrolles. The numbers of the points differ from those of most authors,

Soulié (1994) also numbers Ki 3 as KI 5 and locates this on top of the medial side of the heel, in the angle between the posterior edge of the medial malleolus and the tendons running along it (flexor communis, then in front of the flexor proper, then the tibialis posterior); in a hollow. In front of the anterior peroneal arteries, veins and nerves; Two FW (Finger Width) above KI 5 and two small FW below KI 4.

Lawson-Wood (1973) locates IV 3 on the internal aspect of the foot, 1cm below and behind the internal malleolus. Masayoshi (1975) locates KI 3 on the rear side of the medial malleolus of the foot: in the pulse region of the posterior femoral artery.

Ki 4 DA ZHONG – GREAT BELL

⊥ ***0.2 TO 0.3 CUN*** ∆ ***3 TO 7***

- JUNCTION/Luo/Connecting/Passage/Lo/Lê
- RE-UNION/Crossing/Meeting Point of the Kidney Channel with the Bladder Channel – Foot Shao Yin Channel with the Foot Tai Yang Channel.
- HOST/GUEST COMBINATION – Source Point with the Junction Point of its Paired Official/Organ (Therefore Ki 4 is combined with Bl 64)

Pos: Position of patient: supine or seated.

Loc: a) On the ankle.
b) On the medial aspect of the ankle.
c) Level with the inferior border of the medial malleolus of the tibia.
d) Immediately anterior to the anterior border of the tendocalcaneus (achilles tendon)
e) Halfway between Ki 3 and Ki 5.
f) 0.5 cun inferior and slightly posterior to Ki 3.

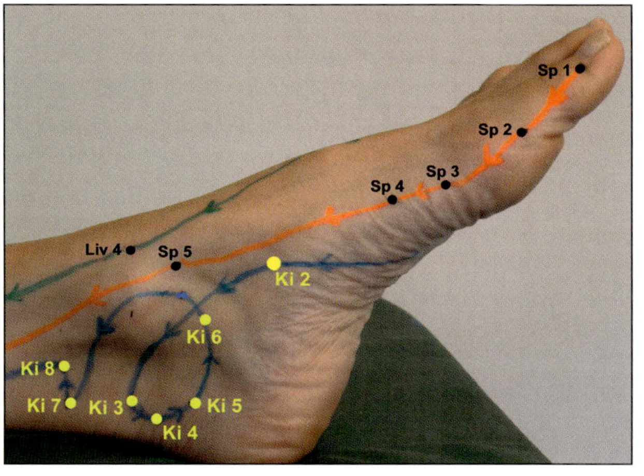

Tip: a) The easiest way of marking and hence needling this point is to have the patients' foot at the end of the couch so they can rest it against your body.
b) Locating Ki 4 may be difficult with the patient in the supine position as the tendo-calcaneus rests on the couch and may be partially occluded. Ask the patient to rotate their leg outwards slightly to enable palpation and accurate point location and needling.
c) To accurately locate the prominence of the medial malleolus, stand at the opposite side of the patient, i.e. stand on the left side for the prominence of the right medial malleolus and vice versa. Look directly over the anterior surface of the leg for the contour of the medial malleolus. From the prominence of the medial malleolus draw a line towards the tendo-calcaneus.
d) The groove may not be apparent if the person has swollen ankles but the point is often easier to palpate.
e) Place the flat of your finger in the groove between the prominence of the medial malleolus and the tendocalcaneus and palpate for the point on the drawn line. Ki 3 is located in the deepest part of the groove, not necessarily halfway between the malleolus and the tendocalcaneus.
f) Locate the inferior border of the medial malleolus and draw a straight line posteriorly towards the tendocalcaneus.

g) Place the flat of your finger in the groove between the medial malleolus and the tendocalcaneus and then palpate for the point on the line you have just drawn at the inferior border of the medial malleolus. The point is located anterior to the anterior border of the tendocalcaneus, therefore it is slightly more posterior than Ki 3 and is tight up against the tendon, still in the groove, but not in the deepest part.
h) The point is easier to locate and needle with the patient supine rather than seated.
i) If the patient is in a supine position, the proximity of the couch to the tendocalcaneus can make this point difficult to locate. Therefore ask the patient to rotate their leg slightly outwards, so you can reach the area for accurate point location. You will also need to needle the point in this position.
j) There should be no need for you to mark out 0.5 cun as the landmark for this is the inferior border of the medial malleolus. If you cannot feel the inferior border of the medial malleolus, try palpating the deepest part of the groove towards the heel with the flat of your finger. Eventually you should feel a depression where the achilles tendon inserts in to the calcaneus. which is 1 cun inferior to Ki 3 (at Ki 5) in the deepest part of the groove. The point lies halfway between Ki 3 and Ki 5, but slightly more posterior than both these points.
k) Although the position of the patient can be supine or seated, it is easier to locate with the patient supine as you are not having to bend down to the ground to locate and needle this.

Note: There are texts that locate this point level with the prominence of the medial malleolus in the deepest part of the groove where Ki 3 is located. Worsley (1982) locates IV 4 (our Ki 3) on the medial surface of the ankle, posterior to the prominence of the medial malleolus, upon the posterior tibial artery, 1 ACI (Anatomical Chinese Inch) distal to IV 3.

Soulié (1994) numbers Ki 4 as KI 6. He locates this on the medial side of the ankle; in the angle between the upper edge of the medial malleolus and the tibia; in the angle between the edge of the tendon that runs along the malleolus (tibialis posterior muscle) and the superior edge of a ligament at an angle (achillo-malleolar); on the flexor communis and the edge of the flexor pollicis longus between the tibialis posterior and the Achilles tendon; in a hollow; two small FW (Finger Width) above KI 3 and two large FW below KI 7. Voisin (1974) numbers Ki 4 as K 6 and locates the point on the medial aspect of the foot: 1.5 fb (finger breadth) behind the medial malleolus. on the upper border of the calcaneum.

Voisin modified the pathway of the Kidney meridian between K 3 and K 7, in accordance with observations made by Dr. Ferreyrolles. The numbers of the points differ from those of most authors. Lawson-Wood (1973) locates IV 4 at 1cm behind the internal malleolus at the horizontal level of the most prominent part of the malleolus.

Wu (1973) locates KI 4 upon the internal side of the foot, at one-half pouce below KI 3, between the tendons. Lavier (1974) in an illustration locates KI 4 directly inferior to KI 3 and directly superior to Ki 5, in a groove approximately at the attachment of the achilles tendon to the calcaneus. Shandong (1982) locate Dazhong inferior and posterior to the medial malleolus, in the depression medial to the insertion of the achilles tendon.

Ki 5 HUI QUAN – WATER SPRING

⊥ ***0.3 TO 0.5 CUN*** Δ 5

- ACCUMULATION/Xi Cleft/Gueki Point

Pos: Position of patient: supine or seated.

Loc:
a) On the ankle.
b) On the medial aspect of the ankle.
c) Anterior and superior to the tuberosity of the medial side of the calcaneus.
d) Where the tendocalcaneus (achilles tendon) inserts into the calcaneus
e) 1 cun directly inferior to Ki 3.

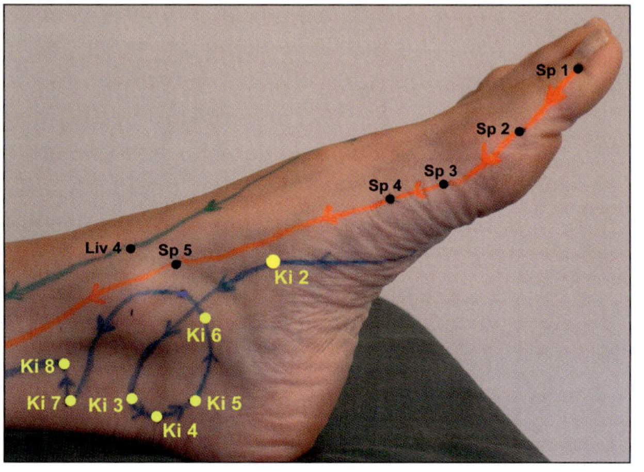

Tip:
a) The easiest way of marking and hence needling this point is to have the patients' foot at the end of the couch so they can rest it against your body.
b) Locating Ki 5 may be difficult with the patient in the supine position as the tendo-calcaneus rests on the couch and may be partially occluded. Ask the patient to rotate their leg outwards slightly to enable palpation and accurate point location and needling.
c) To accurately locate the prominence of the medial malleolus, stand at the opposite side of the patient, i.e. stand on the left side for the prominence of the right medial malleolus and vice versa. Look directly over the anterior surface of the leg for the contour of the medial malleolus. From the prominence of the medial malleolus draw a line towards the tendo-calcaneus.
d) The groove may not be apparent if the person has swollen ankles but the point is often easier to palpate.
e) Place the flat of your finger in the groove between the prominence of the medial malleolus and the tendocalcaneus and palpate for the point on the drawn line. Ki 3 is located in the deepest part of the groove, not necessarily halfway between the malleolus and the tendocalcaneus.
f) Ki 5 is located in a depression on or just superior to the border of the calcaneus.
g) If you are unable to locate the point, locate the inferior border of the medial malleolus which is 0.5 cun inferior to the prominence of the medial malleolus. Double this measurement to add another 0.5 cun from the inferior border of the medial malleolus (1 cun). Palpate for Ki 5 in this area.
h) Draw a mark at the 1 cun measurement directly inferior to Ki 3 and palpate from the posterior border of the calcaneus until your finger goes over the tuberosity of the calcaneus and then palpate for the point.
i) The Kidney channel from Ki 3 to Ki 5 seems to be a semi circle with Ki 4 located slightly posterior to Ki 3 and Ki 5.

j) The point is easier to locate and needle with the patient supine rather than seated.
k) If the patient is in a supine position, the proximity of the couch to the tendocalcaneus can make this point difficult to locate. Therefore ask the patient to rotate their leg slightly outwards, so you can reach the area for accurate point location. You will also need to needle the point in this position.
l) Although the position of the patient can be supine or seated, it is easier to locate with the patient supine as you are not having to bend down to the ground to locate and needle this point.

Note: Voisin (1974) locates K 4 (our Ki 5) on the medial aspect of the foot: calcaneum, 1 fb (finger breadth) below Kidney 6 (Ki 3). Voisin modified the pathway of the Kidney meridian between K 3 and K 7, in accordance with observations made by Dr. Ferreyrolles. The numbers of the points differ from those of most authors.

Soulié (1994) locates KI 4 (our Ki 5) on the heel, medial face: one large FW (Finger Width) below and slightly behind the medial malleolus; in the angle between the inferior edge of the transverse superior edge of the calcaneus and the posterior edge of the vertical tendons (flexor communis, then flexor pollicis longus, then tibialis posterior); in a hollow; One FW posterior to KI 3 (Ki 6) and two FW under KI 5 (Ki 3).

Worsley (1982) locates IV 5 on the medial surface of the ankle, 1 ACI (Anatomical Chinese Inch) distal to IV 4 (our Ki 3), on the superior edge of the calcaneus. Lavier (1974) in an illustration locates KI 5 directly inferior to KI 4 on the calcaneus. Wu (1973) locates KI 5 upon the internal side of the foot, at one pouce below Ki 3.

Ki 6 ZHAO HAI – ILLUMINATED SEA

⊥ ***0.3 TO 0.5 CUN*** ***Δ 3 TO 5***

- 8 EXTRAORDINARY VESSEL/Coalescent Point of Yin Heel/Yin Motility Vessel (Yin Qiao Mai)
- 8 EXTRAORDINARY CHANNELS CONFLUENT/8 Extraordinary Meridians Confluent/8 Extraordinary Vessels Opening/Master Point of the Yin Heel/Yin Motility Vessel (Yin Qiao Mai)
- 8 EXTRAORDINARY VESSEL/Coupled Point of the Ren Mai (Conception/Directing Vessel)

Pos: Position of patient: supine or seated.

Loc: a) On the foot.
b) On the medial aspect of the foot.
c) Approximately 1 cun inferior to the prominence of the medial malleolus.
d) Approximately 0.4 cun inferior to the inferior border of the medial malleolus.
e) On the superior border of the sustentaculum tali of the calcaneus.
f) Immediately inferior to the talus bone.
g) Between the tendons of the tibialis posterior and flexor digitorum longus (see tip f).

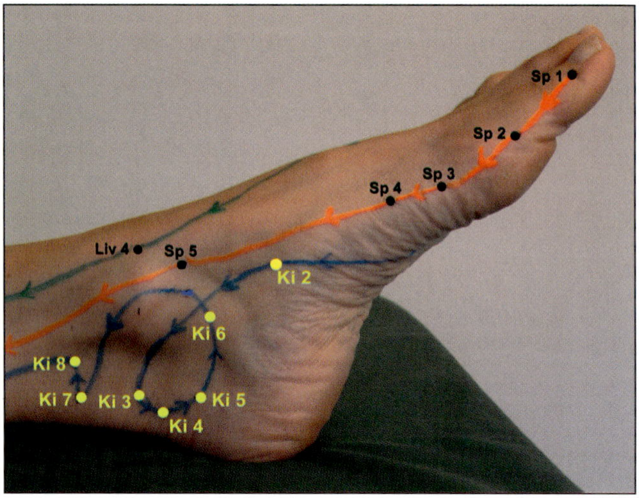

Tip:

a) The easiest way of marking and hence needling this point is to have the patients' foot at the end of the couch so they can rest it against your body.

b) To accurately locate the prominence of the medial malleolus, stand at the opposite side of the patient, i.e. stand on the left side for the prominence of the right medial malleolus and vice versa. Look directly over the anterior surface of the leg for the contour of the medial malleolus.

c) Place your thumb on the posterior border and the middle finger on the anterior border of the medial malleolus. Place your index finger on the prominence of the medial malleolus which is half way between the two borders. If the medial malleolus is flat this method is particularly useful in locating Ki 6 which is inferior to the medial malleolus.

d) Run your index finger down from the prominence of the medial malleolus towards the sustentaculum tali. This may feel like a "shelf-like" prominence directly inferior to the inferior border of the medial malleolus. The sustentaculum tali is a piece of bone that protrudes from the calcaneus bone. (The talus bone is deeper lying and cannot usually be palpated.)

e) If you cannot feel the sustentaculum tali this may be due to oedema or a small sustentaculum tali. If so mark 1 cun inferior to the prominence of the medial malleolus or 0.4 cun inferior to the inferior border of the medial malleolus.

f) Locate the inferior border of the medial malleolus which is 0.5 cun inferior to the prominence of the medial malleolus. Double this measurement to add another 0.5 cun from the inferior border of the medial malleolus (1 cun). Palpate for Ki 6 in this area.

g) Once you have the cun measurement inferior to the medial malleolus, draw in a mark at the cun measurment, and palpate from the prominenence of the medial malleolus towards the mark. The point may or may not be at 1 cun or 0.4 cun as palpation will give you ultimate accuracy.

h) Ki 6 is usually located between the tendons of the tibialis posterior and flexor digitorum longus however the sustentaculum tali always takes precedence. If they can be palpated, the tibialis posterior tendon is the closest to the medial malleolus.

i) It is easier to locate with the patient supine as you do not have to bend down to locate and needle the point. It is important to locate and needle the point with the patient's foot in the same position.

Note: Voisin (1974) locates K 3 (our Ki 6) on the medial aspect of the foot: 1 fb (finger breadth) below the summit of the medial malleolus. Voisin modified the pathway of the Kidney meridian between K 3 and K 7, in accordance with observations made by Dr. Ferreyrolles. The numbers of the points differ from those of most authors. Soulié (1994) locates KI 3 (our Ki 6) on the foot, medial face: just under the medial malleolus; in the angle between the inferior edge of the calcaneus and the posterior edge of the tendons of the flexor digitorum and flexor pollicis longus muscle; in a hollow; slightly above the plantar cushion; three FW (Finger Width) above KI 2 and one FW below KI 4 (our Ki 5).

Wu (1973) locates KI 6 upon the internal side of the leg, at four fen below the internal malleus, between two tendons, and above the bony prominence. So (1985) locates KI 6 1/3 division below the medial malleolus, anterior to the big tendon, or between the two tendons. Worsley (1982) locates IV 6 on the medial surface of the ankle, 4 fen distal to the inferior border of the medial malleolus. Eachou (1995) locates KI 6 in the fossa below the medial malleolus of the tibia, between the medial malleolus and the talus. Qiu (1996) locates K 6 in the depression at the lower border of the medial malleolus. Masayoshi (1975) locates KI 6 on the lower part of the medial malleolus of the foot at the depression on the rough surface of the calcaneus.

Cun Measurements of the Medial Aspect of the Leg

The distance from the prominence of the medial malleolus to the popliteal crease on the medial side of the knee flexure is measured as 15 cun. This must be measured with the patient in a supine position with the leg flat. This method may seem more user friendly than using the 13 cun measurement as it should be easier to divide the 15 cun measurement in to 3 sections of 5 and then to divide the 5 in to 1 cun measurements.

The distance from the prominence of the medial malleolus to the inferior border of the medial condyle of the tibia bone (Sp 9) is measured as 13 cun. This must be measured with the patient in a seated position with the knee bent at 90 degrees. The difficulty of measuring 13 cun is not just dividing 13 cun in to equal 1 cun measurements but to accurately mark the inferior border of the medial condyle of the tibia where Sp 9 is located can be difficult.

Note: There are approximately 2 cun between the inferior border of the medial condyle of the tibia and the popliteal crease on the medial flexure of the knee, If you were to measure 13 cun in the supine position and measure 2 cun to the popliteal crease of the medial flexure of the knee, the 2 cun measurement would seem greater compared when locating the cun measurments in the seated position.

Ki 7-9 are on the medial aspect of the lower leg, Ki 10 at the medial extremity of the knee flexure.

Ki 7 FU LIU – RETURNING CURRENT

⊥ ***0.3 TO 0.5 CUN*** Δ ***3 TO 7***

- METAL
- TONIFICATION/Reinforcing
- MOTHER
- JING – RIVER/Shu – Transporting/Antique

Pos: Position of patient: supine (at 15 cun), or in a seated position with the leg bent at 90 degrees (at 13 cun).

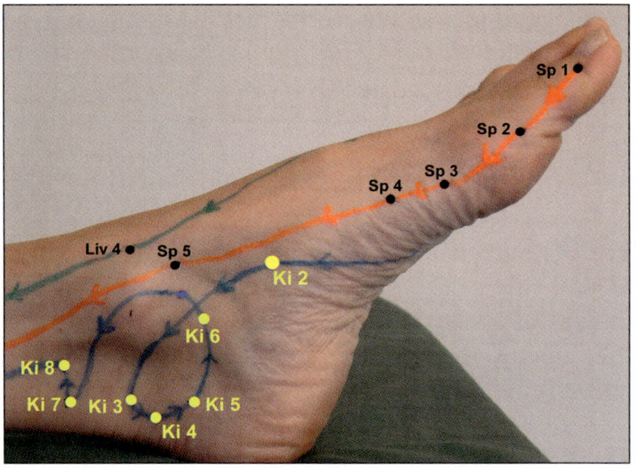

Loc: a) On the lower leg.
b) On the medial aspect of the lower leg.
c) On the anterior border of the tendocalcaneus (achilles tendon).
d) 2 cun superior to the prominence of the medial malleolus.
e) 2 cun superior to Ki 3.

Cun: a) In the supine position, the distance from the prominence of the medial malleolus to the popliteal crease on the medial side of the knee flexure is measured as 15 cun.
b) 15 cun is measured with the patient in a supine position with the leg flat.
c) This method may seem more user friendly than using the 13 cun measurement as it should be easier to divide 15 cun measurement in to 3 sections of 5 and then to divide the 5 in to 1 cun measurements.

Tip: a) Measure 2 cun superior to the prominence of the medial malleolus (2 cun superior to Ki 3). As the foot naturally relaxes, it may be difficult measuring 2 cun from Ki 3 than from the prominence of the medial malleolus. This is because Ki 3 may seem more superior to the prominence of the medial malleolus rather than level to it.
b) Palpate for Ki 7 at 2 cun. The point should lie in the deepest part of the groove formed by the posterior border of the tibia and the anterior border of the tendocalcaneus. The deepest part of the groove is nearer to the anterior border of the tendocalcaneus than the posterior border of the medial border of the tibia.
c) Although Ki 7 is located at 2 cun, it is only an approximation. Palpation will give you overall accuracy.

d) If the patient is in a supine position, the proximity of the couch to the tendocalcaneus can make this point difficult to locate. Therefore ask the patient to rotate their leg slightly outwards, so you can reach the area for accurate point location. You will also need to needle the point in this position.

Note: Lawson-Wood (1973) locates IV 7 about 6 cm above the internal malleolus, and 1 cm posterior to the tibia. Lavier (1974) in an illustration locates KI 7 at 3 pouce proximal to the prominence of the medial malleolus, immediately anterior to the anterior border of the achilles tendon. Voisin (1974) locates K 7 in relation to the tibia, 0.5-1 fb (finger breadth) behind its posterior border, 3 fb above the medial malleolus.

Wu (1973) locates KI 7 upon the internal surface of the leg, at 3 pouce above the internal malleus and behind the flexor digitorum longus, on the posterior tibial artery. Worsley (1982) locates IV 7 on the medial surface of the leg, 3 ACI (Anatomical Chinese Inch) proximal to the level of the prominence of the medial malleolus, posterior to the flexor digitorum longus.

Soulié (1994) locates KI 7 on the medial lower leg; two FW (Finger Width) above the medial malleolus; one half FW posterior to the posterior edge of the tibia, between two muscles; on the posterior edge of the tibialis posterior muscle; on the anterior edge of the flexor communis; on the lower edge of a transverse mass; in a hollow; two FW above KI 4; one FW inferior and posterior to KI 8. Masayoshi (1975) locates KI 7 at 3 sun above the lower edge of the medial malleolus between the posterior edge of the tibia and the achilles tendon.

Ki 8 JIAO XIN – EXCHANGE PLEDGES

⊥ ***0.3 TO 0.5 CUN*** ∆ ***3 TO 5***

- ACCUMULATION/Xi Cleft/Gueki Point of the Yin Heel/Yin Motility Vessel (Yin Qiao Mai)
- 8 EXTRAORDINARY VESSEL/Coalescent Point of the Yin Heel/Yin Motility Vessel (Yin Qiao Mai)

Pos: Position of patient: supine (at 15 cun), or in a seated position with the leg bent at 90 degrees (at 13 cun).

Loc:
a) On the lower leg.
b) On the medial aspect of the lower leg.
c) Posterior to the medial border of the tibia.
d) 2 cun superior to the prominence of the medial malleolus.
e) 2 cun superior to Ki 3.
f) 0.5 cun anterior to Ki 7.

Cun:
a) In the supine position, the distance from the prominence of the medial malleolus to the popliteal crease on the medial side of the knee flexure is measured as 15 cun.
b) 15 cun is measured with the patient in a supine position with the leg flat.
c) This method may seem more user friendly than using the 13 cun measurement as it should be easier to divide 15 cun measurement in to 3 sections of 5 and then to divide the 5 in to 1 cun measurements.

Tip: a) Measure 2 cun superior to the prominence of the medial malleolus (2 cun superior to Ki 3). As the foot naturally relaxes, it may be difficult measuring 2 cun from Ki 3 than from the prominence of the medial malleolus. This is because Ki 3 may seem more superior to the prominence of the medial malleolus rather than level to it.

b) Palpate for Ki 8 at 2 cun. The point should lie slightly anterior to Ki 7 which is in the deepest part of the groove formed by the posterior border of the tibia and the anterior border of the tendocalcaneus.

c) This point is located nearer to the posterior border of the medial border of the tibia than Ki 7 which is nearer to the tendocalcaneus. The point is still located in the groove but at the anterior aspect of it.

d) Although Ki 8 is located at 2 cun, it is only an approximation. Palpation will give you overall accuracy.

e) If the patient is in a supine position, the proximity of the couch to the tendocalcaneus can make this point difficult to locate. Therefore ask the patient to rotate their leg slightly outwards, so you can reach the area for accurate point location. You will also need to needle the point in this position.

Note: Wu (1973) locates KI 8 upon the internal surface of the leg, at three pouce above the internal malleus, between the tibia and the flexor digitorum longus and in front of KI 7. Voisin (1974) locates K 8 in relation to the tibia, just behind its posterior border, 4 fb (finger breadth) above the medial malleolus. Worsley (1982) locates IV 8 on the medial surface of the leg, 3 ACI (Anatomical Chinese Inch) proximal to the prominence of the medial malleolus, 0.5 ACI anterior to IV 7, and anterior to the flexor digitorum longus. Lavier (1974) in an illustration locates KI 8 at 3 pouce proximal to the prominence of the medial malleolus, on the posterior border of the tibia.

So (1985) locates KI 8 proximal from the edge of the medial malleolus 2 divisions, behind the tibia, between two small muscles. Lotan (2000) locates K 8 posterior to the tibia, level with 2 cun superior to the medial malleolus peak.

Soulié (1994) locates KI 8 on the medial lower leg: three FW (Finger Width) above the medial malleolus. Just on the posterior edge of the tibia; in the upper part of a hollow; between bone and muscle (flexor communis muscle). Slightly above the transverse edge of the muscle which disappears under the tibia (tibialis posterior muscle); on the lower edge of a transverse mass (fibres of the flexor communis); one FW above and in front of KI 7; one FW under SP 6; four FW inferior and anterior to KI 9.

Ki 9 ZHU BIN – BUILDING GUEST

⊥ ***0.3 TO 0.7 CUN*** **Δ** ***3 TO 7***

- ACCUMULATION/Xi Cleft/Gueki Point of the Yin Linking Vessel (Yin Wei Mai)

Pos: Position of patient: supine (at 15 cun), or in a seated position with the leg bent at 90 degrees (at 13 cun).

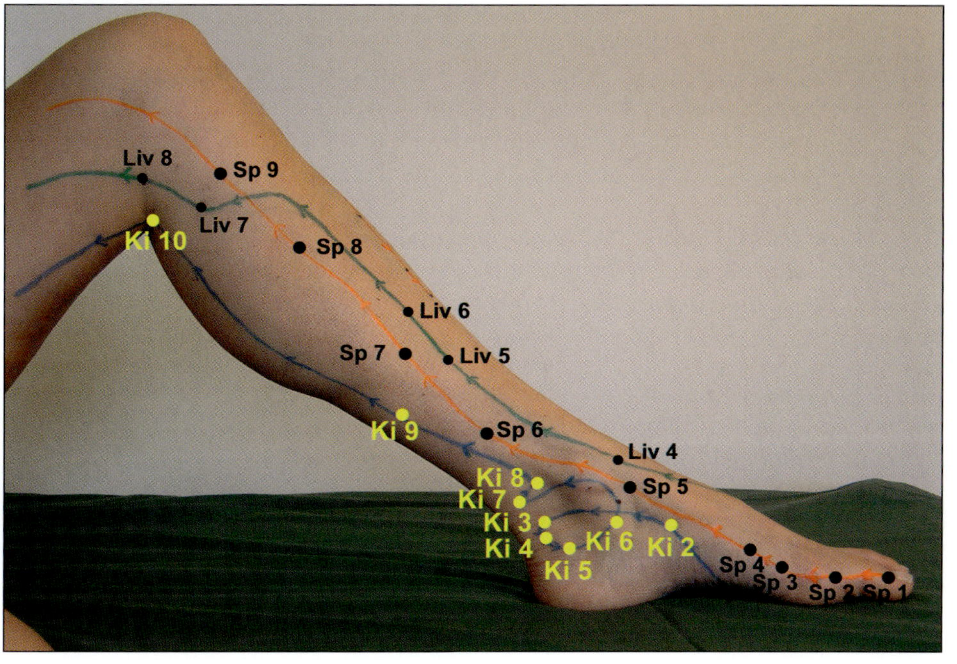

Loc: a) On the lower leg.
b) On the medial aspect of the lower leg.
c) On a line from Ki 3 to Ki 10.
d) In a seam between the medial border of the gastrocnemius (calf) and the soleus muscles, or on some people between the medial border of the tendocalcaneus (achilles tendon) and the soleus muscle.
e) 5 cun superior to the prominence of the medial malleolus.
f) 5 cun superior to Ki 3.
g) Level with Liv 5 (see separate location).

Cun: a) In the supine position, the distance from the prominence of the medial malleolus to the popliteal crease on the medial side of the knee flexure is measured as 15 cun.
b) 15 cun is measured with the patient in a supine position with the leg flat.
c) This method may seem more user friendly than using the 13 cun measurement as it should be easier to divide 15 cun measurement in to 3 sections of 5 and then to divide the 5 in to 1 cun measurements.

Tip: a) Measure 5 cun superior to the prominence of the medial malleolus (5 cun superior to Ki 3). As the foot naturally relaxes, it may be difficult measuring 5 cun from Ki 3 than from the prominence of the medial malleolus. This is because Ki 3 may seem more superior to the prominence of the medial malleolus rather than level to it.

b) Palpate for Ki 9 with the flat of your finger from Ki 3 with the flow of the channel to 5 cun.

c) The point lies in a seam from Ki 3 towards the knee, but at 5 cun the seam will be formed either by the medial border of the gastrocnemius muscle and the soleus muscle or by the medial border of the tendocalcaneus and the soleus muscle.

d) Although Ki 9 is located at 5 cun, it is only an approximation. Palpation will give you overall accuracy.

e) If the patient is in a supine position, the proximity of the couch to the tendocalcaneus can make this point difficult to locate. Therefore ask the patient to rotate their leg slightly outwards, so you can reach the area for accurate point location. You will also need to needle the point in this position.

Note: Worsley (1982) locates IV 9 on the medial surface of the leg, 6.5 ACI (Anatomical Chinese Inch) proximal to the level of the prominence of the medial malleolus, on the medial edge of the tendon of the gastrocnemius, directly proximal to IV 7. Voisin (1974) locates K 9 in relation to the tibia, at 1.5 fb (finger breadth) behind its posterior border, 9 fb above the medial malleolus.

Wu (1973) locates KI 9 upon the internal surface of the leg, at six pouce above the internal malleus, inside of the tendon of the gastrocnemius muscle. So (1985) locates KI 9 at 5 divisions above the medial malleolus, 3 divisions above KI 7, between two muscles.

Legge (1999) locates Ki 9 in the hollow inferior to the belly of the gastrocnemius, 5 cun above Ki 3. Lavier (1974) in an illustration locates KI 9 at 6.5 pouce proximal to the prominence of the medial malleolus, on the anterior border of the achilles tendon/gastrocnemius muscle, level with LI 5 (Liv 5).

Eachou (1995) locates KI 9 at 5 inches above the medial malleolus of the tibia, on the line between KI 3 and KI 10, at the inferior part of the medial side of the gastrocnemius muscle; or 5 inches above KI 3.

Soulié (1994) locates KI 9 on the medial lower leg: about mid-height, mid-width; seven FW (Finger Width) above the medial malleolus. In the anterior angle between the large posterior tendon (Achilles) and the lower edge of the medial gastrocnemius, at its union with the Achilles tendon; in a hollow; on the soleus muscle; two FW anterior and behind SP 6 where the meridian passes; seven FW below KI 10.

Deadman (1998) locates KID 9 on the medial aspect of the lower leg, 5 cun superior to KID 3, on the line drawn between KID 3 and KID 10, about 1 cun posterior to the medial border of the tibia (on the same level as LIV 5). Academy (1975) locates K 9 at 5 cun above K 3, about 1 cun posterior to the medial border of the tibia.

Cheng (1987) locates K 9 at 5 cun directly above K 3 at the lower end of the belly of the m. gastrocnemius, on the line drawn from K 3 to K 10. Shanghai (1981) locates K 9 about 5 units above K 3 and 2 units posterior to the medial margin of the tibia. Below the medial belly of the gastrocnemius muscle where it forms the calcaneus tendon. Underneath is the soleus muscle.

Shanghai (1993) locates KI 9 on the middle part of the medial aspect of the leg, 5 cun above the medial malleolus, at the junction of the middle and posterior thirds of the line connecting the medial border of the tibia and the posterior midline of the leg. Masayoshi (1975) locates KI 9 at the lower third of the inner side of the lower leg, between the gastrocnemic tendon and the soleus. Katsusuke (1983) locates KI 9 in the muscle that is the width of the index finger inward from the edge of the shin at a point five sun above the inner side of the ankle.

Qiu (1996) locates K 9 at 5 cun above K 3, on the line linking K 3 and K 10. At the lower end of the belly of the m. gastrocnemius, tendo calcaneus, m. soleus. Lotan (2000) locates K 9 between the soleus and the gastrocnemius, level with 5 cun superior to the mediasl malleolus peak. Ellis (1991) locates KI 9 on the line drawn from KI 3 to KI 10, at the lower end of the body of the gastrocnemius muscle, on the anteromedial edge of the muscle, about 5 inches above KI 3. Shandong (1982) locate Zhubin on the line between Pt. Taixi (Ki 3) and Pt. Yingu (Ki 10), on the lower border of the medial belly of the m. gastrocnemius.

Ki 10 can be located with the patient in a prone position and the knees semi-flexed, or with the patient in a supine position with the knees semi-flexed.

Ki 10 YIN GU – YIN VALLEY

⊥ ***0.4 TO 0.8 CUN*** **Δ *3***

- WATER
- HORARY from 5 p.m. to 7 p.m.
- SEASONAL HORARY – Winter
- HE – SEA/Shu – Transporting/Antique

Pos: Position of patient: prone with the knees semi-flexed, or supine with the knees semi-flexed.

Loc: a) On the posterior surface of the leg.
b) On the posterior aspect of the popliteal crease (flexure) of the knee.
c) On the tendon of the semimembranosus muscle.
d) On the medial border of the tendon of the semitendinosus muscle.

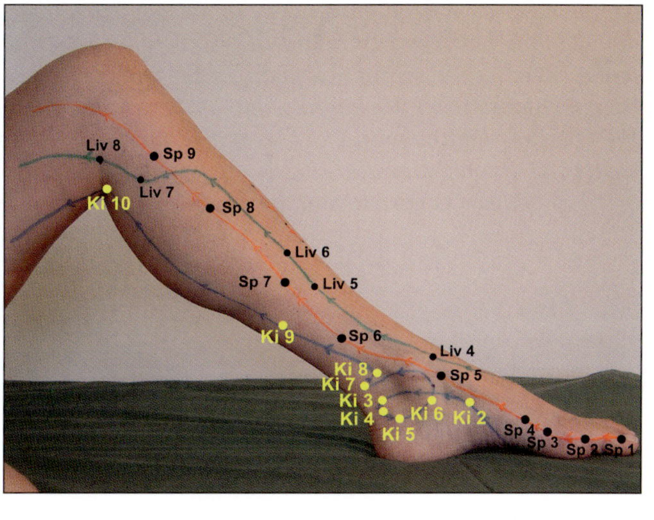

Tip: a) With the patient in the PRONE position, and the knees semi flexed feel for the tendons of the semimembranosus and semitendinosus muscles on the posterior aspect of the popliteal crease. If you cannot feel them, you may need to ask the patient to flex their leg against resistance, then when you can feel the tendons, ask them to relax again.

b) The tendon of the semitendinosus muscle is a thin tight tendon that is located on top of the tendon of the semimembranosus muscle. The tendon of the semimembranosus muscle has been described as thin but it is a wide flat tendon that lies under the tendon of the semitendinosus.

c) If you can feel two tight bands you are feeling the medial aspect of the tendon of the semimembranosus and the medial border of the tendon of the semitendinosus.

d) Ki 10 is located on the medial aspect of the popliteal crease.

e) With the patient in the SUPINE position with the knees semi-flexed and with you at their side, ask the patient to rest their knee on your torso.so you can access the point more easily.

f) You should be able to feel two tight tendons (like guitar strings) when you palpate the posterior aspect of the popliteal crease at the medial end. The tight medial tendon is the medial aspect of the tendon of the semimembranosus muscle. This wide flat tendon lies across and under the tendon of the semitendinosus, therefore Ki 10 lies on top of the semimembranosus, on the medial border of the semitendinosus.

g) It is important to locate and needle Ki 10 in the same position.

h) If you are having difficulty locating the posterior aspect of the popliteal crease ask the patient to flex their leg, and then mark in the crease.

Note: Wu (1973) locates KI 10 upon the internal surface of the leg, just below the tendon which lies at the extremity of the popliteal crease. Voisin (1974) locates K 10 in relation to the knee, at its medial aspect, posterior part: tibial plateau. So (1985) locates KI 10 in between BL 54 (Bl 40) and LV 8 at the same level as BL 54 (Bl 40), between the two tendons at the medial edge of the inner knee crease. Eachou (1995) locates KI 10 at the medial end of the skin crease of the popliteal fossa between the tendons of the semimembranosus and semitendinosus muscles, or at the midpoint between LIV 8 and BL 40. Soulié (1994) locates KI 10 on the posteromedial face of the knee: on the medial extremity of the transverse crease; on the lateral edge of the tendon (semitendinosis); on the lateral edge of the medial gastrocnemius; in a hollow; around eleven FW (Finger Width) above KI 8; seven FW above KI 9; three large FW under SP 9. Ellis (1991) locates KI 10 on the medial side of the popliteal fossa, level with BL 40, between the tendons of the semitendinosus muscle and the semimembranosus muscle when the knee is flexed.

Ki 11-27 are on the anterior torso, (Ki 11-15 in the lower jiao, 16-21 in the middle jiao, Ki 22-27 in the upper jiao).

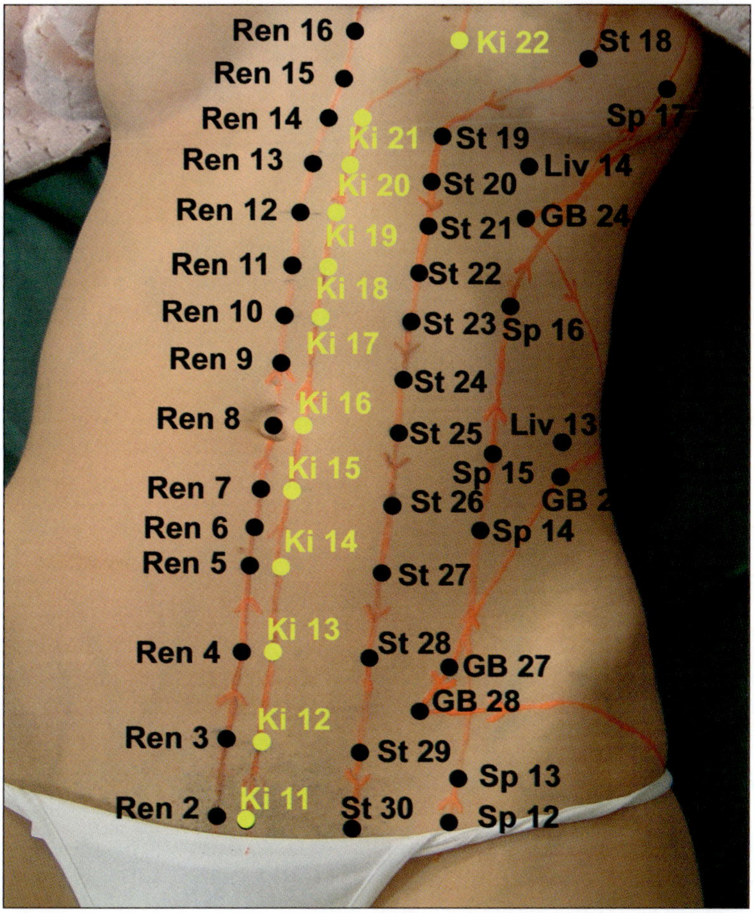

The transverse measurement for the middle and lower abdomen (middle and lower jiao) is calculated as 2 cun, between the anterior median line (at the centre of the umbilicus) and the lateral border of the rectus abdominis muscle (at St 25) Alternatively the cun measurements between the anterior median line (at the centre of the umbilicus) and the medial border of the anterior superior iliac spine which is part of the iliac crest of the ilium (one of three parts of the in nominate or hip bone) is 4 cun.

The lateral border of the rectus abdominis muscle is not the actual edge of the muscle but the most prominent surface of the rectus abdominis muscle before it begins to 'slope' in to the torso, eg. the corner of an inverted 'L', just before you go on to the lateral aspect from the anterior surface. When the muscle is contracted by asking your patient to raise their head slightly, the muscle forms a curved ridge that can be palpated. The lateral border of the rectus abdominis muscle is on the most lateral part of the palpable curve which makes it more medial than the actual edge of the muscle.

The transverse cun measurements for the middle and lower abdomen (middle and lower jiao) which includes the Kidney, Stomach, Spleen, Gall Bladder and Liver channels (lateral to the anterior median line) are as follows:

Ki 11 to Ki 21 = 0.5 cun
St 19 to St 30 = 2 cun
Sp 13 to Sp 16 = 4 cun (Sp 12 = 3.5 cun)
GB 24 = 4 cun
Liv 14 = 4 cun

Note: Some acupuncture schools have used different transverse cun measurements at the level of the umbilicus: the Kidney channel has been put at 0.5, 1 and 1.5 pouce/ACI, the Stomach channel at 2.5 or 3 pouce/ACI and the Spleen channel at 4 or 4.5 pouce/ACI. A few schools still do use these transverse measurements, but they still mainly have the same longitudinal measurements for their point locations as the majority use.

Ki 16, St 25 and Sp 15 are all transversely level with the centre of the umbilicus and are used as reference points for marking their channels cun measurements.

The longitudinal measurements of the anterior torso are:

9 cun from the xiphisternal joint to the suprasternal fossa (with the space between 2 ribs measuring approximately 1.6 cun in the lower chest, and 1 cun in the upper chest)

8 cun from the centre of the umbilicus to the xiphisternal joint

For the descriptions relating to the channels in the middle jiao, the longitudinal cun measurements are given from the centre of the umbilicus superiorly or from the xiphisternal joint inferiorly , depending on the direction of the flow of the channel.

5 cun from the centre of the umbilicus to the superior border of the symphysis pubis bone

For the descriptions relating to the channels in the lower jiao, the longitudinal cun measurements are given from the centre of the umbilicus inferiorly or from the superior border of the symphysis pubis bone superiorly, depending on the direction of the flow of the channel.

Note: These transverse distances have traditionally varied. The Kidney channel has appeared as 0.5/1/1.5 cun lateral to the median line. 0.5 cun is the accepted opinion in modern China (and some Japanese texts).

Ki 11 HENG GU – TRANSVERSE BONE

⊥ ***0.3 TO 0.5 CUN*** Δ ***5 TO 15***
FORBIDDEN TO NEEDLE AND MOXA THIS POINT DURING PREGNANCY.

- 8 EXTRAORDINARY VESSEL/Coalescent Point of Penetrating Vessel (Chong Mai)
- RE-UNION/Crossing/Meeting Point of the Kidney Channel with the Penetrating Vessel – Foot Shao Yin Channel with the Chong Mai.

Pos: Position of patient: supine.

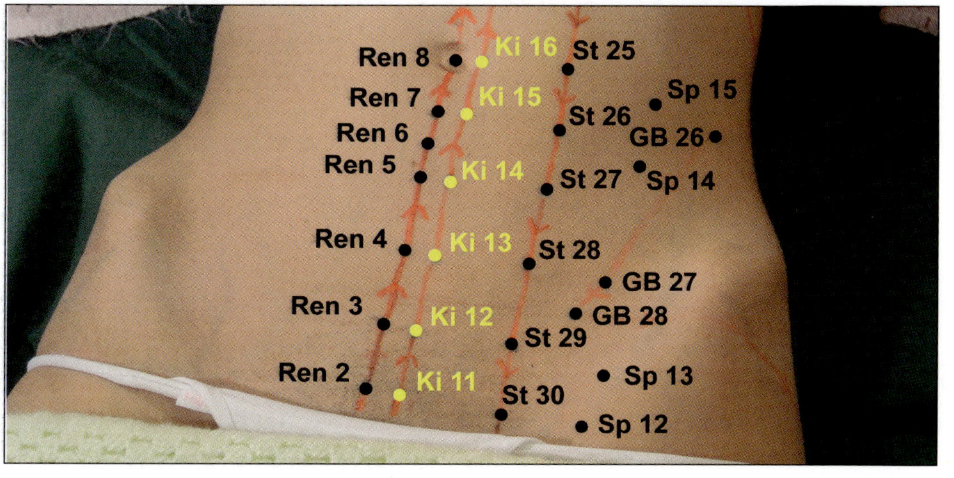

Loc: a) On the anterior aspect of the torso.
b) On the lower abdomen (in the lower jiao).
c) On the superior border of the symphysis pubis.
d) 0.5 cun lateral to the anterior median line (Ren Mai).
e) 5 cun inferior to the level of the centre of the umbilicus.
f) Level with Ren 2 (which is on the anterior median line, at 5 cun inferior to the level of centre of the umbilicus and is on the superior border of the symphysis pubis.

Cun: a) The transverse measurement for the middle and lower abdomen (middle and lower jiao) is 2 cun between the anterior median line (at the centre of the umbilicus) and the lateral border of the rectus abdominis muscle (at St 25).
b) The lateral border of the rectus abdominis muscle is not the actual edge of the muscle but the most prominent surface of the muscle before it begins to 'slope' in to the torso. By visualising the corner of an inverted 'L', the point is located on the antero-lateral edge of the muscle. To locate this muscle ask the patient to slightly raise their head. The lateral border of the rectus abdominis muscle is on the most lateral part of the palpable curve which is more medial than the actual edge of the muscle. The edge of the rectus abdominis muscle is measured as 4 cun. Once established you can then divide the 4 cun into other cun measurements for use on the Stomach and Kidney and Spleen channels etc.

c) Another way to mark out the transverse cun measurements at the level of the umbilicus is to locate the medial border of the anterior superior iliac spine (part of the iliac crest). To locate the 4 cun line of the Spleen channel, place a pen longitudinally on the medial border of the anterior superior iliac spine approximately halfway between the centre of the umbilicus and the superior border of the symphysis pubis. For the Stomach channel divide the 4 cun measurement in half to get 2 cun. For the Kidney channel divide the 2 cun in to half cun divisions. The Kidney channel is at 0.5 cun lateral to the anterior median line

d) The transverse cun measurements for the middle and lower abdomen (middle and lower jiao) includes the Kidney, Stomach, Spleen, Gall Bladder and Liver channels (lateral to the anterior median line): Ki 11 to Ki 21 = 0.5 cun; St 19 to St 30 = 2 cun; Sp 12 = 3.5 cun; Sp 13 to Sp 16 = 4 cun; GB 24 = 4 cun; Liv 14 = 4 cun.

e) The longitudinal measurement of the lower abdomen is 5 cun from the centre of the umbilicus to the superior border of the symphysis pubis.

Tip:

a) Locate 0.5 cun measurement lateral to the anterior median line and on the superior border of the symphysis pubis.

b) If you cannot feel the superior border of the symphysis pubis, ask the patient to semi-flex their legs to relax the abdominal muscles to enable you to palpate the superior border.

c) Ki 11 may be slightly less than 0.5 cun lateral to the anterior median line as the rectus abdominis muscle begins to narrow towards the groin and inserts at the pubic tubercles.

d) Place your finger on the anterior median line, (on Ren 2) 5 cun inferior to the level of the centre of the umbilicus, and palpate laterally to 0.5 cun.

e) Palpation in this area should reveal the accurate location for Ki 11.

Note: Some acupuncture schools have used different transverse cun measurements at the level of the umbilicus: the Kidney channel has been put at 1.5 pouce/ACI, the Stomach channel at 2.5 or 3 pouce/ACI and the Spleen channel at 4 or 4.5 pouce/ACI. A few schools still do use these transverse measurements, but they still mainly have the same longitudinal measurements for their point locations as the majority use.Voisin (1974) locates K 11 on the abdomen, onthe upper border of the pubis, 2 fb (finger breadth) from the midline. Worsley (1982) locates IV 11 at 1.5 ACI (Anatomical Chinese Inch) lateral to the median line, at the level of the superior edge of the pubic symphysis, 5 ACI inferior to the level of the umbilicus.

Wu (1973) locates KI 11 above the superior edge of the pubis, at one and one-half pouce from the median line of the abdomen. Lavier (1973) illustrates KI 11 as being located on the superior border of the pubis and transversley level with VC 2 (Ren 2), at 5 pouce below the level of the umbilicus, at 1.5 pouce lateral to the anterior median line. Soulié (1994) locates KI 11 on the lower abdomen: just at the upper edge of the transverse bone (pubis); one large FW (Finger Width) on either side of the median line; in a hollow; mid-width on a large vertical muscle (rectus abdominus muscle); on the lateral edge of a vertical artery (superficial abdominal); one FW below KI 12; one large FW on either side of CV 2 (Ren 2); three FW medial to ST 30.

Lawson-Wood (1973) locates IV 11 at 4 cm from the centre line of the pubic symphysis, almost on the superior border of the os pubis. Stiefvater places it at 2 cm. He lists this point as an Alarm point for V – the Circulation-Sexfield (Pericardium) as well as V 1.(Pc 1).

Ki 12 DA HE – GREAT BRIGHTNESS

⊥ ***0.5 TO 1.0 CUN*** Δ ***5 TO 10***
FORBIDDEN TO NEEDLE AND MOXA THIS POINT DURING PREGNANCY.

- 8 EXTRAORDINARY VESSEL/Coalescent Point of Penetrating Vessel (Chong Mai)
- RE-UNION/Crossing/Meeting Point of the Kidney Channel with the Penetrating Vessel – Foot Shao Yin Channel with the Chong Mai

Pos: Position of patient: supine.

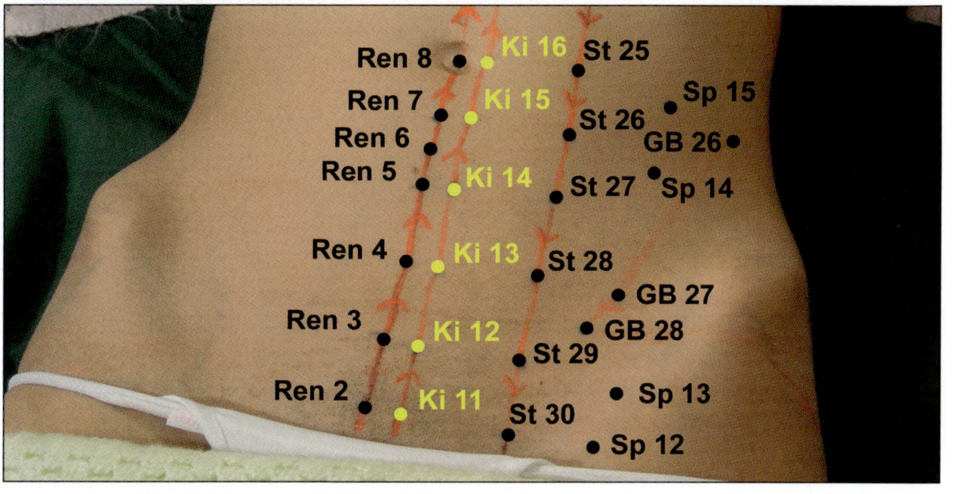

Loc: a) On the anterior aspect of the torso.
b) On the lower abdomen (in the lower jiao).
c) 0.5 cun lateral to the anterior median line (Ren Mai).
d) 1 cun superior to the superior border of the symphysis pubis.
e) 1 cun superior to Ki 11.
f) 4 cun inferior to the level of the centre of the umbilicus.
g) Level with Ren 3 (see separate location).

Cun: a) The transverse measurement for the middle and lower abdomen (middle and lower jiao) is 2 cun between the anterior median line (at the centre of the umbilicus) and the lateral border of the rectus abdominis muscle (at St 25).
b) The lateral border of the rectus abdominis muscle is not the actual edge of the muscle but the most prominent surface of the muscle before it begins to 'slope' in to the torso. By visualising the corner of an inverted 'L', the point is located on the antero-lateral edge of the muscle. To locate this muscle ask the patient to slightly raise their head. The lateral border of the rectus abdominis muscle is on the most lateral part of the palpable curve which is more medial than the actual edge of the muscle. The edge of the rectus abdominis muscle is measured as 4 cun. Once established you can then divide the 4 cun into other cun measurements for use on the Stomach and Kidney and Spleen channels etc.

c) Another way to mark out the transverse cun measurements at the level of the umbilicus is to locate the medial border of the anterior superior iliac spine (part of the iliac crest). To locate the 4 cun line of the Spleen channel, place a pen longitudinally on the medial border of the anterior superior iliac spine approximately halfway between the centre of the umbilicus and the superior border of the symphysis pubis. For the Stomach channel divide the 4 cun measurement in half to get 2 cun. For the Kidney channel divide the 2 cun in to half cun divisions. The Kidney channel is at 0.5 cun lateral to the anterior median line

d) The transverse cun measurements for the middle and lower abdomen (middle and lower jiao) includes the Kidney, Stomach, Spleen, Gall Bladder and Liver channels (lateral to the anterior median line): Ki 11 to Ki 21 = 0.5 cun; St 19 to St 30 = 2 cun; Sp 12 = 3.5 cun; Sp 13 to Sp 16 = 4 cun; GB 24 = 4 cun; Liv 14 = 4 cun.

e) The longitudinal measurement of the lower abdomen is 5 cun from the centre of the umbilicus to the superior border of the symphysis pubis.

Tip: a) Mark out 5 equal cun measurements longitudinally from the superior border of the symphysis pubis to the centre of the umbilicus at the anterior median line.

b) If you cannot feel the superior border of the symphysis pubis, ask the patient to semi-flex their legs to relax the abdominal muscles to enable you to palpate the superior border.

c) Place your finger on the anterior median line, (on Ren 3) at 1 cun superior to the border of the symphysis pubis or 4 cun inferior to the centre of the umbilcus, and palpate laterally to 0.5 cun.

d) Palpate along the Kidney channel with the direction of the flow towards the umbilicus from the superior border of the symphysis pubis until you are at 4 cun inferior to the umbilicus.

e) Palpation in this area should reveal the accurate location for Ki 12.

Note: Some acupuncture schools have used different transverse cun measurements at the level of the umbilicus: the Kidney channel has been put at 1.5 pouce/ACI, the Stomach channel at 2.5 or 3 pouce/ACI and the Spleen channel at 4 or 4.5 pouce/ACI. A few schools still do use these transverse measurements, but they still mainly have the same longitudinal measurements for their point locations as the majority use.

Voisin (1974) locates K 12 on the abdomen: 2 fb (finger breadth) above the pubis, 2 fb (finger breadth) from the midline. Worsley (1982) locates IV 12 on the abdomen, 1.5 ACI (Anatomical Chinese Inch) lateral to the median line, 4 ACI inferior to the level of the umbilicus, at the level of XIII 3 (Ren 3). Wu (1973) locates KI 12 upon the abdomen, (at one and one-half pouce from the median line), at one pouce above K 11.

Lavier (1973) illustrates KI 12 as being located on the abdomen, transversely level with VC 3 (Ren 3), at 4 pouce below the level of the umbilicus, and at 1.5 pouce lateral to the anterior median line. Soulié (1994) locates KI 12 on the lower abdomen: about one FW (Finger Width) above the pubis and two FW on either side of the median line; mid-width on the large vertical muscle (rectus abdominus); in a hollow; on the lateral edge of the vertical artery (superficial abdominal artery); one FW above KI 11; one FW below KI 13; one large FW on either side of CV 3 (Ren 3); two FW medial to ST 29.

Ki 13 QI XUE – DOOR OF INFANTS

⊥ ***0.5 TO 1.0 CUN*** Δ ***5 TO 10***
FORBIDDEN TO NEEDLE AND MOXA THIS POINT DURING PREGNANCY.

- 8 EXTRAORDINARY VESSEL/Coalescent Point of Penetrating Vessel (Chong Mai)
- RE-UNION/Crossing/Meeting Point of the Kidney Channel with the Penetrating Vessel – Foot Shao Yin Channel with the Chong Mai

Pos: Position of patient: supine.

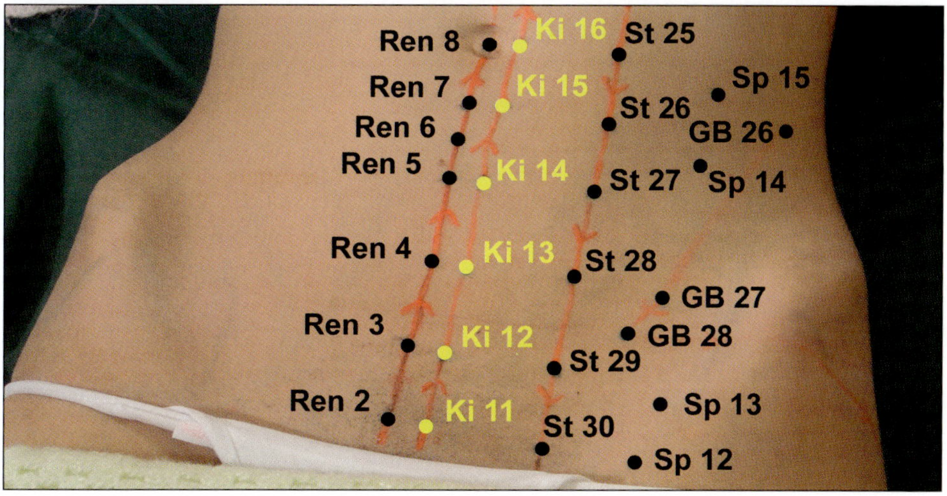

Loc: a) On the anterior aspect of the torso.
b) On the lower abdomen (in the lower jiao).
c) 0.5 cun lateral to the anterior median line (Ren Mai).
d) 2 cun superior to the superior border of the symphysis pubis.
e) 2 cun superior to Ki 11.
f) 3 cun inferior to the level of the centre of the umbilicus.
g) Level with Ren 4 (see separate location).

Cun: a) The transverse measurement for the middle and lower abdomen (middle and lower jiao) is 2 cun between the anterior median line (at the centre of the umbilicus) and the lateral border of the rectus abdominis muscle (at St 25).
b) The lateral border of the rectus abdominis muscle is not the actual edge of the muscle but the most prominent surface of the muscle before it begins to 'slope' in to the torso. By visualising the corner of an inverted 'L', the point is located on the antero-lateral edge of the muscle. To locate this muscle ask the patient to slightly raise their head. The lateral border of the rectus abdominis muscle is on the most lateral part of the palpable curve which is more medial than the actual edge of the muscle. The edge of the rectus abdominis muscle is measured as 4 cun. Once established you can then divide the 4 cun into other cun measurements for use on the Stomach and Kidney and Spleen channels etc.

c) Another way to mark out the transverse cun measurements at the level of the umbilicus is to locate the medial border of the anterior superior iliac spine (part of the iliac crest). To locate the 4 cun line of the Spleen channel, place a pen longitudinally on the medial border of the anterior superior iliac spine approximately halfway between the centre of the umbilicus and the superior border of the symphysis pubis. For the Stomach channel divide the 4 cun measurement in half to get 2 cun. For the Kidney channel divide the 2 cun in to half cun divisions. The Kidney channel is at 0.5 cun lateral to the anterior median line

d) The transverse cun measurements for the middle and lower abdomen (middle and lower jiao) includes the Kidney, Stomach, Spleen, Gall Bladder and Liver channels (lateral to the anterior median line): Ki 11 to Ki 21 = 0.5 cun; St 19 to St 30 = 2 cun; Sp 12 = 3.5 cun; Sp 13 to Sp 16 = 4 cun; GB 24 = 4 cun; Liv 14 = 4 cun.

e) The longitudinal measurement of the lower abdomen is 5 cun from the centre of the umbilicus to the superior border of the symphysis pubis.

Tip:
a) Mark out 5 equal cun measurements longitudinally from the superior border of the symphysis pubis to the centre of the umbilicus at the anterior median line.
b) If you cannot feel the superior border of the symphysis pubis, ask the patient to semi-flex their legs to relax the abdominal muscles to enable you to palpate the superior border.
c) Place your finger on the anterior median line, (on Ren 4) at 2 cun superior to the border of the symphysis pubis or 3 cun inferior to the centre of the umbilcus, and palpate laterally to 0.5 cun.
d) Palpate along the Kidney channel with the direction of the flow towards the umbilicus from the superior border of the symphysis pubis until you are at 3 cun inferior to the umbilicus.
e) Palpation in this area should reveal the accurate location for Ki 13.

Note: Some acupuncture schools have used different transverse cun measurements at the level of the umbilicus: the Kidney channel has been put at 1.5 pouce/ACI, the Stomach channel at 2.5 or 3 pouce/ACI and the Spleen channel at 4 or 4.5 pouce/ACI. A few schools still do use these transverse measurements, but they still mainly have the same longitudinal measurements for their point locations as the majority use. Voisin (1974) locates K 13 on the abdomen: 4 fb (finger breadth) above the pubis, 2.5 fb (finger breadth) from the midline. Worsley (1982) locates IV 13 on the abdomen, 1.5 ACI (Anatomical Chinese Inch) lateral to the median line, 3 ACI inferior to the level of the umbilicus, at the level of XIII 4 (Ren 4).

Wu (1973) locates KI 13 upon the abdomen, (at one and one-half pouce from the median line), at two pouce above K 11. Lavier (1973) illustrates KI 13 as being located on the abdomen, transversely level with VC 4 (Ren 4), at 3 pouce below the level of the umbilicus, and at 1.5 pouce lateral to the anterior median line. Soulié (1994) locates KI 13 on the abdomen: about two FW (Finger Width) above the pubis (three FW below the level of the navel). Two FW on either side of the median line. Mid-width on the large vertical muscle (rectus abdominis) ; in a hollow; on the medial edgeof the vertical artery (superficial abdominal artery);one FW above KI 12; one FW below KI 14; two FW on either side of CV 4 (Ren 4); two FW medial to ST 28. Shandong (1982) locate Qixue at 1 cun above Pt. Dahe (Ki 12).

Ki 14 SI MAN – FOUR FULL

⊥ ***0.5 TO 1.0 CUN*** ***Δ 5 TO 30***
FORBIDDEN TO NEEDLE AND MOXA THIS POINT DURING PREGNANCY.

- 8 EXTRAORDINARY VESSEL/Coalescent Point of Penetrating Vessel (Chong Mai)
- RE-UNION/Crossing/Meeting Point of the Kidney Channel with the Penetrating Vessel – Foot Shao Yin Channel with the Chong Mai

Pos: Position of patient: supine.

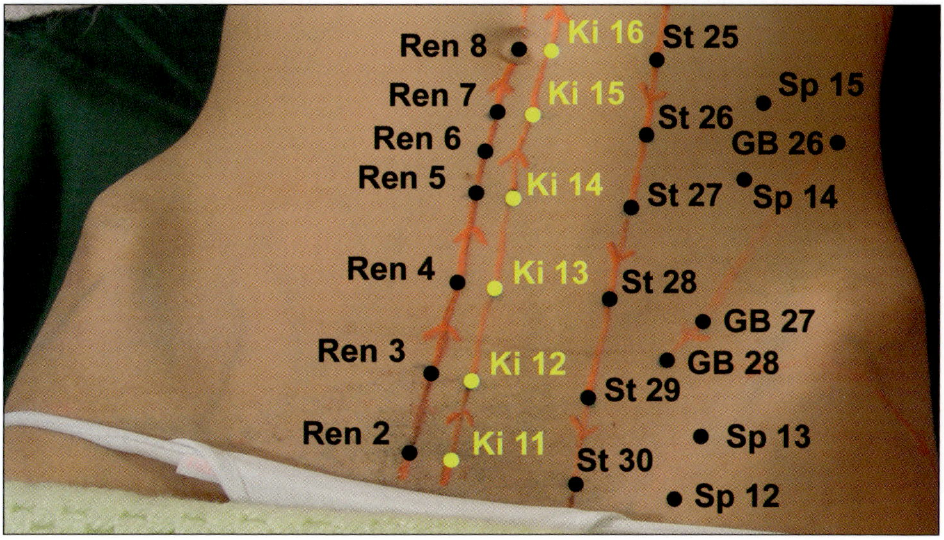

Loc: a) On the anterior aspect of the torso.
b) On the lower abdomen (in the lower jiao).
c) 0.5 cun lateral to the anterior median line (Ren Mai).
d) 3 cun superior to the superior border of the symphysis pubis.
e) 3 cun superior to Ki 11.
f) 2 cun inferior to the level of the centre of the umbilicus.
g) Level with Ren 5 (see separate location).

Cun: a) The transverse measurement for the middle and lower abdomen (middle and lower jiao) is 2 cun between the anterior median line (at the centre of the umbilicus) and the lateral border of the rectus abdominis muscle (at St 25).
b) The lateral border of the rectus abdominis muscle is not the actual edge of the muscle but the most prominent surface of the muscle before it begins to 'slope' in to the torso. By visualising the corner of an inverted 'L', the point is located on the antero-lateral edge of the muscle. To locate this muscle ask the patient to slightly raise their head. The lateral border of the rectus abdominis muscle is on the most lateral part of the palpable curve which is more medial than the actual edge of the muscle. The edge of the rectus abdominis muscle is measured as 4 cun. Once established you can then divide the 4 cun into other cun measurements for use on the Stomach and Kidney and Spleen channels etc.

c) Another way to mark out the transverse cun measurements at the level of the umbilicus is to locate the medial border of the anterior superior iliac spine (part of the iliac crest). To locate the 4 cun line of the Spleen channel, place a pen longitudinally on the medial border of the anterior superior iliac spine approximately halfway between the centre of the umbilicus and the superior border of the symphysis pubis. For the Stomach channel divide the 4 cun measurement in half to get 2 cun. For the Kidney channel divide the 2 cun in to half cun divisions. The Kidney channel is at 0.5 cun lateral to the anterior median line

d) The transverse cun measurements for the middle and lower abdomen (middle and lower jiao) includes the Kidney, Stomach, Spleen, Gall Bladder and Liver channels (lateral to the anterior median line): Ki 11 to Ki 21 = 0.5 cun; St 19 to St 30 = 2 cun; Sp 12 = 3.5 cun; Sp 13 to Sp 16 = 4 cun; GB 24 = 4 cun; Liv 14 = 4 cun.

e) The longitudinal measurement of the lower abdomen is 5 cun from the centre of the umbilicus to the superior border of the symphysis pubis.

Tip:

a) Mark out 5 equal cun measurements longitudinally from the superior border of the symphysis pubis to the centre of the umbilicus at the anterior median line.

b) If you cannot feel the superior border of the symphysis pubis, ask the patient to semi-flex their legs to relax the abdominal muscles to enable you to palpate the superior border.

c) Place your finger on the anterior median line, (on Ren 5) at 3 cun superior to the border of the symphysis pubis or 2 cun inferior to the centre of the umbilcus, and palpate laterally to 0.5 cun.

d) Palpate along the Kidney channel with the direction of the flow towards the umbilicus from the superior border of the symphysis pubis until you are at 2 cun inferior to the umbilicus.

e) Palpation in this area should reveal the accurate location for Ki 14.

Note: Some acupuncture schools have used different transverse cun measurements at the level of the umbilicus: the Kidney channel has been put at 1.5 pouce/ACI, the Stomach channel at 2.5 or 3 pouce/ACI and the Spleen channel at 4 or 4.5 pouce/ACI. A few schools still do use these transverse measurements, but they still mainly have the same longitudinal measurements for their point locations as the majority use.Voisin (1974) locates K 14 on the abdomen: 3 fb (finger breadth) below the umbilical plane, 3 fb (finger breadth) from the midline. Worsley (1982) locates IV 14 on the abdomen, 1.5 ACI (Anatomical Chinese Inch) lateral to the median line, 2 ACI inferior to the level of the umbilicus, at the level of XIII 5 (Ren 5).

Wu (1973) locates KI 14 upon the abdomen, (at one and one-half pouce from the median line). at three pouce above K 11. Lavier (1973) illustrates KI 14 as being located on the abdomen, transversely level with VC 5 (Ren 5), at 2 pouce below the level of the umbilicus, and at 1.5 pouce lateral to the anterior median line. Soulié (1994) locates KI 14 on the abdomen: about two FW (Finger Width) below the level of the umbilicus (three FW above the pubis). About two FW on either side of the median line; at the mid-width of a large vertical muscle (rectus abdominis muscle); in a hollow; one FW above KI 13; one FW below KI 15; two FW on either side of CV 5 (Ren 5). Shandong (1982) locate Siman at 1 cun above Pt. Qixue (Ki 13).

Ki 15 ZHONG ZHU – MIDDLE FLOWING OUT

⊥ ***0.5 TO 1.0 CUN*** Δ ***5 TO 15***
FORBIDDEN TO NEEDLE AND MOXA THIS POINT DURING PREGNANCY.

- 8 EXTRAORDINARY VESSEL/Coalescent Point of Penetrating Vessel (Chong Mai)
- RE-UNION/Crossing/Meeting Point of the Kidney Channel with the Penetrating Vessel – Foot Shao Yin Channel with the Chong Mai

Pos: Position of patient: supine.

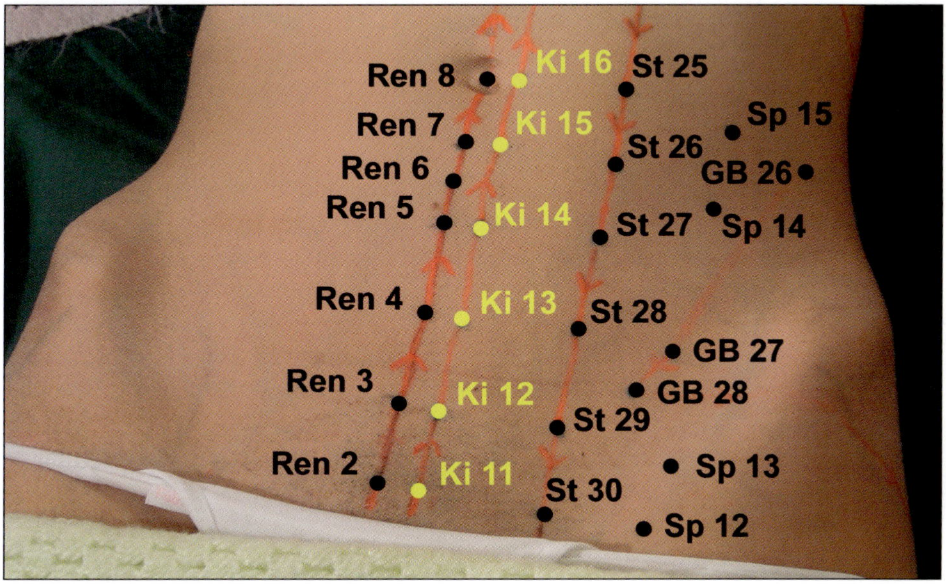

Loc: a) On the anterior aspect of the torso.
b) On the lower abdomen (in the lower jiao).
c) 0.5 cun lateral to the anterior median line (Ren Mai).
d) 4 cun superior to the superior border of the symphysis pubis bone.
e) 4 cun superior to Ki 11.
f) 1 cun inferior to the level of the centre of the umbilicus.
g) Level with Ren 7 (see separate location).

Cun: a) The transverse measurement for the middle and lower abdomen (middle and lower jiao) is 2 cun between the anterior median line (at the centre of the umbilicus) and the lateral border of the rectus abdominis muscle (at St 25).
b) The lateral border of the rectus abdominis muscle is not the actual edge of the muscle but the most prominent surface of the muscle before it begins to 'slope' in to the torso. By visualising the corner of an inverted 'L', the point is located on the antero-lateral edge of the muscle. To locate this muscle ask the patient to slightly raise their head. The lateral border of the rectus abdominis muscle is on the most lateral part of the palpable curve which is more medial than the actual edge of the muscle. The edge of the rectus abdominis muscle is measured as 4 cun. Once established you can then divide the 4 cun into other cun measurements for use on the Stomach and Kidney and Spleen channels etc.

c) Another way to mark out the transverse cun measurements at the level of the umbilicus is to locate the medial border of the anterior superior iliac spine (part of the iliac crest). To locate the 4 cun line of the Spleen channel, place a pen longitudinally on the medial border of the anterior superior iliac spine approximately halfway between the centre of the umbilicus and the superior border of the symphysis pubis. For the Stomach channel divide the 4 cun measurement in half to get 2 cun. For the Kidney channel divide the 2 cun in to half cun divisions. The Kidney channel is at 0.5 cun lateral to the anterior median line

d) The transverse cun measurements for the middle and lower abdomen (middle and lower jiao) includes the Kidney, Stomach, Spleen, Gall Bladder and Liver channels (lateral to the anterior median line): Ki 11 to Ki 21 = 0.5 cun; St 19 to St 30 = 2 cun; Sp 12 = 3.5 cun; Sp 13 to Sp 16 = 4 cun; GB 24 = 4 cun; Liv 14 = 4 cun.

e) The longitudinal measurement of the lower abdomen is 5 cun from the centre of the umbilicus to the superior border of the symphysis pubis.

Tip: a) Mark out 5 equal cun measurements longitudinally from the superior border of the symphysis pubis to the centre of the umbilicus at the anterior median line.

b) If you cannot feel the superior border of the symphysis pubis, ask the patient to semi-flex their legs to relax the abdominal muscles to enable you to palpate the superior border.

c) Place your finger on the anterior median line, (on Ren 7) at 4 cun superior to the border of the symphysis pubis or 1 cun inferior to the centre of the umbilcus, and palpate laterally to 0.5 cun.

d) Palpate along the Kidney channel with the direction of the flow towards the umbilicus from the superior border of the symphysis pubis until you are at 1 cun inferior to the umbilicus.

e) Palpation in this area should reveal the accurate location for Ki 15.

Note: Some acupuncture schools have used different transverse cun measurements at the level of the umbilicus: the Kidney channel has been put at 1.5 pouce/ACI, the Stomach channel at 2.5 or 3 pouce/ACI and the Spleen channel at 4 or 4.5 pouce/ACI. A few schools still do use these transverse measurements, but they still mainly have the same longitudinal measurements for their point locations as the majority use.

Voisin (1974) locates K 15 on the abdomen: 1.5 fb (finger breadth) below the umbilical plane, 3 fb (finger breadth) from the midline. Worsley (1982) locates IV 15 on the abdomen, 1.5 ACI (Anatomical Chinese Inch) lateral to the median line, 1 ACI inferior to the level of the umbilicus, at the level of XIII 7 (Ren 7). Wu (1973) locates KI 15 upon the abdomen, (at one and one-half pouce from the median line), at four pouce above K 11. Lavier (1973) illustrates KI 15 as being located on the abdomen, transversely level with VC 7 (Ren 7), at 1 pouce below the level of the umbilicus, and at 1.5 pouce lateral to the anterior median line.

Soulié (1994) locates KI 15 on the abdomen: at the level of one FW (Finger Width) below the umbilicus; two large FW on either side of the median line; mid-width on the large vertical muscle (rectus abdominis); in a hollow; one FW above KI 14; one FW below KI 16; two large FW on either side of CV 6 (Ren 6); two large FW medial to ST 26. Shandong (1982) locate Abdomen-Zhongzhu at 1 cun above Pt. Siman (Ki 14).

The transverse measurement for the middle and lower abdomen (middle and lower jiao) is calculated as 2 cun, between the anterior median line (at the centre of the umbilicus) and the lateral border of the rectus abdominis muscle (at St 25). Alternatively the cun measurements between the anterior median line (at the centre of the umbilicus) and the medial border of the anterior superior iliac spine which is part of the iliac crest of the ilium (one of three parts of the in nominate or hip bone) is 4 cun.

The lateral border of the rectus abdominis muscle is not the actual edge of the muscle but the most prominent surface of the rectus abdominis muscle before it begins to 'slope' in to the torso, eg. the corner of an inverted 'L', just before you go on to the lateral aspect from the anterior surface. When the muscle is contracted by asking your patient to raise their head slightly, the muscle forms a curved ridge that can be palpated. The lateral border of the rectus abdominis muscle is on the most lateral part of the palpable curve which makes it more medial than the actual edge of the muscle.

The transverse cun measurements for the middle and lower abdomen (middle and lower jiao) which includes the Kidney, Stomach, Spleen, Gall Bladder and Liver channels (lateral to the anterior median line) are as follows:

Ki 11 to Ki 21 = 0.5 cun
St 19 to St 30 = 2 cun
Sp 13 to Sp 16 = 4 cun (Sp 12 = 3.5 cun)
GB 24 = 4 cun
Liv 14 = 4 cun

Note: Some acupuncture schools have used different transverse cun measurements at the level of the umbilicus: the Kidney channel has been put at 0.5, 1 and 1.5 pouce/ACI, the Stomach channel at 2.5 or 3 pouce/ACI and the Spleen channel at 4 or 4.5 pouce/ACI. A few schools still do use these transverse measurements, but they still mainly have the same longitudinal measurements for their point locations as the majority use.

Ki 16, St 25 and Sp 15 are all transversely level with the centre of the umbilicus and are used as reference points for marking their channels cun measurements.

The longitudinal measurements of the anterior torso are:

9 cun from the xiphisternal joint to the suprasternal fossa (with the space between 2 ribs measuring approximately 1.6 cun in the lower chest, and 1 cun in the upper chest)
8 cun from the centre of the umbilicus to the xiphisternal joint

For the descriptions relating to the channels in the middle jiao, the longitudinal cun measurements are given from the centre of the umbilicus superiorly or from the xiphisternal joint inferiorly, depending on the direction of the flow of the channel.

5 cun from the centre of the umbilicus to the superior border of the symphysis pubis bone. For the descriptions relating to the channels in the lower jiao, the longitudinal cun measurements are given from the centre of the umbilicus inferiorly or from the superior border of the symphysis pubis bone superiorly, depending on the direction of the flow of the channel.

Ki 16 HUANG SHU – VITALS CORRESPONDENCE

⊥ ***0.5 TO 1.0 CUN*** Δ ***5 TO 7***
FORBIDDEN TO NEEDLE AND MOXA THIS POINT DURING PREGNANCY.

- 8 EXTRAORDINARY VESSEL/Coalescent Point of Penetrating Vessel (Chong Mai)
- RE-UNION/Crossing/Meeting Point of the Kidney Channel with the Penetrating Vessel – Foot Shao Yin Channel with the Chong Mai

Pos: Position of patient: supine.

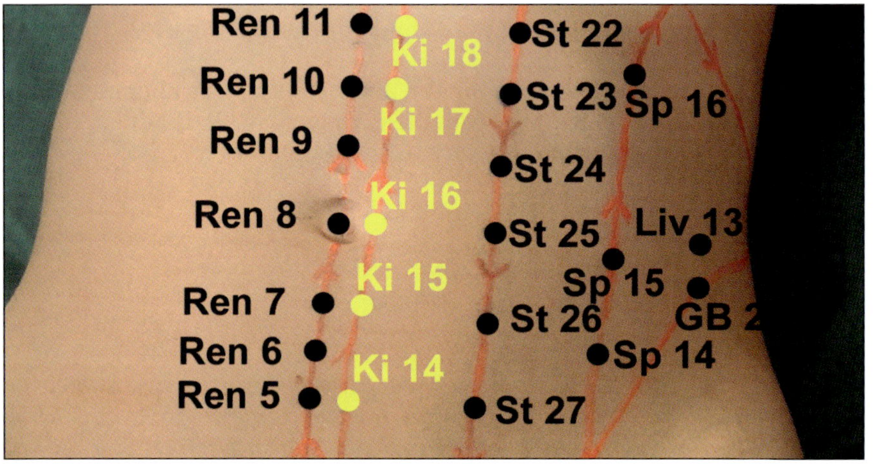

Loc: a) On the anterior aspect of the torso.
b) In between the mid-abdomen and lower abdomen (in between the middle and lower jiao).
c) 0.5 cun lateral to the anterior median line (Ren Mai).
d) Level with the centre of the umbilicus.
e) Level with Ren 8 (which is at the level of the centre of the umbilicus).

Cun: a) The transverse measurement for the middle and lower abdomen (middle and lower jiao) is 2 cun between the anterior median line (at the centre of the umbilicus) and the lateral border of the rectus abdominis muscle (at St 25).
b) The lateral border of the rectus abdominis muscle is not the actual edge of the muscle but the most prominent surface of the muscle before it begins to 'slope' in to the torso. By visualising the corner of an inverted 'L', the point is located on the antero-lateral edge of the muscle. To locate this muscle ask the patient to slightly raise their head. The lateral border of the rectus abdominis muscle is on the most lateral part of the palpable curve which is more medial than the actual edge of the muscle. The edge of the rectus abdominis muscle is measured as 4 cun. Once established you can then divide the 4 cun into other cun measurements for use on the Stomach and Kidney and Spleen channels etc.

c) Another way to mark out the transverse cun measurements at the level of the umbilicus is to locate the medial border of the anterior superior iliac spine (part of the iliac crest). To locate the 4 cun line of the Spleen channel, place a pen longitudinally on the medial border of the anterior superior iliac spine approximately halfway between the centre of the umbilicus and the superior border of the symphysis pubis. For the Stomach channel divide the 4 cun measurement in half to get 2 cun. For the Kidney channel divide the 2 cun in to half cun divisions. The Kidney channel is at 0.5 cun lateral to the anterior median line

d) The transverse cun measurements for the middle and lower abdomen (middle and lower jiao) which includes the Kidney, Stomach, Spleen, Gall Bladder and Liver channels (lateral to the anterior median line) are: Ki 11 to Ki 21 = 0.5 cun; St 19 to St 30 = 2 cun; Sp 13 to Sp 16 = 6 cun (Sp 12 = 3.5 cun); GB 24 = 4 cun; Liv 14 = 4 cun.

e) Ki 16, St 25 and Sp 15 are all transversely level with the centre of the umbilicus and are used as reference points for marking their channels cun measurements.

f) The longitudinal measurement of the mid abdomen is 8 cun from the centre of the umbilicus to the xiphisternal joint. The longitudinal measurement of the lower abdomen is 5 cun from the superior border of the symphysis pubis bone to the centre of the umbilicus.

Tip:
a) Locate 0.5 cun lateral to the anterior median line and transversely level with the centre of the umbilicus.
b) Place your finger just lateral to the centre of the umbilicus and run it slightly laterally to locate the point and the 0.5 cun measurement.
c) Lightly place the flat of your finger with the direction of the flow of the channel towards the umbilicus from the superior border of the symphysis pubis until you are at the level of the centre of the umbilicus (0.5 cun lateral to the anterior median line).
d) Palpation in this area should reveal the accurate location for Ki 16.

Note: Some acupuncture schools have used different transverse cun measurements at the level of the umbilicus: the Kidney channel has been put at 1.5 pouce/ACI, the Stomach channel at 2.5 or 3 pouce/ACI and the Spleen channel at 4 or 4.5 pouce/ACI. A few schools still do use these transverse measurements, but they still mainly have the same longitudinal measurements for their point locations as the majority use.Voisin (1974) locates K 16 on the abdomen: at the level of the umbilical plane, 3.5 fb (finger breadth) from the midline.

Worsley (1982) locates IV 16 on the abdomen, 1.5 ACI (Anatomical Chinese Inch) lateral to the centre of the umbilicus. Wu (1973) locates KI 16 upon the abdomen at the height of the umbilicus (at one and one-half pouce from the median line), at five pouce above K 11. Lavier (1973) illustrates KI 16 as being located on the abdomen, transversely level with the umbilicus, and at 1.5 pouce lateral to the anterior median line.

Soulié (1994) locates KI 16 on the abdomen: two large FW (Finger Width) on either side and at the level of the umbilicus; mid-width of the large vertical muscle (rectus abdominis); in a hollow; one FW above KI 15; two FW below KI 17; two large FW on either side of CV 8 (Ren 8); two large FW medial to ST 25. Shandong (1982) locate Huangshu (Ki 16) at 1 cun above Pt. Abdomen-Zhongzhu, 0.5 cun lateral to the umbilicus.

Ki 17 SHANG QU – MERCHANT CROOKED

⊥ ***0.5 TO 1.0 CUN*** ***Δ 5 TO 7***
FORBIDDEN TO NEEDLE AND MOXA THIS POINT DURING PREGNANCY.

- 8 EXTRAORDINARY VESSEL/Coalescent Point of Penetrating Vessel (Chong Mai)
- RE-UNION/Crossing/Meeting Point of the Kidney Channel with the Penetrating Vessel – Foot Shao Yin Channel with the Chong Mai

Pos: Position of patient: supine.

Loc: a) On the anterior aspect of the torso.
b) On the mid-abdomen (in the middle jiao).
c) 0.5 cun lateral to the anterior median line (Ren Mai).
d) 2 cun superior to the level of the centre of the umbilicus.
e) Level with Ren 10 (which is on the anterior median line, at 2 cun superior to the level of the centre of the umbilicus).

Cun: a) The transverse measurement for the middle and lower abdomen (middle and lower jiao) is 2 cun between the anterior median line (at the centre of the umbilicus) and the lateral border of the rectus abdominis muscle (at St 25).
b) The lateral border of the rectus abdominis muscle is not the actual edge of the muscle but the most prominent surface of the muscle before it begins to 'slope' in to the torso. By visualising the corner of an inverted 'L', the point is located on the antero-lateral edge of the muscle. To locate this muscle ask the patient to slightly raise their head. The lateral border of the rectus abdominis muscle is on the most lateral part of the palpable curve which is more medial than the actual edge of the muscle. The edge of the rectus abdominis muscle is measured as 4 cun. Once established you can then divide the 4 cun into other cun measurements for use on the Stomach and Kidney and Spleen channels etc.
c) Another way to mark out the transverse cun measurements at the level of the umbilicus is to locate the medial border of the anterior superior iliac spine (part of the iliac crest). To locate the 4 cun line of the Spleen channel, place a pen longitudinally on the medial border of the anterior superior iliac spine approximately halfway between the centre of the umbilicus and the superior border of the symphysis pubis. For the Stomach channel divide the 4 cun measurement in half to get 2 cun. For the Kidney channel divide the 2 cun in to half cun divisions. The Kidney channel is at 0.5 cun lateral to the anterior median line.
d) The transverse cun measurements for the middle and lower abdomen (middle and lower jiao) which includes the Kidney, Stomach, Spleen, Gall Bladder and Liver channels (lateral to the anterior median line) are: Ki 11 to Ki 21 = 0.5 cun; St 19 to St 30 = 2 cun; Sp 13 to Sp 16 = 6 cun (Sp 12 = 3.5 cun); GB 24 = 4 cun; Liv 14 = 4 cun.
e) Ki 16, St 25 and Sp 15 are all transversely level with the centre of the umbilicus and are used as reference points for marking their channels cun measurements.
f) The longitudinal measurement of the mid abdomen is 8 cun from the centre of the umbilicus to the xiphisternal joint.

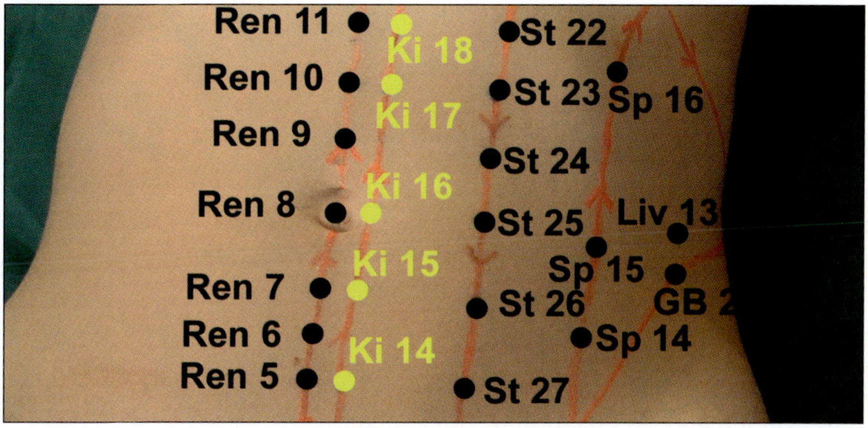

Tip:
a) Locate 0.5 cun lateral to the anterior median line at the level of the centre of the umbilicus and mark out the longitudinal measurement 2 cun superior to the centre of the umbilicus.
b) Place your finger on the anterior median line, (on Ren 10) at 2 cun superior to the level of the umbilicus, and run it laterally to 0.5 cun.
c) Lightly place the flat of your finger with the direction of the flow of the channel from the level of the centre of the umbilicus superiorly towards the chest (0.5 cun lateral to the anterior median line) to 2 cun (superior to the level of the centre of the umbilicus).
d) Palpation in this area should reveal the accurate location for Ki 17.

Note: Some acupuncture schools have used different transverse cun measurements at the level of the umbilicus: the Kidney channel has been put at 1.5 pouce/ACI, the Stomach channel at 2.5 or 3 pouce/ACI and the Spleen channel at 4 or 4.5 pouce/ACI. A few schools still do use these transverse measurements, but they still mainly have the same longitudinal measurements for their point locations as the majority use.

Voisin (1974) locates K 17 on the abdomen: 2 fb (finger breadth) above the umbilical plane, 3.5 fb (finger breadth) from the midline. Worsley (1982) locates IV 17 on the abdomen, 1.5 ACI (Anatomical Chinese Inch) lateral to the median line., 2 ACI superior to the level of the umbilicus, at the level of XIII 10 (Ren 10). Wu (1973) locates KI 17 upon the abdomen (at one and one-half pouce from the median line), at two pouce above K 16.

Lavier (1973) illustrates KI 17 as being located on the abdomen, transversely level with VC 10 (Ren 11), at 2 pouce above the level of the umbilicus, and at 1.5 pouce lateral to the anterior median line. Soulié (1994) locates KI 17 on the Epigastrium: about one and one half FW (Finger Width) above the umbilicus. About one FW on either side of the median line; mid-width on the large vertical muscle (rectus abdominis); in a hollow; at a level of the mid-height of the tenth rib; two FW above KI 16; one FW below KI 18; about one FW above and on either side of CV 10; about one FW above and medial to ST 24; one FW under and medial to ST 23. Shandong (1982) locate Shangqu at 1 cun above Pt. Huangshu (Ki 16). (This point is 1 cun above the centre of the umbilicus in the description but at 2 cun above the umbilicus in the illustration)

Ki 18 SHI GUAN – STONE BORDER

⊥ ***0.5 TO 1.0 CUN*** **Δ** ***5 TO 7***
FORBIDDEN TO NEEDLE AND MOXA THIS POINT DURING PREGNANCY.

- 8 EXTRAORDINARY VESSEL/Coalescent Point of Penetrating Vessel (Chong Mai)
- RE-UNION/Crossing/Meeting Point of the Kidney Channel with the Penetrating Vessel – Foot Shao Yin Channel with the Chong Mai

Pos: Position of patient: supine.

Loc:
a) On the anterior aspect of the torso.
b) On the mid-abdomen (in the middle jiao).
c) 0.5 cun lateral to the anterior median line (Ren Mai).
d) 3 cun superior to the level of the centre of the umbilicus.
e) Level with Ren 11 (which is on the anterior median line, at 3 cun superior to the level of the centre of the umbilicus).

Cun:
a) The transverse measurement for the middle and lower abdomen (middle and lower jiao) is 2 cun between the anterior median line (at the centre of the umbilicus) and the lateral border of the rectus abdominis muscle (at St 25).
b) The lateral border of the rectus abdominis muscle is not the actual edge of the muscle but the most prominent surface of the muscle before it begins to 'slope' in to the torso. By visualising the corner of an inverted 'L', the point is located on the antero-lateral edge of the muscle. To locate this muscle ask the patient to slightly raise their head. The lateral border of the rectus abdominis muscle is on the most lateral part of the palpable curve which is more medial than the actual edge of the muscle. The edge of the rectus abdominis muscle is measured as 4 cun. Once established you can then divide the 4 cun into other cun measurements for use on the Stomach and Kidney and Spleen channels etc.
c) Another way to mark out the transverse cun measurements at the level of the umbilicus is to locate the medial border of the anterior superior iliac spine (part of the iliac crest). To locate the 4 cun line of the Spleen channel, place a pen longitudinally on the medial border of the anterior superior iliac spine approximately halfway between the centre of the umbilicus and the superior border of the symphysis pubis. For the Stomach channel divide the 4 cun measurement in half to get 2 cun. For the Kidney channel divide the 2 cun in to half cun divisions. The Kidney channel is at 0.5 cun lateral to the anterior median line
d) The transverse cun measurements for the middle and lower abdomen (middle and lower jiao) which includes the Kidney, Stomach, Spleen, Gall Bladder and Liver channels (lateral to the anterior median line) are: Ki 11 to Ki 21 = 0.5 cun; St 19 to St 30 = 2 cun; Sp 13 to Sp 16 = 6 cun (Sp 12 = 3.5 cun); GB 24 = 4 cun; Liv 14 = 4 cun.
e) Ki 16, St 25 and Sp 15 are all transversely level with the centre of the umbilicus and are used as reference points for marking their channels cun measurements.
f) The longitudinal measurement of the mid abdomen is 8 cun from the centre of the umbilicus to the xiphisternal joint.

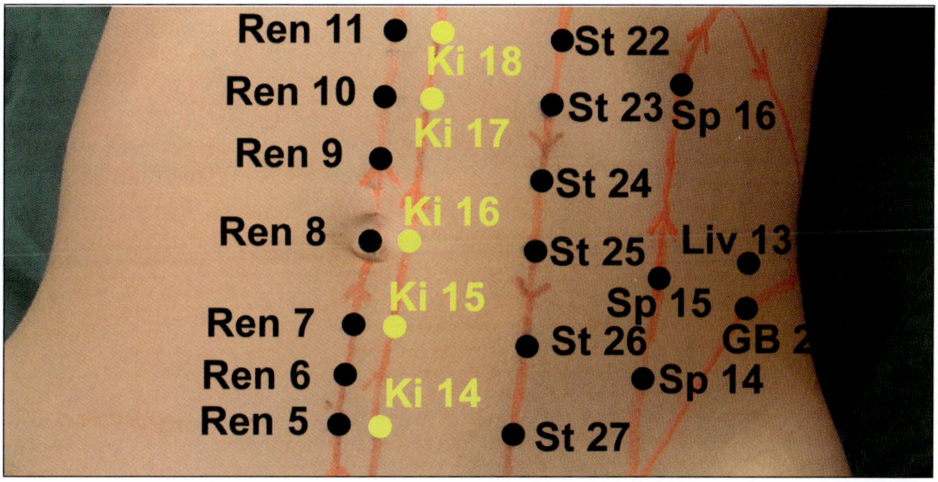

Tip:
a) Locate 0.5 cun lateral to the anterior median line at the level of the centre of the umbilicus and mark out the longitudinal measurement 3 cun superior to the centre of the umbilicus.
b) Place your finger on the anterior median line, (on Ren 11) at 3 cun superior to the level of the umbilicus, and run it laterally to 0.5 cun.
c) Lightly place the flat of your finger with the direction of the flow of the channel from the level of the centre of the umbilicus superiorly towards the chest (0.5 cun lateral to the anterior median line) to 3 cun (superior to the level of the centre of the umbilicus).
d) Palpation in this area should reveal the accurate location for Ki 18.

Note: Some acupuncture schools have used different transverse cun measurements at the level of the umbilicus: the Kidney channel has been put at 1.5 pouce/ACI, the Stomach channel at 2.5 or 3 pouce/ACI and the Spleen channel at 4 or 4.5 pouce/ACI. A few schools still do use these transverse measurements, but they still mainly have the same longitudinal measurements for their point locations as the majority use.

Voisin (1974) locates K 18 on the abdomen: 3 fb (finger breadth) above the umbilical plane, on the lateral border of the rectus abdominis. Worsley (1982) locates IV 18 on the abdomen, 1.5 ACI (Anatomical Chinese Inch) lateral to the median line., 3 ACI superior to the level of the umbilicus, at the level of XIII 11 (Ren 11). Wu (1973) locates KI 18 upon the abdomen (at one and one-half pouce from the median line), at three pouce above K 16. Lavier (1973) illustrates KI 18 as being located on the abdomen, transversely level with VC 11 (Ren 11), at 3 pouce above the level of the umbilicus, and at 1.5 pouce lateral to the anterior median line.

Soulié (1994) locates KI 18 on the Epigastrium: about three small FW (Finger Width) above the umbilicus. at the mid-distance from the medial edge of mid-height of the ninth rib and of the median line; in a hollow; mid-width of the rectus abdominis muscle; one FW above KI 17; one FW below KI 19; about one FW below and on either side of CV 12 (Ren 12); one FW medial and above ST 23; one FW medial and below ST 22. Shandong (1982) locate Shiguan at 1 cun above Pt. Shangqu (Ki 17).

Ki 19 YIN DU – YIN CAPITAL

⊥ ***0.5 TO 1.0 CUN*** Δ ***5 TO 10***
FORBIDDEN TO NEEDLE AND MOXA THIS POINT DURING PREGNANCY.

- 8 EXTRAORDINARY VESSEL/Coalescent Point of Penetrating Vessel (Chong Mai)
- RE-UNION/Crossing/Meeting Point of the Kidney Channel with the Penetrating Vessel – Foot Shao Yin Channel with the Chong Mai

Pos: Position of patient: supine.

Loc: a) On the anterior aspect of the torso.
b) On the mid-abdomen (in the middle jiao).
c) 0.5 cun lateral to the anterior median line (Ren Mai).
d) 2 cun superior to the level of the centre of the umbilicus.
e) Level with Ren 12 (which is on the anterior median line, at 4 cun superior to the level of the centre of the umbilicus).

Cun: a) The transverse measurement for the middle and lower abdomen (middle and lower jiao) is 2 cun between the anterior median line (at the centre of the umbilicus) and the lateral border of the rectus abdominis muscle (at St 25).
b) The lateral border of the rectus abdominis muscle is not the actual edge of the muscle but the most prominent surface of the muscle before it begins to 'slope' in to the torso. By visualising the corner of an inverted 'L', the point is located on the antero-lateral edge of the muscle. To locate this muscle ask the patient to slightly raise their head. The lateral border of the rectus abdominis muscle is on the most lateral part of the palpable curve which is more medial than the actual edge of the muscle. The edge of the rectus abdominis muscle is measured as 4 cun. Once established you can then divide the 4 cun into other cun measurements for use on the Stomach and Kidney and Spleen channels etc.
c) Another way to mark out the transverse cun measurements at the level of the umbilicus is to locate the medial border of the anterior superior iliac spine (part of the iliac crest). To locate the 4 cun line of the Spleen channel, place a pen longitudinally on the medial border of the anterior superior iliac spine approximately halfway between the centre of the umbilicus and the superior border of the symphysis pubis. For the Stomach channel divide the 4 cun measurement in half to get 2 cun. For the Kidney channel divide the 2 cun in to half cun divisions. The Kidney channel is at 0.5 cun lateral to the anterior median line
d) The transverse cun measurements for the middle and lower abdomen (middle and lower jiao) which includes the Kidney, Stomach, Spleen, Gall Bladder and Liver channels (lateral to the anterior median line) are: Ki 11 to Ki 21 = 0.5 cun; St 19 to St 30 = 2 cun; Sp 13 to Sp 16 = 6 cun (Sp 12 = 3.5 cun); GB 24 = 4 cun; Liv 14 = 4 cun.
e) Ki 16, St 25 and Sp 15 are all transversely level with the centre of the umbilicus and are used as reference points for marking their channels cun measurements.
f) The longitudinal measurement of the mid abdomen is 8 cun from the centre of the umbilicus to the xiphisternal joint.

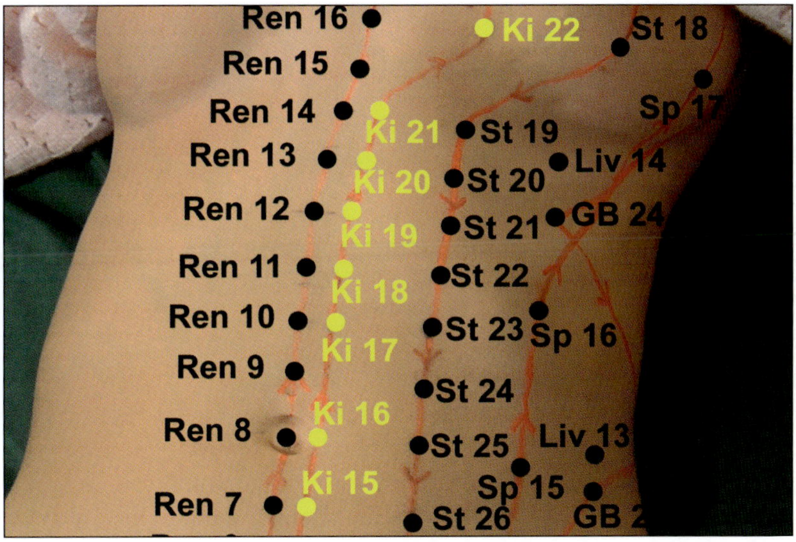

Tip:
a) Locate 0.5 cun lateral to the anterior median line at the level of the centre of the umbilicus and mark out the longitudinal measurement 4 cun superior to the centre of the umbilicus.
b) Place your finger on the anterior median line, (on Ren 12) at 4 cun superior to the level of the umbilicus, and run it laterally to 0.5 cun.
c) Lightly place the flat of your finger with the direction of the flow of the channel from the level of the centre of the umbilicus superiorly towards the chest (0.5 cun lateral to the anterior median line) to 4 cun (superior to the level of the centre of the umbilicus).
d) Palpation in this area should reveal the accurate location for Ki 19.

Note: Some acupuncture schools have used different transverse cun measurements at the level of the umbilicus: the Kidney channel has been put at 1.5 pouce/ACI, the Stomach channel at 2.5 or 3 pouce/ACI and the Spleen channel at 4 or 4.5 pouce/ACI. A few schools still do use these transverse measurements, but they still mainly have the same longitudinal measurements for their point locations as the majority use.

Voisin (1974) locates K 19 on the abdomen: 4 fb (finger breadth) above the umbilical plane, on the lateral border of the rectus abdominis. Worsley (1982) locates IV 19 on the abdomen, at 1.5 ACI (Anatomical Chinese Inch) lateral to the median line., 4 ACI superior to the level of the umbilicus, at the level of XIII 12 (Ren 12).

Wu (1973) locates KI 19 upon the abdomen (at one and one-half pouce from the median line), at four pouce above K 16. Lavier (1973) illustrates KI 19 as being located on the abdomen, transversely level with VC 12 (Ren 12), at 4 pouce above the level of the umbilicus, and at 1.5 pouce lateral to the anterior median line. Soulié (1994) locates KI 19 on the Epigastrium: about three FW (Finger Width) below the lower extremity of the sternum. at the level of the mid-height of the eighth rib, and at mid-distance from the rib to the median line ; aboutr mid-width of the vertical muscle (rectus abdominis); in a hollow; one FW above KI 18; two FW below KI 20; about one FW on either side and above CV 12 (Ren 12); one FW medial and above ST 22; one FW medial and below ST 21. Shandong (1982) locate Yindu at 1 cun above Pt. Shiguan (Ki 18).

Ki 20 FU TONG GU – THROUGH THE VALLEY

⊥ ***0.5 TO 0.7 CUN*** Δ ***7 TO 10***
FORBIDDEN TO NEEDLE AND MOXA THIS POINT DURING PREGNANCY.

- 8 EXTRAORDINARY VESSEL/Coalescent Point of Penetrating Vessel (Chong Mai)
- RE-UNION/Crossing/Meeting Point of the Kidney Channel with the Penetrating Vessel – Foot Shao Yin Channel with the Chong Mai

Pos: Position of patient: supine.

Loc: a) On the anterior aspect of the torso.
b) On the mid-abdomen (in the middle jiao).
c) 0.5 cun lateral to the anterior median line (Ren Mai).
d) 5 cun superior to the level of the centre of the umbilicus.
e) Level with Ren 13 (which is on the anterior median line, at 5 cun superior to the level of the centre of the umbilicus).

Cun: a) The transverse measurement for the middle and lower abdomen (middle and lower jiao) is 2 cun between the anterior median line (at the centre of the umbilicus) and the lateral border of the rectus abdominis muscle (at St 25).
b) The lateral border of the rectus abdominis muscle is not the actual edge of the muscle but the most prominent surface of the muscle before it begins to 'slope' in to the torso. By visualising the corner of an inverted 'L', the point is located on the antero-lateral edge of the muscle. To locate this muscle ask the patient to slightly raise their head. The lateral border of the rectus abdominis muscle is on the most lateral part of the palpable curve which is more medial than the actual edge of the muscle. The edge of the rectus abdominis muscle is measured as 4 cun. Once established you can then divide the 4 cun into other cun measurements for use on the Stomach and Kidney and Spleen channels etc.
c) Another way to mark out the transverse cun measurements at the level of the umbilicus is to locate the medial border of the anterior superior iliac spine (part of the iliac crest). To locate the 4 cun line of the Spleen channel, place a pen longitudinally on the medial border of the anterior superior iliac spine approximately halfway between the centre of the umbilicus and the superior border of the symphysis pubis. For the Stomach channel divide the 4 cun measurement in half to get 2 cun. For the Kidney channel divide the 2 cun in to half cun divisions. The Kidney channel is at 0.5 cun lateral to the anterior median line
d) The transverse cun measurements for the middle and lower abdomen (middle and lower jiao) which includes the Kidney, Stomach, Spleen, Gall Bladder and Liver channels (lateral to the anterior median line) are: Ki 11 to Ki 21 = 0.5 cun; St 19 to St 30 = 2 cun; Sp 13 to Sp 16 = 6 cun (Sp 12 = 3.5 cun); GB 24 = 4 cun; Liv 14 = 4 cun.
e) Ki 16, St 25 and Sp 15 are all transversely level with the centre of the umbilicus and are used as reference points for marking their channels cun measurements.
f) The longitudinal measurement of the mid abdomen is 8 cun from the centre of the umbilicus to the xiphisternal joint.

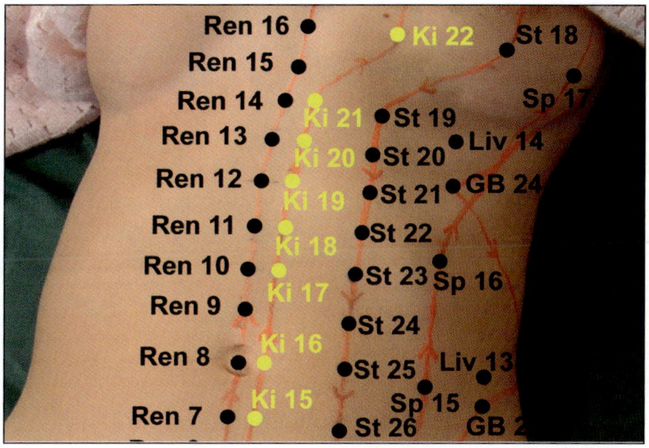

Tip: a) Locate 0.5 cun lateral to the anterior median line at the level of the centre of the umbilicus and mark out the longitudinal measurement 5 cun superior to the centre of the umbilicus.

b) Place your finger on the anterior median line, (on Ren 13) at 5 cun superior to the level of the umbilicus, and run it laterally to 0.5 cun.

c) Lightly place the flat of your finger with the direction of the flow of the channel from the level of the centre of the umbilicus superiorly towards the chest (0.5 cun lateral to the anterior median line) to 5 cun (superior to the level of the centre of the umbilicus).

d) Palpation in this area should reveal the accurate location for Ki 20.

e) If the patient has a long xiphoid process then palpate for the point level with the cun measurement rather than with the Ren point (the length of the xiphoid affects only the Ren channel).

Note: Some acupuncture schools have used different transverse cun measurements at the level of the umbilicus: the Kidney channel has been put at 1.5 pouce/ACI, the Stomach channel at 2.5 or 3 pouce/ACI and the Spleen channel at 4 or 4.5 pouce/ACI. A few schools still do use these transverse measurements, but they still mainly have the same longitudinal measurements for their point locations as the majority use.

Voisin (1974) locates K 20 on the abdomen: 2 fb (finger breadth) below the costal border, 3 fb from the midline. Worsley (1982) locates IV 20 on the abdomen, 1.5 ACI (Anatomical Chinese Inch) lateral to the median line, 5 ACI superior to the level of the umbilicus, at the level of XIII 13 (Ren 13). Shandong (1982) locate Abdomen-Tonggu at 1 cun above Pt. Yindu (Ki 20).

Wu (1973) locates KI 20 upon the abdomen (at one and one-half pouce from the median line), at five pouce above K 16. Lavier (1973) illustrates KI 20 as being located on the abdomen, transversely level with VC 13 (Ren 13), at 5 pouce above the level of the umbilicus, and at 1.5 pouce lateral to the anterior median line.

Soulié (1994) locates KI 20 on the Epigastrium: one large FW (Finger Width) below the lower edge of the sternum (without the xyphoid process).One FW medial and above the union between the seventh and eighth ribs; one FW on either side of the median line ; mid-width of the rectus abdominis; in a hollow; two FW above KI 19; one FW below KI 21; one FW above and on either side of CV 14 (Ren 14); one FW medial and above ST 21; two FW medial to ST 20.

Ki 21 YOU MEN – DARK GATE

⊥ ***0.3 TO 0.5 CUN*** **Δ** ***5 TO 10***
FORBIDDEN TO NEEDLE AND MOXA THIS POINT DURING PREGNANCY.

- 8 EXTRAORDINARY VESSEL/Coalescent Point of Penetrating Vessel (Chong Mai)
- RE-UNION/Crossing/Meeting Point of the Kidney Channel with the Penetrating Vessel – Foot Shao Yin Channel with the Chong Mai

Pos: Position of patient: supine.

Loc: a) On the anterior aspect of the torso.
b) On the mid-abdomen (in the middle jiao).
c) 0.5 cun lateral to the anterior median line (Ren Mai).
d) 6 cun superior to the level of the centre of the umbilicus.
e) Level with Ren 14 (which is on the anterior median line, at 5 cun superior to the level of the centre of the umbilicus).

Cun: a) The transverse measurement for the middle and lower abdomen (middle and lower jiao) is 2 cun between the anterior median line (at the centre of the umbilicus) and the lateral border of the rectus abdominis muscle (at St 25).
b) The lateral border of the rectus abdominis muscle is not the actual edge of the muscle but the most prominent surface of the muscle before it begins to 'slope' in to the torso. By visualising the corner of an inverted 'L', the point is located on the antero-lateral edge of the muscle. To locate this muscle ask the patient to slightly raise their head. The lateral border of the rectus abdominis muscle is on the most lateral part of the palpable curve which is more medial than the actual edge of the muscle. The edge of the rectus abdominis muscle is measured as 4 cun. Once established you can then divide the 4 cun into other cun measurements for use on the Stomach and Kidney and Spleen channels etc.
c) Another way to mark out the transverse cun measurements at the level of the umbilicus is to locate the medial border of the anterior superior iliac spine (part of the iliac crest). To locate the 4 cun line of the Spleen channel, place a pen longitudinally on the medial border of the anterior superior iliac spine approximately halfway between the centre of the umbilicus and the superior border of the symphysis pubis. For the Stomach channel divide the 4 cun measurement in half to get 2 cun. For the Kidney channel divide the 2 cun in to half cun divisions. The Kidney channel is at 0.5 cun lateral to the anterior median line
d) The transverse cun measurements for the middle and lower abdomen (middle and lower jiao) which includes the Kidney, Stomach, Spleen, Gall Bladder and Liver channels (lateral to the anterior median line) are: Ki 11 to Ki 21 = 0.5 cun; St 19 to St 30 = 2 cun; Sp 13 to Sp 16 = 6 cun (Sp 12 = 3.5 cun); GB 24 = 4 cun; Liv 14 = 4 cun.
e) Ki 16, St 25 and Sp 15 are all transversely level with the centre of the umbilicus and are used as reference points for marking their channels cun measurements.
f) The longitudinal measurement of the mid abdomen is 8 cun from the centre of the umbilicus to the xiphisternal joint.

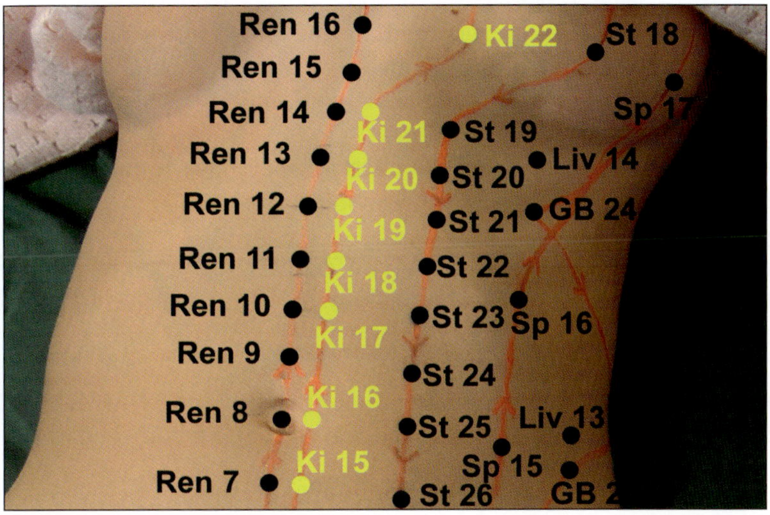

Tip:

a) Locate 0.5 cun lateral to the anterior median line at the level of the centre of the umbilicus and mark out the longitudinal measurement 6 cun superior to the centre of the umbilicus.

b) Place your finger on the anterior median line, (on Ren 14) at 6 cun superior to the level of the umbilicus, and run it laterally to 0.5 cun.

c) Lightly place the flat of your finger with the direction of the flow of the channel from the level of the centre of the umbilicus superiorly towards the chest (0.5 cun lateral to the anterior median line) to 6 cun (superior to the level of the centre of the umbilicus).

d) Palpation in this area should reveal the accurate location for Ki 21.

e) If the patient has a long xiphoid process then palpate for the point level with the cun measurement rather than with the Ren point (the length of the xiphoid affects only the Ren channel).

Note: Some acupuncture schools have used different transverse cun measurements at the level of the umbilicus: the Kidney channel has been put at 1.5 pouce/ACI, the Stomach channel at 2.5 or 3 pouce/ACI and the Spleen channel at 4 or 4.5 pouce/ACI. A few schools still do use these transverse measurements, but they still mainly have the same longitudinal measurements for their point locations as the majority use. Voisin (1974) locates K 21 on the Hypochondrium: a little below and laterally to the tip of the xiphoid process, below the cartilage uniting sixth and seventh ribs. Worsley (1982) locates IV 21 on the abdomen, 1.5 ACI (Anatomical Chinese Inch) lateral to the median line, 6 ACI superior to the level of the umbilicus, at the level of XIII 14 (Ren 14).

Wu (1973) locates KI 21 upon the abdomen (at one and one-half pouce from the median line), at six pouce above K 16. Lavier (1973) illustrates KI 21 as being located on the abdomen, transversely level with VC 14 (Ren 14), at 6 pouce above the level of the umbilicus, and at 1.5 pouce lateral to the anterior median line. Soulié (1994) locates KI 21 on the Epigastrium, base of the sternum: about one FW (Finger Width) on either side of the median line. Just at the lower opening of the joint of the seventh rib on the lower extremity of the sternum; in a hollow; on the rectus abdominis muscle.; one FW above KI 20; two FW under KI 22; three FW medial to ST 19; one FW lateral to CV 15 (Ren 15). Shandong (1982) locate Youmen at 1 cun above Pt. Abdomen-Tonggu (Ki 20).

The distance between the anterior median line and the contour linking the mid-point of the clavicle with the centre of the nipple (on a man) is 4 cun. The Kidney channel in the upper jiao is 2 cun lateral to the anterior median line.

The transverse measurement for the chest (upper jiao) is calculated as 8 cun from the anterior median line to the tip of the acromion process.

The transverse distance between the two nipples (on a man) is 8 cun. The distance between the bilateral Stomach channels at St 12 is also 8 cun, and can be used as a substitute measurement.

The transverse cun measurements for the upper jiao (chest) which includes the Kidney, Stomach, Spleen and Lung channels (lateral to the anterior median line) are as follows:

Ki 22 to Ki 27 = 2 cun
St 13 to St 18 = 4 cun
Sp 17 to Sp 20 = 6 cun
Lu 1 to Lu 2 = 6 cun

The longitudinal measurements of the anterior torso are:

9 cun from the xiphisternal joint to the suprasternal fossa (with the space between 2 ribs measuring approximately 1.6 cun in the lower chest, and 1 cun in the upper chest)
8 cun from the centre of the umbilicus to the xiphisternal joint

For the descriptions relating to the channels in the middle jiao, the longitudinal cun measurements are given from the centre of the umbilicus superiorly or from the xiphisternal joint inferiorly, depending on the direction of the flow of the channel.

5 cun from the centre of the umbilicus to the superior border of the symphysis pubis.

For the descriptions relating to the channels in the lower jiao, the longitudinal cun measurements are given from the centre of the umbilicus inferiorly or from the superior border of the symphysis pubis superiorly, depending on the direction of the flow of the channel.

Ki 22 BU LANG – WALKING ON THE VERANDAH

⊥ ***0.3 CUN*** Δ ***5***

- EXIT
- RE-UNION/Crossing/Meeting Point of the Kidney Channel with the Pericardium Channel – Foot Shao Yin Channel with the Hand Jue Yin Channel.

Pos: Position of patient: supine.

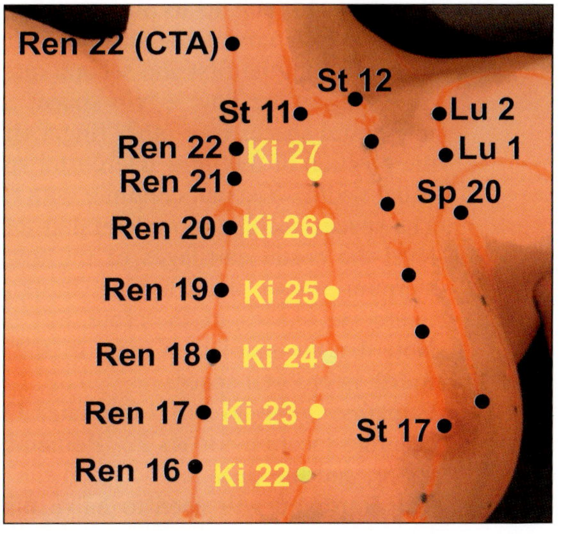

Loc:
a) On the anterior aspect of the torso.
b) On the chest (in the upper jiao).
c) In the fifth intercostal space.
d) 2 cun lateral to the anterior median line (Ren Mai).
e) Level with Ren 16 (Xiphisternal joint).

Cun:
a) The transverse cun measurements for the upper jiao (chest) includes the Kidney, Stomach, Spleen and Lung channels (lateral to the anterior median line). The cun measurements are as follows:
Ki 22 to Ki 27 = 2 cun; St 13 to St 18 = 4 cun; Sp 17 to Sp 20 = 6 cun and Lu 1 to Lu 2 = 6 cun.
b) The transverse measurement for the upper jiao is calculated using the anterior median line and the mid point of the clavicle.
c) Identify the mid point of the clavicle by locating the medial end of the clavicle at the sterno-clavicular joint and the lateral end of the acromioclavicular joint, and divide the distance by half.
d) The distance from the anterior median line to the mid point of the clavicle is 4 cun.
e) From the mid point of the clavicle divide in half again to give 2 cun and 6 cun measurements. The Kidney channel is 2 cun lateral to the anterior median line.
f) The transverse distance between the two nipples (on a man) is 8 cun, thus the distance from the anterior median line to the nipple is 4 cun.

Tip:
a) Without using cun measurements Ki 22 is located approximately halfway between the anterior median line and the nipples. Draw a vertical line from the halfway mark.
b) Locate the xiphisternal joint by simultaneously palpating along and up the medial borders of the left and right rib cages. The xiphisternal joint is located where the finger tips meet (on the anterior median line) at Ren 16.
c) Draw a horizontal line laterally from the xiphisternal joint. The fifth intercostal space is located where the vertical and horizontal lines intersect.

d) Palpate for Ki 22 in the deepest part of the fifth intercostal space.
e) If using the cun measurements locate 2 cun lateral to the anterior median line.
f) The Kidney channel follows the contours of the chest, especially the curvature of the breast on a woman as it travels down towards the nipple. The more 'flat chested' a person is the lesser the curvature is.
g) Place your finger in the fifth intercostal space between the fifth and sixth ribs and run laterally 2 cun. As you run your finger laterally the intercostal space begins to curve slightly upwards and you should be in the deepest part of the intercostal space
h) Palpation will locate the point accurately.
i) It can be difficult to locate the third intercostal space onwards as the pectoralis major muscle covers the surface of the ribs. To assist with point location place a finger in both the first and second intercostal space.
j) Your fingers are now a "rib space" apart. If you place one finger in the second intercostal space, your other finger should then give you a good approximation of the position of the third intercostal space (intercostal spaces are approximately of equal width). You can continue with this method of locating the intercostal spaces. The spaces become more lateral at the level of the fourth intercostal space. At this level the costal cartilages of the lower ribs can merge together to attach to the sternum rather than having individual articulations with the sternum. The intercostal spaces are therefore only easily palpable more laterally.
k) Note that the nipples on men or 'flat chested' women are generally located at the fourth intercostal space.
l) Palpation in the area of 2 cun lateral to the anterior median line should reveal the accurate location for Ki 22. Remember that the nipple lies in the 4th intercostal space, and the distance between the anterior median line to the nipple is 4 cun. Therefore you will need to halve this distance for Ki 22. There will be a slight lateral curvature on the Kidney channel as you mark the points from Ki 22 to Ki 27 towards the breast area.
m) Another way of identifying the intercostal spaces is to count them from the bottom of the rib cage upwards. For the 9th intercostal space (there are 9 intercostal spaces in total) palpate for the inferior border of the rib cage which will be the 10th rib. Place your finger in the intercostal space superior to this rib. You will now be in the 9th intercostal space.
n) When the 9th intercostal space has been established, place the flat of your index or middle finger in the 9th intercostal space and palpate for the 8th intercostal space by feeling for the superior border of the 9th rib. Once you have located the 9th rib, palpate superiorly until you feel a softness, which will be the 8th intercostal space. Use this procedure to palpate and locate the fifth intercostal space.
o) An easy way to remember which Kidney point lies in which intercostal space is to remember the formula: 27 minus Kidney point X equals intercostal space X. For example, 27 – Ki 22 = 5th intercostal space; 27 – Ki 26 = 1st intercostal space etc.
p) When needling Ki 22 do not be concerned with insertion in to breast tissue as the mammary gland will be further lateral. Be careful not to needle past the maximum needle depth as there is a risk of a pneumothorax.

Note: Voisin (1974) locates K 22 in relation to the sixth rib, upper border, 2-3 fb (finger breadth) from the midline. Huang (1993) locates Ki 22 in a depression one cun and six fen under Spirit Seal (Ki 23).

Ki 23 SHEN FENG – SPIRIT SEAL

⊥ *0.3 CUN* Δ *5*

Pos: Position of patient: supine.

Loc: a) On the anterior aspect of the torso.
b) On the chest (in the upper jiao).
c) In the fourth intercostal space.
d) 2 cun lateral to the anterior median line (Ren Mai).
e) Level with Ren 17.

Cun: a) The transverse cun measurements for the upper jiao (chest) includes the Kidney, Stomach, Spleen and Lung channels (lateral to the anterior median line). The cun measurements are as follows: Ki 22 to Ki 27 = 2 cun; St 13 to St 18 = 4 cun; Sp 17 to Sp 20 = 6 cun and Lu 1 to Lu 2 = 6 cun.

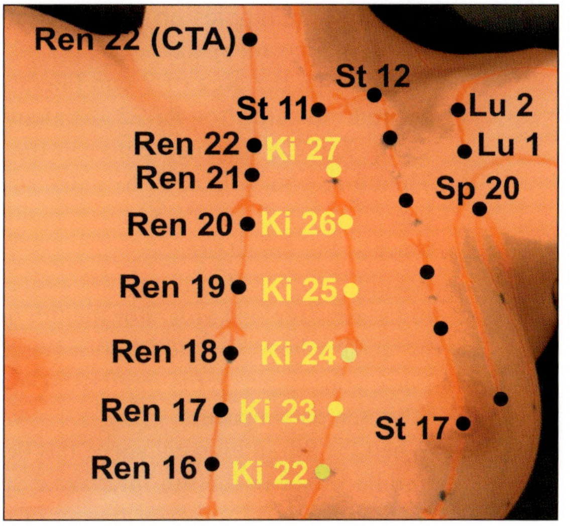

b) The transverse measurement for the upper jiao is calculated using the anterior median line and the mid point of the clavicle.
c) Identify the mid point of the clavicle by locating the medial end of the clavicle at the sterno-clavicular joint and the lateral end of the acromioclavicular joint, and divide the distance by half.
d) The distance from the anterior median line to the mid point of the clavicle is 4 cun.
e) From the mid point of the clavicle divide in half again to give 2 cun and 6 cun measurements. The Kidney channel is 2 cun lateral to the anterior median line.
f) The transverse distance between the two nipples (on a man) is 8 cun, thus the distance from the anterior median line to the nipple is 4 cun.

Tip: a) Without using cun measurements Ki 23 is located approximately halfway between the anterior median line and the nipples. Draw a vertical line from the halfway mark.
b) Palpate for Ki 23 in the deepest part of the fourth intercostal space.
c) If using the cun measurements locate 2 cun lateral to the anterior median line.
d) The Kidney channel follows the contours of the chest, especially the curvature of the breast on a woman as it travels down towards the nipple. The more 'flat chested' a person is the lesser the curvature is.
e) Place your finger in the fourth intercostal space between the fourth and fifth ribs and run laterally 2 cun. As you run your finger laterally the intercostal space begins to curve slightly upwards and you should be in the deepest part of the intercostal space
f) Palpation will locate the point accurately.

g) It can be difficult to locate the third intercostal space onwards as the pectoralis major muscle covers the surface of the ribs. To assist with point locationplace a finger in both the first and second intercostal space.

h) Your fingers are now a "rib space" apart. If you place one finger in the second intercostal space, your other finger should then give you a good approximation of the position of the third intercostal space (intercostal spaces are approximately of equal width). You can continue with this method of locating the intercostal spaces. The spaces become more lateral at the level of the fourth intercostal space. At this level the costal cartilages of the lower ribs can merge together to attach to the sternum rather than having individual articulations with the sternum. The intercostal spaces are therefore only easily palpable more laterally.

i) Note that the nipples on men or 'flat chested' women are generally located at the fourth intercostal space.

j) Palpation in the area of 2 cun lateral to the anterior median line should reveal the accurate location for Ki 22. Remember that the nipple lies in the 4th intercostal space, and the distance between the anterior median line to the nipple is 4 cun. Therefore you will need to halve this distance for Ki 23. There will be a slight lateral curvature on the Kidney channel as you mark the points from Ki 22 to Ki 27 towards the breast area.

k) Another way of identifying the intercostal spaces is to count them from the bottom of the rib cage upwards. For the 9th intercostal space (there are 9 intercostal spaces in total) palpate for the inferior border of the rib cage which will be the 10th rib. Place your finger in the intercostal space superior to this rib. You will now be in the 9th intercostal space.

l) When the 9th intercostal space has been established, place the flat of your index or middle finger in the 9th intercostal space and palpate for the 8th intercostal space by feeling for the superior border of the 9th rib. Once you have located the 9th rib, palpate superiorly until you feel a softness, which will be the 8th intercostal space. Use this procedure to palpate and locate the fifth intercostal space.

m) An easy way to remember which Kidney point lies in which intercostal space is to remember the formula: 27 minus Kidney point X equals intercostal space X.
For example, 27 – Ki 23 = 4th intercostal space; 27 – Ki 26 = 1st intercostal space etc.

n) When needling Ki 23 do not be concerned with insertion in to breast tissue as the mammary gland will be further lateral. Be careful not to needle past the maximum needle depth as there is a risk of a pneumothorax.

Note: Voisin (1974) locates K 23 in relation to the fifth rib, upper border, 2-3 fb (finger breadth) from the midline. Huang (1993) locates Ki 23 in a depression one cun and six fen under Spirit Homeland (Ki 24 – Spirit Buriel Ground).

Ki 24 LING SHU – SPIRIT BURIAL GROUND

⊥ ***0.3 CUN*** Δ ***5***

Pos: Position of patient: supine.

Loc:
a) On the anterior aspect of the torso.
b) On the chest (in the upper jiao).
c) In the third intercostal space.
d) 2 cun lateral to the anterior median line (Ren Mai).
e) Level with Ren 18.

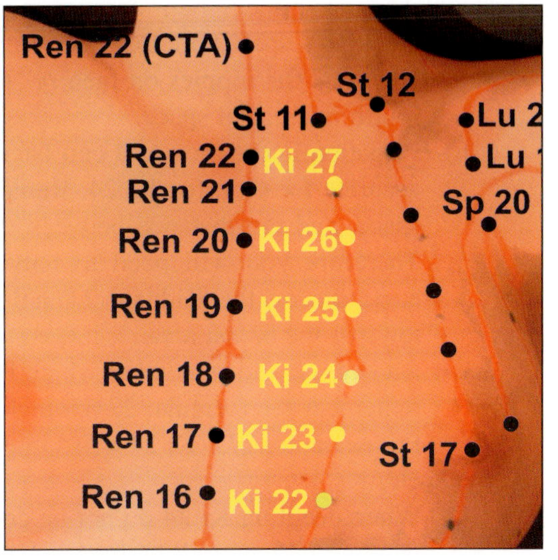

Cun:
a) The transverse cun measurements for the upper jiao (chest) includes the Kidney, Stomach, Spleen and Lung channels (lateral to the anterior median line). The cun measurements are as follows: Ki 22 to Ki 27 = 2 cun; St 13 to St 18 = 4 cun; Sp 17 to Sp 20 = 6 cun and Lu 1 to Lu 2 = 6 cun.
b) The transverse measurement for the upper jiao is calculated using the anterior median line and the mid point of the clavicle.
c) Identify the mid point of the clavicle by locating the medial end of the clavicle at the sterno-clavicular joint and the lateral end of the acromioclavicular joint, and divide the distance by half.
d) The distance from the anterior median line to the mid point of the clavicle is 4 cun.
e) From the mid point of the clavicle divide in half again to give 2 cun and 6 cun measurements. The Kidney channel is 2 cun lateral to the anterior median line.
f) The transverse distance between the two nipples (on a man) is 8 cun, thus the distance from the anterior median line to the nipple is 4 cun.

Tip:
a) Locate 2 cun lateral to the anterior median line and palpate for Ki 24 in the deepest part of the third intercostal space.
b) The Kidney channel follows the contours of the chest, especially the curvature of the breast on a woman as it travels down towards the nipple. The more 'flat chested' a person is the lesser the curvature is.
c) Place your finger in the third intercostal space between the third and fourth ribs and run laterally 2 cun. As you run your finger laterally the intercostal space begins to curve slightly upwards and you should be in the deepest part of the intercostal space
d) Palpation will locate the point accurately.
e) It can be difficult to locate the third intercostal space onwards as the pectoralis major muscle covers the surface of the ribs. To assist with point locationplace a finger in both the first and second intercostal space.

f) Your fingers are now a "rib space" apart. If you place one finger in the second intercostal space, your other finger should then give you a good approximation of the position of the third intercostal space (intercostal spaces are approximately of equal width). You can continue with this method of locating the intercostal spaces. The spaces become more lateral at the level of the fourth intercostal space. At this level the costal cartilages of the lower ribs can merge together to attach to the sternum rather than having individual articulations with the sternum. The intercostal spaces are therefore only easily palpable more laterally.
g) Note that the nipples on men or 'flat chested' women are generally located at the fourth intercostal space.
h) Palpation in the area of 2 cun lateral to the anterior median line should reveal the accurate location for Ki 24. Remember that the nipple lies in the 4th intercostal space, and the distance between the anterior median line to the nipple is 4 cun. Therefore you will need to halve this distance. There will be a slight lateral curvature on the Kidney channel as you mark the points from Ki 22 to Ki 27 towards the breast area.
i) An easy way to remember which Kidney point lies in which intercostal space is to remember the formula: 27 minus Kidney point X equals intercostal space X.
For example, 27 – Ki 24 = 3rd intercostal space; 27 – Ki 26 = 1st intercostal space etc.
j) When needling Ki 24 do not be concerned with insertion in to breast tissue as the mammary gland will be further lateral. Be careful not to needle past the maximum needle depth as there is a risk of a pneumothorax.

Note: Voisin (1974) locates K 24 in relation to the fourth rib, upper border, 2-3 fb (finger breadth) from the midline. Huang (1993) locates Ki 24 in a depression one cun and six fen below Spirit Storehouse (Ki 25).

Ki 25 SHEN CANG – SPIRIT STOREHOUSE

⊥ ***0.3 CUN*** **Δ *5***

Pos: Position of patient: supine.

Loc: a) On the anterior aspect of the torso.
b) On the chest (in the upper jiao).
c) In the second intercostal space.
d) 2 cun lateral to the anterior median line (Ren Mai).
e) Level with Ren 19.

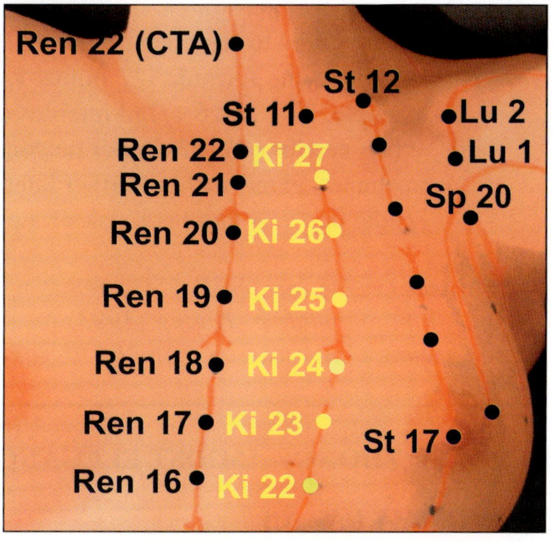

Cun: a) The transverse cun measurements for the upper jiao (chest) includes the Kidney, Stomach, Spleen and Lung channels (lateral to the anterior median line). The cun measurements are as follows:
Ki 22 to Ki 27 = 2 cun; St 13 to St 18 = 4 cun; Sp 17 to Sp 20 = 6 cun and Lu 1 to Lu 2 = 6 cun.
b) The transverse measurement for the upper jiao is calculated using the anterior median line and the mid point of the clavicle.
c) Identify the mid point of the clavicle by locating the medial end of the clavicle at the sterno-clavicular joint and the lateral end of the acromioclavicular joint, and divide the distance by half.
d) The distance from the anterior median line to the mid point of the clavicle is 4 cun.
e) From the mid point of the clavicle divide in half again to give 2 cun and 6 cun measurements. The Kidney channel is 2 cun lateral to the anterior median line.
f) The transverse distance between the two nipples (on a man) is 8 cun, thus the distance from the anterior median line to the nipple is 4 cun.

Tip: a) Locate 2 cun lateral to the anterior median line and palpate for Ki 25 in the deepest part of the second intercostal space.
b) The Kidney channel follows the contours of the chest, especially the curvature of the breast on a woman as it travels down towards the nipple. The more 'flat chested' a person is the lesser the curvature is.
c) Place your finger in the second intercostal space between the second and third ribs and run laterally 2 cun. As you run your finger laterally the intercostal space begins to curve slightly upwards and you should be in the deepest part of the intercostal space
d) Palpation will locate the point accurately.

e) Note that the nipples on men or 'flat chested' women are generally located at the fourth intercostal space.

f) Palpation in the area of 2 cun lateral to the anterior median line should reveal the accurate location for Ki 25. Remember that the nipple lies in the 4th intercostal space, and the distance between the anterior median line to the nipple is 4 cun. Therefore you will need to halve this distance. There will be a slight lateral curvature on the Kidney channel as you mark the points from Ki 22 to Ki 27 towards the breast area.

g) An easy way to remember which Kidney point lies in which intercostal space is to remember the formula: 27 minus Kidney point X equals intercostal space X. For example, 27 – Ki 25 = 2nd intercostal space; 27 – Ki 26 = 1st intercostal space etc.

h) When needling Ki 25 do not be concerned with insertion in to breast tissue as the mammary gland will be further lateral. Be careful not to needle past the maximum needle depth as there is a risk of a pneumothorax.

Note: Voisin (1974) locates K 25 in relation to the third rib, upper border, 2-3 fb (finger breadth) from the midline. Huang (1993) locates Ki 25 in a depression one cun and six fen below Thriving Center (Ki 26 – Amidst Elegance).

Ki 26 YU ZHONG – AMIDST ELEGANCE

⊥ ***0.3 CUN*** Δ 5

Pos: Position of patient: supine.

Loc:
a) On the anterior aspect of the torso.
b) On the chest (in the upper jiao).
c) In the first intercostal space.
d) 2 cun lateral to the anterior median line (Ren Mai).
e) Level with Ren 20.

Cun:
a) The transverse cun measurements for the upper jiao (chest) includes the Kidney, Stomach, Spleen and Lung channels (lateral to the anterior median line). The cun measurements are as follows: Ki 22 to Ki 27 = 2 cun; St 13 to St 18 = 4 cun; Sp 17 to Sp 20 = 6 cun and Lu 1 to Lu 2 = 6 cun.
b) The transverse measurement for the upper jiao is calculated using the anterior median line and the mid point of the clavicle.

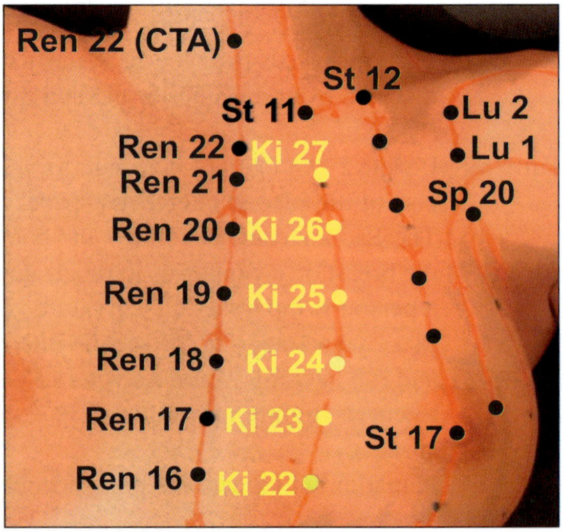

c) Identify the mid point of the clavicle by locating the medial end of the clavicle at the sterno-clavicular joint and the lateral end of the acromioclavicular joint, and divide the distance by half.
d) The distance from the anterior median line to the mid point of the clavicle is 4 cun.
e) From the mid point of the clavicle divide in half again to give 2 cun and 6 cun measurements. The Kidney channel is 2 cun lateral to the anterior median line.
f) The transverse distance between the two nipples (on a man) is 8 cun, thus the distance from the anterior median line to the nipple is 4 cun.

Tip: a) Locate 2 cun lateral to the anterior median line and palpate for Ki 26 in the deepest part of the first intercostal space.
b) The Kidney channel follows the contours of the chest, especially the curvature of the breast on a woman as it travels down towards the nipple. The more 'flat chested' a person is the lesser the curvature is.
c) Place your finger in the first intercostal space between the first and second ribs and run laterally 2 cun. As you run your finger laterally the intercostal space begins to curve slightly upwards and you should be in the deepest part of the intercostal space
d) Palpation will locate the point accurately.
e) Note that the nipples on men or 'flat chested' women are generally located at the fourth intercostal space.
f) Palpation in the area of 2 cun lateral to the anterior median line should reveal the accurate location for Ki 26. Remember that the nipple lies in the 4th intercostal space, and the distance between the anterior median line to the nipple is 4 cun. Therefore you will need to halve this distance. There will be a slight lateral curvature on the Kidney channel as you mark the points from Ki 22 to Ki 27 towards the breast area.
g) An easy way to remember which Kidney point lies in which intercostal space is to remember the formula: 27 minus Kidney point X equals intercostal space X.
For example, 27 – Ki 26 = 1st intercostal space; 27 – Ki 22 = 5th intercostal space; etc.
h) When needling Ki 26 do not be concerned with insertion in to breast tissue as the mammary gland will be further lateral. Be careful not to needle past the maximum needle depth as there is a risk of a pneumothorax.

Note: Voisin (1974) locates K 26 in relation to the second rib, upper border, 2-3 fb (finger breadth) from the midline. Huang (1993) locates Ki 26 in a depression one cun and six fen below Transport Mansion (Ki 27 – Store House).

Ki 27 SHU FU – STORE HOUSE

⊥ ***0.3 CUN*** Δ ***5***

Pos: Position of patient: supine.

Loc: a) On the anterior aspect of the torso.
b) On the chest (in the upper jiao).
c) In the depression between the lower border of the sternal end of the clavicle and the upper border of the first rib.
d) 2 cun lateral to the anterior median line (Ren Mai).
e) Level with Ren 21.

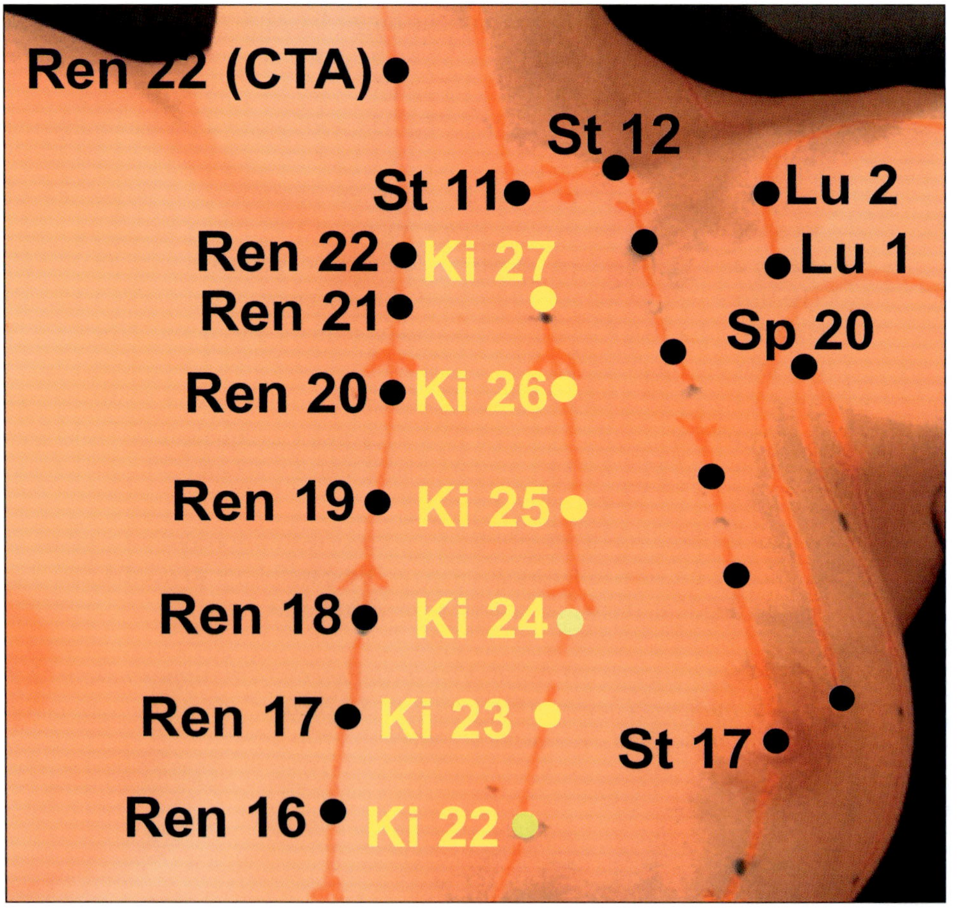

Cun: a) The transverse cun measurements for the upper jiao (chest) includes the Kidney, Stomach, Spleen and Lung channels (lateral to the anterior median line). The cun measurements are as follows:
Ki 22 to Ki 27 = 2 cun; St 13 to St 18 = 4 cun; Sp 17 to Sp 20 = 6 cun and Lu 1 to Lu 2 = 6 cun.

b) The transverse measurement for the upper jiao is calculated using the anterior median line and the mid point of the clavicle.

c) Identify the mid point of the clavicle by locating the medial end of the clavicle at the sterno-clavicular joint and the lateral end of the acromioclavicular joint, and divide the distance by half.

d) The distance from the anterior median line to the mid point of the clavicle is 4 cun.

e) From the mid point of the clavicle divide in half again to give 2 cun and 6 cun measurements. The Kidney channel is 2 cun lateral to the anterior median line.

f) The transverse distance between the two nipples (on a man) is 8 cun, thus the distance from the anterior median line to the nipple is 4 cun.

Tip: a) Locate 2 cun lateral to the anterior median line.

b) Place your finger on the sternal end of the clavicle and run your finger laterally along the superior border of the clavicle until you are able to palpate a notch which is to cun lateral to the anterior median line.

c) Place the finger between the clavicle and the first rib and run laterally 2 cun level with the notch (on the sternal aspect of the superior border of the clavicle).

d) It may be difficult feeling for the first rib as it only palpable at the sternal end of the clavicle.

e) Palpation 2 cun lateral to the anterior median line should reveal a small gap between the inferior border of the clavicle and the superior border of the first rib.

f) An easy way to remember which Kidney point lies in which intercostal space is to remember the formula: 27 minus Kidney point X equals intercostal space X.
For example, 27 – Ki 27 = no intercostal space; 27 – Ki 22 = 5th intercostal space; etc.

g) When needling Ki 27 be careful not to needle past the maximum needle depth as there is a risk of a pneumothorax.

Note: Voisin (1974) locates K 27 in relation to the clavicle, lower border, 2 fb (finger breadth) from the midline. Huang (1993) locates Ki 27 in a depression under the clavicle two cun bilateral to Turning Pivot (Ren 21 – Pearl Jade).

REFERENCES FOR THE KIDNEY CHANNEL

Wu, Wei-P'ing 1973 Chinese Acupuncture – KI 1: 98; KI 2: 98; KI 3: 98; KI 4: 99; KI 5: 99; KI 6: 99; KI 7: 99; KI 8: 99; KI 9: 99; KI 10: 100; KI 11: 100; KI 12: 100; KI 13: 100; KI 14: 100; KI 15: 100; KI 16: 101; KI 17: 101; KI 18: 101; KI 19: 101; KI 20: 101; KI 21: 101

Worsley, J R 1982 Traditional Chinese Acupuncture Volume 1 – Meridians and Points. IV 1: 95; IV 3: 95; IV 4: 95; IV 5: 95; IV 6: 97; IV 7: 97; IV 8: 97; IV 9: 97; IV 11: 99; IV 12: 99; IV 13: 99; IV 14: 99; IV 15: 101; IV 16: 101; IV 17: 101; IV 18: 101; IV 19: 103; IV 20: 103; IV 21: 103

Voisin, Dr. H 1974 Essentials of Acupuncture – K 1: 70; K 2: 70; K 5 (Ki 3): 70; K 6 (Ki 4): 70; K 4 (Ki 5): 70; K 3 (Ki 6): 70; K 7: 70; K 8: 70; K 9: 70; K 10: 70; K 11: 70; K 12: 70; K 13: 70; K 14: 72; K 15: 72; K 16: 72; K 17: 72; K 18: 72; K 19: 72; K 20: 72; K 21: 72; K 22: 72; K 23: 72; K 23: 72; K 24: 72; K 25: 72; K 26: 72; K 27: 72

Legge, David 1999 Acupuncture Points and Meridians – Ki 1: 63;

Soulié De Morant, George. 1994 Chinese Acupuncture – KI 1: 442; KI 2: 443; KI 5 (Ki 3): 445; KI 6 (Ki 4): 446; KI 4 (Ki 5): 445; KI 3 (Ki 6): 444; KI 7: 447; KI 8 447; KI 9: 448; KI 10: 449; KI 11: 449; KI 12: 450; KI 13: 450; KI 14: 451; KI 15: 451; KI 16: 452; KI 17: 452; KI 18: 453; KI 19: 454; KI 20: 454; KI 21: 454

Li Ding (Prof.). 1991. Acupuncture, Meridian Theory and Acupuncture Points – K 1: 323

So, James Tin Yau (Dr) 1985 The Book of Acupuncture Points: KI 1: 141; KI 6: 144; KI 8: 146; KI 9: 196; KI 10: 197

Yang Jiasan (Prof) 1982 The Way to Locate Acu-Points – K 1: 58; K 2: 58

Lawson-Wood 1973 Acupuncture Handbook – IV 1: 36; IV 3: 44; IV 4: 52; IV 7: 28; IV 11: 17

Huang-fu Mi. Trans: Yang Shou-zhong and Charles Chace 1993 The Systematic Classic of Acupuncture & Moxibustion – Ki 1: 188; Ki 22: 157; Ki 23: 157; Ki 24: 156: Ki 25: 156; Ki 26: 156; Ki 27: 156

Masayoshi Hyodo 1975 Ryodoraku Acupuncture – KI 1: 51; KI 2: 51; KI 3: 51; KI 6: 51; KI 7: 51; KI 9: 51

Deadman, Peter; Al-Khafaji, Mazin; Baker, Kevin 1998 Manual of Acupuncture, An – KID 2: 338; KID 9: 349

Eachou Chen 1995 Cross-sectional Anatomy of Acupoints – KI 2: 91; KI 6: 87; KI 9: 78; KI 10: 64/65

Shanghai College of Traditional Chinese Medicine. 1993 Applied Anatomical Charts of Acupuncture and Moxibustion – KI 2: 102; KI 9: 106

Academy of Traditional Chinese Medicine, The. 1975 – Outline of Chinese Acupuncture, An. K 2: 157; K 9: 158

Lavier, Dr. J 1974 Points of Chinese Acupuncture – KI 3: 47; KI 4: 47; KI 5: 47; KI 7: 39; KI 8: 39; KI 9: 39; KI 11: 53; KI 12: 53; KI 13: 53; KI 14: 53; KI 15: 53; KI 16: 51/53; KI 17: 51; KI 18: 51; KI 19: 51; KI 20: 51; KI 21: 51

Shandong Medical College and Shandong College of Traditional Chinese Medicine 1982 Anatomical Atlas of Chinese Acupuncture Points – Dazhong (Ki 4): 39; Zhubin (Ki 9): 39; Qixue (Ki 13): 39; Siman (Ki 14): 39; Abdomen-Zhongzhu (Ki 15): 39; Huangshu (Ki 16): 40; Shangqu (Ki 17): 40 (Illustration: 37); Shiguan (Ki 18): 40; Yindu (Ki 19): 40; Abdomen-Tonggu (Ki 20): 40; Youmen (Ki 21): 40

Lotan, Alon 2000 Acupoint Location Guide – K 8: 105; K 9: 105

Qiu Mao-Liang 1996 – Chinese Acupuncture and Moxibustion – K 6: 120; K 9: 120

Cheng Xinnong (Editor) 1987 Chinese Acupuncture and Moxibustion – K 9: 183

Shanghai College of Traditional Medicine 1981 Acupuncture – A Comprehensive Text – K 9: 294;

Ellis, Wiseman and Boss. 1991 Fundamentals of Chinese Acupuncture – KI 9: 253; KI 10: 253

Katsusuke Serizawa 1983 Tsubo – Vital Points for Oriental Therapy – KI 9: 211;

THE PERICARDIUM CHANNEL OF THE HAND (JUE YIN)

Primary Channel

The Pericardium channel starts deep in the thorax, attached to the pericardium. A deep channel enters the heart tissue then travels to Ren 17 and down the median line, connecting with Ren 12 and Ren 7 (i.e. the upper/middle/lower regions of the Triple Heater).

A lateral deep branch travels from the pericardium across the chest, to emerge at Pc 1 where the channel becomes superficial. It ascends to the axilla, then follows the medial aspect of the arm down to Pc 8 on the palm. One branch goes from Pc 8 to the radial side of the middle finger (Pc 9), one channel connects with TH 1 at the ulnar side of the ring finger.

(Some texts also mention a deep branch rising from the pericardium up through the throat to the ear, to join the Triple Heater channel at TH 16.)

Divergent Channel

After leaving the primary channel at a point 3 cun inferior to the axilla, it enters the chest and communicates with the Triple Heater channel. A branch ascends to pass across the throat and emerge behind the ear, where it joins the Triple Heater channel again.

Connecting Channel

This leaves the primary channel at Pc 6, and spreads out between the tendons of the forearm, following the Pericardium channel up to the pericardium and then to the heart.

Muscle Channel

This begins on the palmar aspect of the third digit and accompanies the Lung muscle channel upwards, binding at the medial aspect of the elbow and again below the axilla. It then descends to spread over the ribs, both front and back. A branch enters the body below the axilla, and spreads over the chest, binding with the diaphragm.

THE PERICARDIUM CHANNEL OF THE HAND

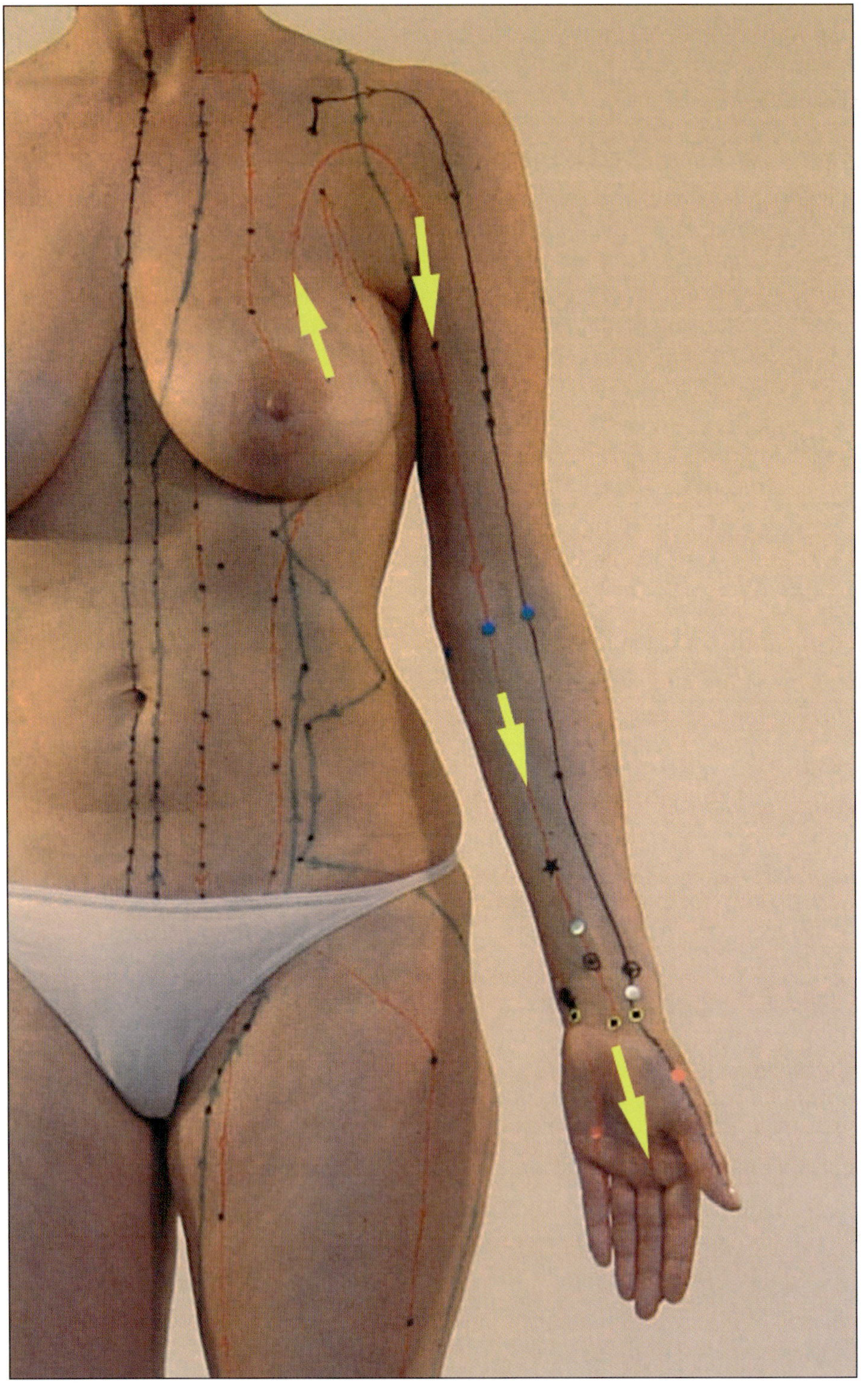

Points of the Pericardium Channel – Hand Jue Yin

(Pc/P/Per/PC/HP/HC/Cx/V) Also known as Heart Protector, Circulation-Sex and Heart Constrictor Channels

To locate the Pericardium channel the arm must be in the anatomical position. Pc 1 is on the anterior torso, Pc 2 on the anterior aspect of the upper arm.

Pc 1 TIAN CHI – HEAVENLY POND

⊥ ***0.3 CUN (MEN)*** **Δ** ***3 TO 5 (MEN)***
FORBIDDEN TO NEEDLE AND MOXA ON WOMEN

- ENTRY (On Males Only)
- WINDOW OF THE SKY/Window of Heaven (On Males Only)
- RE-UNION/Crossing/Meeting Point of the Pericardium Channel with the Kidney, Gall Bladder and Liver Channels – Hand Jue Yin Channel with the Foot Shao Yin, Foot Shao Yang and Foot Jue Yin Channels.

Pos: Position of patient: supine, in the anatomical position (arms at the side and flat on the couch with the palms facing upwards).

Loc: a) On the anterior torso.
b) On the chest (in the upper jiao).
c) 1 cun lateral to the centre of the nipple.
d) In the 4th intercostal space.

Tip: a) Forbidden to needle on women (mammary gland).
b) Sometimes this point is not level with the nipple as the 4th intercostal space may begin to curve upwards as it runs laterally toward the spine. On some men the point is located higher than the centre of the nipple.
c) The transverse measurement between the two nipples (on a man) is 8 cun, therefore you can divide down to 1 cun and use this to mark 1 cun lateral to the centre of the nipple.
d) 1 cun lateral to the centre of the nipple is a guide for locating this point but palpation is more important for accuracy.

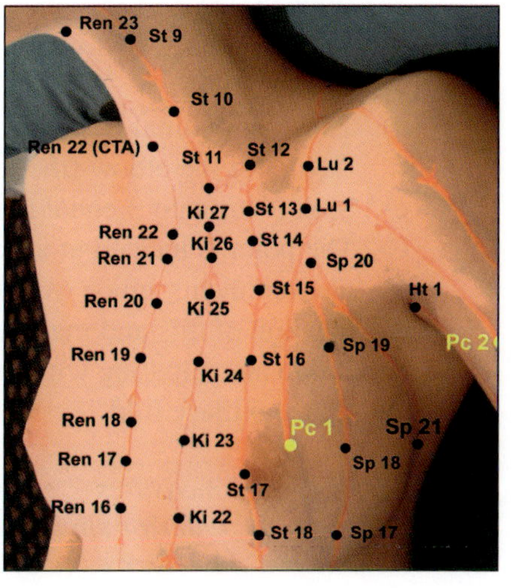

Note: Lawson-Wood (1973) lists this point as an Alarm point for V – the Circulation-Sexfield (Pericardium) as well as IV 11 (Ki 11). Shandong (1982) locate Tianchi as our location for men. They also include a location for women: In the 4th intercostal space, 1 cun lateral to the mid-clavicular line.

Pc 2 TIAN QUAN – HEAVENLY SPRING

⊥ ***0.5 TO 0.7 CUN*** Δ ***3***

- ENTRY (On Women Only)
- WINDOW OF THE SKY/Window of Heaven

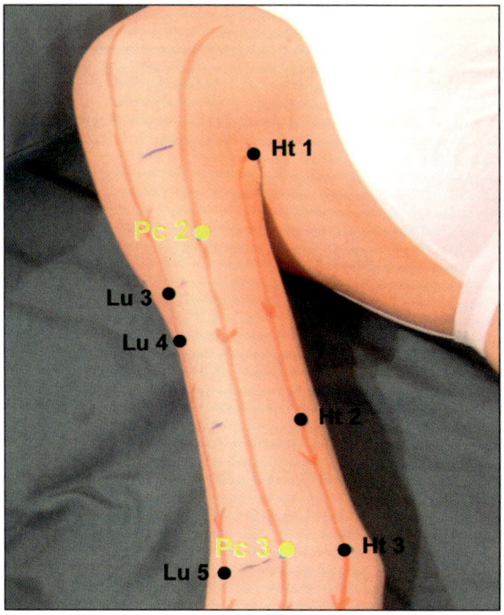

Pos: Position of patient: supine, in the anatomical position (arms at the side and flat on the couch with the palms facing upwards).

Loc:
a) On the anterior surface of the upper arm.
b) Between the two muscle bellies of the biceps brachii muscle.
c) 7 cun proximal to the flexure of the elbow (transverse cubital crease).
d) 2 cun distal to the axillary fold.

Tip:
a) Flexing the elbow against resistance should expose the two heads of the biceps brachii muscle.
b) Once you have felt for this muscle, relax the arm and run your finger down from the shoulder towards the elbow, you should be able to feel the two separate heads of the biceps brachii.
c) With the arm in the anatomical position, run your finger along the Pericardium channel with the direction of flow along the centre of the anterior surface of the upper arm.
d) The longitudinal distance between the anterior end of the axillary fold and the flexure of the elbow (the transverse cubital crease) is measured as 9 cun.
e) Split 9 cun into 3 equal measurements.
f) The point is located at approximately 7 cun proximal to the elbow crease. The cun measurements guide you to the area, then palpation gives you the accuracy for location of this and many other points.
g) If you are palpating with the flow of the channel, Pc 2 is approximately 2 cun distal to the axillary fold.

Note: Lavier (1974) measures 7 pouce from the elbow fold to the deltoid 'V'. Soulié (1994) locates PC 2 on the anterior shoulder: one FW (Finger Width) medial to the axillary fold; at the angle between the lower edge of the second rib (under the clavicle) and the lateral edge of the pectoralis major and, deeper, the pectoralis minor; in a hollow; on the lateral edge of a vertical muscle (coracobrachialis); two FW below LU 1. Voisin (1974) locates P 2 on the biceps, medial border; slightly below the nipple level.

Pc 3 on the anterior aspect of the flexure of the elbow and is usually medial to the tendon of the biceps brachii muscle.

Pc 3 QU ZE – CROOKED MARSH

⊥ ***0.3 TO 0.5 CUN*** Δ ***3 TO 5***

- WATER
- HE – SEA/Shu – Transporting/Antique

Pos: Position of patient: supine, in the anatomical position (arms at the side and flat on the couch with the palms facing upwards).

Loc: a) On the anterior surface of the forearm.
b) On the anterior flexure of the elbow.
c) At the mid-point of the elbow crease (transverse cubital crease).
d) Medial to the tendon of the biceps brachii muscle, when the arm is slightly flexed.

Tip: a) To expose the flexure of the elbow (transverse cubital crease) flex the arm and then draw a line along the formed crease.
b) If more than one crease is exposed, it is usually the most prominent one that is used.
c) To expose the tendon of the biceps brachii muscle, flex the elbow against resistance.
d) If you run your finger with the flow of the channel along the medial border of the biceps brachii, your finger should naturally fall into a hollow at the elbow flexure which is medial to the tendon of the biceps brachii .
e) Where the channel follows the anatomy this will determine the position of the point relative to the medial aspect of the tendon and the medial epicondyle of the humerus.
f) To reduce patient discomfort when needling this point it is important that you support the arm slightly flexed.

Note: Worsley (1982) locates as above, he also states that on some people the point can be lateral to the tendon of the biceps brachii muscle. Wu (1973) locates HC 3 in the crease formed by the flexure of the arm, inside the tendon of the biceps.

Pc 4-6 are located on the anterior aspect of the forearm.

Pc 4-7 should always lie between the ulna and radius bones and between the tendons of the palmaris longus and flexor carpi radialis muscles.

The distance between the flexure of the elbow and the flexure of the wrist is measured as 12 cun. To find the flexure of the wrist, flex and extend the hand and palpate for the articulation.

Pc 4 XI MEN – GATE OF QI RESERVE

⊥ ***0.3 TO 0.5 CUN*** **Δ** ***3 TO 5***

- ACCUMULATION/Xi Cleft/Gueki

Pos: Position of patient: supine, in the anatomical position (arms at the side and flat on the couch with the palms facing upwards).

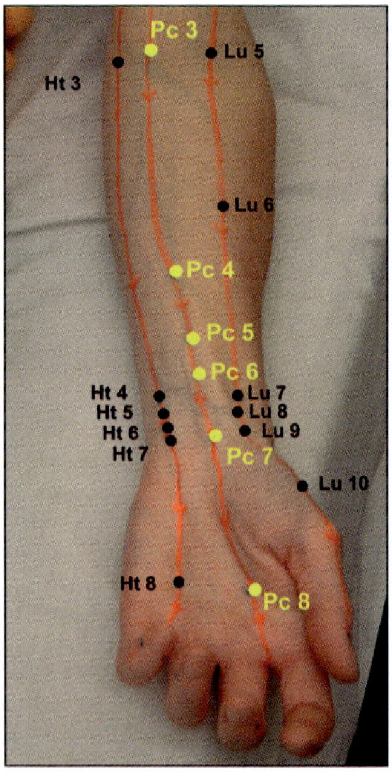

Loc:
a) On the anterior surface of the forearm.
b) Between the ulna and radius bones.
c) On the line connecting Pc 3 to Pc 7.
d) Between the tendons of the flexor carpi radialis and palmaris longus muscles.
e) 5 cun proximal to the flexure of the wrist at Pc 7.

Tip:
a) The tendons of the flexor carpi radialis and the palmaris longus muscles run parallel to each other along the anterior forearm. These tendons lie at the anterior midline of the wrist flexure but diverge medially where they insert at the flexure of the elbow (medial epicondyle of the humerus).
b) The tendon of the flexor carpi radialis muscle is lateral to the tendon of the palmaris longus muscle.
c) You will be in between these two tendons if you run your finger with the flow of the channel from Pc 3 on the elbow flexure to the wrist flexure.
d) You may be able to feel the seam formed by these muscles as these tendons are not always palpable this far proximal as they graduate in to muscle.
e) The tendon of the palmaris longus muscle is absent in a small percentage of the population. If this is the case then you will need to locate the medial border of the tendon of the flexor carpi radialis muscle as a landmark.
f) The distance between Pc 3 and Pc 7 is 12 cun, this point is 5 cun proximal to Pc 7.
g) Once you have marked the 5 cun measurement, palpate for the point.

Note: Soulié (1994) locates PC 4 on the anterior part of the forearm (palm up, in supination): six FW (Finger Width) above the wrist; about mid-width; at the angle between the lower edge of a transverse mass and the radial (lateral) edge of a large tendon of the flexor; ulnar edge of the flexor carpi radialis; in a hollow; six FW below PC 3; two FW above PC 5; one FW medial to LU 6; three FW lateral to SI 8. voisin (1974) locates P 4 on the forearm, anterior aspect: slightly above centre between folds of elbow flexion and wrist flexion.

Pc 5 JIAN SHI – THE INTERMEDIARY

⊥ ***0.3 TO 0.5 CUN*** **Δ** ***3 TO 5***

- METAL
- JING – RIVER/Shu – Transporting/Antique
- RE-UNION/Crossing/Meeting Point of the Three Yin (Arm) Channels: Pericardium, Heart and Lung Hand Jue Yin, Hand Shao Yin and Hand Tai Yin Channels
- SUN SI-MIAO GHOST (Gui) – Ghost Point Name: Gui Cu – Ghost in the Cave or Ghost Road (Pc 8 is commonly known as Gui Cu)

Pos: Position of patient: supine, in the anatomical position (arms at the side and flat on the couch with the palms facing upwards).

Loc: a) On the anterior surface of the forearm.
b) Between the ulna and radius bones.
c) On the line connecting Pc 3 to Pc 7.
d) Between the tendons of the flexor carpi radialis and palmaris longus muscles.
e) 3 cun proximal to the flexure of the wrist at Pc 7.

Tip: a) The tendons of the flexor carpi radialis and the palmaris longus muscles run parallel to each other along the anterior forearm. These tendons lie at the anterior midline of the wrist flexure but diverge medially where they insert at the flexure of the elbow (medial epicondyle of the humerus) .
b) To demonstrate the tendon of the flexor carpi radialis muscle and the tendon of the palmaris longus muscle, ask the patient to contract the muscles of the hand by making a claw shape, or to attempt to raise the forearm against resistance applied to the palm of the hand, all the while keeping the wrist straight.
c) The tendon of the flexor carpi radialis muscle is lateral to the tendon of the palmaris longus muscle.
d) You will be in between these two tendons if you run your finger with the flow of the channel from Pc 3 on the elbow flexure to the wrist flexure .
e) You may be able to feel the seam formed by these muscles as these tendons are not always palpable this far proximal as they graduate in to muscle.
f) The tendon of the palmaris longus muscle is absent in a small percentage of the population. If this is the case then you will need to locate the medial border of the tendon of the flexor carpi radialis muscle as a landmark.
g) The distance between Pc 3 and Pc 7 is 12 cun, this point is 3 cun proximal to Pc 7.
h) Once you have marked the 3 cun measurement, palpate for the point.

Pc 6 NEI GUAN – INNER FRONTIER GATE

⊥ ***0.3 TO 0.5 CUN*** **Δ** ***3 TO 5***

- JUNCTION/Luo/Connecting/Passage/Lo/Lê
- 8 EXTRAORDINARY CHANNELS CONFLUENT/8 Extraordinary Meridians Confluent/8 Extraordinary Vessels Opening/Master Point of the of the Yin Linking Vessel (Yin Wei Mai)
- 8 EXTRAORDINARY VESSEL/Coupled Point of the Penetrating Vessel (Chong Mai)
- RE-UNION/Crossing/Meeting Point of the Pericardium Channel with the Triple Heater Channel – Hand Jue Yin Channel with the Hand Shao Yang Channel
- HOST/GUEST COMBINATION – Source Point with the Junction Point of its Paired Official/Organ Therefore Pc 6 is combined with TH 4

Pos: Position of patient: supine, in the anatomical position (arms at the side and flat on the couch with the palms facing upwards).

Loc: a) On the anterior surface of the forearm.
b) Between the ulna and radius bones.
c) On the line connecting Pc 3 to Pc 7.
d) Between the tendons of the flexor carpi radialis and palmaris longus muscles.
e) 2 cun proximal to the flexure of the wrist at Pc 7.

Tip: a) The tendons of the flexor carpi radialis and the palmaris longus muscles run parallel to each other along the anterior forearm. These tendons lie at the anterior midline of the wrist flexure but diverge medially where they insert at the flexure of the elbow (medial epicondyle of the humerus) .
b) To demonstrate the tendon of the flexor carpi radialis muscle and the tendon of the palmaris longus muscle, ask the patient to contract the muscles of the hand by making a claw shape, or to attempt to raise the forearm against resistance applied to the palm of the hand, all the while keeping the wrist straight.
c) The tendon of the flexor carpi radialis muscle is lateral to the tendon of the palmaris longus muscle.
d) You will be in between these two tendons if you run your finger with the flow of the channel from Pc 3 on the elbow flexure to the wrist flexure.

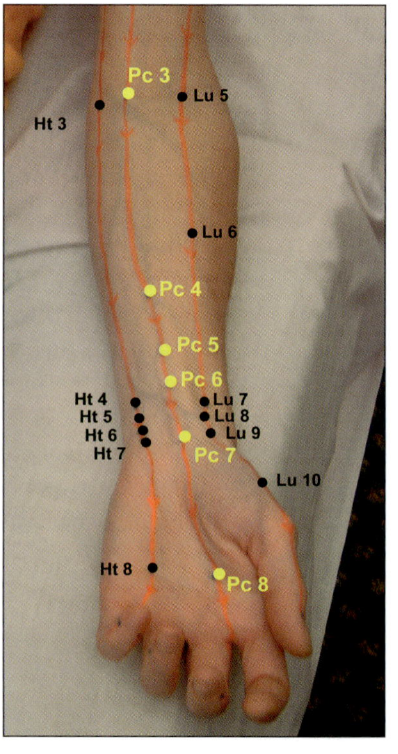

e) You may be able to feel the seam formed by these muscles as these tendons are not always palpable this far proximal as they graduate in to muscle.
f) The tendon of the palmaris longus muscle is absent in a small percentage of the population. If this is the case then you will need to locate the medial border of the tendon of the flexor carpi radialis muscle as a landmark.
g) The distance between Pc 3 and Pc 7 is 12 cun, this point is 2 cun proximal to Pc 7.
h) Once you have marked the 2 cun measurement, palpate for the point.

Note: Voisin (1974) locates P 6 on the forearm, anterior aspect: 3 fb above the wrist flexion fold.

Pc 7 on the anterior aspect of the flexure of the wrist.

Pc 7 DA LING – GREAT MOUND

⊥ ***0.3 CUN*** **Δ *3***

- SOURCE/Yuan/Regulator/Primary
- EARTH
- SEDATION/Reducing/Dispersing
- CHILD
- SHU – STREAM/Shu – Transporting/Antique
- HOST/GUEST COMBINATION – Source Point with the Junction Point of its Paired Official/Organ Therefore Pc 7 is combined with TH 5
- SUN SI-MIAO GHOST (Gui) – Ghost Point Name: Gui Xin – Ghost Heart (Less common is Lu 9)

Pos: Position of patient: supine, in the anatomical position (arms at the side and flat on the couch with the palms facing upwards).

Loc: a) On the anterior surface of the forearm.
b) On the line connecting Pc 3 to Pc 7.
c) At the centre of the flexure of the wrist.
d) Between the tendons of the flexor carpi radialis and palmaris longus muscles.
e) On the proximal ulnar corner of the scaphoid bone.

Tip: a) The tendons of the flexor carpi radialis and the palmaris longus muscles run parallel to each other along the anterior forearm. These tendons lie at the anterior midline of the wrist flexure but diverge medially where they insert at the flexure of the elbow (medial epicondyle of the humerus).
b) To demonstrate the tendon of the flexor carpi radialis muscle and the tendon of the palmaris longus muscle, ask the patient to contract the muscles of the hand by making a claw shape, or to attempt to raise the forearm against resistance applied to the palm of the hand, all the while keeping the wrist straight.

c) The tendon of the flexor carpi radialis muscle is lateral to the tendon of the palmaris longus muscle.
d) You will be in between these two tendons if you run your finger with the flow of the channel from Pc 3 on the elbow flexure to the wrist flexure .
e) You may be able to feel the seam formed by these muscles as these tendons are not always palpable this far proximal as they graduate in to muscle.
f) The tendon of the palmaris longus muscle is absent in a small percentage of the population. If this is the case then you will need to locate the medial border of the tendon of the flexor carpi radialis muscle as a landmark.
g) To locate the flexure of the wrist, flex and extend the hand (sometimes near the centre of the most distal skin crease) to find the hinge of the joint.
h) You may need to flex and extend the patients hand when you are palpating for this point.

Note: Soulié (1994) locates PC 7 on the anterior wrist (pal up, in supination): about mid-width; one FW above the wrist, at the angle between the upper edge of the transverse head of the radius and the lateral (radial) edge of the large tendon of the flexor; in a hollow; medial side of the strong tendon of the flexor carpi radialis.

Pc 8 is located on the palmar aspect of the hand.

Pc 8 LAO GONG – PALACE OF WEARINESS

⊥ ***0.2 TO 0.3 CUN*** Δ ***3 (NOT DIRECTLY ON PALM)***

- FIRE
- EXIT
- HORARY from 7 p.m. to 9 p.m.
- SEASONAL HORARY – Summer
- YING – SPRING/Shu – Transporting/Antique
- RE-UNION/Crossing/Meeting Point of the Pericardium Channel with the Triple Heater Channel – Hand Jue Yin Channel with the Hand Shao Yang Channel
- SUN SI-MIAO GHOST (Gui) – Ghost Point Name: Gui Cu – Ghost in the Cave or Ghost Road (Pc 5 is also known as Gui Cu)

Pos: Position of patient: supine, in the anatomical position (arms at the side and flat on the couch with the palms facing upwards).

Loc: a) On the palmar surface of the hand.
b) Between the second and third metacarpal bones (closer to the third).
c) Proximal to the head of the third metacarpal bone.

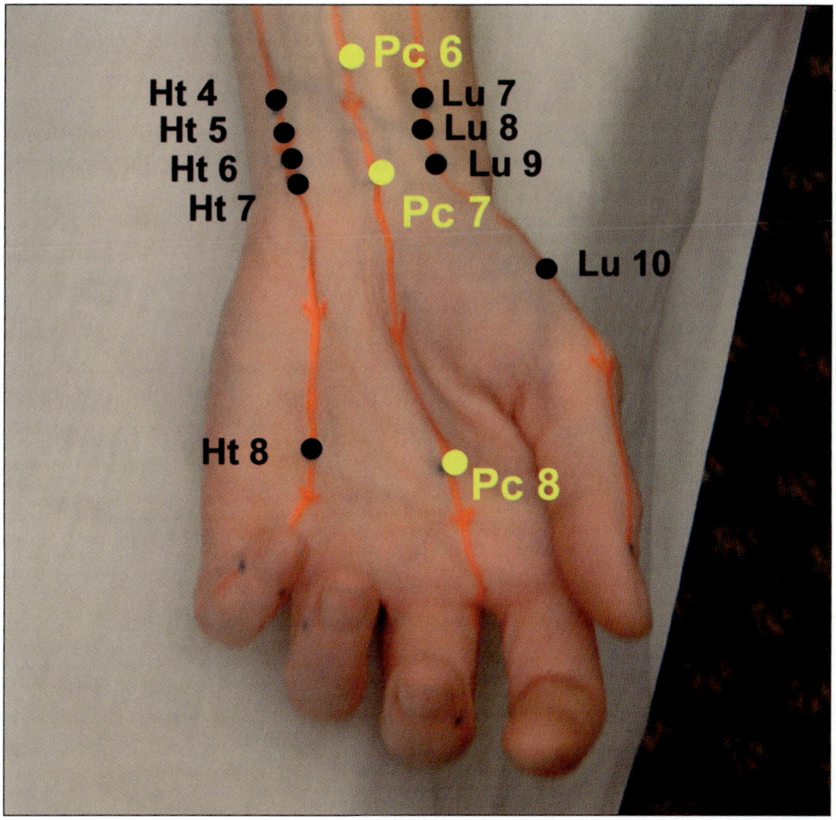

Tip:
a) This point normally lies just proximal to the proximal transverse crease (head line) of the hand, but the definitive location is in relation to the bone rather than the crease.
b) To help with the location of this point run your finger with the flow of the channel from the flexure of the wrist at Pc 7 towards the radial side of the third digit .
c) You can also place one finger on the posterior surface of the hand and feel for the second and third metacarpo-phalangeal joints (knuckles).
d) Place your finger still on the posterior surface of the hand, and feel the bones so that you are proximal to the heads of the second and third metacarpal bones and press in, this will push the bones nearer to the palmar surface of the hand and make the palpation of the anatomy much easier. Then relax the hand in the anatomical position to palpate for the point.
e) The point lies on the palmar surface of the hand just proximal to the flares formed by the heads of the second and third metacarpal bones but slightly nearer the third metacarpal bone than the second because the Pericardium channel ends on the radial side of the third digit.
f) To reduce needle sensation support the patient's hand in a relaxed position.

Note: Many texts use an alternative location as well as the location above, eg. Wu (1973) locates HC 8 on the palm of the hand upon the " line of the head", at the middle of the third metacarpal. Soulié (1994) locates PC 8 in the centre of the palm: on the line of the medius-annular joint; on the transverse line (the "head line" of palmistry); at the medial angle near the head and body of the third metacarpal ; on the lateral edge of a tendon running along the metacarpal (annular flexor); in a hollow; (therefore between the third and fourth metacarpal bones but nearer to the third). Lavier (1974) in an illustration locates the point between the third and fourth metacarpal bones on the proximal transverse crease ("head line").

Worsley (1982) locates V 8 on the palmar surface of the hand, between the third and fourth metacarpal bones, on the proximal transverse crease, or the "head line" of the hand. Voisin (1974) has two Pc 8's; one on the palm, on the lateral border of the third metacarpal, P8b is located 2mm more distally and has the same function, (i.e. one point on each palmar crease). Low (1988) locates PC 8 between the third/fourth metacarpals and 1 cun below the metacarpo-phalangeal crease, this would appear to be an Extra point given both as AR17 and OAR15. Jayasuriya (1982) locates Pc 8 between the tips of the middle and ring fingers as these touch the central region of the palm when the fist is lightly clenched

Yang (1982) locates this point posterior to the third metacarpophalangeal joint, on the radial side of the third metacarpal, on the transverse palmar crease. Deadman (1998) locates PC 8 between the second and third metacarpal bones, but an illustration places it on the "life line" of the hand which seems to place it half-way between the head and base of the second and third metacarpal bones, although the description does place it proximal to the metacarpo-phalangeal joint. In the location note it states that in some classical sources Pc 8 is on the ulnar side of the third metacarpal bone, where the tip of the fourth finger lands on the hand when a fist is made.

Shanghai (1981) locates P 8 with the fingers cupped in the palm in a half fist, then where the front of the tip of the middle finger lies is where the point can be located between the 2nd and 3rd metacarpal bones. Shandong (1982) locate Laogong in the middle of the paln. between the middle and the index (between the 3rd and 4th ossa metacarpole) when the hand is grasped. Legge (1999) locates P 8 on the palm between the 2nd and 3rd metacarpal bones, proximal to the metacarpophlangeal joints. Lotan (2000) locates P 8 in the depression, between the 2nd and 3rd metacarpal bones, proximal to the bone heads.

Pc 9 on the posterior surface of the third digit.

Pc 9 ZHONG CHONG – RUSHING INTO THE MIDDLE

⊥ ***0.1 CUN*** Δ ***1 TO 3***

- WOOD
- TONIFICATION/Reinforcing
- MOTHER
- JING – WELL/Shu – Transporting/Antique

Pos: Position of patient: supine or seated.

Loc: a) On the hand.
b) On the posterior aspect of the third digit (middle finger).
c) The radial nail point of the third digit.
d) Approximately 0.1 cun proximal to the corner of the nail.
e) Just distal to the flare of the distal phalanx.

Tip: a) The point is level with the nail bed (where the nail attaches to the skin) rather than the cuticle.
b) Draw a horizontal line across the nail bed.
c) Draw a vertical line from the radial border of the nail towards the nail bed.
d) The lines drawn from b) and c) (vertical and horizontal) form an intersection. This is approximately where the point is located.

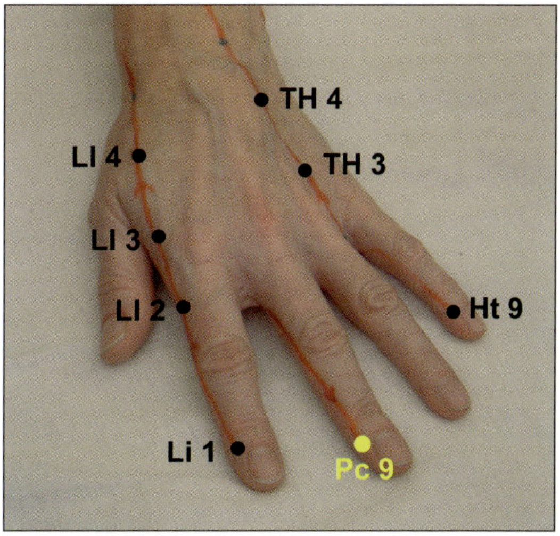

Note: Ellis (1991) in a Classical description locates PC 9 at the tip of the middle finger, in the depression the width of a Chinese leek leaf from the corner of the nail (The Great Compendium). Huang (1993) locates Per 9 at the tip of the middle finger in a depression the distance of a leek leaf from the corner of the nail. Shanghai (1984) Shandong (1982) locate Zhong-chong at the tip of the middle finger. – The location however, at the centre of the tip of the third digit, has historically been one of the ten Shixuan points (M-UE-9). Legge (1999) locates P 9 in the centre of the tip of the middle finger. Lotan (2000) locates P 9 at the middle (3rd) finger tip.

REFERENCES FOR THE PERICARDIUM CHANNEL

Lawson – Wood 1973 Acupuncture Handbook – V 1: 17

Shandong Medical College and Shandong College of Traditional Chinese Medicine 1982 Anatomical Atlas of Chinese Acupuncture Points – Tianchi (Pc 1) – Female Location Only: 42; Laogong (Pc 8): 43; Zhong-chong (Pc 9): 43

Soulie De Morant, George. 1994 Chinese Acupuncture – PC 2: 460; PC 7: 463; PC 8: 463

Voisin, Dr. H 1974 Essentials of Acupuncture – P 2: 80; P 4: 80; P 6: 80; P 8: 80

Worsley, J R 1982 Traditional Chinese Acupuncture Volume 1 – Neridians and Points. V 3: 113; V 8: 117

Wu, Wei-P'ing 1973 Chinese Acupuncture – HC 3: 103; HC 8: 104

Lavier, Dr. J 1974 Points of Chinese Acupuncture – Upper Arm Pouce Measurement: 8/9; HC 8: 21

Low, Royston. 1988 The Non-Meridial Points of Acupuncture – Pc 8: Unknown; M-UE-9: Unknown

Yang Jiasan (Prof) 1982 The Way to Locate Acu-Points – P 8: 12

Shanghai College of Traditional Medicine 1981 Acupuncture – A Comprehensive Text – Pc 8: 251

Deadman, Peter; Al-Khafaji, Mazin; Baker, Kevin 1998 Manual of Acupuncture, An – P 8: 380/381

Legge, David 1999 Acupuncture Points and Meridians – P 8: 69; P 9: 69

Lotan, Alon 2000 Acupoint Location Guide – P 8: 115; P 9: 115

Ellis, Wiseman and Boss. 1991 Fundamentals of Chinese Acupuncture – PC 9 (Classical Location): 275

Huang-fu Mi. Trans: Yang Shou-zhong and Charles Chace 1993 The Systematic Classic of Acupuncture & Moxibustion – Per 9: 173

THE TRIPLE HEATER CHANNEL OF THE HAND (SHAO YANG)

Primary Channel

The Triple Heater channel starts at a superficial level at TH 1 on the ulnar aspect of the fourth digit, and continues up the posterior surface of the forearm and upper arm to TH 14 at the shoulder.

From TH 14 a deep channel travels to TH 15 (via SI 12), meets the posterior median line at Du 14, then passes over the shoulder to GB 21, and to St 12 in the supraclavicular fossa. From St 12 it travels down to Ren 17 to connect with the pericardium and upper jiao, then penetrates the diaphragm and travels into the middle and lower jiaos, connecting with Ren 12 and Ren 7.

A second deep branch leaves Ren 17, travels back up to St 12, then continues up the lateral aspect of the neck to TH 16 at the posterior border of the ear. The channel runs superficially behind the ear to TH 20. Here a deep channel passes to GB 6-4 on the forehead, then loops over the cheek to link with SI 18.

A deep branch leaves TH 17 and runs through the ear to emerge at SI 19, linking with GB 3 and TH 21-22, and crossing over to TH 23 and GB 1 at the lateral canthus of the eye.

(Historical texts say that the Triple Heater channel connects with Bl 53, and follows the course of the Bladder channel to link with the bladder itself.)

Divergent Channel

This separates from the primary channel at the vertex, descends into the supraclavicular fossa, travels across the upper/middle/lower burners of the Triple Heater, and finally disperses in the chest.

Connecting Channel

This leaves the primary channel at TH 5 and passes up the posterior aspect of the arm and shoulder, joining the Pericardium channel in the chest.

Muscle Channel

This starts at the tip of the fourth digit and binds at the dorsum of the wrist. From here it passes up along the forearm, binding with the olecranon and continuing up the lateral aspect of the upper arm. It passes over the shoulder to the neck, joining the Small Intestine muscle channel. A branch separates at the angle of the mandible and binds with the root of the tongue. Another branch passes up anterior to the ear to the lateral canthus of the eye, then travels across the temple where it binds at the corner of the forehead.

THE TRIPLE HEATER CHANNEL OF THE HAND

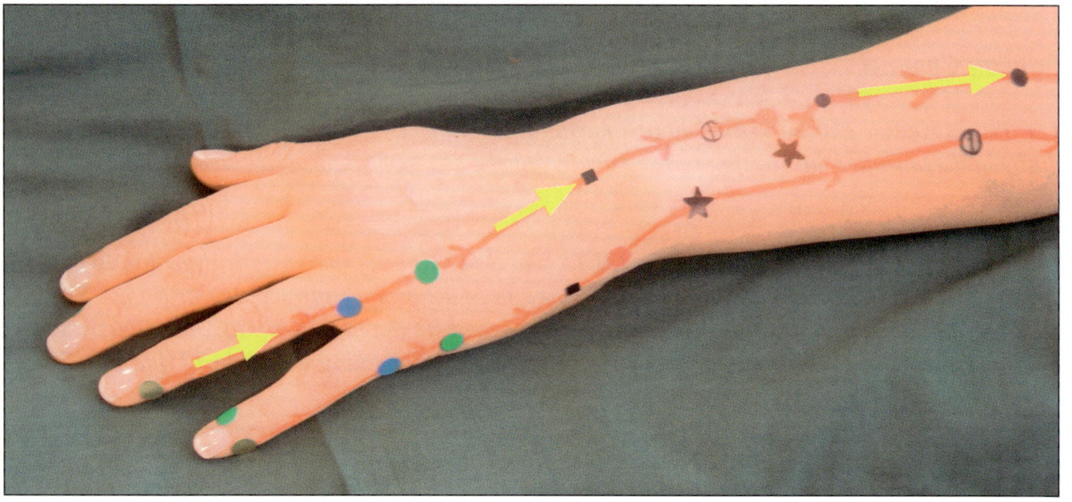

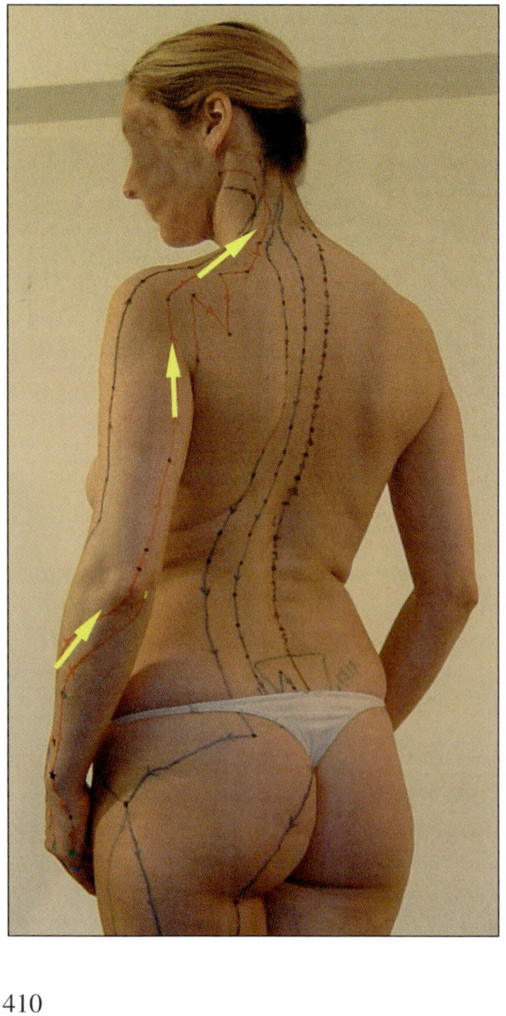

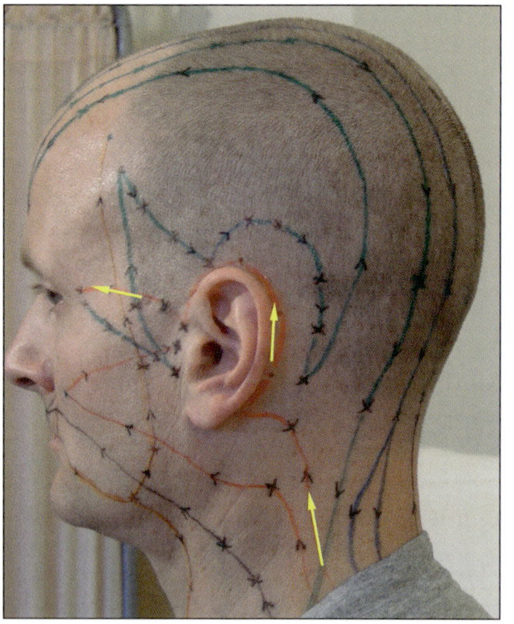

Points of the Triple Heater Channel-Hand Shao Yang
(TH/TB/SJ/TW/TE/T/VI) Also known as Tri-Heater, Triple Burner, San Jiao, Triple Warmer and Triple Energiser Channels

To locate TH 1-9, pronate the forearm. The distance between the wrist and elbow flexures is measured as 12 cun.

TH 1 is on the ulnar aspect of the fourth digit.

TH 1 GUAN CHONG – RUSHING THE FRONTIER GATE

⊥ ***0.1 CUN*** Δ ***3***

- METAL
- ENTRY
- JING – WELL/Shu – Transporting/Antique
- RE-UNION/Crossing/Meeting Point of the Triple Heater Channel with the Pericardium Channel – Hand Shao Yang Channel with the Hand Jue Yin Channel

Pos: Position of patient: supine or seated.

Loc: a) On the hand.
b) On the posterior aspect of the fourth digit (ring finger).
c) The ulnar nail point of the fourth digit.
d) Approximately 0.1 cun proximal to the corner of the nail.
e) Just distal to the flare of the distal phalanx.

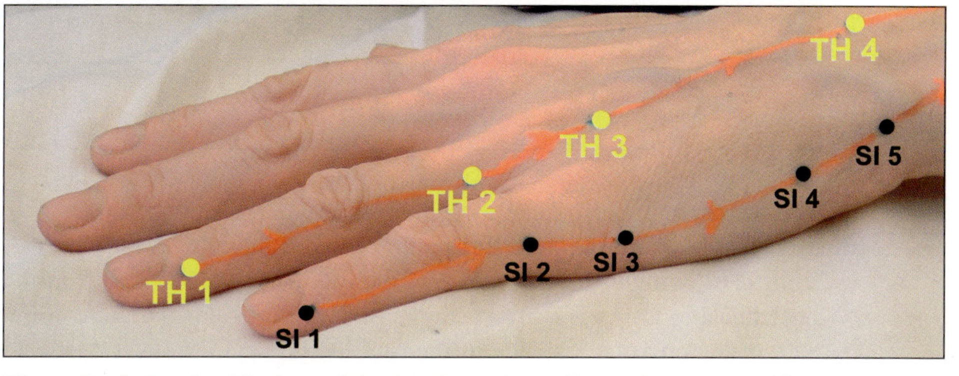

Tip: a) The point is level with the nail bed (where the nail attaches to the skin) rather than the cuticle.
b) Draw a horizontal line across the nail bed.
c) Draw a vertical line from the ulnar border of the nail towards the nail bed.
d) The lines drawn from b) and c) (vertical and horizontal) form an intersection. This is approximately where the point is located.

Note: Ellis (1991) in a Classical description locates TB 1 on the outer side of the finger next to the little finger, the width of a Chinese leek leaf away from the nail (The Great Compendium). Huang (1993) locates TH 1 at the tip of the finger next to the small one (i.e., the ring finger), the distance of a leek leaf from the corner of the nail.

TH 2-3 are on the posterior surface of the hand.

TH 2 YE MEN – FLUID SECRETION GATE

⊥ ***0.1 TO 0.3 CUN*** Δ ***3***

- WATER
- YING – SPRING/Shu – Transporting/Antique

Pos: Position of patient: supine with the forearm fully pronated (palms facing downwards).

Loc: a) On the postero-ulnar surface of the fourth digit (ring finger).
b) Distal to the metacarpo-phalangeal joint
c) Just distal to the flare of the base of the proximal phalanx of the fourth digit.
d) Proximal to the web margin.

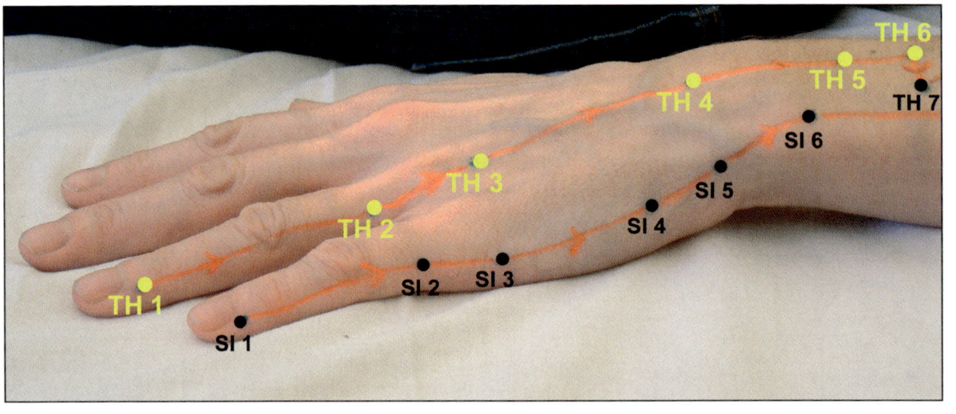

Tip: a) The web margin can be made visible with the digits spread out.
b) To help with the location of this point, run your finger with the flow of the channel from TH 1 along the ulnar surface of the fourth digit towards the fourth metacarpo-phalangeal joint. As you approach the metacarpo-phalangeal joint you will feel the base of the proximal phalanx of the fourth digit begin to flare.
c) Just distal to where the base of the proximal phalanx flares and proximal to the web margin between the fourth and fifth digits is where the point is located.

Note: Wu (1973) locates TH 2 upon the dorsal surface of the hand, between the fourth and fifth metacarpals, at the height of the creases formed by the metacarpo-phalangeal articulation. Jayasuriya (1982) and Deadman (1998) locate TH 2 0.5 cun proximal to the margin of the web between the 4th and 5th metacarpal bones. Deadman (1998) also states that if a loose fist is made the point can be located at the proximal end of a crease formed by the web space. Voisin (1974) T 2 on the hand, dorsum: between MCP joints 4 and 5, close to metacarpal 4.

Cheng (1987) locates TH 2 with the fist clenched the point is in the depression proximal to the margin of the web between the ring and small fingers. Shandong (1982) locate Yemen in the web between the ring and the small fingers. Legge (1999) locates SJ 2 on the back of the hand, proximal to the margin of the web between the 4th and 5th fingers. The point is needled with the fist loosely clenched. Lotan (2000) locates TW (SJ) 2, when the hand is fisted, between the ring and little fingers, distal to the 4th and 5th proximal phalanges bone bases.

TH 3 ZHONG ZHU – MIDDLE ISLET

⊥ ***0.2 TO 0.3 CUN*** Δ ***3 TO 5***

- WOOD
- TONIFICATION
- MOTHER
- SHU – STREAM/Shu – Transporting/Antique

Pos: Position of patient: supine with the forearm fully pronated (palms facing downwards).

Loc: a) On the posterior surface of the hand.
b) On the ulnar side of the fourth metacarpal bone.
c) Proximal to the fourth metacarpo-phalangeal joint.
d) Proximal to the flare of the head of the fourth metacarpal bone.

Tip: a) If a loose fist is made the point lies in a hollow proximal to the head of the fourth metacarpal bone.
b) The heads of the metacarpal bones are the "knuckles" of the hand.
c) To help with the location of this point, run your finger with the flow of the channel from TH 1 along the ulnar surface of the fourth digit towards the flexure of the wrist. You should be able to feel your finger go over the fourth metacarpo-phalangeal joint into a hollow. To locate accurately, palpate for the point in this hollow.
d) This point can be needled with the hand either in a loose fist position or with the hand flat. Whatever the position you use to locate the point should also be used to needle it.

Note: Voisin (1974) locates T 3 on the hand, dorsum: just distal to the junction of metacarpals 4 and 5, close to metacarpal 4. Shandong (1982) locate Hand-Zhongzhu with the hand clenched, between the ossa metacarpale IV and V, in the depression 1 cun above the art. metacarpophalangae. Legge (1999) locates SJ 3 on the back of the hand, between the 4th and 5th metacarpals, in the depression proximal to the metacarpo-phalangeal joints. Lotan (2000) locates TW (SJ) 3, when the hand is fisted, between the 4th and 5th metacarpal bones, proximal to the bone heads.

TH 4 is on the posterior flexure of the wrist.

TH 4 YANG CHI – YANG POND

⊥ ***0.3 CUN*** Δ ***3***

- SOURCE/Yuan/Regulator/Primary
- HOST/GUEST COMBINATION – Source Point with the Junction Point of its Paired Official/Organ Therefore TH 4 is combined with Pc 6

Pos: Position of patient: supine with the forearm fully pronated (palms facing downwards).

Loc: a) On the posterior surface of the flexure of the wrist.
b) In the depression between the tendons of the extensor digitorum and the extensor digiti minimi muscles.
c) On the ulnar side of the tendon of the extensor digitorum muscle.
d) Between the ulna and radius bones of the arm, and the triquetrum and lunate bones (two of the carpals) of the hand.

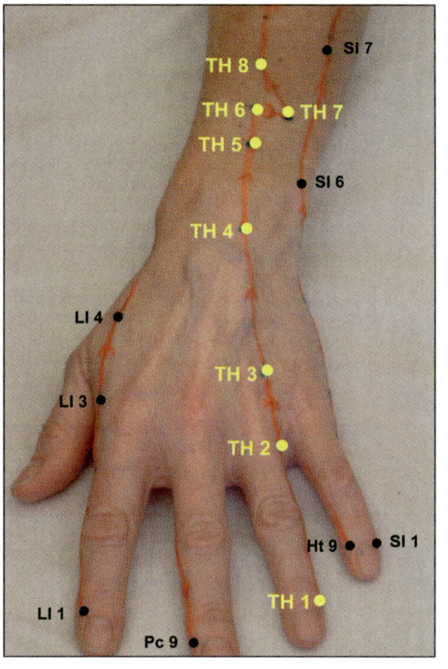

Tip: a) To expose the tendons of the extensor digitorum and the extensor digiti minimi muscles, flex and extend the hand.
b) To palpate the space between the ulnar and the carpal bones of the hand, again flex and extend the hand so that a gap widens and narrows between the bones. The point is located in the hollow formed by the bones and the tendons.
c) To help with the location of this point, run your finger with the flow of the channel from TH 1 along the ulnar surface of the fourth digit and fourth metacarpal bone towards the flexure of the wrist.
d) TH 4 lies on the ulnar side of the tendon of the extensor digitorum.
e) Make sure you do not locate the point too close to the head of the ulna. Try to visualise the continuation of the TH channel which does not flow over the ulna nor does it divert sharply to the median of the posterior surface of the arm (it does not follow the contour of the bone). Neither does the TH channel flow at the median aspect of the wrist, it lies just medial (ulnar) to the median line.

Note: Wu (1973) locates TH 4 at the centre of the dorsal surface of the wrist. Shandong (1982) locate Yangchi between the ossa metacarpale III and IV, just above the dorsal crease of the wrist, the depression at the ulnar aspect of the tendon of m. extensor digitorum. Legge (1999) locates SJ 4 on the doral aspect of the wrist, in the depression found distal to the ulnar styloid process and the ulnar side of the tendon of the extensor digitorum. Lotan (2000) locates TW (SJ) 4 on the wrist joint, ulnar to the extensor digitorum tendon.

TH 5-9 are on the posterior aspect of the forearm.

TH 5 WAI GUAN – OUTER FRONTIER GATE

⊥ ***0.3 TO 0.5 CUN*** **Δ** ***3 TO 7***

- JUNCTION/Luo/Connecting/Passage/Lo/Lê
- 8 EXTRAORDINARY CHANNELS CONFLUENT/8 Extraordinary Meridians Confluent/8 Extraordinary Vessels Opening/Master Point of the Yang Linking Vessel (Yang Wei Mai)
- 8 EXTRAORDINARY VESSEL/Coupled Point of the Girdle Vessel (Dai Mai)
- RE-UNION/Crossing/Meeting Point of the Triple Heater Channel with the Pericardium Channel – Hand Shao Yang Channel with the Hand Jue Yin Channel
- HOST/GUEST COMBINATION – Source Point with the Junction Point of its Paired Official/Organ Therefore TH 5 is combined with Pc 7

Pos: Position of patient: supine with the forearm fully pronated (palms facing downwards).

Loc: a) On the posterior surface of the forearm.
b) On the posterior median line of the forearm.
c) Between the radius and ulna bones.
d) Between the tendons of the extensor digitorum and extensor pollicis longus muscles.
e) 2 cun proximal to the flexure of the wrist at TH 4.

Tip: a) The distance between TH 4 and the transverse cubital crease (which is at the same level as the tip of the olecranon) is 12 cun, this point is 2 cun proximal to TH 4.
b) To expose the tendons of the extensor digitorum muscle, flex and extend the digits (wiggle the fingers), you will feel the tendons move.
c) The tendon of the extensor pollicis longus muscle is one of the deep extensor muscles, and therefore can be difficult to feel for as it goes deep in to the forearm. Sometimes by flexing and extending the thumb (to which it attaches) you can feel it under the tendons of the extensor digitorum muscle.
d) If you are able to feel the tendon of the extensor pollicis longus muscle the point is located on the ulnar (medial) border between this and the 4 tendons of the extensor digitorum muscle.
e) If you cannot feel the tendon of the extensor pollicis longus muscle then you need to make sure you are between the radius and ulna bones and on the posterior median line of the forearm radial (lateral) to the 4 tendons of the extensor digitorum muscle to locate this point.
f) Location of this point is made more simple by placing your finger on the posterior surface of the wrist and to feel for a narrow gap between the ulna and radius bones, then run your finger along the posterior surface of the forearm and you should be running along the median line.
g) At 2 cun proximal to TH 4, palpation of the point will give the greater accuracy.

Note: In some texts this point is described as being between the border of the radius bone and the tendons of the extensor digitorum muscles, (which may or may not be on the posterior median line of the forearm). Voisin (1974) locates T 5 on the forearm, dorsal aspect: 3 fb (finger breadth) above the wrist dorsiflexion fold, ulnar border of radius (hand kept in supination).

TH 6 ZHI GOU – BRANCH DITCH

⊥ ***0.3 TO 0.5 CUN*** Δ ***3 TO 5***

- FIRE
- HORARY from 9 p.m. to 11 p.m.
- SEASONAL HORARY – Summer
- JING – RIVER/Shu – Transporting/ Antique

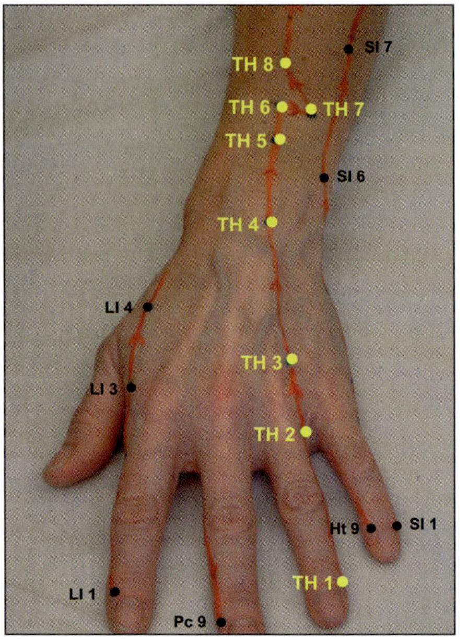

Pos: Position of patient: supine with the forearm fully pronated (palms facing downwards).

Loc: a) On the posterior surface of the forearm.
b) On the posterior median line of the forearm.
c) Between the radius and ulna bones.
d) Between the tendons of the extensor digitorum and extensor pollicis longus muscles.
e) 3 cun proximal to the flexure of the wrist at TH 4.

Tip: a) The distance between TH 4 and the transverse cubital crease (which is at the same level as the tip of the olecranon) is 12 cun, this point is 3 cun proximal to TH 4.
b) To expose the tendons of the extensor digitorum muscle, flex and extend the digits (wiggle the fingers), you will feel the tendons move.
c) The tendon of the extensor pollicis longus muscle is one of the deep extensor muscles, and therefore can be difficult to feel for as it goes deep in to the forearm. Sometimes by flexing and extending the thumb (to which it attaches) you can feel it under the tendons of the extensor digitorum muscle.
d) If you are able to feel the tendon of the extensor pollicis longus muscle the point is located on the ulnar (medial) border between this and the 4 tendons of the extensor digitorum muscle.
e) If you cannot feel the tendon of the extensor pollicis longus muscle then you need to make sure you are between the radius and ulna bones and on the posterior median line of the forearm radial (lateral) to the 4 tendons of the extensor digitorum muscle to locate this point.
f) Location of this point is made more simple by placing your finger on the posterior surface of the wrist and to feel for a narrow gap between the ulna and radius bones, then run your finger along the posterior surface of the forearm and you should be running along the median line.
g) At 3 cun proximal to TH 4, palpation of the point will give the greater accuracy.

Note: In some texts this point is described as being on medial (radial) side the extensor digitorum muscle, (which may or may not be on the posterior median line of the forearm). Voisin (1974) locates T 6 on the forearm, dorsal aspect: 4 fb (finger breadth) above the wrist dorsiflexion fold, ulnar border of radius. Shandong (1982) locate Zhigou at 1 cun above Pt. Waiguan (TH 5), between the ulna and the radius.

TH 7 HUI ZONG – ASSEMBLY OF ANCESTORS

⊥ ***0.3 CUN*** Δ ***3 TO 7***

- ACCUMULATION/Xi Cleft/Gueki

Pos: Position of patient: supine with the forearm fully pronated (palms facing downwards).

Loc: a) On the posterior surface of the forearm.
b) Between the radius and ulna bones.
c) On the lateral (radial) border of the ulna
d) Between the tendons of the extensor carpi ulnaris and extensor digiti minimi muscles.
e) 3 cun proximal to the flexure of the wrist at TH 4, on a level with TH 6.
f) Approximately one finger width medial (ulnar) to TH 6.

Tip: a) The distance between TH 4 and the transverse cubital crease (which is at the same level as the tip of the olecranon) is 12 cun, this point is 3 cun proximal to TH 4.
b) To expose the tendon of the extensor carpi ulnaris muscle extend and adduct the wrist against resistance.
c) To expose the tendon of the extensor digiti minimi muscle, flex and extend the fifth digit (wiggle the finger), you will feel the tendon move.
d) Location of this point is made more simple by placing your finger on the posterior surface of the wrist and to feel for a narrow gap between the ulna and radius bones, then run your finger along the posterior surface of the forearm and you should be running along the median line.
e) At 3 cun proximal to TH 4 at TH 6 run your finger medially (ulnar/little finger side) to TH 7 until you feel a seam that is formed by the tendon of the extensor carpi ularis and the extensor digiti minimi muscles, the point should be on the lateral (radial) border of the ulna bone.
f) Palpation of the point will give you the most accurate location of the point.

Note: Worsley (1982) locates TH 7 as above but instead of one finger width medial to TH 6, a measurement of 0.5 ACI (Anatomical Chinese Inch) medial to TH 6 is stated. Soulié (1994) locates TW 7 on the posterior forearm: three FW (Finger Width) above the wrist; two tight FW above the prominence of the ulnar process; at the angle between the lateral (radial) edge of the ulna and the tendon of the posterior ulna bone and the lower edge of a tendon, in an angle (insertion of the extensor pollicis longus); in a hollow; between the posterior ulnar artery and the ulnar edge of the extensor of the little finger; one FW above TW 5; one ulnar FW from TW 6; one FW below TW 8. Voisin (1974) locates T 7 on the forearm, dorsal aspect: same level (as T 6), but radial border of ulna (hand in supination).

TH 8 SAN YANG LUO – THREE YANG JUNCTION

⊥ *0.3 TO 0.5 CUN* Δ *7 TO 9*

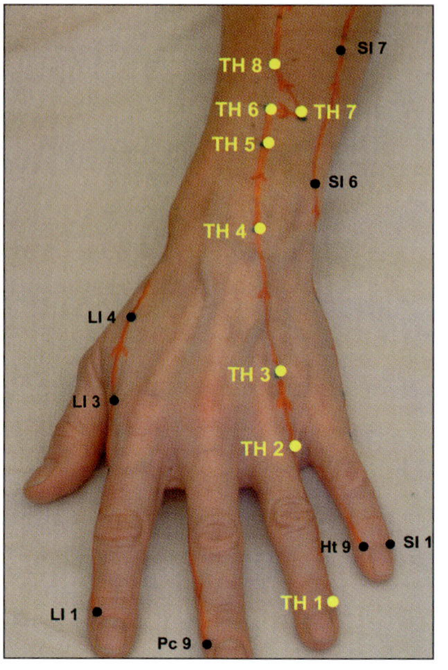

- RE-UNION/Crossing/Meeting Point of the Three Yang (Arm) Channels: Triple Heater, Small Intestine and Large Intestine – Hand Shao Yang, Hand Tai Yang and Hand Yang Ming Channels

Pos: Position of patient: supine with the forearm fully pronated (palms facing downwards).

Loc: a) On the posterior surface of the forearm.
b) Between the radius and ulna bones.
c) Between the tendons of the extensor digitorum and abductor pollicis longus muscles.
d) 4 cun proximal to the flexure of the wrist at TH 4.

Tip: a) The distance between TH 4 and the transverse cubital crease (which is at the same level as the tip of the olecranon) is 12 cun, this point is 4 cun proximal to TH 4.
b) To expose the tendons of the extensor digitorum muscle, flex and extend the digits (wiggle the fingers).
c) The tendon of the abductor pollicis longus muscle is one of the deep extensor muscles and lies beneath the tendons of the extensor digitorum muscle. It is difficult feeling for it as it goes deep in to the forearm, and therefore is not particularly helpful when locating this point.
d) To locate this point, mark out your 4 cun measurement. flex and extend the digits to demonstrate the tendons of the extensor digitorum muscle and make sure you are in between the ulna and radius bones by visualising the posterior median line of the arm and by palpating the borders of the bones.
e) For accuracy of location, palpate for the point. Make sure that when you are needling TH 8, you are not needling into one of the tendons of the extensor digitorum muscle.

Note: Soulié (1994) locates TW 8 on the posterior side of the forearm, palm down (in pronation): four large FW (Finger Width) above the wrist; at the angle between the medial (ulnar) edge of the median tendons (extensor of the extensor digiti muscle) and of the lower edge of the tendon on an angle of the extensor pollicis longus muscle; in a hollow; on the radial edge of the posterior ulnar artery and ulna; one FW above TW 7; one FW below TW 9. Voisin (1974) locates T 8 on the forearm, dorsal aspect: midwidth: 6 fb (finger breadth) above the wrist dorsiflexion fold. Shandong (1982) locate Sanyangluo at 1 cun above Pt. Zhigou (TH 6).

TH 9 SI DU – FOURTH GUTTER

⊥ ***0.5 TO 0.7 CUN*** Δ ***3 TO 7***

Pos: Position of patient: supine with the forearm fully pronated (palms facing downwards).

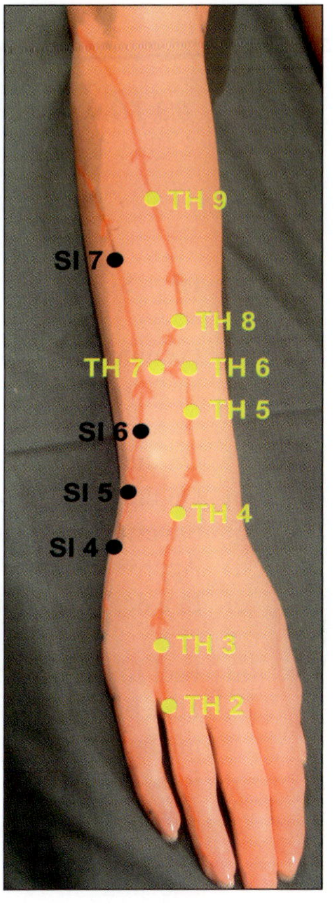

Loc:
a) On the posterior surface of the forearm.
b) Between the radius and ulna bones.
c) In the seam between the extensor digitorum and extensor carpi ulnaris muscles.
d) 7 cun proximal to the flexure of the wrist at TH 4.

Tip:
a) The distance between TH 4 and the transverse cubital crease (which is at the same level as the tip of the olecranon) is 12 cun, this point is 7 cun proximal to TH 4.
b) To expose the tendons of the extensor digitorum muscle, flex and extend the digits (wiggle the fingers).
c) To expose the extensor carpi ulnaris muscle extend and adduct the wrist against resistance.
d) To locate this point, make sure you are in the seam between the extensor carpi ulnaris and the extensor digitorum muscles. As you place the flat part of your finger in the middle of the arm from the flexure of the wrist and run it up towards the flexure of the elbow, these muscles begin to run medially. You should be able to feel a seam between these two muscles.
e) At approximately 7 cun proximal to TH 4 you should be able to palpate for the point.

Note: Soulié (1994) locates TW 9 on the posterior forearm: about mid-width; palm down (in pronation); six FW above the wrist; at the angle between the medial (ulnar) edge of the median tendons (extensors: extensor digiti minimi) and of the lower edge of one tendon at an angle of the extensor pollicis brevis; on the radial edge of the posterior ulnar artery and ulna; in a hollow; one FW above TW 8; eight FW below TW 10; at the level of LI 7, LU 6, PC 4 and SI 7.

Voisin (1974) locates T 9 on the forearm, dorsal aspect: midwidth: 6 fb (finger breadth) below the tip of the elbow (olecranon). Shandong (1982) locate Sidu at 5 cun above Pt. Waiguan (TH 5), between the radius and the ulna. Lotan (2000) locates TW (SJ) 9, when the hand rests on the belly, 7 cun proximal to the wrist (carpal) joint, radial to the extensor digitorum.

To locate TH 10-14 have the patient in a seated position, with the elbow flexed. TH 10 -14 are on the posterior aspect of the upper arm.

There are 9 cun between the axillary fold and the transverse cubital crease/tip of the olecranon of the ulna bone.

TH 10 TIAN JING – HEAVENLY WELL

⊥ ***0.3 TO 0.5 CUN*** **Δ *3 TO 5***

- EARTH
- SEDATION/Reducing/Dispersing
- CHILD
- HE – SEA/Shu – Transporting/Antique

Pos: Position of patient: seated with the elbow flexed at 90 degrees and with the palmar surface of the hand facing upwards (holding a tray position).

Loc: a) On the posterior surface of the upper arm.
b) On the posterior midline of the upper arm.
c) Superior to the superior border of the olecranon.
d) Approximately 1 cun proximal to the tip of the olecranon of the ulna bone.
e) In a depression that is in the tendon of the triceps brachii muscle.

Tip: a) Feel for the tip of the olecranon of the ulna bone, and draw in the posterior midline of the upper arm (vertical line).
b) Run your finger superiorly until you reach the superior border of the olecranon, then draw in a horizontal line along it. You should have a vertical line and a horizontal line.
c) If you gently palpate just superior to your horiztontal line on the vertical line you should feel a depression on the tendon of the triceps brachii muscle. The depression can be quite large on some people.
d) There are 9 cun between the axillary fold and the transverse cubital crease/tip of the olecranon of the ulna bone. Even though 1 cun is described in the location of this point, it is only an approximation, therefore palpation of the point takes precedence.

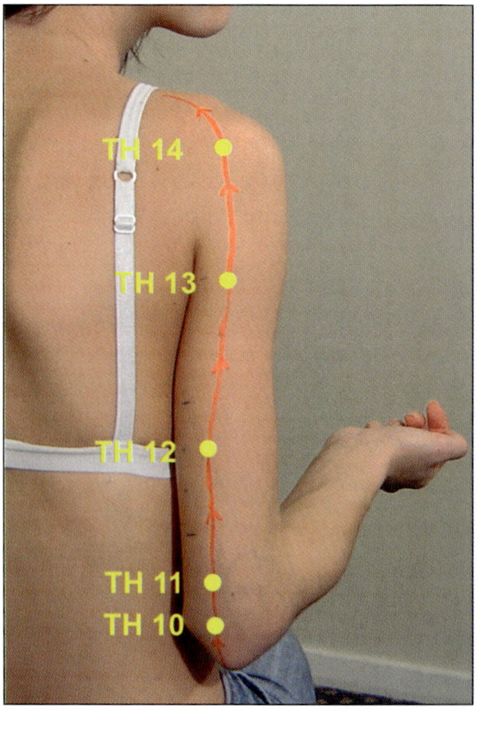

Note: Worsley (1982) locates TH 10 sligthly medial to the posterior midline of the upper arm. This may suggest that the point is in a seam formed by the medial and long heads of the triceps brachii muscle as they are joining to form a common tendon of insertion along with the lateral head. Wu (1973) again locates TH 10 as above, but places it outside the tendon of the triceps brachii muscle. Lavier (1974) measures 7 pouce from the elbow fold to the deltoid 'V'. Lotan (2000) locates TW 10 (SJ) 10, when the elbow is flexed and the palm faces the superior (supination), lateral to the triceps brachii tendon, about 1 cun proximal to the olecranon peak.

TH 11 QING LENG YUAN – PURE COLD ABYSS

⊥ *0.3 TO 0.5 CUN* Δ *3 TO 7*

Pos: Position of patient: seated with the forearm positioned so that the medial surface of the upper arm is against the torso with the elbow flexed at an angle of 90 degrees.

Loc:
a) On the posterior surface of the upper arm.
b) On the posterior midline of the upper arm.
c) Superior to the superior border of the olecranon.
d) Approximately 2 cun proximal to the tip of the olecranon of the ulna bone.
e) In a depression in the tendon of the triceps brachii muscle, in the midline.
f) 1 cun superior to TH 10.

Tip:
a) Feel for the tip of the olecranon of the ulna bone, and draw in the posterior midline of the upper arm (vertical line).
b) If you gently palpate on the vertical line you should feel a depression in the tendon of the triceps brachii muscle at approximately 2 cun superior to the olecranon of the ulna bone.
c) There are 9 cun measurements between the axillary fold and the transverse cubital crease / tip of the olecranon of the ulna bone. Split your 9 cun measurement in to 3 to make three 3 cun measurements and then split these in to thirds to make 1 cun measurements.
d) As the cun measurement for this point is only an approximation, palpation of the point would take precedence.

Note: Lavier (1974) measures 7 pouce from the elbow fold to the deltoid 'V'. Soulié (1994) locates TW 11 on the posterior arm: five FW (Finger Width) above the olecranon process; posterior edge of the humerus and anterior edge of the triceps; on the lower edge of a transverse mass; in a hollow; three FW above TW 10; six FW below TW 12; about three FW posterior to LI 13. Voisin (1974) locates T 11 on the arm, posterior aspect: 1.5 fb (finger breadth) above the preceding point. Lotan (2000) locates TW (SJ) 11, when the elbow is flexed and the point faces the superior (supination), lateral to the triceps brachii tendon, 2 cun proximal to the olecranon peak.

TH 12 XIAO LUO – RELAX AND JOY

⊥ ***0.5 TO 0.7 CUN*** Δ ***3 TO 7***

Pos: Position of patient: seated with the forearm positioned so that the medial surface of the upper arm is against the torso with the elbow flexed at an angle of 90 degrees.

Loc: a) On the posterior surface of the upper arm.
b) On the posterior midline of the upper arm.
c) On the triceps brachii muscle.
d) Approximately 5 cun proximal to the tip of the olecranon of the ulna bone.
e) Midway between TH 11 and TH 13 (please see separate descriptions).

Tip: a) Feel for the tip of the olecranon of the ulna bone, and draw in the posterior midline of the upper arm (vertical line).
b) If you gently palpate on the vertical line you should feel a depression on the triceps brachii muscle at approximately 5 cun superior to the olecranon of the ulna bone.
c) There are 9 cun measurements between the axillary fold and the transverse cubital crease /tip of the olecranon of the ulna bone. Split your 9 cun measurement in to 3 to make three 3 cun measurements and then split these in to thirds to make 1 cun measurements.
d) Alternative method of locating TH 12: On the posterior midline of the upper arm, feel for the inferior border of the deltoid muscle and make a mark (TH 13).

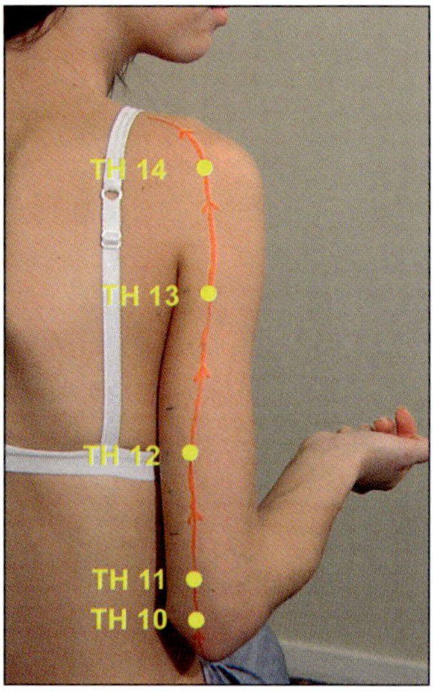

e) Then mark out 2 cun proximal to the tip of the olecranon of the ulna bone on the posterior midline of the upper arm (TH 11).
f) Halve these two marks (d and e), this should give you the approximate area of the location of the point (Approximately 5 cun). When you have established this, palpate for the point.
g) As the cun measurement is only an approximation, palpation of the point would take precedence.

Note: Wu (1973) locates TH 12 on the posterior surface of the upper arm, 5 pouce above the point of the elbow and 4 pouce below the posterior extremoity of the crease of the axilla. Located by halving the distance between TH 10 and TH 14. Deadman (1998) locate SJ 12 by measuring 10 cun between SJ 10 and SJ 14. and then to measure 4 cun proximal to SJ 10 and 6 cun distal to SJ 14 , between the muscle bellies of the long and lateral heads of the triceps. Voisin (1976) locates T 12 on the posterior aspect of the arm, midwidth, and on the posterior border of the deltoid. Eachou (1995) locates TB 12 4.5 inches above the olecranon process of the ulna, midway between TB 11 and TB 13.

Lavier (1974) measures 7 pouce from the elbow fold to the deltoid 'V'. Soulié (1994) locates TW 12 on the lateral, posterior arm; five FW (Finger Width) below the acromion; on the posterior edge of the humerus; on the lower edge of the insertion of the deltoid; in a hollow; six FW above TW 11; three FW below TW 13.

TH 13 NAO HUI – SHOULDER MEETING

⊥ ***0.5 TO 0.7 CUN*** Δ ***5 TO 7***

- RE-UNION/Crossing/Meeting Point of the Triple Heater Channel with the Yang Linking Vessel – Hand Shao Yang Channel with the Yang Wei Mai

Pos: Position of patient: seated with the forearm positioned so that the medial surface of the upper arm is against the torso with the elbow flexed at an angle of 90 degrees.

Loc: a) On the posterior surface of the upper arm.
b) On the posterior midline of the upper arm.
c) On the inferior border of the deltoid muscle.
d) Approximately 3 cun inferior to TH 14 (acromial angle).

Tip: a) Draw in the posterior midline of the upper arm (vertical line).
b) On the posterior midline of the upper arm, feel for the inferior border of the deltoid muscle.
c) To demonstrate the deltoid muscle ask the person to resist their arm by getting them to push their elbow backwards against your hand.
d) Alternative way using the cun measurements: There are 9 cun measurements between the axillary fold and the transverse cubital crease /tip of the olecranon of the ulna bone. Split your 9 cun measurement in to 3 to make three 3 cun measurements.
e) Feel for the tip of the olecranon of the ulna bone, and draw in the posterior midline of the upper arm (vertical line).
f) Gently palpate towards the shoulder on the posterior midline of the upper arm, you should be able to feel a depression on the inferior border of the deltoid muscle at approximately 3 cun inferior to TH 14 (at the acromial angle).
g) Transfer your 3 cun measurement you made earlier to TH 14 (acromial angle) and mark in 3 cun distal to it on the posterior midline of the arm.
h) Palpate for the point on the inferior border of the deltoid muscle.

Note: Wu (1973) locates TH 13 on the dorsal surfcae of the shoulder, 3 pouce below the acromion eminence, on the humerus. Voisin (1976) locates T 13 on the posterolateral aspect of the arm, 3 fb (finger breadth) below the most prominent point or angle of the shoulder. Deadman (1998) locate the point as above but also say that it is approximately two thirds of the distance between SJ 10 and SJ 14. Qiu (1996) locates SJ 13 3 cun below SJ 14 on the posterior border of the m. deltoideus.

Soulié (1994) locates TW 13 on the posterolateral side of the arm: three FW (Finger Width) below the acromion; on the posterior edge of the humerus; at the angle of the lower edge of the transverse insertion (infraspinatus); in a hollow; just above the insertion of the teres minor; three FW above TW 12; four FW below and a little before TW 14; three FW behind LI 15. Shandong (1982) locate Naohui at the junction between the line connecting Pt. Jianliao (TH 14) and olecranon and the posterior border of m. deltoideus.

TH 14 JIAN LIAO – SHOULDER BONE

⊥ *0.7 CUN* Δ *3 TO 7*

Pos: Position of patient: seated with the forearm positioned so that the medial surface of the upper arm is against the torso with the elbow flexed at an angle of 90 degrees.

Loc:
a) On the posterior surface of the shoulder.
b) Posterior and inferior to the acromion process of the scapula.
c) At the inferolateral corner of the acromion process of the scapula.
d) At the acromial angle.
e) Approximately 1 cun posterior to LI 15 when the arm is abducted.

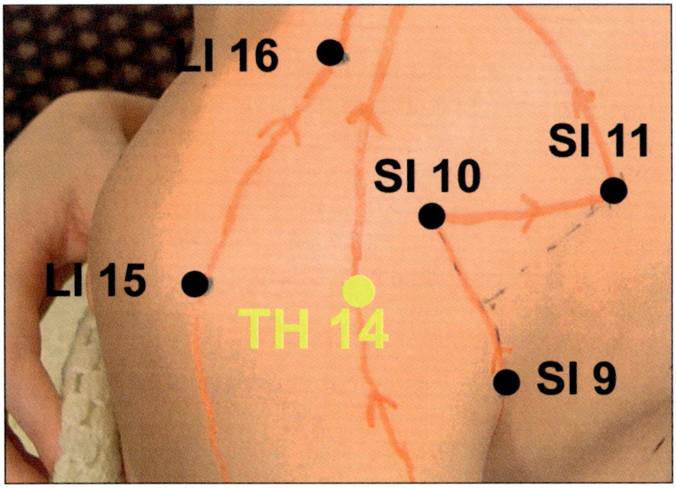

Tip:
a) Draw in the posterior midline of the upper arm (vertical line).
b) Run your finger from the elbow superiorly along the posterior median line of the upper arm to the posterior surface of the shoulder until you meet some resistance, this will be the inferolateral corner of the acromion process where you will need to palpate for this point.
c) When the arm is abducted a depression is formed by the space between the origin of the deltoid muscle and the extremity of the acromion of the scapula.
d) SI 10, TH 14 and LI 15 are located in relation to the acromion process of the scapula, SI 10 being inferior to the neck of the acromion, TH 14 is on the inferolateral corner of the acromion process, at the acromion angle, and LI 15 is inferior to the acromion, between the acromion and the greater tuberosity of the humerus. LI 15 is the most lateral point. 1 cun posterior to this point is TH14 and 1 cun medial to TH 14 is SI 10, so these points are all approximately equidistant from each other. The acromion forms a scallop shape and these three points lie inferior to it.

Note: Lotan (2000) locates TW (SJ) 14 in the depression, about 0.3 cun inferior (and distal) to the acromion posterior-lateral corner

TH 15 is superior to the superior aspect of the scapula.

TH 15 TIAN LIAO – HEAVENLY BONE

⊥ *0.3 TO 0.5 CUN* Δ *3 TO 7*

- 8 EXTRAORDINARY VESSEL/Coalescent Point of the Yang Linking Vessel (Yang Wei Mai)
- 8 EXTRAORDINARY VESSEL/Coalescent Point of the Yang Heel/Yang Motility Vessel (Yang Qiao Mai) – see note
- RE-UNION/Crossing/Meeting Point of the Triple Heater Channel with the Gall Bladder Channel and the Yang Linking Vessel – Hand Shao Yang Channel with the Foot Shao Yang Channel and Yang Wei Mai

Pos: Position of patient: seated with the shoulders in a relaxed position.

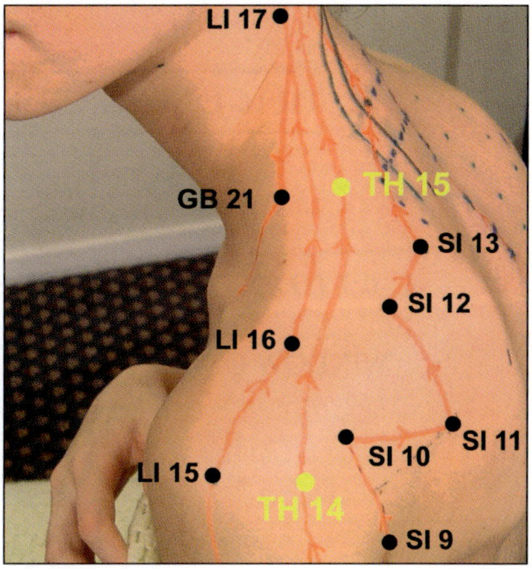

Loc: a) On the shoulder.
b) On the trapezius muscle.
c) At the transverse mid-point between Du 14 (at the posterior median line) and the lateral tip of the acromion of the scapula.
d) Also midway between SI 13 (at the medial end of the supraspinous fossa) and GB 21 (at the highest point of the shoulder).
e) On a vertical line from SI 13 to TH 15, ending at GB 21.

Tip: a) Measure your mid-point between Du 14 and the lateral tip of the acromion of the scapula.
b) Alternatively mark out SI 13 (see separate description) and then draw a vertical line from this point over the shoulder.
c) On the highest surface of the shoulder you can feel a transverse tight band of muscle (from the neck laterally) that is part of the trapezius muscle. This part of the trapezius muscle is tighter than the rest of the muscle as it maintains the level and the poise of the shoulder. If the person were to 'hunch' their shoulder, this band of muscle would feel more prominent.
d) If you were to feel the posterior border of this band of muscle on your vertical line or on the mid-point marked earlier (a) you will then be able to palpate for this point. GB 21 is on the anterior border of this band of muscle (which is at the highest point of the shoulder).
e) To feel the posterior and anterior borders of this tight band of muscle you should be able to 'pinch' it. TH 15 and GB 21 lie on the posterior and anterior borders respectively. TH 15 is approximately midway between SI 13 and GB 21, so for accuracy, palpation for this point is extremely important.

Note: Cheng (1987) locates this point as above but also says that the point is on the superior angle of the scapula bone. Soulié (1994) locates TH 15 about mid-width of the posterior part of the shoulder: just on the upper edge of the swelling of the transverse spine of the scapula; between the bone and the supraspinatus; in a hollow; five FW medial to TW 14; two FW lateral to SI 13; behind GB 21.

Wu (1973) locates TH 15 upon the posterior surface of the shoulder, at one pouce behind GB 21 upon a vertical line passing through SI 13. Worsley (1982) locates VI 15 on the posterior surface of the shoulder, superior to the scapula, mid-way between the spinous process of the seventh cervical vertebra and the tip of the acromion, in line with VII 21 and II 13. Shandong (1982) locate Tianliao at the superior angle of the scapula, between Pt. Jianjing (GB 21) and Pt. Quyuan (SI 13)

Note: In some texts TH 15 is listed as an 8 EXTRAORDINARY VESSEL/Coalescent Point of Yang Qiao Mai (Yang Heel/Yang Motility Vessel), whereas in others it is omitted.

TH 16-19 are posterior to the posterior border of the ear.

TH 16 TIAN YOU – HEAVENLY WINDOW

⊥ ***0.3 TO 0.5 CUN*** ***∆ FORBIDDEN TO MOXA***

- WINDOW OF THE SKY/Window of Heaven

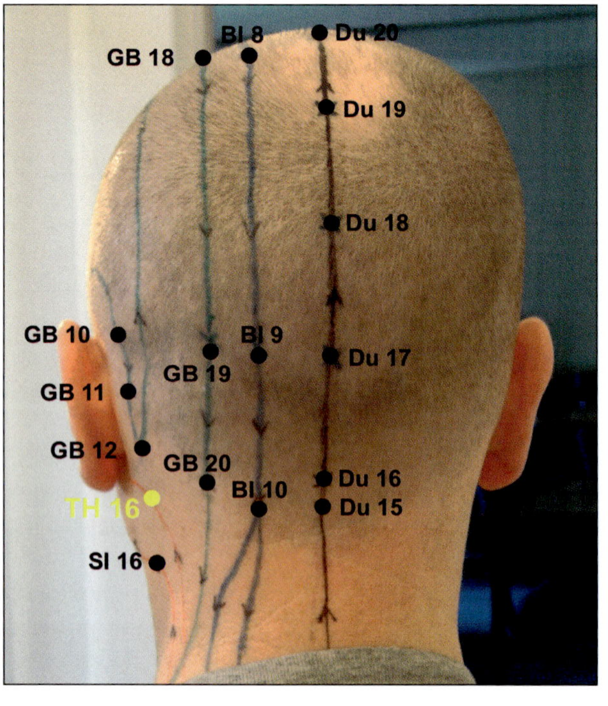

Pos: Position of patient: seated.

Loc:
a) On the posterior aspect of the neck.
b) On the posterior border of the sternocleidomastoid muscle.
c) Posterior and inferior to the mastoid process of the temporal bone.
d) Inferior to the inferior border of the medial aspect of the temporal bone
e) Approximately 1 cun inferior to GB 12 (see tip e for location).
f) Level with the angle of the mandible (SI 17)
g) Approximately level with Bl 10.

Tip:
a) Feel for the posterior border of the sternocleidomastoid muscle by palpation. If you cannot feel the border, then ask the patient to rotate their head against resistance when the hand is applied to the opposite side of the face.
b) Feel for the attachment of the posterior border of the sternocleidomastoid muscle to the mastoid process, you should be able to feel for the point which is posterior and inferior to the mastoid process.
c) When palpating for this point you need to feel for resistance, where your finger cannot go any more lateral than the posterior border of the sternocleidomastoid muscle and where you cannot go any more superior than the inferior border of the temporal bone. This is more inferior than GB 12 (approximately 1 cun inferior).
d) Make sure you are close to the posterior border of the sternocleidomastoid muscle otherwise you may stray too medially towards the seam formed by the lateral border of the trapezius muscle and the posterior border of the sternocleidomastoid muscle which is in the proximity of GB 20.
e) TH 16 is on the neck and off the skull and level with the angle of the mandible (jaw) as opposed to GB 12, which is on the skull, at the articulation of the occipital bone and the mastoid process of the temporal bone.
f) The prominence of the mastoid process is a little like feeling for the prominences of the malleoli (ankles), where you feel the contour of the bone. Where it protudes outwards most is the prominence. GB 12 is level with the prominence and posterior to the mastoid process.
g) Approximately 1 cun inferior to GB 12, and level with the angle of the mandible should give you the correct level for palpation of this point. If you are not level with the angle of the mandible you may be too superior.

Note: Soulié (1994) locates TW 16 on the lateral side of the neck: one large FW below and behind the bulge behind the ear (mastoid); at the angle between the posterior edge of a large muscle, on an angle towards the front (sternocleidomastoid muscle) and the lower edge of a deep, transverse prominence (transverse process of the first cervical vertebra – atlas). In front of a muscle on a posterior angle (splenius of the head); two FW below and behind TW 17; one FW behind SI 17.

TH 17 YI FENG – WIND SCREEN

⊥ *0.3 TO 0.5 CUN* Δ *3 TO 7*

- RE-UNION/Crossing/Meeting Point of the Triple Heater Channel with the Gall Bladder Channel – Hand Shao Yang Channel with the Foot Shao Yang Channel

Pos: Position of patient: seated.

Loc: a) On the neck.
b) Posterior to the ear lobe.
c) Half-way between the ramus of the mandible and the mastoid process of the temporalbone.

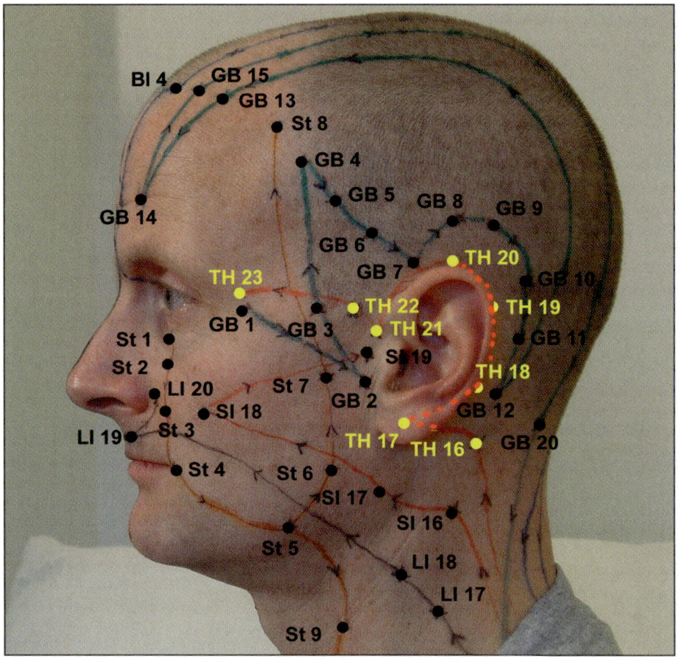

Tip: a) Open the mouth to expose a hollow between the ramus of the mandible and the mastoid process of the temporal bone.
b) As this point is posterior to the ear lobe, you will need to either push the ear lobe forwards or to lift up the ear lobe to expose the point.
c) Palpation of this point will reveal quite a large hollow.

Note: Worsley (1982) also includes the point as being adjacent to the cartilage of the external auditory canal. Cheng (1987) locates this point posterior to the lobule of the ear, between the mandible and mastoid process. Soulié (1994) locates TW 17 on the head: behind the lobe of the ear; at the posterior angle between the lower point of the bony protrusion (mastoid) and the upper edge of the insertion on it of a large muscle (sternocleidomastoid muscle); in a hollow; two FW (Finger Width) above and in front of TW 16; two FW below TW 18; one FW behind SI 17; two FW below and in front of GB 12.

Voisin (1974) locates T 17 in the retroauricular groove, lower part: anterior border of the mastoid process, 1 fb (finger breadth) above its tip. Wu (1973) locates TH 17 upon the head, behind the lobe of the ear, and in front of the point of the mastoid. Shandong (1982) locate Yifeng posterior to the inferior border of the lobolus auriculae in the depression antero-inferior to the processus mastoideus.

TH 18 QI MAI – FEEDING MERIDIANS

⊥ ***0.1 TO 0.2 CUN*** Δ ***FORBIDDEN TO MOXA***

Pos: Position of patient: seated.

Loc:
a) On the lateral aspect of the head.
b) On the mastoid bone.
c) Directly posterior to the helix of the ear when this is flattened against the skull.
d) One third of the distance from TH 17 to TH 20.

Tip:
a) Press the helix of the ear against the skull and draw a line around the contour it.
b) The point will either be on this line or will just disappear under the helix of the ear when it is flattened against the skull.
c) Draw two marks indicating the base and the apex of the pinna of the ear, which is at the approximate location of TH 17 and the location of TH 20 (please see separate descriptions for these points).
d) Divide these two marks in to thirds, following the contour of the helix of the ear.
e) At the one third mark from the base of the helix of the ear (from approximately TH 17) on the line or just beneath the helix of the ear when flattened against the skull is where the point is approximately located.
f) Palpation of this point reveals a good depression on the mastoid bone.
g) Be careful not to press too strongly as the patient may feel light headed or faint.

Note: Worsley (1982) uses the curve of the hair line to locate VI 17. Academy (1975) locates SJ 17 posterior to the ear, in the centre of the mastoid process, at the junction of the lower and middle third of the curve-line connecting SJ 20 with SJ 17 along the helix. Soulié (1994) locates TW 18 on the head: behind the mid-height of the ear; at the angle between the upper edge of a transverse bulge and the anterior edge of the mastoid process; on the posterior edge of a vertical artery; two FW above TW 17; one FW below TW 19; two FW in front of GB 11. Vosin (1974) locates T 18 in the retroauricular groove, at the level of the centre of the tragus. Wu (1973) locates TH 18 upon the head, behind the pinna of the ear, at one pouce above TH 17, at the hairline. Shandong (1982) locate Qimai in the centre of the pars mastoideus.

TH 19 LU XI – SKULL BREATHING

⊥ ***0.1 TO 0.3 CUN*** Δ ***3 TO 7***

Pos: Position of patient: seated.

Loc:
- a) On the lateral aspect of the head.
- b) On the mastoid bone.
- c) Directly posterior to the helix of the ear when this is flattened against the skull.
- d) Two thirds of the distance from TH 17 to TH 20.

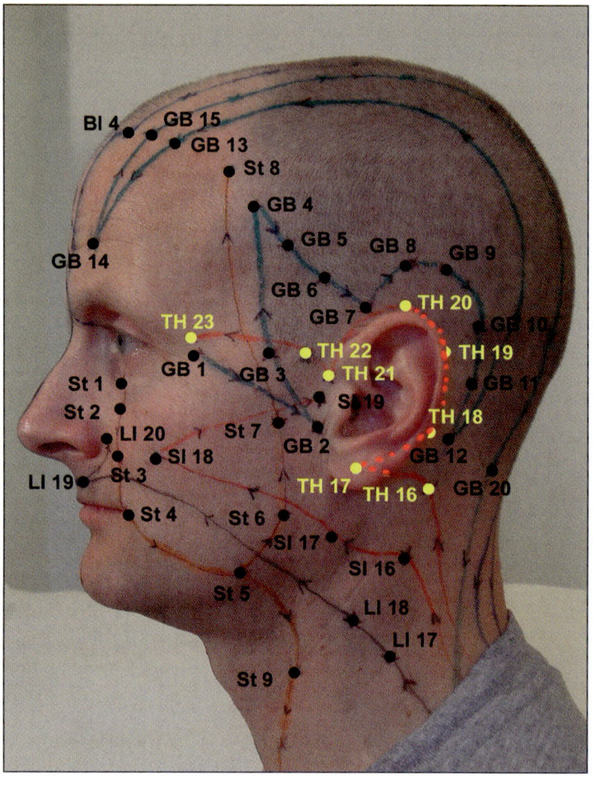

Tip:
- a) Press the helix of the ear against the skull and draw a line around the contour it.
- b) The point will either be on this line or will just disappear under the helix of the ear when it is flattened against the skull.
- c) Draw two marks indicating the base and the apex of the pinna of the ear, which is at the approximate location of TH 17 and the location of TH 20 (please see separate descriptions for these points).
- d) Divide these two marks in to thirds, following the contour of the helix of the ear.
- e) At the two thirds mark from the base of the helix of the ear (from approximately TH 17) on the line or just beneath the helix of the ear when flattened against the skull is where the point is approximately located.
- f) Palpation of this point reveals a good depression on the mastoid bone.
- g) Be careful not to press too strongly as the patient may feel light headed or faint.

Note: Worsley (1982) uses the curve of the hair line to locate this point. Soulié (1994) locates TW 19 on the head: between the posterosuperior attachment of the ear and the anterior edge of the upper point of the mastoid process. In the anterior upper angle of the two flat reliefs; on the anterior edge of an artery. The ears vary considerably in their attachments; one FW (Finger Width) above TW 18; two FW under and behind TW 20. Vosin (1974) locates T 19 in the retroauricular groove, upper part: slightly below the level of the uppermost attachment of the auricle. Wu (1973) locates TH 19 behind the pinna of the ear, at two pouce above TH 17, at the hairline. Shandong (1982) locate Luxi midway of the curve between Pt. Qimai (TH 17) and Pt. Jiaosun (TH 20).

TH 20 JIAO SUN – SMALL ANGLE OF EAR

⊥ ***0.1 TO 0.3 CUN*** Δ ***3 TO 7***

- RE-UNION/Crossing/Meeting Point of the Triple Heater Channel with the Gall Bladder and Small Intestine Channels.- Hand Shao Yang Channel with the Foot Shao Yang and Hand Tai Yang Channels

Pos: Position of patient: seated.

Loc: a) On the lateral aspect of the head.
b) On the temporal bone.
c) Level with or immediately superior to the superior border of the helix (apex of the ear) when the ear is bent forward.

Tip: a) Press the helix of the ear against the skull and draw a mark at the apex (highest part) of the helix (auricle).
b) The point may be on the contour line of the helix of the ear or immediately superior to it, but palpation will give you the accurate location of the point.
c) When you bend the helix of the ear forward, make sure it only the helix and not the main body of the ear.

Note: There are various traditions that use the hair line as a reference to locating this point. Worsley (1982) locates VI 20 as being on the hair line and immediately superior to the level of the apex of the pinna. Wu (1973) locates TH 20 upon the side of the cranium, at the highest point of the curve of the hair line which contours the ear. Deadman (1998) locates SJ 20 by folding the ear forwards, then it is level with the apex of the ear. Academy (1975) also use the folding of the ear forward, and where the tip touches within the hairline is where the point is located. Voisin (1974) locates T 20 on the hair line, at the upper tip of the auricle.

Yang (1982) folds the auricle, then the point is level with the ear apex. Cheng (1987) locates the point directly above the ear apex, within the hair line. Eachou (1995) locates the point in the superior auricular sulcus and superior to the tip of the ear. Qiu (1996) places this point within the hair line and directly above the ear apex. Jayasuriya (1982) locates SJ 20 at the level of the apex of the ear.

Soulié (1994) locates TW 20 above the ears: one FW (Finger Width) posterior to the vertical anterior to the lobe (about mid-width of the ear). At the level of three FW above the transverse prominence of the zygomatic arch; on the superior, posterior edge of a bulge on an angle; on the upper edge of an artery (auricular artery); two FW in front of TW 19; one half FW above TW 22 and TW 23, on the extremity of the eyebrow; one FW below and posterior to GB 8.

TH 21-23 are on the lateral aspect of the head and face.

TH 21 ER MEN – EAR GATE

⊥ *0.3 CUN* Δ *3 TO 7*

Pos: Position of patient: supine.

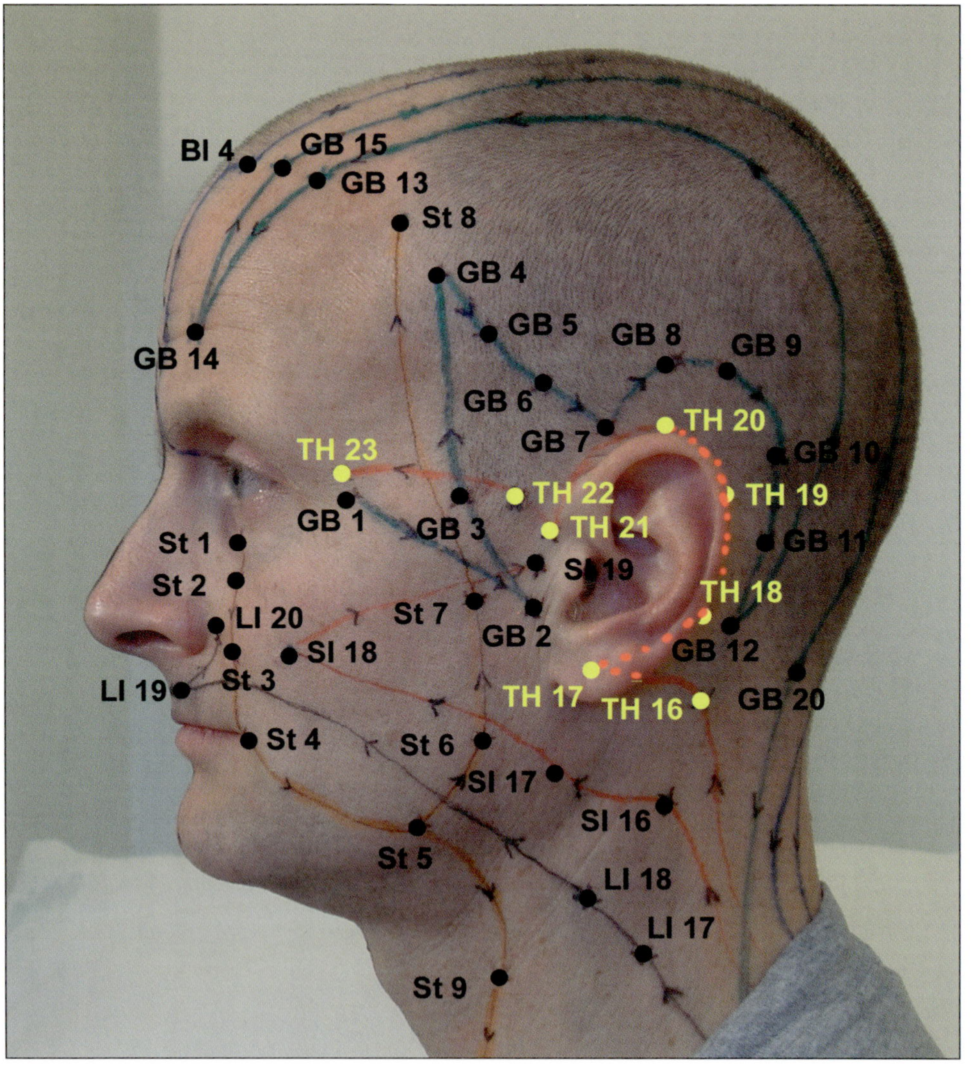

Loc: a) On the lateral aspect of the face.
b) Anterior to the superior edge of the tragus of the ear.
c) At the posterior border of the condyle of the mandible bone.
d) This point lies superior to SI 19.

Tip: a) This point is located with the mouth open as the movement of the condyle of the mandible reveals a depression where you would locate TH 21.
b) Make sure you are locating this point anterior to the superior edge of the tragus of the ear and not anterior to the middle of the tragus of the ear otherwise you could drift to SI 19 (inferior to TH 21).
c) If you were to place your finger anterior and superior to the middle of the tragus of the ear, when the mouth is opened you will feel a depression.
d) Perhaps draw a line out from the middle of the tragus of the ear to give you your level, then palpate for the point that is superior to it.
e) Needle the point with the mouth open.

Note: Jayasuriya (1982) locates the point in front of the supra-tragic notch when the mouth is slightly open. Qiu (1996) Locates it anterior to the supratragic notch, at the posterior border of the condylar process of the mandible. Soulié (1996) locates TW 23 (our TH 21) on the cheek: just anterior to the tragus and at the level of the ear hollow, between the tragus and the vertical artery (auricular artery and nerve). Between two small deep bones; one half FW (Finger Width) posterior to the rising portion of the maxilla; in a hollow; two FW under TW 22; two FW above and anterior to SI 19.

Cheng (1987), anterior to the supratragic notch and slightly superior to the condyloid process of the mandible with the mouth opened. Yang (1982) also locates the point anterior to the supratragic notch. Academy (1975) locates it with the mouth open, in front of the anterior notch of the auricle and slightly superior to the condyloid process of the manidble. Wu (1973) locates TH 21 before the ear at the apex of the angle formed by the tragus and helix.

Voisin (1974) locates T 21 between the helix and tragus, just in front and above the tragus. (He goes on to say that this point is Triple Heater 23 according to most authors.) Shandong (1982) locate Ermen above Pt. Tinggong, in front of the anterior notch of the auricula, in the depression when the mouth is open.

Legge (1999) locates SJ 21 with the mouth slightly open, the point is in the top of the depression anterior to the supratragic notch, superior to the condyloid process of the mandible. Lotan (2000) locates TW (SJ) 21, when the mouth is slightly open, between the ear cartilage and the condylar process, level with the tragus superior edge.

TH 22 HE LIAO – HARMONY BONE

⊥ *0.3 CUN* Δ *3 TO 5*

- EXIT
- RE-UNION/Crossing/Meeting Point of the Triple Heater Channel with the Gall Bladder and Small Intestine Channels.- Hand Shao Yang Channel with the Foot Shao Yang and Hand Tai Yang Channels

Pos: Position of patient: supine or seated.

Loc: a) On the temporal region of the head.
b) 0.5-1.5 cun anterior to the superior root of the pinna of the ear.
c) Just posterior to the superficial temporal artery.
d) At the mid-point between GB 7 and GB 3 (see separate descriptions).

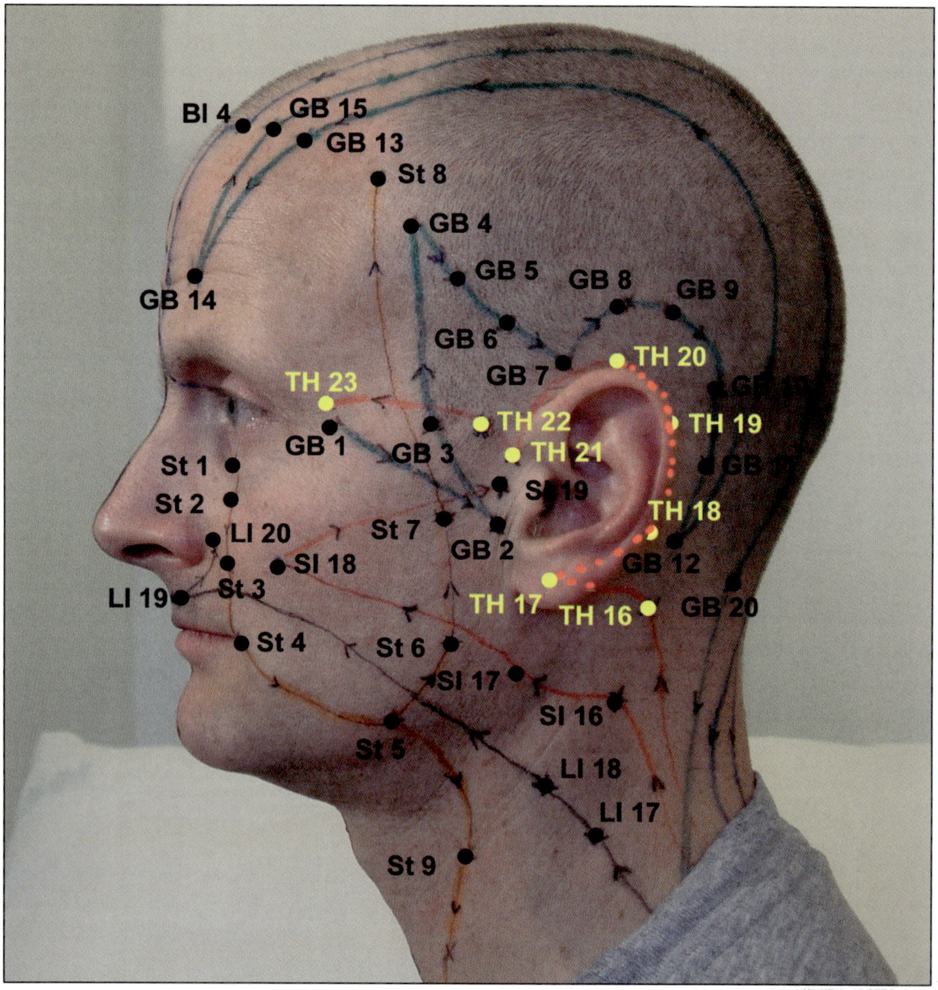

Tip: a) Feel for the superior root of the pinna of the ear.
b) Then with your finger on the superior root of the pinna move it anteriorly towards the lateral aspect of the eye so that you are in the hairline.
c) You should be able to feel a pulsation from the superficial temporal artery in the hairline, and the point lies just posterior to it.
d) On some people this point may be just posterior to the hairline.

Note: Deadman (1998) locate SJ 22 at 0.5 cun anterior to the upper border of the root of the ear, on the posterior border of the hairline of the temple. Jayasuriya (1982) also makes reference to the posterior border of the hairline but does not refer to a measurement anterior to the hairline. Voisin (1974) locates T 22 in front of the auricle, on the upper border of the zygomatic arch. Wu (1973) locates TH 22 in front of the ear, before the helix, between TH 21 and GB 7, at the insertion of the helix. Yang (1982) locates the point 1 cun anterior to the root of the auricle. Academy of Traditional Chinese Medicine (1975) locates SJ 22 on the hairline anterior and superior to SJ 21, anterior to and level with the root of the auricle, posterior to the superficial temporal artery.

TH 23 SI ZHU KONG – SILK BAMBOO HOLLOW

⊥ ***0.3 CUN*** △ ***FORBIDDEN TO USE MOXA***

Pos: Position of patient: supine or seated.

Loc: a) On the temporal region of the head.
b) At the lateral extremity of the eyebrow.
c) Just posterior to the supraorbital ridge of the frontal bone.

Tip: a) When you palpate for this point make sure that you are level with the lateral extremity of the eyebrow otherwise you may be palpating GB 1 or other points in the vicinity.
b) When you have established the level of the extremity of the eyebrow, feel posterior to the supraorbital ridge of the frontal bone (sometimes called the orbit bone) and palpate for the point.

Note: Soulié (1994) locates TW 21 (our TH 23) above and in front of the ear: two FW (Finger Width) above a transverse relief of the zygomatic arch; on the extremity of the eyebrow; in a hollow; one FW above GB 1; two FW anterior and slightly above GB 7. Voisin (1974) locates T 23 on the temple: the hollow is slightly above and lateral to the lateral extremity of the eyebrow. (He goes on to say that this is the location of Triple Heater 21 according to most authors.) Shandong (1982) locate Sizhukong in the depression lateral to the lateral tip of the supercilium.

REFERENCES FOR THE TRIPLE HEATER CHANNEL

Ellis, Wiseman and Boss. 1991 Fundamentals of Chinese Acupuncture – TB 1: 280

Huang-fu Mi. Trans: Yang Shou-zhong and Charles Chace 1993 The Systematic Classic of Acupuncture & Moxibustion – TH 1: 180

Wu, Wei-P'ing 1973 Chinese Acupuncture – TH 2: 105; TH 4: 105; TH 10: 107; TH 12: 107; TH 13: 107; TH 15: 108; TH 17: 108; TH 18: 108; TH 19: 108; TH 20: 108; TH 21: 109

Jayasuriya, Anton 1982 Clinical Acupuncture – SJ 2: 401; SJ 20: 402; SJ 21:402; SJ 22: 402

Deadman, Peter; Al-Khafaji, Mazin; Baker, Kevin 1998 Manual of Acupuncture, An – SJ 2: 392; SJ 12: 404; SJ 13: 404; SJ 20:410; SJ 22: 411

Voisin, Dr. H 1974 Essentials of Acupuncture – T 2: 92; T 3: 92; T 5: 92; T 6: 92; T 7: 92; T 8: 92; T 9: 92; T 11: 92; T 12: 92; T 13: 92; T 17: 92; T 18: 92; T 19: 94; T 20: 94; T 21: 94; T 22: 94; T 23: 94

Cheng Xinnong (Editor) 1987 Chinese Acupuncture and Moxibustion – SJ 2: 192; SJ 15: 196; SJ 17: 196; SJ 20: 198

Shandong Medical College and Shandong College of Traditional Chinese Medicine 1982 Anatomical Atlas of Chinese Acupuncture Point – Yemen (TH 2): 46; Hand-Zhongzhu (TH 3): 46; Yangchi (TH 4): 46; Zhigou (TH 6): 46; Sanyangluo (TH 8): 46; Sidu (TH 9): 46; Naohui (TH 13): 46; Tianliao (TH 15): 46; Yifeng (TH 17): 47; Qimai (TH 18): 47; Luxi (TH 19): 47; Ermen (TH 21): 47; Sizhukong (TH 23): 47

Legge, David 1999 Acupuncture Points and Meridians – SJ 2: 73; SJ 3: 73; SJ 4: 73; SJ21: 74

Lotan, Alon 2000 Acupoint Location Guide – TW (SJ) 2: 117; TW (SJ) 3: 117; TW (SJ) 4: 119; TW (SJ) 9: 119; TW (SJ) 11: 119; TW (SJ) 14: 123; TW (SJ) 21: 127

Worsley, J R 1982 Traditional Chinese Acupuncture Volume 1 – Meridians and Points. VI 7: 129;
VI 10: 129; VI 15: 131; VI 17: 133; VI 18: 133; VI 19: 133; VI 20: 135

Soulié De Morant, George. 1994 Chinese Acupuncture – TW 7: 469; TW 8: 469; TW 9: 470; TW 11: 471; TW 12: 471; TW 13: 472; TW 15: 472; TW 16: 473; TW 17: 473; TW 18: 474; TW 19: 474; TW 20: 474; TW 23 (TH 21): 476; TW 21 (TH 23): 475

Eachou Chen 1995. Cross-sectional Anatomy of Acupoints – TB 12: 14; TB 20: 110

Qiu Mao-Liang 1996 – Chinese Acupuncture and Moxibustion – SJ 13: 132; SJ 20:134

Yang Jiasan (Prof) 1982 The Way to Locate Acu-Points – SJ 20: 24; SJ 21: 24; SJ 22: 24

Academy of Traditional Chinese Medicine, The. 1975 – Outline of Chinese Acupuncture, An. SJ 20: 171; SJ 21: 171; SJ 22: 172

Lavier, Dr. J 1974 Points of Chinese Acupuncture – Upper Arm Pouce Measurement: 10/11

THE GALLBLADDER CHANNEL OF THE FOOT (SHAO YANG)

Primary channel

The Gallbladder channel starts superficially at the lateral canthus of the eye (GB 1) and zig-zags up and down the lateral aspects of the face and head, finally descending (from GB 15) to GB 20 inferior to the occiput and GB 21 on the shoulder.

(There are connections from GB 3 to TH 22 to St 8 to GB 4-7 to TH 20 and back to GB 8. Some texts refer to a connection between GB 14 and Bl 1).

One deep branch of the primary channel goes from GB 1 down the cheek to the mandible, (connecting with St 5), then up to the inferior border of the zygomatic bone (crossing the Triple Heater channel and joining SI 18), and down the angle of the mandible to join St 6, finally passing on down the neck to reach St 12 where it reconnects with the main channel.

Another branch leaves GB 12, travels to TH 17 behind the mastoid process, enters the ear, then emerges in front of the ear at SI 19, passing St 7 on its way back to GB 1 at the lateral canthus.

At GB 21, the channel runs posteriorly across the shoulder to Du 14, down to Bl 11, laterally to SI 12, then back across the shoulder to St 12 in the supraclavicular fossa, where the channel becomes superficial again.

At this point a deep channel travels through the thorax, crossing the superficial channel at GB 24, and comes down through the diaphragm, connecting with Liv 13, then passes through the liver and Gallbladder organs. It continues to the lower abdomen and inguinal region, passes the pubic area, and turns backwards to the hip (to GB 30).

The superficial channel from St 12 passes in front of the axilla and zig-zags down the lateral aspect of the chest and floating ribs to the greater trochanter of the femur at GB 30, (via Liv 13/14 and St 30 according to Japanese texts).

Meanwhile at GB 29 a deep channel goes round the back and across to the sacrum, connecting with Bl 31 to 34, then down to Du 1 and back across to GB 30.

The superficial channel runs from GB 30 down the lateral side of the leg/foot to GB 41, (where a deep channel runs between the first and second metatarsals to the medial aspect of the first digit, and crosses under the toenail to connect with Liv 1). The Gallbladder channel continues, to end at GB 44 on the lateral aspect of the fourth digit.

Divergent Channel

This leaves the primary channel on the thigh and crosses over the hip joint to enter the lower abdomen in the pelvic region, where it links with the divergent channel of the Liver. It then crosses between the lower ribs, connects with the gallbladder and diffuses through the liver, before passing up to the heart and oesophagus, dispersing in the face. It connects with the eye, rejoining the primary channel at the lateral canthus.

Connecting Channel

This leaves the primary channel at GB 37 on the lateral aspect of the lower leg to connect with the Liver channel, then passes downwards to disperse over the dorsum of the foot.

Muscle Channel

This begins on the fourth digit, binds with the lateral malleolus and passes up the lateral aspect of the leg, binding with the knee. A branch leaves the head of the fibula and ascends the thigh. One sub-branch travels anteriorly, binding with the thigh above St 32. Another travels posteriorly to bind with the sacrum.

The main channel passes upwards across the ribs to the anterior border of the axilla, binding first in the breast region and then superior to the clavicle.

Another branch of the main channel runs from the axilla across the clavicle, emerging anterior to the Bladder muscle channel, and continues up posterior to the ear to the temple. It then crosses to the vertex, where it joins its bilateral counterpart.

A branch descends from the temple across the cheek, and binds at the bridge of the nose; a sub branch binds with the lateral canthus of the eye.

THE GALLBLADDER CHANNEL OF THE FOOT

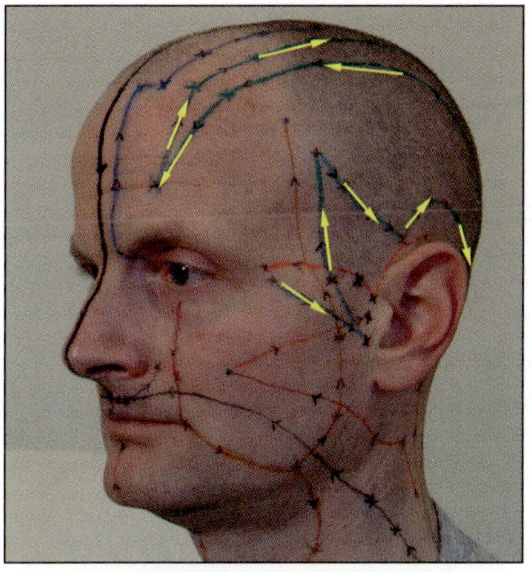

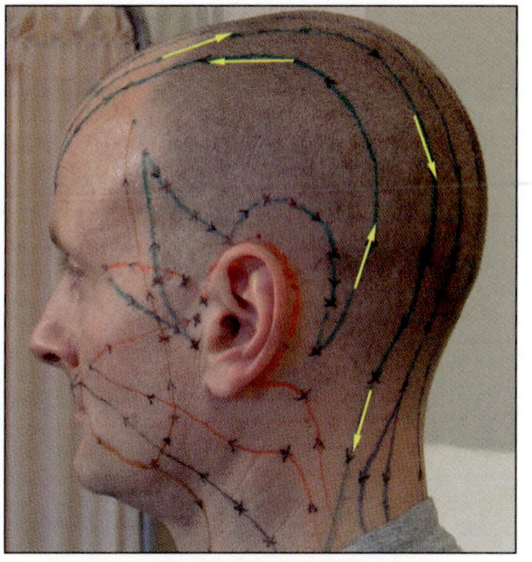

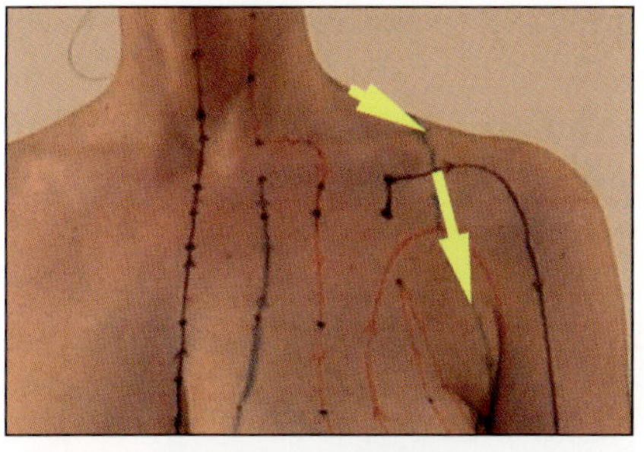

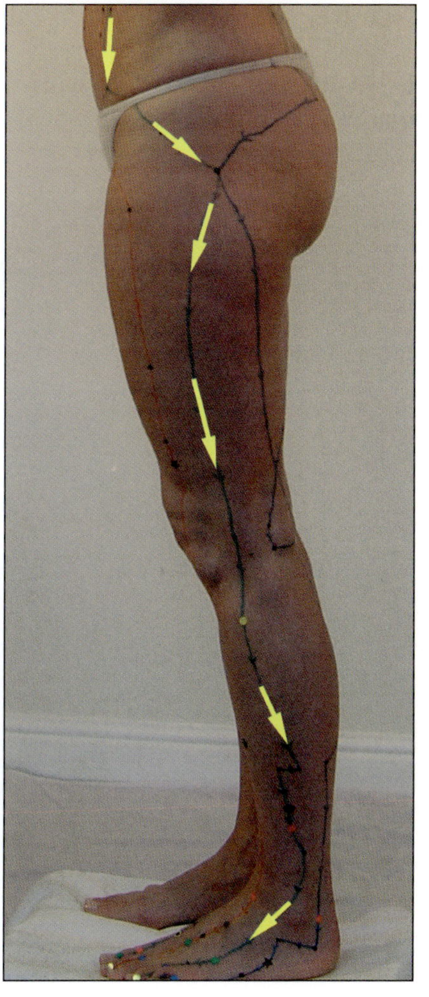

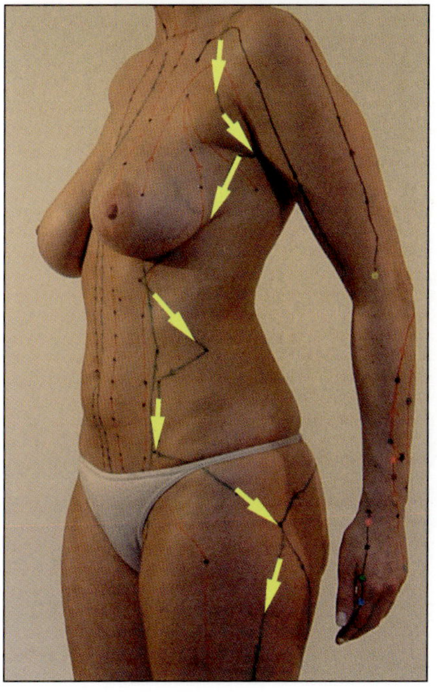

Points of the Gall Bladder Channel – Foot Shao Yang (GB/Gb/G/VII)

Longitudinal bone proportional measurements of the head:

- **3 cun from between the two eyebrows (M-HN-3, Du 24.5 or Yin Tang) to the natural anterior hairline on the anterior median line.**
- **12 cun from the natural anterior hairline to the posterior hairline on the median line.**
- **3 cun from the posterior hairline to the space between the 7th cervical and 1st thoracic vertebrae (Du 14) on the posterior median line.**
- **15 cun (anterior natural hairline to the space between C7/T1);**
- **18 cun (between the two eyebrows at Du 24.5 or Yin Tang to the space between C7/T1).**

Transverse bone proportional measurements of the head:

- **(Anterior) 9 cun between the two corners of the forehead (St 8).**
- **(Posterior) 9 cun between the bilateral mastoid processes.**

It may be easier to use a length of paper so that you can draw on the cun measurements as opposed to drawing the measurements on the scalp itself.

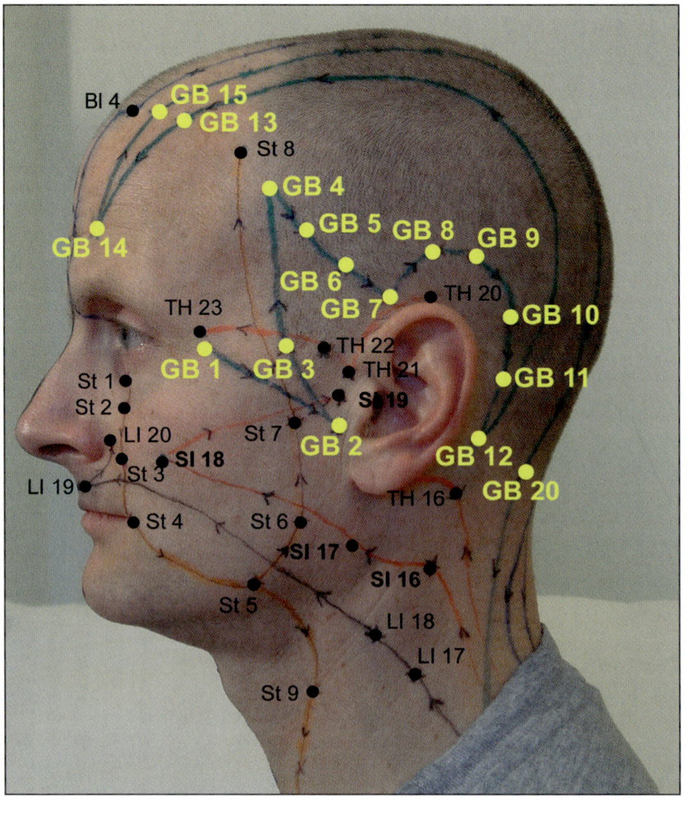

GB 1-20 are on the lateral aspect of the face, head and neck.

GB 1 TONG ZI LIAO – ORBIT BONE

⊥ ***0.3 CUN*** **Δ** ***3 TO 5***

- ENTRY
- RE-UNION/Crossing/Meeting Point of the Gall Bladder Channel with the Triple Heater and Small Intestine Channels – Foot Shao Yang Channel with the Hand Shao Yang and Hand Tai Yang Channels

Pos: Position of patient: supine or seated.

Loc: a) On the temporal region of the head.
b) Just lateral to the orbital ridge of the zygomatic bone.
c) Approximately 0.5 cun lateral and level to the lateral canthus of the eye.

Tip: a) Ensure that you are level with the lateral canthus otherwise you may be palpating TH 23 or other points in the vicinity, particularly if palpating too superiorly.
b) When you have established the level of the lateral canthus, run your finger from the lateral canthus laterally going over the orbital ridge of the zygomatic bone.
c) As you go over the orbital ridge of the zygomatic bone, you should be able to palpate GB 1, which is approximately 0.5 cun lateral to the lateral canthus of the eye.
d) On some people, the orbital ridge of the the zygomatic bone may seem quite wide. As long as you palpate over this ridge (which may be more than 0.5 cun), you will be able to palpate GB 1.

Note: Soulié (1994) locates GB 1 on the cheek: lower temple; two FW (Finger Width) lateral to the lateral corner of the eye. One FW above the angle of the posterior edge of the vertical suture (temporosphenoid) and the upper edge of the transverse prominence of the zygomatic arch; three FW in front of GB 3; separated from GB 4 by a horizontal suture; two FW above and lateral to ST 1. Voisin (1974) locates G 1 in relation to the orbite: 1 fb (finger breadth) lateral to its lateral border.

GB 2 TING HUI – HEARING ASSEMBLY

⊥ ***0.3 TO 0.5 CUN*** Δ ***3 TO 5***

Pos: Position of patient: supine or seated.

Loc: a) On the lateral aspect of the face.
b) Anterior to the ear.
c) On the posterior border of the condyle of the mandible bone.
d) Anterior and just inferior to the inferior border of the tragus of the ear.
e) Anterior to the intertragic incisure.
f) Inferior to SI 19.
g) Located with the mouth open.

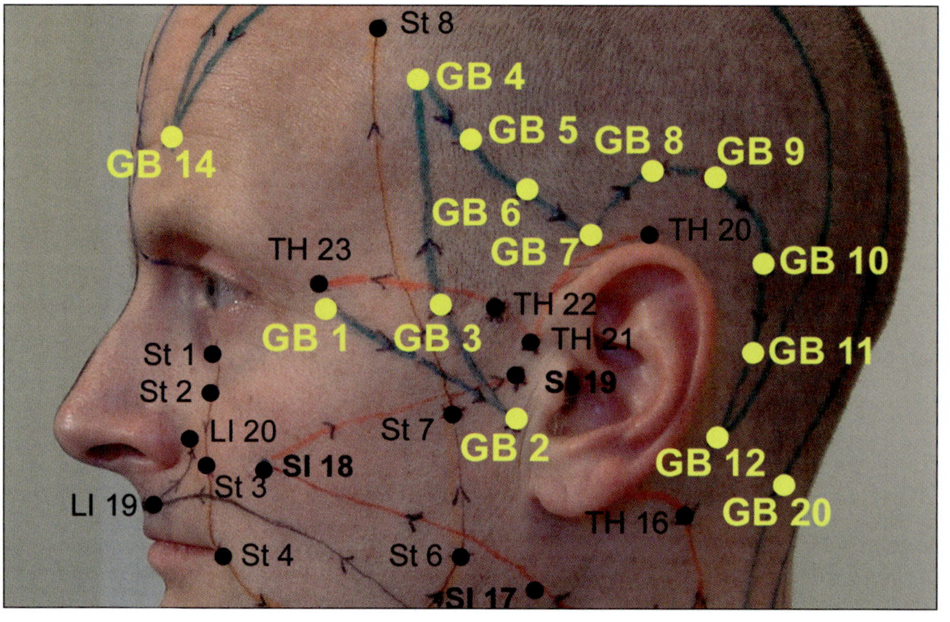

Tip: a) It is important that this point is always located with the mouth open. The movement of the mandibular condyle reveals a depression where GB 2 is located.
b) With the patient's mouth slightly open locate SI 19 which is level with the middle of the tragus of the ear, on the posterior border of the mandiblar condyle.
c) Palpate inferiorly from SI 19 to the inferior border of the tragus of the ear.
d) The intertragic incisure is just inferior to the inferior border of the tragus of the ear. GB 2 is located between the anterior border of the intertragic incisure and the posterior border of the mandibular condyle.
e) This point is always needled with the mouth open.

Note: Gray (1978) The intertragic incisure is inferior to base of the tragus of the ear and lies superior to the lobule of the ear. Voisin (1974) locates G 2 in relation to the ear lobule, at the anteroinferior part of its attachment to the cheek. Soulié (1994) locates GB 2 on the cheek: one half FW (Finger Width) in front of the hole of the ear. A little under the posterior angle of the head and body of the maxilla; on the superior edge of an insertion on the bone (risorius); between the bone and the vessels (superficial temporal artery and vein); two tightened FW (Finger Width) above and posterior to TW 21.

So (1985) locates GB 2 out 1/3 division horizontally from the "V" formed by the tragus and the earlobe, in the crossing hollow of the jaw bone. Worsley (1982) locates VII 2 on the posterior margin of the condyle of the mandible, anterior to the inferior border of the tragus. When the mouth is opened, a depression appears at this point. Masayoshi (1975) locates GB 2 medial to the edge of the temple. Wu (1973) locates GB 2 in front of the lbe of the ear, behind the condyle of the mandible.

GB 3 SHANG GUAN – UPPER PASS

⊥ ***0.3 CUN*** Δ ***3 TO 5***

- RE-UNION/Crossing/Meeting Point of the Gall Bladder Channel with the Triple Heater and Stomach Channels – Foot Shao Yang Channel with the Hand Shao Yang and Foot Yang Ming Channels

Pos: Position of patient: supine or seated.

Loc:
a) On the lateral aspect of the face.
b) Anterior to the ear.
c) On the upper border of the zygomatic arch of the temporal bone.
d) Directly superior to St 7 (which is in the middle of the lower border of the zygomatic arch of the temporal bone).
e) Superior to the anterior border of the condyle of the mandible.
f) Superior to GB 2 and SI 19(see separate descriptions).

Tip:
a) First locate St 6 and St 7.
b) Locate the prominence of the masseter muscle (location of St 6), on the mandible bone and ask the patient to clench their teeth.
c) Run your finger directly superior until you feel the inferior border of the zygomatic arch of the temporal bone.
d) To locate the mandibular condyle ask the patient to open their mouth but closing the mouth when locating GB 3. The point is in a depression which disappears when the mouth is opened.
e) St 7 is located just superior to the anterior border of the mandibular condyle, inferior to the zygomatic arch and directly superior to St 6 (the prominence of the masseter bone).
f) From St 7 palpate superiorly over the zygomatic arch of the temporal bone and you should be able to feel a notch. GB 3 is in the notch.

Note: So (1985) Locates GB 3 at 1 and 1/2 eye divisions in front of TW 21, on the upper edge of the cheek bone, directly above ST 7. Wu (1973) locates GB 3 upon the face, at mid-distance between the ear and the external edge of the orbit, above the zygomatic arch. Soulié (1994) locates GB 3 on the face: about mid-distance from the ear to the edge of the orbit; at the angle between the transverse edge of the zygomatic arch and the posterior edge of the upper prominence of the arch; above the anterior edge of the condyle of the maxilla; three FW (Finger Width) under and behind GB 1; two tightened FW lateral. to SI 19; two FW under and anterior to TW 21; three FW under GB 7. Voisin (1974) locates G 3 in relation to the zygomatic arch, the upper border, at 1 fb (finger breadth) lateral to its centre. Lotan (2000) locates GB 3 superior to the vertical slit on the zygomatic arch superior border.

GB 4 HAN YAN – LOATHSOME JAWS

⊥ ***0.3 TO 0.5 CUN*** **Δ** ***3***

- RE-UNION/Crossing/Meeting Point of the Gall Bladder Channel with the Triple Heater and Stomach Channels – Foot Shao Yang Channel with the Hand Shao Yang and Foot Yang Ming Channels

Pos: Position of patient: supine or seated.

Loc: a) On the temporal region of the head.
b) Posterior to the natural hairline.
c) Approximately 1 cun inferior to St 8.
d) Between St 8 and GB 7.
e) One quarter of the distance between St 8 and GB 7.
f) Three quarters of the distance between GB 7 and St 8.

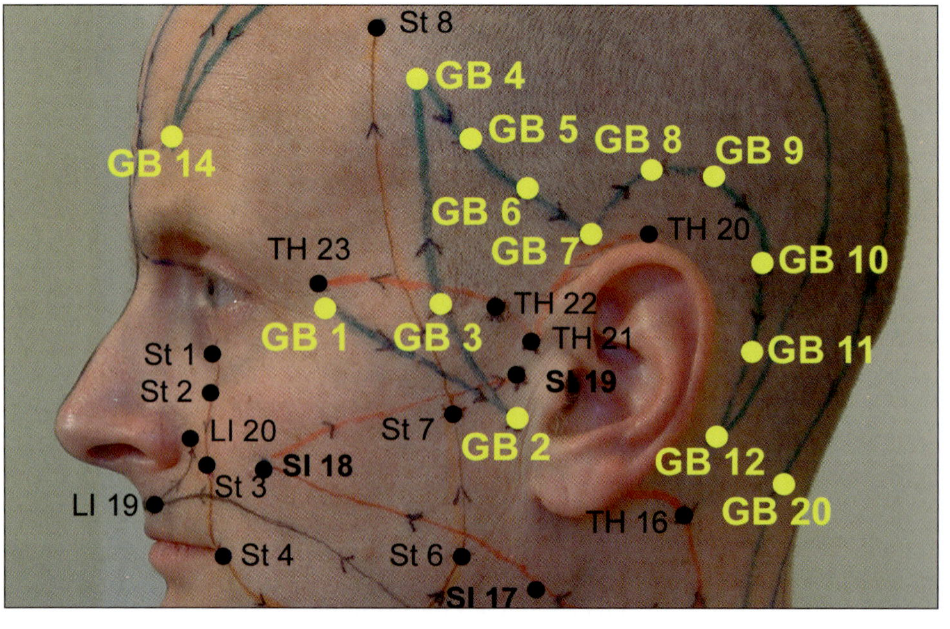

Tip:
a) The easiest method of locating GB 4 is to locate St 8 which is at the corner of the forehead, 0.5 cun posterior to the natural anterior hairline, on the medial border of the temporalis muscle (See St 8 tips section for more information).
b) Once you have located St 8, palpate approximately 1 cun inferiorly until you can feel a good *men* (depression) – this may or may not be at 1 cun inferior to St 8 as palpation takes precedence.
c) Another method of locating GB 4 is locate TH 20, GB 7 and St 8. TH 20 is on the lateral aspect of the head, on the temporal bone, and level with or immediately superior to the apex of the pinna of the ear (See TH 20 tips section for more information).
d) GB 7 is on the lateral aspect of the head, on the temporal bone, level with and approximately one finger width anterior to TH 20 (See GB 7 location and tips sections for more information).
e) St 8 is at the corner of the forehead, 0.5 cun posterior to the natural anterior hairline, on the the medial border of the temporalis muscle (See St 8 location and tips sections for more information).
f) You need to locate GB 7 and St 8 as these are two reference points when locating GB 4, GB 5 and GB 6.
g) Divide the distance between GB 7 and St 8 in to four equal parts.
h) GB 4 is located one quarter of the distance inferior to St 8 or three quarters of the distance superior to GB 7.
i) Asking the patient to chew can often make this point easier to palpate and locate.

Note: Wu (1973) locates GB 4 upon the temple, upon a horizontal line passing through GB 14, GB 8, GB 9, at mid-distance between TH 23 and TH 22. Voisin (1974) locates G 4 on the temporal area, upper part: on the coronal suture. Worsley (1982) locates VII 4 on the temple, 0.5 ACI (Anatomical Chinese Inch) posterior to the natural hairline, 1 ACI inferior to XI 8 (St 8). Soulié (1994) locates GB 4 on the temple: approximately 2 FW (Finger Width) lateral to the extremity of the eyebrow. A little above the lateral edge of the prominence (between the parietal-sphenoid suture and the upper edge of the horizontal prominence (the temporoparietal suture); on the point of the parietal bone; separated from GB 1 by a horizontal mass; one medial (anterior) FW to GB 5; two FW under GB 16; three tightened FW under and lateral to ST 8.

Academy (1975) locates GB 4 at 1 cun below St 8, on the hairline of the temporal region. Masayoshi (1975) locates GB 4 in the temporal region 1 finger width inside from the hairline. Eachou (1995) locates GB 4 at the anterior temporal region, one quarter of the distance between ST 8 and GB 7; or 1 inch inferior and posterior to ST 8 and 0.5 inch inside the temporal hairline. So (1985) locates GB 4 at 2 divisions above XF 3 Yin Tang, lateral one division past the hairline in the horizontal and vertical cleft. Lavier (1974) in an illustration locates GB 4 on the cranium, the temple, superior to a line drawn from GV 24 (Du 24) through ST 8, GB 5 and GB 7 to the external auditory meatus of the ear. The point is located in a suture (not labelled) superior to this line and superior to GB 5. Shandong (1982) locate Hanyan on the hairline of the temporal region, between Pt. Touwei (St 8) and Pt. Xuanlu (GB 5).

GB 5 XUAN LU – SUSPENDED SKULL

⊥ ***0.3 CUN*** Δ ***3***

- RE-UNION/Crossing/Meeting Point of the Gall Bladder Channel with the Triple Heater and Stomach Channels – Foot Shao Yang Channel with the Hand Shao Yang and Foot Yang Ming Channels

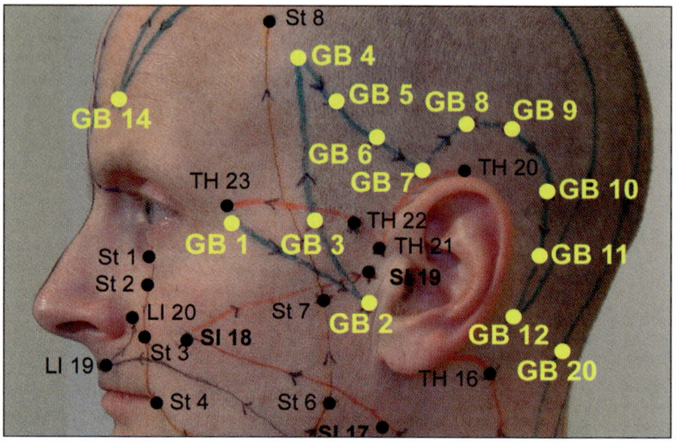

Pos: Position of patient: supine.

Loc: a) On the temporal region of the head.
b) Posterior to the natural hairline.
c) Halfway between St 8 and GB 7.

Tip: a) The easiest method of locating GB 5 is to locate TH 20, GB 7 and St 8. TH 20 is on the lateral aspect of the head, on the temporal bone, and level with or immediately superior to the apex of the pinna of the ear (See TH 20 tips section for more information).
b) GB 7 is on the lateral aspect of the head, on the temporal bone, level with and approximately one finger width anterior to TH 20 (See GB 7 location and tips sections for more information).
c) St 8 is at the corner of the forehead, 0.5 cun posterior to the natural anterior hairline, on the the medial border of the temporalis muscle (See St 8 location and tips sections for more information).
d) You need to locate GB 7 and St 8 as these are two reference points when locating GB 4, GB 5 and GB 6.
e) GB 5 is located approximately halfway between St 8.
f) Palpation of this area will accurately locate the point.

Note: Wu (1973) locates GB 5 upon the temple, at one pouce below GB 4, upon a horizontal line passing through TH 23. Worsley (1982) locates VII 5 on the temple, 0.5 ACI (Anatomical Chinese Inch) posterior to the natural hairline, one third of the distance from VII 4 (GB 4) to VII 7 (GB 7). Voisin (1974) locates G 5 in relation to the temporal area, 1 fb (finger breadth) posterior to Gallbladder 4. Soulié (1994) locates GB 5 on the temple: three FW (Finger Width) lateral (posterior) to the extremity of the eyebrow, two FW above the horizontal prominence of the zygomatic arch; at the angle between the anterior edge of the vertical mass (temporal-parietal suture) and the upper edge of the horizontal suture of the same bones; on the point of the parietal bone; one FW lateral to (behind) GB 4; one FW medial (anterior) to GB 6; one Fw under and a bit medial (anterior) to GB 13; two FW above and lateral to GB 3; one FW above and lateral to GB 1.

Academy (1975) locates GB 5 in the line connecting GB 4 and GB 7, at the junction of the anterior and middle third of the line. Masayoshi (1975) locates GB 5 midway between GB 4 and GB 6. So (1985) locates GB 5 at one division above XF 3, Yin Tang, between the eyebrows; lateral one division past the hairline in the horizontal and vertical cleft. Lavier (1974) in an illustration locates GB 5 on the cranium, the temple, in a suture (not labelled) and on a line drawn from GV 24 (Du 24) through (ST 8, GB 5 and GB 7) to the external auditory meatus of the ear.

GB 6 XUAN LI – SUSPENDED REGULATOR

⊥ ***0.3 CUN*** **Δ *3***

- RE-UNION/Crossing/Meeting Point of the Gall Bladder Channel with the Triple Heater and Stomach Channels – Foot Shao Yang Channel with the Hand Shao Yang and Foot Yang Ming Channels

Pos: Position of patient: supine or seated.

Loc: a) On the temporal region of the head.
b) Posterior to the hairline.
c) Between St 8 and GB 7.
d) Three quarters of the distance between St 8 and GB 7.
e) One quarter of the distance between GB 7 and St 8.

Tip: a) The easiest method of locating GB 6 is locate TH 20, GB 7 and St 8. TH 20 is on the lateral aspect of the head, on the temporal bone, and level with or immediately superior to the apex of the pinna of the car (See TH 20 tips section for more information).
b) GB 7 is on the lateral aspect of the head, on the temporal bone, level with and approximately one finger width anterior to TH 20 (See GB 7 location and tips sections for more information).
c) St 8 is at the corner of the forehead, 0.5 cun posterior to the natural anterior hairline, on the the medial border of the temporalis muscle (See St 8 location and tips sections for more information).
d) You need to locate GB 7 and St 8 as these are two reference points when locating GB 4, GB 5 and GB 6.
e) Divide the distance between GB 7 and St 8 in to four equal parts.
f) GB 6 is located three quarters of the distance superior to St 8 or one quarter of the distance inferior to GB 7.
g) Palpation of this area will accurately locate this point.

Note: Wu (1973) locates GB 6 upon the temple, one pouce below GB 5. Legge (1999) locates GB 6 within the hairline inferior to the corner of the temporal region, midway between GB 5 and GB 7. Voisin (1974) locates G 6 on the temporal area, 1.5 fb (finger breadth) posterior and inferior to Gallbladder 4. Masayoshi (1975) locates GB 6 at 3 sun below GB 4. So (1985) locates GB 6 directly lateral to the end of the eyebrow; one division past the hairline at the horizontal/vertical cleft. Worsley (192) locates VII 6 on the temple, 0.5 ACI (Anatomical Chinese Inch) posterior to the natural hairline, one third of the distance between VII 4 (GB 4) to VII 7 (GB 7). Jayasuriya (1982) locates GB 6 within the lateral hairline, midway between GB 5 and GB 7.

Academy (1975) locates GB 6 in the line connecting GB 4 and GB 7, at the junction of the inferior and middle third of the line. Ellis (1991) locates GB 6 within the hairline of the temporal region, midway between GB 5 and GB 7. Soulié (1994) locates GB 6 on the temple: one FW (Finger Width) anterior to the vertical line from the anterior edge of the ear. Two FW above the transverse relief of the zygomatic arch. At the angle of the superior edge of a slight transverse relief (on the inferior curve) and the posterior edge of a vertical relief. In a notch of the temporal-parietal suture.; one FW lateral (posterior) to GB 5; one half FW anterior to GB 7; two large FW under GB 17.

Lavier (1974) in an illustration locates GB 6 on the cranium, the temple, inferior to a line drawn from GV 24 (Du 24) through ST 8, GB 5 and GB 7 to the external auditory meatus of the ear. The point is located in a suture (not labelled) inferior to this line and inferior to GB 5. Shandong (1982) locate Xuanli on the hairline of the temporal region, between Pt. Xuanlu (GB 5) and Pt. Qubin (GB 7).

GB 7 QU BIN – CROOKED HAIR ON THE TEMPLES

⊥ ***0.3 CUN*** **Δ** ***3 TO 5***

- RE-UNION/Crossing/Meeting Point of the Gall Bladder Channel with the Bladder Channel – Foot Shao Yang Channel with the Foot Tai Yang Channel

Pos: Position of patient: supine or seated.

Loc: a) On the temporal region of the head.
b) On the temporal bone.
c) Posterior to the hairline.
d) On a transverse level with TH 20 and the apex of the the pinna of the ear.
e) Approximately 1 finger width anterior to TH 20.

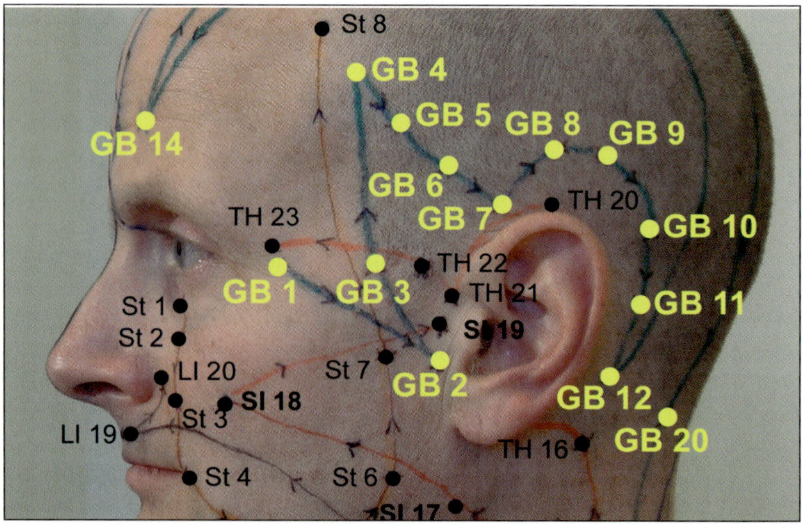

Tip:
a) Locate TH 20 first as this is a reference point.
b) TH 20 is on the lateral aspect of the head, on the temporal bone, and level with or immediately superior to the apex of the pinna of the ear (See TH 20 tips section for more information).
c) Draw a horizontal line anteriorly from TH 20 (towards the eye) and palpate for GB 7 approximately 1 finger width anterior to TH 20 on this line.
d) On some people this point may be slightly inferior to the horizontal line. It is important to palpate the area for accurate point location which may or may not be at one finger width.

Note: Lavier (1974) in an illustration locates GB 7 on the cranium, the temple, on a line drawn from GV 24 (Du 24) through ST 8 (GB 5 and GB 7) to the external auditory meatus of the ear. In another illustration GB 7 is located anterior to TH 20, anterior to the apex of the pinna of the ear. Lotan (2000) locates GB 7 vertically superior to the ear cartilage anterior border, level with the auricle apex superior border. About 1 finger breadth anterior to TW (SJ) 20. Academy (1975) locates GB 7 at the crossing point of the horizontal line of the auricle and the line that projects from the anterior auricle. Masayoshi (1975) locates GB 7 anterior to the upper extremity of the auricle, about 1 finger width above the cheekbone.

Worsley (1982) locates VII 7 on the temple, 0.5 ACI (Anatomical Chinese Inch) posterior to the natural hairline, at the level of the apex of the pinna, approximately 1 ACI anterior to and slightly inferior to VI 20 (TH 20). So (1985) locates GB 7 lateral to a point midway between the outer canthus and the end of the eyebrow, one division past the hairline in the horizontal cleft, Cheng (1987) locates GB 7 directly above the posterior border of the pre-auricular hairline, about one finger-breadth anterior to Jiaosun (SJ 20). Shanghai (1993) locates GB 7 on the head, at a crossing point of the vertical posterior border of the temples and the horizontal line through the ear apex (1 cun anterior to Jiaosun -SJ 20).

Soulié (1994) locates GB 7 on the lateral side of the head: three FW (Finger Width) above the transverse relief of the zygomatic arch; one FW anterior to the vertical from the anterior edge of the ear. At the angle of the superior edge of a slight horizontal relief (inferior curve) and the anterior edge of a vertical relief. Between two horizontal reliefs; one half FW posterior to GB 6; one FW in front of and a bit under GB 8; two large FW under and posterior to GB 17; two large FW under and anterior to GB 18; one FW above and a bit anterior to TW 23; one FW above and very much anterior to TW 20. Wu (1973) locates GB 7 in front of the ear, at one pouce before TH 20, upon the hairline.

Voisin (1974) locates G 7 in the temporal area, 1 fb (finger breadth) in front and above the upper attachment of the ear to the cheek.. Eachou (1995) locates GB 7 by drawing a horizontal line from Jiaosun (TB 20) and a vertical line from the anterior helix of the ear, the point is located at the intersection of the two lines (approximately one finger width anterior to Jiaosun (TB 20)). Qiu (1996) locates GB 7 directly above the posterior border of the pre-auricular hairline, about the level of Jiaosun (SJ 20). Katsusuke (1983)locates GB 7 one sun above the highest part of the cheekbone in front of the ear.

GB 8 SHUAI GU – FLOWING VALLEY

⊥ ***0.3 CUN*** **Δ** ***3 TO 5***

- RE-UNION/Crossing/Meeting Point of the Gall Bladder Channel with the Bladder Channel – Foot Shao Yang Channel with the Foot Tai Yang Channel

Pos: Position of patient: supine or seated.

Loc: a) On the lateral aspect of the head.
b) On the parietal bone.
c) 1 to 1.5 cun superior to the apex of the pinna of the ear.
d) Directly superior TH 20.

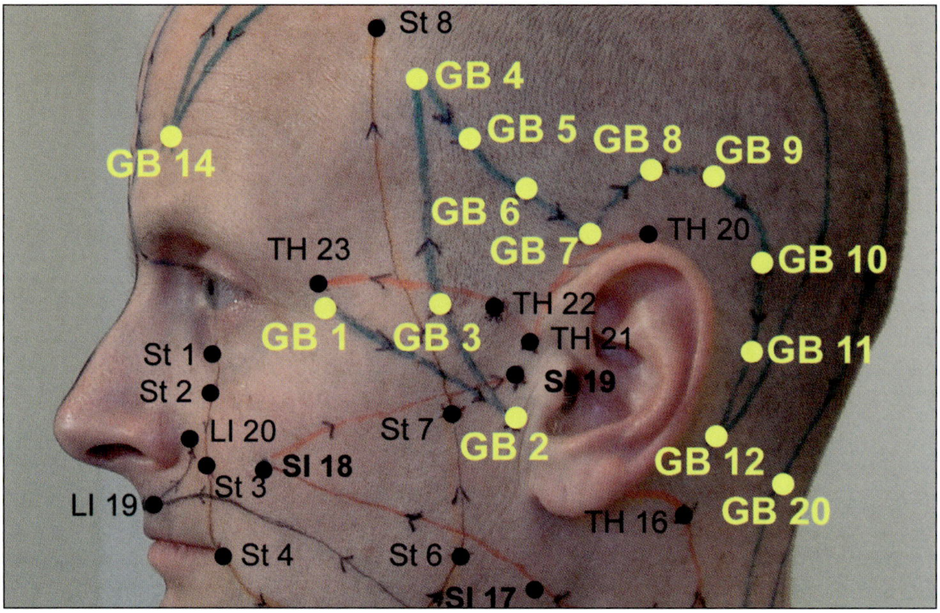

Tip: a) First locate TH 20 as a point of reference.
b) TH 20 is on the lateral aspect of the head, on the temporal bone, and level with or immediately superior to the apex of the pinna of the ear.
c) Press the helix of the ear against the skull and draw a mark on the skull at the apex (highest part) of the pinna.
d) When the helix of the ear is bent forward, make sure it is only the helix and not the main body of the ear.
e) TH 20 may be on the contour line of the helix of the ear or immediately superior to it. Palpation of the point will ensure accuracy.
f) Palpation is easiest method to locate GB 8, see g). If you prefer to use cun measurements, see h) and i)
g) Palpate superiorly from the apex of the pinna of the ear from TH 20, until you feel a depression which is GB 8.

h) To use the 1.5 cun measurement locate St 8 and the anterior median line which will give 4.5 cun. St 8 is at the corner of the forehead, 0.5 cun posterior to the natural anterior hairline, on the the medial border of the temporalis muscle (See St 8 location and tips sections for more information).
i) Divide 4.5 cun in to 3 equal measurements to give 1.5 cun. Use this 1.5 cun measurement to locate GB 8 which is approximately 1 to 1.5 cun superior to the apex of the pinna of the ear and directly superior to TH 20.

Note: Soulié (1974) locates GB 8 on the lateral side of the head: three FW (Finger Width) above the level of the zygomatic arch at the vertical of the anterior of the ear; at the angle between the upper edge of the transverse mass (inferior curve) and the anterior edge of the vertical prominence; one FW posterior to GB 7; three large FW lateral to GB 13; one half FW under GB 18; two above and anterior to GB 9; one above and anterior to TW 20. So (1985) locates GB 8: one half the length of the patient's ear directly above the apex of the helix, at the horixontal/vertical cleft.

Voisin (1974) locates G 8 in the temporal area, 2 fb (finger breadth) above and slightly in front of the highest point of the ear. Lavier (1974) in an illustration locates GB 8 directly superior to TH 20 and the apex of the helix of the ear.

GB 9 TIAN CHONG – HEAVEN RUSHING OUT

⊥ ***0.3 CUN*** Δ ***3 TO 5***

- RE-UNION/Crossing/Meeting Point of the Gall Bladder Channel with the Bladder Channel – Foot Shao Yang Channel with the Foot Tai Yang Channel

Pos: Position of patient: supine or seated.

Loc: a) On the lateral aspect of the head.
b) On the parietal bone.
c) Approximately 0.5 cun posterior to GB 8.
d) Directly superior to the posterior border of the root of the pinna of the ear.
e) Approximately 2 cun superior to the natural lateral hairline.

Tip: a) Locate TH 20 and GB 8 first as points of reference.
b) TH 20 is on the lateral aspect of the head, on the temporal bone, and level with or immediately superior to the apex of the pinna of the ear.
c) Press the helix of the ear against the skull and draw a mark on the skull at the apex (highest part) of the pinna.
d) When the helix of the ear is bent forward, make sure it is only the helix and not the main body of the ear.
e) TH 20 may be on the contour line of the helix of the ear or immediately superior to it. Palpation of the point will ensure accuracy.

f) Palpation is easiest method to locate GB 8, see g). If you prefer to use cun measurements, see h) and i)
g) Palpate superiorly from the apex of the pinna of the ear from TH 20, until you feel a depression which is GB 8.
h) To use the 1.5 cun measurement locate St 8 and the anterior median line which will give 4.5 cun. St 8 is at the corner of the forehead, 0.5 cun posterior to the natural anterior hairline, on the the medial border of the temporalis muscle (See St 8 location and tips sections for more information).
i) Divide 4.5 cun in to 3 equal measurements to give 1.5 cun. Use this 1.5 cun measurement to locate GB 8 which is approximately 1 to 1.5 cun superior to the apex of the pinna of the ear and directly superior to TH 20.
j) Palpate just posterior to GB 8 for GB 9 (0.5 cun).
k) Another method is to draw a vertical line superiorly from the posterior border of the root of the pinna of the ear and a horizontal line posteriorly from GB 8. The area of GB 9 is where the two lines intersect.
l) Using the same method as in h) mark 2 cun superior to the lateral natural hairline, and palpate approximately 0.5 cun posterior to GB 8 for GB 9.

Note: Soulié (1994) has a different GB channel layout and numbering system. In his text GB 9 is numbered as GB 15. The point is located on the head: on the posterior and upper edge of the superior point of the mastoid, four FW (Finger Width) above and posterior to the top of the ear, under the prominence of the curved line which ends on the anterior edge of the vertical of the occipital-temporal suture; at the angle of the mastoid suture; one FW posterior to GB 18; two FW above GB 10; two FW posterior to GB 8; two FW below BL 8. Lavier (1974) in an illustration locates GB 9 directly superior to TH 19. Voisin (1974) has a different GB channel layout and numbering system. He locates G 9 in the temporal area, 4.5 fb (finger breadth) above and lateral to the orbit. Eachou (1995) locates GB 9 superior to the ear, 0.5 inch posterior to GB 8; or at the intersection between a vertical line running through the mastoid process of the temporal bone and a horizontal line from GB 8. Yang (1982) locates GB 9 at 1.5 cun posterior and inferior to GB 8. Li (1991) locates GB 9 at 0.5 cun posterior to GB 8 on an extended vertical line drawn from the posterior border of the root of the auricle. Wu (1973) locates GB 9 upon the cranium, at one pouce behind GB 8, in the hair area.

GB 10 FU BAI – FLOATING WHITE

⊥ ***0.3 CUN*** Δ ***3 TO 5***

- RE-UNION/Crossing/Meeting Point of the Gall Bladder Channel with the Bladder Channel – Foot Shao Yang Channel with the Foot Tai Yang Channel

Pos: Position of patient: seated.

Loc: a) On the lateral aspect of the head.
b) Posterior and superior to the mastoid process of the temporal bone.
c) Approximately level with the superior root of the pinna of the ear.

d) Approximately 1 cun posterior to the lateral natural hairline.
e) On the curvature of the Gall Bladder channel from GB 9 to GB 12.
f) Approximately one third of the distance from GB 9 to GB 12.
g) On the curvature of the Gall Bladder channel halfway between GB 9 and GB 11.

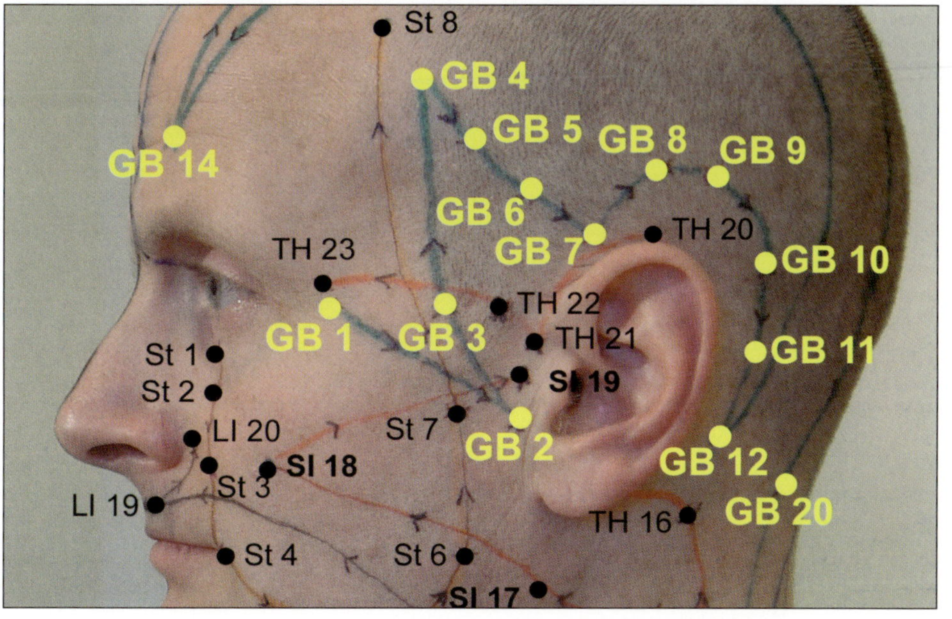

Tip:
a) Draw a horizontal line posteriorly from the superior root of the pinna of the ear.
b) Locate GB 10 by palpating posteriorly from the superior root of the pinna along this line until you are approximately 1 cun posterior to the lateral natural hairline.
c) There are many areas on the head that may feel like a *men* (depression). Ensure that you palpate posteriorly enough as the Triple Heater channel is anterior to the Gall Bladder channel at this level.

Note: Voisin (1974), his Gall Bladder channel flows anteriorly rather than flowing posteriorly towards the mastoid process. His numbering and channel system is different, G 15 in the written description should be G 16 (the illustration is correct but the descriptions of G 15 and G 16 in Voisins book need swapping around): G 15 (GB 10) written description should say the point is located behind the ear: 2.5 fb (finger breadth) behind and slightly below the level of the highest point of the ear. G 16 (GB 11) written description should say the location is in the parietal area: straight above the posterior border of the mastoid process and 1.5 fb above the level of the highest point of the ear. Wu (1973) locates GB 10 behind the ear, at one pouce behind the hairline, at the height of the superior edge of the pinna. Lavier (1974) in an illustration locates GB 10 on a level with and posterior to TH 19. Worsley (1982) locates VII 10, on the head, posterior and slightly superior to the ear, 1 ACI (Anatomical Chinese Inch) posterior to the natural hair line, at the level of the superior edge of the root of the ear.

Soulié (1994) has a different GB channel layout and numbering system. In his text our GB 10 is numbered as GB 16. The point is located on the head: behind the upper edge of the ear; at the angle between the posterior edge of the upper point of the mastoid and the anterior edge of the vertical occipital-temporal suture; Two FW (Finger Width) below GB 9; two FW above GB 12; two FW above and slightly in front of GB 11; one large FW posterior to TW 19. Jayasuriya (1982) locates GB 10 at 1 cun postero-inferior to GB 9, on the superior part of the mastoid process. Eachou (1995) locates GB 10 posterior to the ear, at the superior part of the mastoid process of the temporal bone, 1 inch posterior and inferior to GB 9; or 1 inch posterior to the superior margin of the auricle; or at the midpoint of the slightly curved line between GB 9 and GB 11. Shanghai (1981) locate GB 10 about 1 unit below and posterior to GB 9 on the superior part of the mastoid process.

Yang (1982) locates GB 10 at 1 cun inferior and posterior to GB 9. Academy (1975) locate GB 10 about 1 cun inferior to GB 9, at the upper border of the root of the auricle, 1 cun beyond the hairline. Masayoshi (1975) locates GB 10 at 1 sun below GB 9. So (1985) locates GB 10 in a vertical cleft directly below GB 9 and approximately 3/4 of an eye division from the helix. Li (1991) locates GB 10 posterior to the ear, 1 cun within the hairline at the level of the upper end of the auricle. Shanghai (1993) locate GB 10 on the head, posterior and superior to the mastoid process behind the ear, between GB 9 and GB 11.

GB 11 TOU QIAO YIN – HEAD HOLE YIN

⊥ ***0.3 CUN*** Δ ***3 TO 7***

- RE-UNION/Crossing/Meeting Point of the Gall Bladder Channel with the Bladder Channel – Foot Shao Yang Channel with the Foot Tai Yang Channel

Pos: Position of patient: seated.

Loc:
a) On the lateral aspect of the head.
b) Posterior to the ear.
c) In a depression posterior and superior to the mastoid process of the temporal bone.
d) On a curvature of the Gall Bladder Channel from GB 9 to GB 12.
e) Approximately two thirds of the distance from GB 9 to GB 12.
g) On the curvature of the Gall Bladder channel halfway between GB 10 and GB 12.

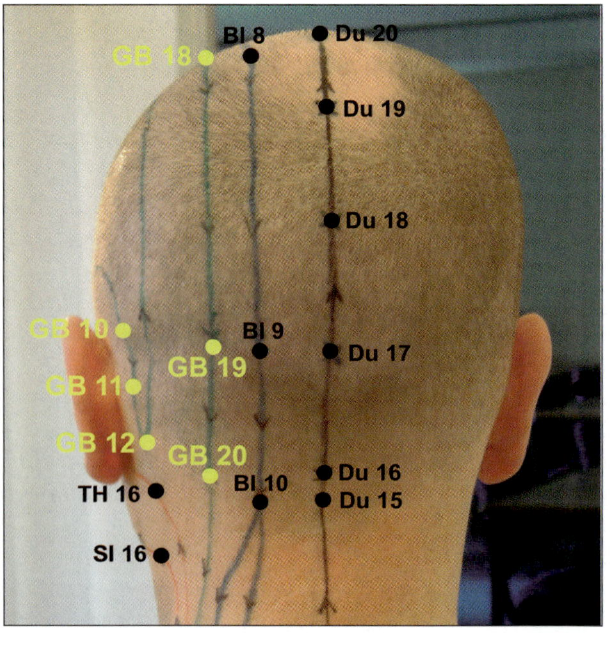

Tip: a) To locate GB 11 palpate superiorly along the posterior aspect of the mastoid process until you are able to palpate a *men* (depression) just superior to the mastoid process.

b) There are many areas on the head that may feel like a depression, therefore ensure that you palpate posteriorly enough as the Triple Heater channel is anterior to the Gall Bladder channel at this level.

Note: Voisin (1974), his Gall Bladder channel flows anteriorly rather than flowing posteriorly towards the mastoid process. His numbering and channel system is different, G 15 in the written description should be G 16 (the illustration is correct but the descriptions of G 15 and G 16 in Voisins book need swapping around): G 15 (GB 10) written description should say the point is located behind the ear: 2.5 fb (finger breadth) behind and slightly below the level of the highest point of the ear. G 16 (GB 11) written description should say the location is in the parietal area: straight above the posterior border of the mastoid process and 1.5 fb above the level of the highest point of the ear. Lavier (1974) in an illustration locates GB 11 on a level with and posterior to TH 18. Wu (1973) locates GB 11 upon the cranium, at the mid-distance between the ear and the posterior median line of the cranium, at one-half pouce above the inferior edge of the occipital. Worsley (1982) locates VII 11, on the head, posterior to the ear, mid-way between VII 10 and VII 12.

Soulié (1994) has a different GB channel layout and numbering system. In his text our GB 11 is numbered as GB 18. The point is located on the posterior lower part of the head: about mid-distance from the ear to the posterior median line. One FW (Finger Width) above the lower edge of the skull; at the angle between the lower edge of a transverse relief (line of the lower curve) and the posterior edge of the insertion of the splenius capitis muscle; one FW posterior to GB 12; one FW lateral to GB 19. Deadman (1998) locate GB 11 posterior to the ear, along a curved line drawn from GB 9 to GB 12 running within the hairline and more or less parallel to the line of the rim of the ear, in a depression slightly greater than two thirds of the distance between GB 9 and GB 12.

Shanghai (1993) locate GB 11 on the head, posterior and superior to the mastoid process, behind the ear, between GB 10 and GB 12. Jayasuriya (1982) locates GB 11 at 1 cun below to GB 10, posterior and superior to the mastoid process. Li (1991) locates GB 11 posterior to the auricle orifice, on the yin aspect of the head, in the depression on the root of the mastoid process. So (1985) locates GB 11 up two-thirds the length of the ear, behind the edge of the helix 2/3 of an eye division, in the horizontal cleft.

Academy (1975) locate GB 11 at the midpoint of the line connecting GB 10 and GB 12. Eachou (1995) locates GB 11 behind the ear in the posterior superior fossa of the mastoid process of the temporal bone, at the midpoint between GB 10 and GB 12, or 1 inch inferior to GB 10. Masayoshi (1975) locates GB 11 at the base of the mastoid process. Shanghai (1981) locate GB 11 at the base of the mastoid process, 1 unit below GB 10. Katsusuke (1983) locates GB 11 behind the ear, directly opposite the ear hole. Shandong (1982) locate Head-Qiaoyin posterior to the processus mastoideus between Pt. Fubai (GB 10) and Pt. Wangu (GB 12).

GB 12 WAN GU – FINAL BONE

⊥ ***0.3 TO 0.5 CUN*** Δ ***3 TO 7***

- RE-UNION/Crossing/Meeting Point of the Gall Bladder Channel with the Bladder Channel – Foot Shao Yang Channel with the Foot Tai Yang Channel

Pos: Position of patient: seated.

Loc: a) On the lateral aspect of the head.
b) In a depression just posterior and inferior to the mastoid process of the temporal bone.
c) Level with the prominence of the mastoid process of the temporal bone.
d) In the articulation between the occipital bone and mastoid process of the temporal bone.
e) Approximately 1 cun superior to TH 16 (see tips).

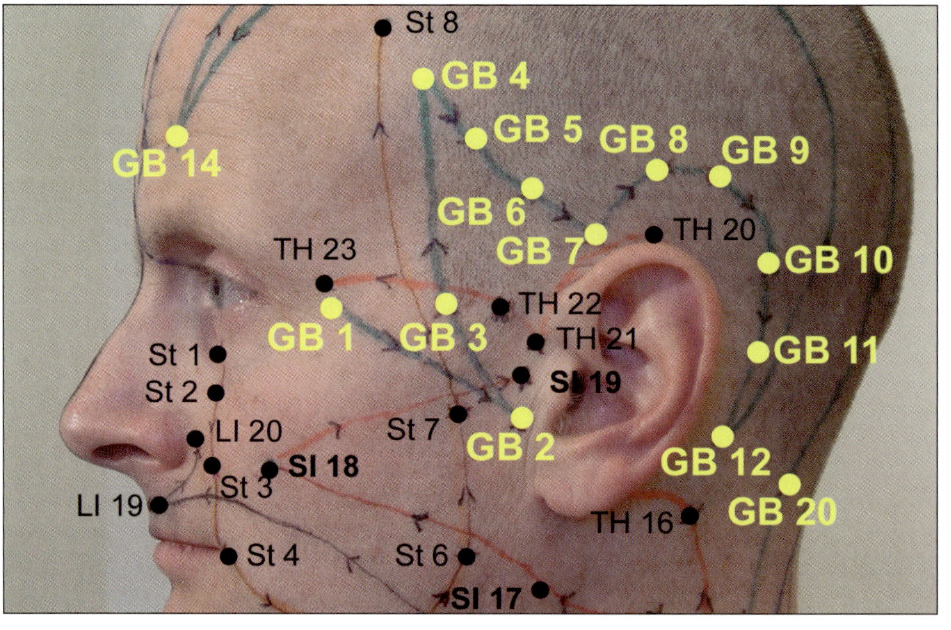

Tip: a) First locate TH 16 by palpating the posterior border of the sternocleidomastoid muscle. If you cannot feel the posterior border, ask the patient to rotate their head against resistance (when the hand is applied to the opposite side of the face).
b) Feel for the posterior border of the sternocleidomastoid muscle by palpation. If you cannot feel the border, then ask the patient to rotate their head against resistance when the hand is applied to the opposite side of the face.
c) Feel for the attachment of the posterior border of the sternocleidomastoid muscle to the mastoid process, you should be able to feel for the point which is posterior and inferior to the mastoid process.

d) When palpating for TH 16 you need to feel for resistance, where your finger cannot go any more lateral than the posterior border of the sternocleidomastoid muscle and where you cannot go any more superior than the inferior border of the temporal bone. This is more inferior than GB 12 (approximately 1 cun inferior).
e) Make sure you are close to the posterior border of the sternocleidomastoid muscle otherwise you may stray too medially towards the seam formed by the lateral border of the trapezius muscle and the posterior border of the sternocleidomastoid muscle which is in the proximity of GB 20.
f) TH 16 is on the neck and off the skull and level with the angle of the mandible (jaw) as opposed to GB 12, which is on the skull, at the articulation of the occipital bone and the mastoid process of the temporal bone.
g) The prominence of the mastoid process is a little like feeling for the prominences of the malleoli (ankles), where you feel the contour of the bone. Where it protudes outwards most is the prominence. GB 12 is level with the prominence and posterior to the mastoid process.
h) Approximately 1 cun inferior to GB 12, and level with the angle of the mandible should give you the correct level for palpation of this point. If you are not level with the angle of the mandible you may be too superior.
i) Ask the patient to slowly raise and lower their head, this opens and closes the articulation between the occipital and temporal bones. GB 12 is located in this articulation and therefore palpation is extremely important.

Note: Voisin (1974), his Gall Bladder channel flows anteriorly rather than flowing posteriorly towards the mastoid process, therefore his numbering and channel system is different. Voisin's G 18 is our GB 12. The description for G 18 is at the mastoid process: on its posterior border, at the level of the lower part of the tragus. Wu (1973) locates GB 12 upon the cranium, on the occiput, within the angle formed by the posterior edge of the mastoid and inferior edge of the occiput. Jayasuriya (1982) locates GB 12 in the depression posterior and inferior to the mastoid process, 0.7 cun below GB 11 and level with Du 16. Worsley (1982) locates VII 12, on the head, within the angle formed by the posterior border of the mastoid process and the inferior edge of the occipital bone when the head is tilted forwards.

Lavier (1974) in an illustration locates GB 12 posterior and inferior to the mastoid process. Soulié (1994) has a different GB channel layout and numbering system. In his text our GB 12 is numbered as GB 17. The point is located on the head: behind the ear: one small FW (Finger Width above the lower edge of the skull; at the lower angle between the posterior edge of the mastoid and the anterior edge of the insertion of the splenius muscle; in a hollow; one FW below GB 10; one FW lateral (anterior) to GB 11. So (1985) locates GB 12 almost one division lateral to GB 20; at the base of the skull between two muscles. Legge (1999) locates GB 12 just posterior to the tip of the mastoid process. Eachou (1995) locates GB 12 posterior to the ear and 0.7 inch inferior to GB 11, the point is located in the posterior inferior fossa of the mastoid process of the temporal bone. Shanghai (1981) locate GB 12 at the posterior border of the mastoid process, 0.7 unit below GB 10. Masayoshi (1975) locates GB 12 one finger width above the tip of the mastoid process. Katsusuke (1983) locates GB 12 in a depression in the back edge of the mastoid process behind the ear, in the depression that is located about the width of one finger above the mastoid process and four bu from the hairline.

Longitudinal bone proportional measurements of the head:

- **3 cun from between the two eyebrows (M-HN-3, Du 24.5 or Yin Tang) to the natural anterior hairline on the anterior median line.**
- **12 cun from the natural anterior hairline to the posterior hairline on the median line.**
- **3 cun from the posterior hairline to the space between the 7th cervical and 1st thoracic vertebrae (Du 14) on the posterior median line.**
- **15 cun (anterior natural hairline to the space between C7/T1);**
- **18 cun (between the two eyebrows at Du 24.5 or Yin Tang to the space between C7/T1).**

Transverse bone proportional measurements of the head:

- **(Anterior) 9 cun between the two corners of the forehead (St 8).**
- **(Posterior) 9 cun between the bilateral mastoid processes.**

It may be easier to use a length of string so that you can draw on the cun measurements as opposed to drawing the measurements on the scalp itself.

GB 13 BEN SHEN – ROOT SPIRIT

⊥ ***0.3 CUN*** Δ ***3 TO 7***

- 8 EXTRAORDINARY VESSEL/Coalescent Point of Yang Linking Vessel (Yang Wei Mai)
- RE-UNION/Crossing/Meeting Point of the Gall Bladder Channel with the Yang Linking Vessel – Foot Shao Yang Channel with the Yang Wei Mai

Pos: Position of patient: supine or seated.

Loc: a) On the anterior aspect of the head.
b) On the frontal bone.
c) Directly superior to the lateral canthus of the eye.
d) Two thirds of the distance from Du 24 to St 8.
e) 3 cun lateral to Du 24 (anterior median line).
f) 0.5 cun posterior to the natural anterior hairline.

Cun: a) First mark the median line on the anterior and posterior aspects of the head at the natural anterior and posterior hairline. Many head points are in relation to the natural hairline. The natural hairline may not be apparent due to the hairline receding. Sometimes you can see a definite change in skin texture from the forehead to the scalp, which is usually where the natural hairline was previously.
b) Measure 12 cun from the natural anterior hairline to the natural posterior hairline on the median line. It may be easier to use a length of string or strip of paper so that you can draw on the cun measurements as opposed to drawing the measurements on the scalp itself.

c) Transverse bone proportional measurements of the head: (anterior) 9 cun between the two corners of the forehead (St 8) and (posterior) 9 cun between the bilateral mastoid processes.

d) Mark in the anterior median line and locate St 8 (see St 8 location and tips section), then divide the distance in to 3 equal measurements from the anterior median line to St 8, this will give you 3 equal divisions of 1.5 cun.

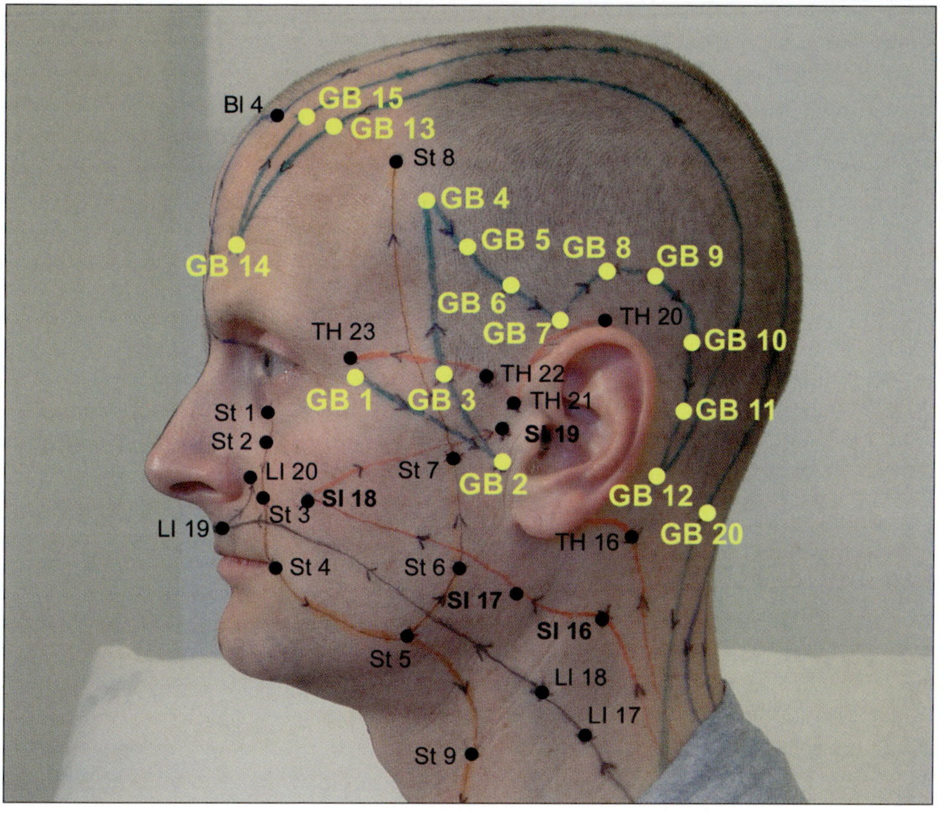

Tip: a) Use the cun guide above to locate GB 13 which is 3 cun lateral to Du 24 (anterior median line).

b) The point is located two thirds of the distance from Du 24 (anterior median line) to St 8 or 3 cun lateral to Du 24 (anterior median line).

c) The *men* (depression) on the head should be relatively easy to palpate. Palpate laterally from the anterior median line at 0.5 cun posterior to the natural anterior hairline from Du 24.

d) The next points in order laterally are Bl 3, Bl 4, GB 15, GB 13 and finally St 8. As you palpate, you may feel tiny ridges on the head. On some people you can visually see these ridges.

e) GB 13 can be located by running your finger directly superior to the lateral canthus of the eye to 0.5 cun posterior to the natural anteror hairline.

f) Palpation takes precedence over cun measurements in relation to 0.5 cun posterior to the natural anterior hairline.

Note: Wu (1973) locates GB 13 upon the upper forehead upon a vertical line passing from the external corner of the eye, at one pouce before the fronto-parietal suture, between St 8 and GB 15. Soulié (1994) has a different GB channel layout and numbering system. He locates our GB 13 (as GB 9), on the upper temple: four FW (Finger Width) above the transverse mass of the zygomatic arch. At the angle between the posterior edge of the frontal parietal suture and the lower edge of the prominence of the superior curve; three FW anterior and above GB 8; two FW posterior to GB 14; one small FW inder GB 16; one FW above GB 4. Voisin (1974), his Gall Bladder channel flows anteriorly rather than flowing posteriorly towards the mastoid process, therefore his numbering and channel system is different. Voisin's G 11 is our GB 13. The description for G 11 is on the frontal area: 4 fb (finger breadth) above the supercilliary arch, straight above the lateral border of the orbit. So (1985) locates GB 13 on a line up from the lateral end of the eyebrow, at the edge of the hair corner in the first straight, hollow cleft. Masayoshi (1975) locates GB 13 on the frontal region of the head, medial to the edge of the temple. Academy (1975) locate GB 13 at 0.5 cun inside the hairline, directly above the outer canthus.

GB 14 YANG BAI – YANG WHITE

⊥ ***0.3 CUN*** **Δ *3***

- 8 EXTRAORDINARY VESSEL/Coalescent Point of Yang Linking Vessel (Yang Wei Mai)
- RE-UNION/Crossing/Meeting Point of the Gall Bladder Channel with the Triple Heater Channel and the Yang Linking Vesse – Foot Shao Yang Channel with the Hand Shao Yang Channel and Yang Wei Mai

Pos: Position of patient: supine or seated.

Loc: a) On the anterior aspect of the head.
b) On the frontal bone.
c) Directly superior to the centre of the pupil of the eye when the person is looking straight ahead.
d) Approximately 1 cun superior to the middle of the eyebrow/supraorbital notch).

Cun: a) Transverse bone proportional measurements of the head: (Anterior) 9 cun between the two corners of the forehead (St 8) and (Posterior) 9 cun between the bilateral mastoid processes.
b) The longitudinal bone proportional measurements of the head are:
3 cun from between the two eyebrows (Du 24.5, M-HN-3 or Yin Tang) to the natural anterior hairline on the anterior median line.
12 cun from the natural anterior hairline to the natural posterior hairline on the median line.
3 cun from the natural posterior hairline to the space between the 7th cervical and 1st thoracic vertebrae (Du 14) on the posterior median line.
c) To locate 0.5 cun posterior to the natural anterior hairline it should be a lot easier to palpate for the point, but you may use any combination of longitudinal measurements, eg.:

12 cun (natural anterior hairline to the natural posterior hairline);
15 cun (anterior natural hairline to the space between C7/T1);
18 cun (between the two eyebrows at Du 24.5, M-HN-3 or Yin Tang to the space between C7/T1).

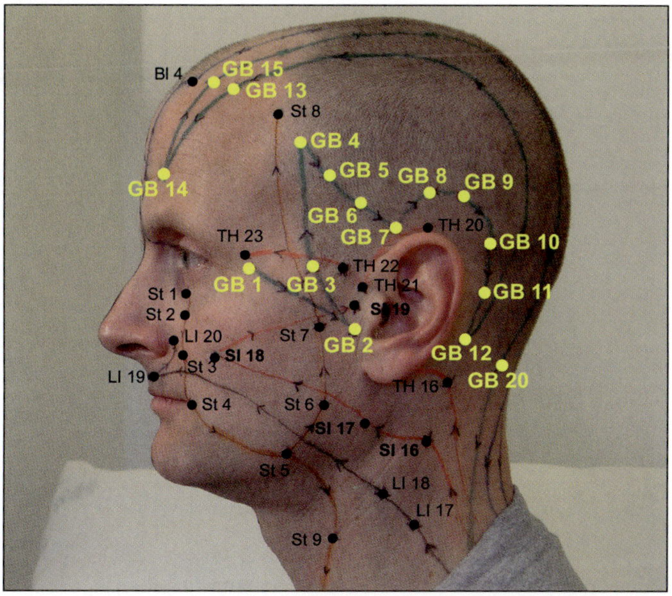

Tip:
a) Measure 3 cun from between the eyebrows (Du 24.5, M-HN-3 or Yin Tang) to the natural anterior hairline on the anterior median line and divide in to 1 cun measurments.
b) Using dividers or other method, transfer 1 cun from the middle of the eyebrow level with the centre of the pupil (with the person looking directly ahead).
c) GB 14 is 1 cun superior to the palpable notch located in the middle of the eyebrow.
d) A common error is to measure 1 cun from the anterior median line by drawing a line laterally towards the eyebrow. The centre of the eyebrow is at a higher level than the cun measurement between the eyebrows.
e) Palpation of this area will accurately locate this point.

Note: Voisin (1974), has GB 14 located as G 10, on the Frontal area: 1.5 fb (finger breadth) above the superciliary arch, straight above the pupil. Soulié (1994) has a different GB channel layout and numbering system. He locates our GB 14 as GB 10, on the forehead: in the angle between the inferior and lateral edge of the frontal prominence and the medial edge of the vertical ridge (frontal crest); two FW (Finger Width) anterior to GB 13; two FW under and lateral to GB 15; one FW above and medial to ST 8. Worsley (1982) locates VII 14 on the forehead, 1 ACI (Anatomical Chinese Inch) superior to the supra-orbital notch, which is found in the middle of the eyebrow. Lotan (2000) locates GB 14 at 1 cun superior to the supraorbital foramen. So (1985) locates GB 14 about one division above the middle of the eyebrow and about 1/2 division lateral in a small hollow. One can feel the nerve with the finger. On high foreheads the point is about 3/4 of a division up from the eyebrow.

GB 15 TOU LIN QI – HEAD ABOVE TEARS

⊥ ***0.3 CUN*** Δ *3*

- 8 EXTRAORDINARY VESSEL/Coalescent Point of Yang Linking Vessel (Yang Wei Mai)
- RE-UNION/Crossing/Meeting Point of the Gall Bladder Channel with the Bladder Channel and the Yang Linking Vesse – Foot Shao Yang Channel with the Foot Tai Yang Channel and the Yang Wei Mai

Pos: Position of patient: supine or seated.

Loc: a) On the anterior aspect of the head.
b) On the frontal bone.
c) Midway between Du24 to St 8.
d) Directly superior to GB 14.
e) 0.5 cun posterior to the natural anterior hairline.
f) 2.25 cun lateral to Du 24 or the anterior median line.

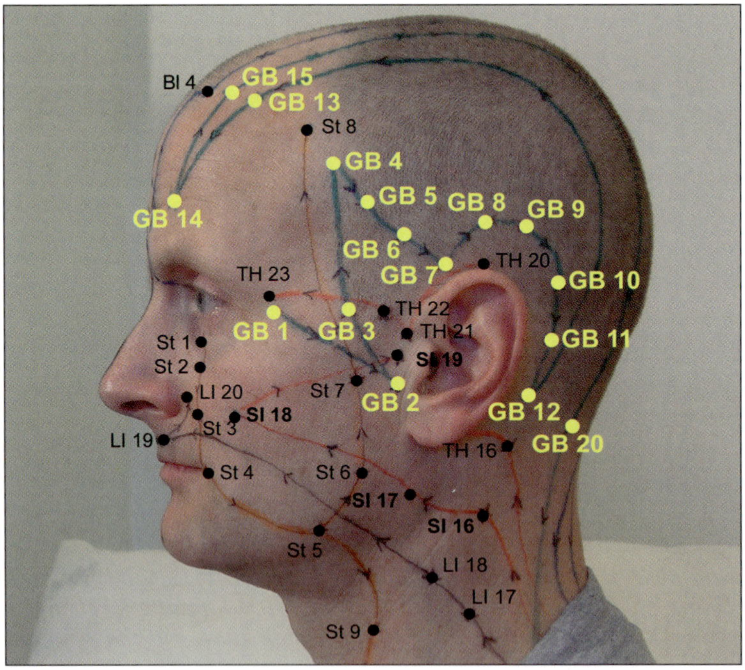

Cun: a) First mark the median line on the anterior and posterior aspects of the head at the natural anterior and posterior hairline. Many head points are in relation to the natural hairline. The natural hairline may not be apparent due to the hairline receding. Sometimes you can see a definite change in skin texture from the forehead to the scalp, which is usually where the natural hairline was previously.

b) Measure 12 cun from the natural anterior hairline to the natural posterior hairline on the median line. It may be easier to use a length of string or strip of paper so that you can draw on the cun measurements as opposed to drawing the measurements on the scalp itself.
c) Transverse bone proportional measurements of the head: (anterior) 9 cun between the two corners of the forehead (St 8) and (posterior) 9 cun between the bilateral mastoid processes.
d) Mark in the anterior median line and locate St 8 (see St 8 location and tips section), then divide the distance in to 3 equal measurements from the anterior median line to St 8, this will give you 3 equal divisions of 1.5 cun.

Tip:
a) To locate GB 15 mark the anterior median line which is the Du (GV) line at the natural anterior hairline.
b) Mark in the anterior median line and locate St 8 (see St 8 separate location and tips section), then divide the distance in to 2 equal measurements from the anterior median line to St 8.
c) The point is located mid-way between Du 24 (anterior median line) and St 8 (or 2.25 cun lateral to Du 24 or the anterior median line).
d) The location description says that GB 15 is directly superior to GB 14 (see separate description), but some skulls may be more 'bulbous' than others. Therefore the point may be superior and slightly lateral rather than directly superior to GB 14. This may be slightly lateral to the centre of the pupil of the eye when the person is looking directly ahead.
e) An alternative method to locate GB 15 is to palpate only:
f) The *men* (depression) on the head should be relatively easy to palpate. Palpating laterally from the anterior median line at 0.5 cun posterior to the natural anterior hairline from Du 24 (anterior median line), the next points in order laterally are Bl 3, Bl 4, GB 15, GB 13 and finally St 8.
g) As you palpate, you may feel tiny ridges on the head. On some people you can visually see these ridges.

Note: Worsley (1982) locates VII 15 on the head, 0.5 ACI (Anatomical Chinese Inch) posterior to the natural hairline, on a vertical line superior to the middle of the pupil when the eye is looking straight ahead. Wu (1973) locates GB 15 upon the upper forehead, at two pouce lateral from the median line of the cranium, and one pouce and a half before the parieto-frontal suture.

Voisin (1974) doesn't locate GB 15 as he has a different channel layout for the Gall Bladder. He seems to go from G 10 (our GB 14) posteriorly and laterally to the next point which he locates as G 11 (our GB 13).

Soulié (1994) has a different GB channel layout and numbering system. He locates our GB 15 as GB 11, on the forehead: upper edge and a bit medial on the frontal prominence; in a notch on the prominence; lateral edge of a vertical flat relief; two tightened FW (Finger Width) above and medial to GB 14; three large FW medial to GB 16; about four FW under BL 4; about two FW inferior and lateral to GV 24 (Du 24).

Note: GB 16-19 lie on the line between GB 15 and GB 20, 2.25 cun lateral to the median line.

GB 16 MU CHUANG – EYE WINDOW

⊥ ***0.3 CUN*** Δ **5**

- 8 EXTRAORDINARY VESSEL/Coalescent Point of Yang Linking Vessel (Yang Wei Mai)
- RE-UNION/Crossing/Meeting Point of the Gall Bladder Channel with the Yang Linking Vessel – Foot Shao Yang Channel with the Yang Wei Mai

Pos: Position of patient: supine or seated.

Loc: a) On the anterior aspect of the head.
b) On the coronal suture.
c) 2 cun posterior to the natural anterior hairline.
d) 1.5 cun posterior to GB 15.
e) 2.25 cun lateral to the anterior median line.
f) One third the distance measured from GB 15 to GB 18 (See Tip 3)

Cun: a) First mark the median line on the anterior and posterior aspects of the head at the natural anterior and posterior hairline. Many head points are in relation to the natural hairline. The natural hairline may not be apparent due to the hairline receding. Sometimes you can see a definite change in skin texture from the forehead to the scalp, which is usually where the natural hairline was previously.

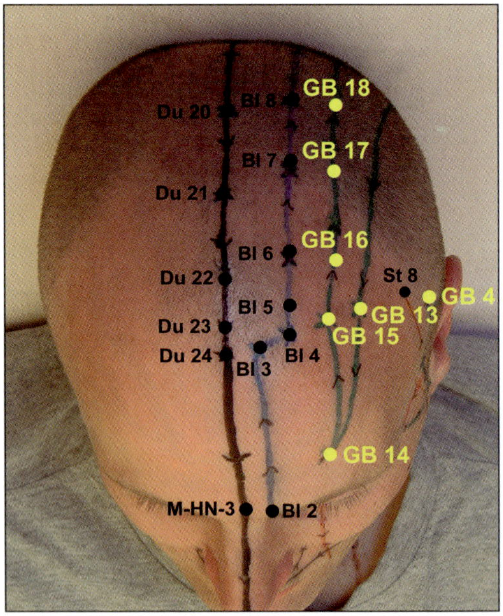

b) Measure 12 cun from the natural anterior hairline to the natural posterior hairline on the median line. It may be easier to use a length of string or strip of paper so that you can draw on the cun measurements as opposed to drawing the measurements on the scalp itself.
c) Transverse bone proportional measurements of the head: (anterior) 9 cun between the two corners of the forehead (St 8) and (posterior) 9 cun between the bilateral mastoid processes.
d) Mark in the anterior median line and locate St 8 (see St 8 location and tips section), then divide the distance in to 3 equal measurements from the anterior median line to St 8, this will give you 3 equal divisions of 1.5 cun.

Tip 1: a) First locate GB 15 which is located 2.25 cun lateral to the anterior median line or half-way between Du 24 and St 8, it is also 0.5 cun posterior to the natural anterior hairline.

b) GB 16 is 1.5 cun posterior to GB 15, or 2 cun posterior to the natural anterior hairline.

c) Measure 1.5 cun posterior to GB 15 or 2 cun posterior to the natural anterior hairline. You should be able to palpate a *men* (depression) which is GB 16. If not you should be able to feel the coronal suture where GB 16 is located – see note below.

d) The cun measurements give an approximation only as the anatomy of the coronal suture takes precedence. Palpation will ensure accurate point location.

Tip 2: a) Another method of locating GB 16 is to use palpation. The *men* (depression) on the head should be relatively easy to palpate for.

b) Palpate laterally from the anterior median line, 0.5 cun posterior to the natural anterior hairline from Du 24 (anterior median line), the next points in order laterally are Bl 3, Bl 4, GB 15, GB 13 and finally St 8. As you palpate, you may feel tiny ridges on the head. On some people you can visually see these ridges.

c) To locate 1.5 cun posterior to the natural anterior hairline or 1 cun posterior to GB 15 (half-way between Du 24 and St 8), palpate the coronal suture, GB 16 is located on the suture.

Tip 3: a) Another method is to locate GB 15, Du 20 and then GB 18. GB 18 lies transversely level with Du 20 – see tips c), d), e) and f) below for the location of these points.

b) GB 15 and GB 18 act as reference points for GB 16 and GB 17.

c) Du 20 is located on the median line of the head, 7 cun superior to the natural posterior hairline, or 5 cun posterior to the natural anterior hairline (for tips, see Du 20).

d) Palpate laterally from Du 20 (2.25 cun) until you can feel a definite *men* (depression). which is GB 18 (see seperate description).

e) GB 15 is located midway between Du 24 and St 8, directly superior to GB 14, 0.5 cun posterior to the natural anterior hairline, 2.25 cun lateral to Du 24 or the anterior median line.

f) GB 18 is located on the parietal bone, 5 cun posterior to the natural anterior hairline, transversely level with Du 20, and at 2.25 cun lateral to the superior median line.

g) Divide the distance in to three equal divisions from GB 15 to GB 18. GB 16 lies at the first third posterior to GB 15, and GB 17 lies at the second third posterior to GB 15 (nearest to GB 18), each at 1.5 cun divisions.

Note: Grays (1978) The coronal suture is formed by the joint between the posterior edge of the frontal bone and the anterior borders of the parietal bones (- coronal suture). Qiu (1996) locates GB 16 at 1 cun posterior to GB 15. Voisin (1974) has a different GB channel layout and numbering system. His G 12 is our GB 16, located on the coronal suture: 4 fb (finger breadth) from the midline of the skull.

Wu (1973) locates GB 16 upon the cranium, at one pouce behind GB 15. Li (1991) locates GB 16 at 1.5 cun posterior to GB 15 and 2.2 cun lateral to the anteroposterior midline of the head. Soulié (1994) has a different GB channel layout and numbering system. He locates GB 12, our GB 16 on the head, top lateral side: four FW (Finger Width) on either side of the medial line; in an angle between the posterior edge of the frontal-parietal suture and the upper edge of a horizontal mass (superior curve); just posterior to the vertical artery and vein; two FW lateral to GB 15; one large FW anterior to GB 17; one half FW above GB 13; two FW under BL 5.

Academy (1975) locate GB 16 at 1 cun above GB 15. Masayoshi (1975) locates GB 16 at 1 sun posterior to GB 15. Shanghai (1993) locate GB 16 on the head, 1.5 cun above the hairline of the forehead, 2,25 cun lateral to the midline of the head, on the line connecting GB 15 and GB 20. Shandong (1982) locate Muchuang at 1 cun posterior to Pt. Head-Linqi (GB 15).

GB 17 ZHEN YING – UPRIGHT LIVING

⊥ ***0.3 CUN*** Δ **5**

- 8 EXTRAORDINARY VESSEL/Coalescent Point of Yang Linking Vessel (Yang Wei Mai)
- RE-UNION/Crossing/Meeting Point of the Gall Bladder Channel with the Yang Linking Vessel – Foot Shao Yang Channel with the Yang Wei Mai

Pos: Position of patient: seated.

Loc: a) On the top of the head.
b) On the parietal bone.
c) 3.5 cun posterior to the natural anterior hairline.
d) 1.5 cun posterior to GB 16/Coronal Suture.
e) 3 cun posterior to GB 15.
f) 2.25 cun lateral to the median line.
g) Two thirds the distance measured from GB 15 to GB 18 (See Tip 3).

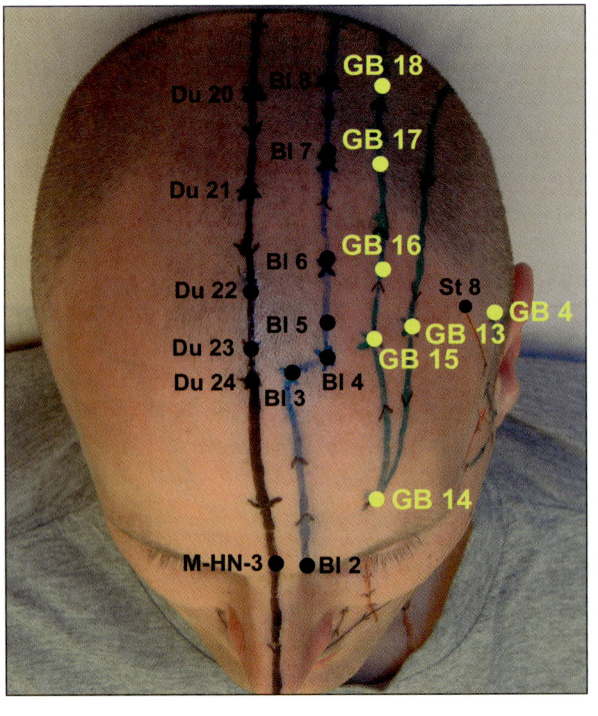

Cun: a) First mark the median line on the anterior and posterior aspects of the head at the natural anterior and posterior hairline. Many head points are in relation to the natural hairline. The natural hairline may not be apparent due to the hairline receding. Sometimes you can see a definite change in skin texture from the forehead to the scalp, which is usually where the natural hairline was previously.

b) Measure 12 cun from the natural anterior hairline to the natural posterior hairline on the median line. It may be easier to use a length of string or strip of paper so that you can draw on the cun measurements as opposed to drawing the measurements on the scalp itself.

c) Transverse bone proportional measurements of the head: (anterior) 9 cun between the two corners of the forehead (St 8) and (posterior) 9 cun between the bilateral mastoid processes.

d) Mark in the anterior median line and locate St 8 (see St 8 location and tips section), then divide the distance in to 3 equal measurements from the anterior median line to St 8, this will give you 3 equal divisions of 1.5 cun.

Tip 1: a) First locate GB 15 which is located 2.25 cun lateral to the anterior median line or half-way between Du 24 and St 8, it is also 0.5 cun posterior to the natural anterior hairline.

b) GB 17 is 3 cun posterior to GB 15, or 3.5 cun posterior to the natural anterior hairline.

c) Measure 1.5 cun posteriorly from GB 15 or 2 cun posterior to the natural anterior hairline and you should be able to palpate a *men* (depression) which is GB 16. If not you should be able to feel the coronal suture where GB 16 is located – see notes below.

d) GB 17 is located 1.5 cun posterior to the coronal suture or 1.5 cun posterior to GB 16.

e) Alternatively measure 3.5 cun posterior to the natural anterior hairline and palpate forGB 17.

f) The cun measurements give an approximation only as the anatomy of the coronal suture takes precedence. Palpation will ensure accurate point location.

Tip 2: a) Another method of locating GB 17 is to use palpation. The *men* (depression) on the head should be relatively easy to palpate for.

b) Palpate laterally from the anterior median line, 0.5 cun posterior to the natural anterior hairline from Du 24 (anterior median line), the next points in order laterally are Bl 3, Bl 4, GB 15, GB 13 and finally St 8. As you palpate, you may feel tiny ridges on the head. On some people you can visually see these ridges.

c) To locate 3.5 cun posterior to the natural anterior hairline or 3 cun posterior to GB 15 (half-way between Du 24 and St 8), palpate the coronal suture, GB 16 is located on the suture (3 cun posterior to GB 15 or 3.5 cun posterior to the natural anterior hairline).

d) GB 17 is located on the parietal bone 2.25 cun lateral to the median line. Use the transverse cun measurements half-way between St 8 and Du 24 only as a guide for 2.25 cun lateral to the superior median line.

e) The cun measurements are only an approximation. Palpation will ensure accurate point location.

Tip 3: a) Another method is to locate GB 15, Du 20 and then GB 18. GB 18 lies transversely level with Du 20 – see tips c), d) and e) below for the location of these points.

b) GB 15 and GB 18 act as reference points for GB 16 and GB 17.

c) Du 20 is located on the median line of the head, 7 cun superior to the natural posterior hairline, or 5 cun posterior to the natural anterior hairline (for tips, see Du 20).

d) Palpate laterally from Du 20 (2.25 cun) until you can feel a definite *men* (depression). which is GB 18. GB 18 is located on the parietal bone, 5 cun posterior to the natural anterior hairline, transversely level with Du 20, and at 2.25 cun lateral to the superior median line.

e) GB 15 is located midway between Du 24 and St 8, directly superior to GB 14, 0.5 cun posterior to the natural anterior hairline, 2.25 cun lateral to Du 24 or the anterior median line.

f) Divide the distance in to three equal divisions from GB 15 to GB 18. GB 16 lies at the first third posterior to GB 15, and GB 17 lies at the second third posterior to GB 15 (nearest to GB 18), each at 1.5 cun divisions.

g) To locate GB 17, palpate 1.5 cun anterior to GB 18.

Note: Gray's (1978) The coronal suture is formed by the joint between the posterior edge of the frontal bone and the anterior borders of the parietal bones. Qiu (1996) locates GB 17 at 1 cun posterior to GB 16. Voisin (1974) has a different GB channel layout and numbering system. His G 13 is near to our GB 17, located in the parietal area: straight above the highest point of the ear, 4 fb (finger breadth) from the midline of the skull. Wu (1973) locates GB 17 upon the cranium, at two pouce behind GB 15.

Worsley (1982) locates VII 17 on the head, 1 ACI (Anatomical Chinese Inch) posterior to VII 16. Li (1991) locates GB 17 at 1.5 cun posterior to GB 16 and 2.2 cun lateral to the anterior and posterior midline of the head. Soulié (1994) has a different GB channel layout and numbering system. He locates GB 13, our GB 17 on the head, lateral side of top: four FW (Finger Width) on either side of the medial line; one FW lateral to the vertical frontal-parietal suture; upper edge of the horizontal mass (superior curve); one FW lateral to GB 16; two FW anterior to GB 18; one FW above GB 8; two FW under BL 6.

Academy (1975) locate GB 17 at 1 cun posterior to GB 16. Masayoshi (1975) locates GB 17 at 1 sun posterior to GB 16. Shanghai (1993) locate GB 17 on the head, 2.5 cun above the hairline of the forehead, 2.25 cun lateral to the midline of the head, on the line connecting GB 15 and GB 20. Shandong (1982) locate Zhengying at 1 cun posterior to Pt. Muchuang (GB 16).

GB 18 CHENG LING – RECEIVING SPIRIT

⊥ ***0.3 CUN*** Δ ***5***

- 8 EXTRAORDINARY VESSEL/Coalescent Point of Yang Linking Vessel (Yang Wei Mai)
- RE-UNION/Crossing/Meeting Point of the Gall Bladder Channel with the Yang Linking Vessel – Foot Shao Yang Channel with the Yang Wei Mai

Pos: Position of patient: seated.

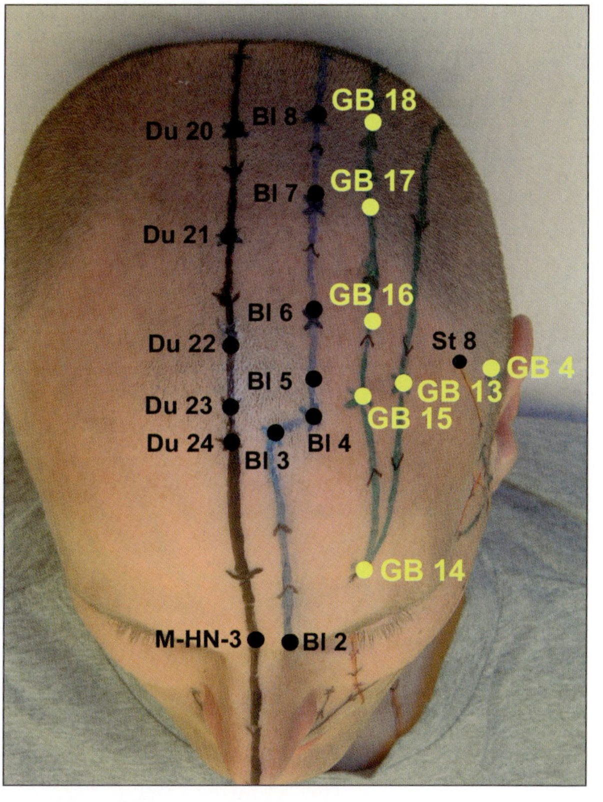

Loc: a) On the top of the head.
b) On the parietal bone.
c) 5 cun posterior to the natural anterior hairline.
d) 4.5 cun posterior to GB 15.,
e) Transversely level with Du 20
f) 1.5 cun posterior to GB 17.
g) 3 cun posterior to GB 16/Coronal Suture.
h) 2.25 cun lateral to the median line.

Cun: a) First mark the median line on the anterior and posterior aspects of the head at the natural anterior and posterior hairline. Many head points are in relation to the natural hairline. The natural hairline may not be apparent due to the hairline receding. Sometimes you can see a definite change in skin texture from the forehead to the scalp, which is usually where the natural hairline was previously.
b) Measure 12 cun from the natural anterior hairline to the natural posterior hairline on the median line. It may be easier to use a length of string or strip of paper so that you can draw on the cun measurements as opposed to drawing the measurements on the scalp itself.
c) Transverse bone proportional measurements of the head: (anterior) 9 cun between the two corners of the forehead (St 8) and (posterior) 9 cun between the bilateral mastoid processes.
d) Mark in the anterior median line and locate St 8 (see St 8 location and tips section), then divide the distance in to 3 equal measurements from the anterior median line to St 8, this will give you 3 equal divisions of 1.5 cun.

Tip 1: a) First locate Du 20 as GB 18 lies transversely level with Du 20.

b) Du 20 is located on the median line of the head, 7 cun superior to the natural posterior hairline or 5 cun posterior to the natural anterior hairline (for tips, see Du 20).

c) Palpate laterally from Du 20 (2.25 cun) until you can feel a definite *men* (depression), which is GB 18.

d) Palpation will ensure accurate point location.

e) GB 15 and GB 18 act as references for GB 16 and GB 17. If you were to divide the distance from GB 15 to GB 18 in to three equak divisions, then GB 16 lies at the first third posterior GB 15, and GB 17 lies at the second third posterior to GB 15 (nearest to GB 18), each at 1.5 cun divisions.

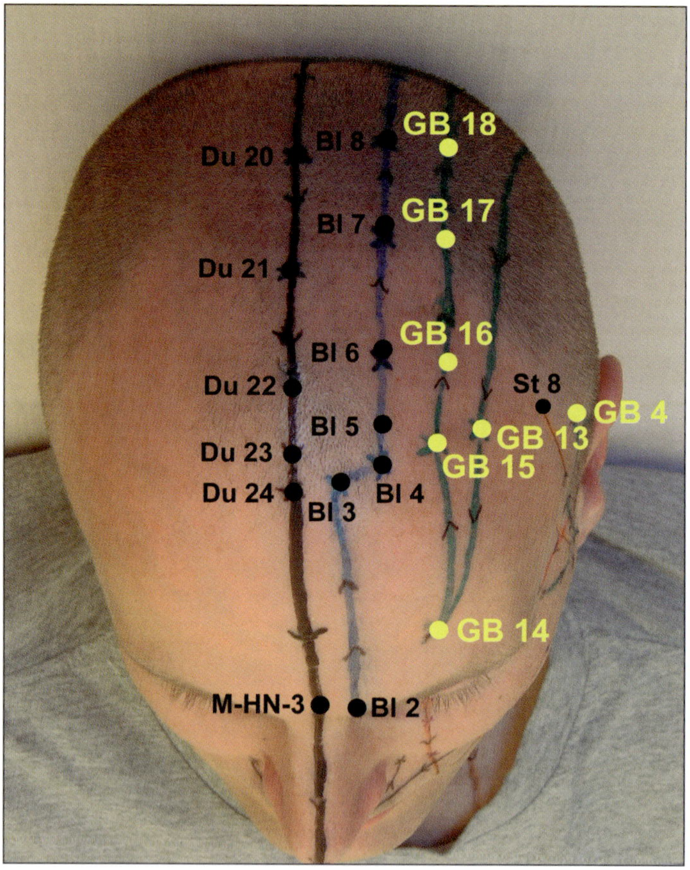

Tip 2: a) An alternative method is to locate GB 15 which is located at 2.25 cun lateral to the anterior median line or half-way between Du 24 and St 8, it is also 0.5 cun posterior to the natural anterior hairline.

b) Once you have located GB 15, GB 18 is 4.5 cun posterior to GB 15, or 5 cun posterior to the natural anterior hairline (1.5 cun posterior to GB 17). Once measured, palpate for the point.

c) Palpation will ensure accurate point location.

Tip 3: a) Another method of locating GB 18 is to use palpation. The *men* (depression) on the head should be relatively easy to palpate for.

b) Palpate laterally from the anterior median line, 0.5 cun posterior to the natural anterior hairline from Du 24 (anterior median line), the next points in order laterally are Bl 3, Bl 4, GB 15, GB 13 and finally St 8. As you palpate, you may feel tiny ridges on the head. On some people you can visually see these ridges.

c) To locate 5 cun posterior to the natural anterior hairline or 4.5 cun posterior to GB 15 (half-way between Du 24 and St 8), palpate the coronal suture, GB 16 is located on the suture (3 cun posterior to GB 15 or 3.5 cun posterior to the natural anterior hairline).

d) GB 17 is located on the parietal bone 2.25 cun lateral to the median line and 1.5 cun posterior to GB 16. Use the transverse cun measurements half-way between St 8 and Du 24 only as a guide for 2.25 cun lateral to the superior median line.

e) GB 18 is 1.5 cun posterior to GB 17 (5 cun posterior to the natural anterior hairline).

f) The cun measurements are only an approximation. Palpation will ensure accurate point location.

Note: Gray's (1978) The coronal suture is formed by the joint between the posterior edge of the frontal bone and the anterior borders of the parietal bones. Qiu (1996) locates GB 18 at 1.5 cun posterior to GB 17 which is the same description as ours, but he describes GB 16 as being 1 cun posterior to GB 15 and GB 17 as being 1 cun posterior to GB 16, this makes his GB 18, 1 cun more anterior than our GB 18.

Academy (1975) locate GB 18 at 1.5 cun posterior to GB 17 which is the same description as ours, but they describe GB 16 as being 1 cun above GB 15 and GB 17 as being 1 cun posterior to GB 16, this makes his GB 18, 1 cun more anterior than our GB 18. Worsley (1982) locates VII 18 on the head, 1.5 ACI (Anatomical Chinese Inch) posterior to VII 17. This point is approximately 0.5 ACI anterior to our location description due to VII 17 only being 1 ACI posterior to VII 16 (our location for GB 17 is 1.5 cun posterior to GB 16).

Voisin (1974) has a different GB channel layout and numbering system. His G 14 is near to our GB 18, located in the parietal area: 4 fb (finger breadth) above and slightly posterior to the base of the mastoid process. Soulié (1994) has a different GB channel layout and numbering system. He locates GB 14 as our GB 18, on the lateral top of the head: four FW (Finger Width) on either side of the medial line; two tightened FW anterior to the vertical occipital-parietal suture; upper edge of the horizontal prominence (superior curve); two FW posterior to GB 17; one FW anterior and a little above GB 9; two FW under BL 7; two FW above GB 8. Wu (1973) locates GB 18 upon the cranium, at three and a half pouce behind GB 15. Li (1991) locates GB 18 at 1.5 cun posterior to GB 17 and 2.2 cun lateral to the anterior and posterior midline.

Masayoshi (1975) locates GB 18 at 1 sun posterior to GB 17. Shanghai (1993) locate GB 18 on the head, 4 cun above the hairline of the forehead, 2.25 cun lateral to the midline of the head, on the line connecting GB 15 and GB 20. Shandong (1982) locate Chengling at 1 cun posterior to Pt. Zhengying (GB 17).

GB 19 NAO KONG – BRAIN HOLLOW

⊥ *0.3 CUN* Δ *5*

- 8 EXTRAORDINARY VESSEL/Coalescent Point of Yang Linking Vessel (Yang Wei Mai)
- RE-UNION/Crossing/Meeting Point of the Gall Bladder Channel with the Yang Linking Vessel – Foot Shao Yang Channel with the Yang Wei Mai

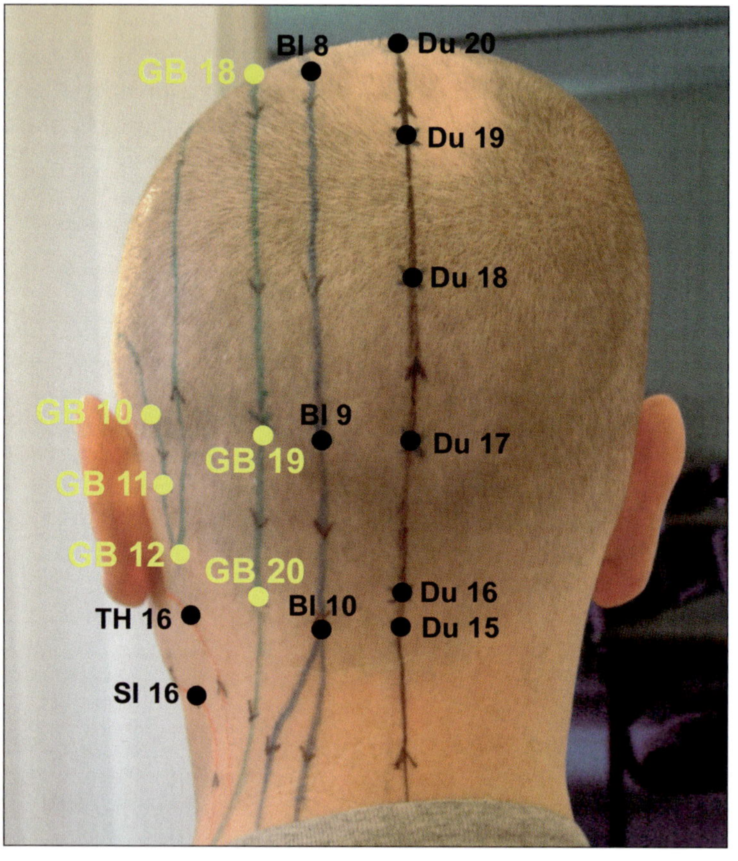

Pos: Position of patient: seated.

Loc:
a) On the posterior aspect of the head.
b) On the level of the upper border of the external occipital protruberance of the occipital bone.
c) Level with Du 17 and Bl 9.
d) 1.5 cun superior to GB 20.
e) 9.5 cun posterior to the natural anterior hairline.
f) 2.5 cun superior to the natural posterior hairline.
g) 2.25 cun lateral to the posterior median line.

Cun: a) First mark the median line on the anterior and posterior aspects of the head at the natural anterior and posterior hairline. Many head points are in relation to the natural hairline. The natural hairline may not be apparent due to the hairline receding. Sometimes you can see a definite change in skin texture from the forehead to the scalp, which is usually where the natural hairline was previously.

b) Measure 12 cun from the natural anterior hairline to the natural posterior hairline on the median line. It may be easier to use a length of string or strip of paper so that you can draw on the cun measurements as opposed to drawing the measurements on the scalp itself.

c) Transverse bone proportional measurements of the head: (anterior) 9 cun between the two corners of the forehead (St 8) and (posterior) 9 cun between the bilateral mastoid processes.

d) Mark in the anterior median line and locate St 8 (see St 8 location and tips section), then divide the distance in to 3 equal measurements from the anterior median line to St 8, this will give you 3 equal divisions of 1.5 cun.

Tip: a) Palpate from the bottom of the neck on to the head. on the posterior median line until your finger feels a resistance formed by the base of the occipital bone. Palpate superiorly until you go over a ridge which is the external occipital protruberance.

b) On the posterior median line and just over this ridge you should be able to palpate Du 17.

c) Palpate laterally from the level of Du 17 (to approximately 2.25 cun), you should be able to feel a *men* (depression) which is GB 19.

d) Using cun measurements to locate GB 19, the distance between a mastoid process and the posterior median line is 4.5 cun. Halve the 4.5 cun lateral to the posterior median line to get 2.25 cun. GB 19 is located at 2.25 cun lateral to the posterior median line.

e) Although the locationof GB 19 is 1.5 cun superior to GB 20, palpating for the point may be easier.

Note: Wu (1973) locates GB 19 upon the cranium, at five pouce behind GB 15. Voisin (1974) locates G 19 behind the ear, on the lambdoid suture, at the level of the highest point of the ear. Masayoshi (1975) locates GB 19 at 1.5 sun posterior to GB 18. His GB 19 is 1 cun anterior to our point due to GB 16 and GB 17 being 1 cun posterior to each other instead of being 1.5 cun from each other. Li (1991) locates GB 19 at 1.5 cun directly above GB 20 midway between the upper border of the mastoid process and the external occpital protruberance.

Yang (1982) locates GB 19 midway between the superior border of the occipital protruberance and the superior border of the mastoid. So (1985) locates GB 19 at 1 and 1/2 divisions above GB 20 in the horizontal/vertical cleft.). Shandong (1982) locate Naokong on the lateral side of the protruberantia occipitalis externa. Pt. Fengchi (GB 20) is just below it.

Soulié (1994) locates GB 19 on the posterior base of the skull: one FW (Finger Width) above the lower edge; two large FW from the posterior medial line; in the angle between the lower edge of a transverse relief (line of the lower curve) and the lateral edge of large muscles (superimposed insertions of the trapezius on the semispinalis capitis muscle); in a marked hollow; one FW medial to GB 11; one large FW above GB 20; two FW lateral and below BL 9. Eachou (1995) locates GB 19 lateral to the occipital protruberance, 1.5 inches auperior to GB 20, and 2 inches lateral to GV 17 (Du 17

GB 20 FENG CHI – WIND POND

⊥ ***0.3 TO 0.5 CUN*** **∆** ***3 TO 10***

- 8 EXTRAORDINARY VESSEL/Coalescent Point of Yang Heel/Yang Motility Vessel (Yang Qiao Mai)
- 8 EXTRAORDINARY VESSEL/Coalescent Point of Yang Linking Vessel (Yang Wei Mai)
- RE-UNION/Crossing/Meeting Point of the Gall Bladder Channel with the Yang Linking and Yang Heel/Motility Vessels – Foot Shao Yang Channel with the Yang Wei Mai and Yang Qiao Mai

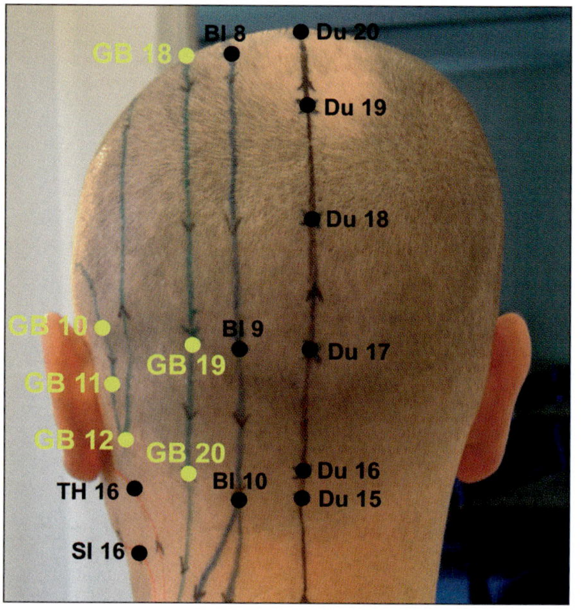

Pos: Position of patient: seated.

Loc: a) On the posterior aspect of the upper neck.
b) Inferior to the occipital bone.
c) Between the lateral border of the trapezius and posterior border of the sternocleidomastoid muscles.
d) Level with Du 16.
e) 2.25 cun lateral to the posterior median line.
f) 11 cun posterior to the natural anterior hairline.
g) 1 cun superior to the natural posterior hairline.

Cun: a) First mark the median line on the anterior and posterior aspects of the head at the natural anterior and posterior hairline. Many head points are in relation to the natural hairline. The natural hairline may not be apparent due to the hairline receding. Sometimes you can see a definite change in skin texture from the forehead to the scalp, which is usually where the natural hairline was previously.
b) Measure 12 cun from the natural anterior hairline to the natural posterior hairline on the median line. It may be easier to use a length of string or strip of paper so that you can draw on the cun measurements as opposed to drawing the measurements on the scalp itself.
c) Transverse bone proportional measurements of the head: (anterior) 9 cun between the two corners of the forehead (St 8) and (posterior) 9 cun between the bilateral mastoid processes.
d) Mark in the anterior median line and locate St 8 (see St 8 location and tips section), then divide the distance in to 3 equal measurements from the anterior median line to St 8, this will give you 3 equal divisions of 1.5 cun.

Tip: a) On the neck, visualise the posterior border of the sternocleidomastoid muscle, the lateral border of the trapezius and the inferior border of the occipital bone.

b) The flow of the channel runs from the skull down to the neck and shoulders. With your thumb pointing downwards from the skull, the end of your thumb should drop in to a deep *men* (depression) between the sternocleidomastoid and trapezius.

c) Palpate for the deepest part of the *men* (depression). Note that this point can be quite large.

d) GB 20 is also level with Du 16 which is on the natural posterior median line and just inferior to the external occipital protuberance of the occipital bone, (1 cun superior to the posterior hairline). If you are having difficulty locating GB 20 from the previous tips you can try palpating for Du 16 first.

e) Once you have located Du 16, palpate laterally until you have gone over the band of the trapezius muscle and in to a deep *men.*

f) It is easier to locate GB 20 by palpation.

Note: Worsley (1982) locates VII 20, inferior to the occipital bone, in the centre of the depression between the external occipital protruberance and the mastoid process, superior to the natural hair line and lateral to the border of the trapezius. Legge (1999) locates GB 20 in the depression under the occiput, between the attachment of the sternocleidomastoid and upper trapezius.

Voisin (1974) locates G 20 on the neck: upper border of trapezius, 2 fb (finger breadth) below occipital bone, at the level of the tip of the mastoid process. Wu (1973) locates GB 20 upon the posterior surface of the neck, one and one-half pouce from the median line, at the height of the point of the mastoid. Jayasuriya (1982) locates GB 20 in the depression immediately inferior and medial to the mastoid process, between the origins of the trapezius and sterno-mastoid muscles. Soulié (1994) locates GB 20 on the nape of the neck: one half FW (Finger Width) below the angle between the lower edge of the skull and the lower edge of the large vertical muscle. Exactly at the angle between the medial edge of the lateral muscle (splenius capitis) and the upper edge of the lateral process of the second cervical vertebra; in a hollow; one large FW below GB 19; about six FW above and medial to GB 21; three tightened FW lateral and slightly above BL 10; one FW inferior and medial to GB 11.

Deadman (1998) locate GB 20 below the occiput, approximately midway between DU 16 and GB 12, in the hollow between the origins of the sternomastoid and trapezius muscles. Yang (1982) locates GB 20 at the midpoint between the inferior border of the mastoid process and Du 16, and 1 cun above the posterior hairline, at the midline. So (1985) locates GB 20 below the occipital bone in the hollow at the lateral edge of the trapezius muscle; this point is at the same level as GV 16 (Du 16). Katsusuke (1983) locates GB 20 in the depressions on the right and left two sun below the central depression at the lower end of the occiput.

Shanghai (1981) locate GB 20 between the hollow below the tuberosity of the occipital bone at the back of the head and the mastoid process, and between the trapezius and sternocleidomastoid muscles. Cheng (1987) locates G 20 in the depression between the upper portion of m. sternocleidomastoideus and m. trapezius, on the same level with Du 16. Eachou (1995) locates GB 20 at the posterior, lateral aspect of the neck at the same height as GV 16(Du 16), in the fossa between the superior margins of the trapezius and sternocleidomastoid muscles. Huang (1993) locates GB 20 posterior to the temple in a depression on the hairline.

GB 21 is on the posterior aspect of the shoulder.

GB 21 JIAN JING – SHOULDER WELL

⊥ ***0.3 TO 0.5 CUN*** **∆** ***5 TO 15***
FORBIDDEN TO NEEDLE AND MOXA THIS POINT IN PREGNANCY – NOT TO BE USED BEFORE THE 2ND STAGE OF LABOUR

Note: Please needle with caution as the apex of the lungs reaches superiorly as far as the shoulder.

- 8 EXTRAORDINARY VESSEL/Coalescent Point of Yang Linking Vessel (Yang Wei Mai)
- RE-UNION/Crossing/Meeting Point of the Gall Bladder Channel with the Triple Heater Channel and the Yang Linking Vesse – Foot Shao Yang Channel with the Hand Shao Yang Channel and Yang Wei Mai

Pos: Position of patient: seated.

Loc:
a) On the shoulder.
b) At the highest point of the shoulder.
c) On the anterior border of the trapezius muscle.
d) Midway between Du 14 and the lateral extremity of the acromion process of the scapula.
e) On a line with SI 13 and TH 15.
f) Directly superior to St 12.

Tip:
a) Locate Du 14, on the posterior median line, between C7 and T1 vertebrae.
b) Place a mark on the lateral extremity of the acromion process. If you are having difficulties feeling for the border, ask the patient to abduct their arm. By taking the weight of their arm, the deltoid muscle will relax enough for you to feel the lateral extremity of the acromion process.
c) Place a mark midway between Du 14 and the lateral extremity of the acromion process, this will be on the highest part of the shoulder.
d) GB 21 will be approximately at this mark. Palpation will accurately locate the point.
e) Another method of locating GB 21 is to palpate from GB 20 which is inferior to the occipital bone and between the trapezius and sternocleidomastoid muscles.
f) From GB 20, palpate inferiorly, following the lateral border of the trapezius muscle on the neck to the anteriior border of the trapezius on the shoulder until you are at the halfway mark on the top of the shoulder.
g) Another way of identifying the anterior border of this band of trapezius muscle is to gently "pinch" the muscle. You should be able to feel two seams identifying the anterior border and posterior seam of the muscle.

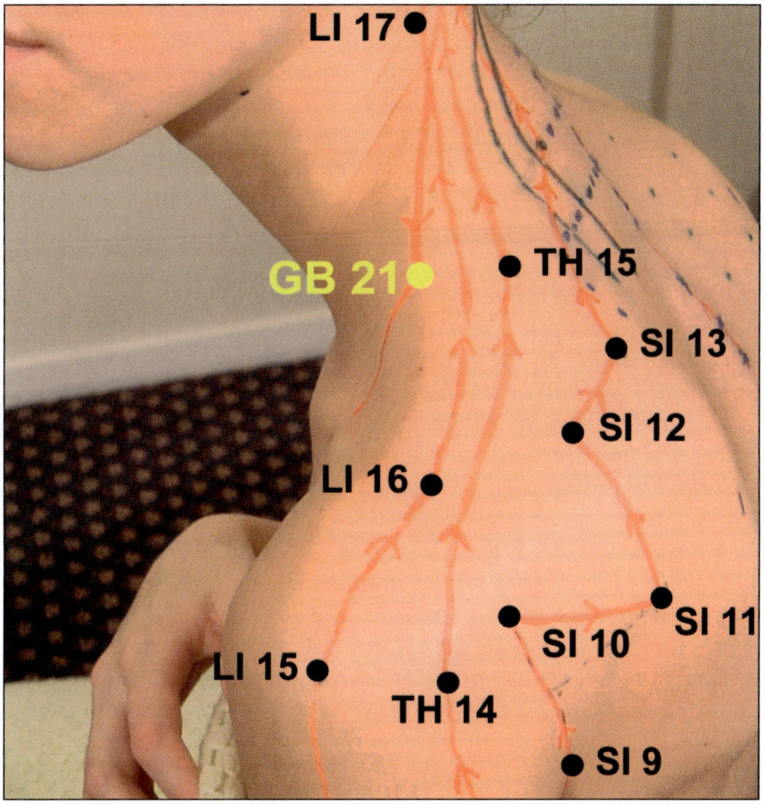

h) Locating the anterior border of the muscle should prevent you from palpating too anteriorly in to the supraclavicular fossa where St 12 is located. Make sure you are on the highest part of the shoulder therefore you should not pinch more than an inch of the trapezius muscle.
i) Another method of locating GB 21 is to locate SI 13 and TH 15 first (see separate locations). These two points are vertically in line with each other, SI 13 being the lower one of the two, GB 21 will be at the highest point of the three points on this line, on the highest part of the shoulder. As SI 13 and TH 15 are not the easiest of points to locate this option of locating GB 21 is not always used.

Note: Wu (1973) locates GB 21 upon the lateral surface of the neck, at the base, before the anterior edge of the trapezius. Legge (1999) locates GB 21 on the belly of the upper trapezius, halfway between the tip of the spinous process of C7 (Du 14) and the acromion process. Voisin (1974) locates G 21 on the neck: in front of the upper border of the trapezius, at the level of the upper border of the thyroid cartilage.

Lavier (1974) in an illustration locates GB 21 on the neck/shoulder, on the anterior border of the trapezius muscle, on a horizontal line running on the neck posteriorly from the laryngeal prominence of the the thyroid cartilage. Jayasuriya (1974) locates GB 21 midway between Du 14 and LI 15, at the highest point of the shoulder.

Shanghai (1993) locates GB 21 on the shoulder, directly above the nipple, on the midpoint of the line connecting DU 14 and the acromion. Li (1991) locates GB 21 midway along a line joining the 7th cervical vertebra and the acromion. Alternatively the operator may stand behind the seated patient, placing his hand on the shoulder, with the transverse crease of the wrist pressing on the lower border of the scapular spine. The thumb is placed on the lower border of the spinous process of the 7th cervical vertebra, while the four fingers closed together, rest on the upper portion of the shoulder with the middle finger slightly curved, the point being located where the finger tip touches.

Worsley (1982) locates VII 21 mid-way between the spinous process of the seventh cervical vertebra and the lateral tip of the clavicle, upon the anterior border of the trapezius, in line with VI 15 (TH 15) and II 13 (SI 13). Soulié (1994) locates GB 21 on the upper shoulder: five FW (Finger Width) medial to the bony extremity (acomion). Just in front of the trapezius muscle, at the angle between the lower edge of a deep transverse mass (first rib) and the posterior edge of a hard vertical muscle (posterior scalenius); in a hollow; four FW medial to LI 16; one large FW lateral to SI 15; two FW posterior to ST 12; three FW anterior to TW 15.

Ellis (1991) locates GB 21 midway between C7 (GV 14/Du 14) and the bony prominence above LI 16, at the highest point of the shoulder. Lotan (2000) locates GB 21 in the trapezius split, midway between C7 spinous process and the acromion peak; at the shoulder highest point; on the superior part of the shoulder but with an anterior aspect; vertically superior to the nipple. Deadman (1998) locate GB21 midway between DU 14 and the tip of the acromion, at the crest of the trapezius muscle (the crest refers to the highest point of the trapezius muscle on the sagittal (anterior-posterior) plane).

So (1985) locates GB 21 one-half way between the end of the clavicle equal with LI 16 and the base of the neck, on the top of the muscle. To locate this point, use the thumb and middle finger to hold the muscle, use the first finger to press down on the middle of the muscle until you feel the muscle divide in half. Between the two halves is the point. Shanghai (1981) locate GB 21 midway between Gv 14 and the acromion of the shoulder (in the posterior margin of the deltoid and trapezius muscles). Yang (1982) locates GB 21 between the midpoint of the clavicle and the superior border of the scapula.

GB 22-28 lie on the lateral aspect of the torso

GB 22 YUAN YE – ARMPIT ABYSS

⊥ ***0.3 TO 0.5 CUN*** ***Δ FORBIDDEN TO USE MOXA***

Pos: Position of patient: supine, seated or lateral recumbent, with the arm raised or abducted.

Loc: a) On the lateral aspect of the torso.
b) On the lateral chest (in the upper jiao).
c) In the fourth intercostal space (occasionally the fifth intercostal space).
d) On the mid-axillary line.
e) Approximately 3 cun inferior to the axillary fold (apex of the axilla).

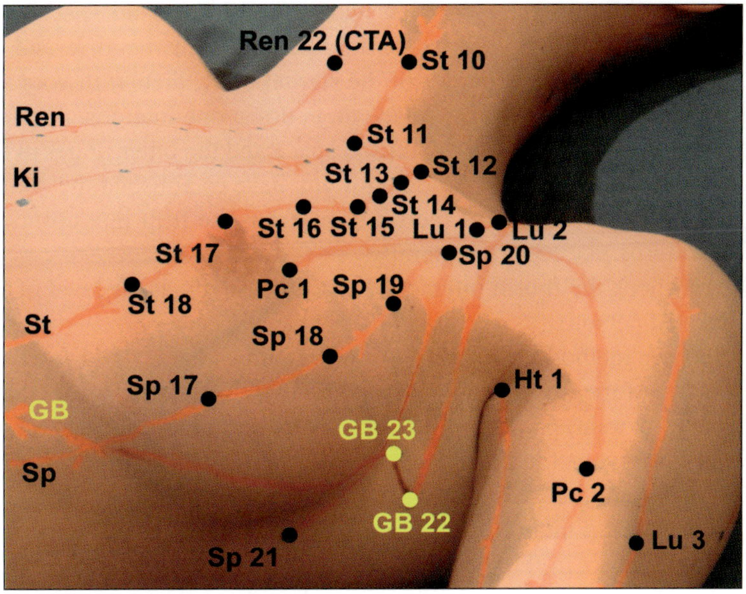

Tip: a) GB 22 is located in the fourth intercostal space. As the fourth intercostal space cannot be palpated effectively due to muscle and breast tissue, the sixth intercostal space is easier to palpate and Sp 21 is used as a reference.

b) Locate the mid-axillary line which runs from the axilla (armpit) longitudinally along the most lateral aspect of the torso. To establish the mid-axillary line ask the patient to place their hands on their waist and locate the posterior border of the pectoralis major muscle (anterior border of the armpit), and the anterior border of the latissimus dorsi muscle (the posterior border of the armpit). Draw two parallel lines longitudinally along the lateral surface of the torso, and the mid-axillary line is half way between these lines. Alternatively you can visualise where the mid-axillary line should be.

c) Draw a transverse line from the centre of the nipple laterally to the mid axillary line as in tip b) above.

d) Sp 21 is used as a reference for GB 22 and GB 23.

e) Sp 21 is located at the intersection of the mid-axillary line and the transverse line in the sixth intercostal space.

f) On a large breasted person you may need to ask them to lift their breast (left breast, right hand; right breast, left hand) to access the point. The nipple is usually in the fourth intercostal space on the anterior aspect of the chest.

g) As Sp 21 may be located in the seventh intercostal space, it is recommended that you use the lines of intersection to locate the sixth intercostal space.

h) Palpate from the sixth intercostal space on the mid-axillary line towards the axilla. As you palpate towards the axilla GB 22 is in the fourth intercostal space, approximately half way between Sp 21 and the apex of the axilla.

i) The pectoralis major muscle covers the surface of the ribs which can make it difficult to locate the intercostal spaces from the third intercostal space downwards.

j) If it is difficult locate the first and second intercostal spaces which are easier to palpate. Place your index and middle finger in the first and second intercostal spaces on the lateral border of the sternal body, then with your two fingers staying at the same distance apart, place them down one intercostal space so that you have one finger in the second intercostal space and the other finger in the third intercostal space. Repeating this method until you have established the sixth intercostal space.
k) Due to the formation of the rib cage, from the fifth intercostal space your fingers need to be placed more laterally.
l) As a check the fourth intercostal space is usually at the level of the nipple (in a flat chested person).
m) Another method of identifying the intercostal spaces is to count them from the bottom of the rib cage upwards. For the 9th intercostal space (there are 9 intercostal spaces in total) palpate for the inferior border of the rib cage which will be the 10th rib. Place your finger in the intercostal space superior to this rib. You will now be in the 9th intercostal space.
n) When the 9th intercostal space has been established, place the flat of your index or middle finger in the 9th intercostal space and palpate for the 8th intercostal space by feeling for the superior border of the 9th rib. Once you have located the 9th rib, palpate superiorly until you feel a softness, which will be the 8th intercostal space. Use this procedure to palpate and locate the other intercostal spaces. Sp 21 is located in the sixth intercostal space, on the mid axillary line.
o) GB 22 is used as a reference to locate GB 23. GB 22 is in the 4th intercostal space on the mid axillary line. On some people GB 22 may be located in the 5th intercostal space. Therefore if you cannot feel a *men* (depression) in 4th intercostal space, palpate in the 5th intercostal space.
p) Palpation will ensure accurate point location.
q) An alternative method is to use cun measurements to locate GB 22 and GB 23. When the arm is abducted the longitudinal distance between the axillary fold or apex of the axilla to the tip of the 11th rib is measured as 12 cun. Divide 12 cun in to 4 equal measurements of 3 cun.
r) GB 22 is located at approximately 3 cun inferior to the axillary fold. This point is located in the 4th (or sometimes 5th) intercostal space so palpation will take overall precedence over the cun measurements.
s) Many people may have more tissue in the area of the tip of the 11th rib. (To locate the tip of the 11th rib, please see Liv 13 tips section).

Note: Voisin (1974) locates G 22 in relation to rib 5, upper border: anterior border of the axillary cavity. Legge (1999) locates GB 22 in the 5th intercostal space, 3 cun below the axilla in the midaxillary line. Jayasuriya (1982) locates GB 22 on the midaxillary line, 3 cun below the axilla, in the 5th intercostal space.

Eachou (1995) locates GB 22 in a seated position with the arm abducted, the point is located 3 inches inferior to the anterior axillary line and in the fifth intercostal space. Shanghai (1981) locate GB 22 on the mid-axillary line 3 units below the axilla and in the 5th intercostal space. So (1985) locates GB 22 at 4 divisions lateral to ST 16, under the armpit between two ribs.

Deadman (1998) locate GB 22 on the mid-axillary line, in the fifth intercostal space, approximately 3 cun inferior to the apex of the axilla, at the level of the nipple. Lotan (2000) locates GB 22 in the 5th intercostal, on the mid-axillary line. Lotan also includes the same location as our description but uses this as an alternative location. Soulié (1994) locates GB 22 on the axilla, mid-length: lower edge of the fourth rib (the third being deep on the axilla); in a hollow; three FW (Finger Width) lateral to PC 1.

GB 23 ZHE JIN – NEGLECTED MUSCLES

⊥ ***0.3 TO 0.5 CUN*** Δ ***3 TO 5***

Pos: Position of patient: supine, seated or lateral recumbent, with the arm raised or abducted.

Loc:
a) On the lateral aspect of the torso.
b) On the lateral chest (in the upper jiao).
c) In the fourth intercostal space (occasionally the fifth intercostal space).
d) 1 cun anterior to GB 22 (or 1 cun anterior to the mid axillary line).
e) 3 cun inferior to the axillary fold (apex of the axilla).

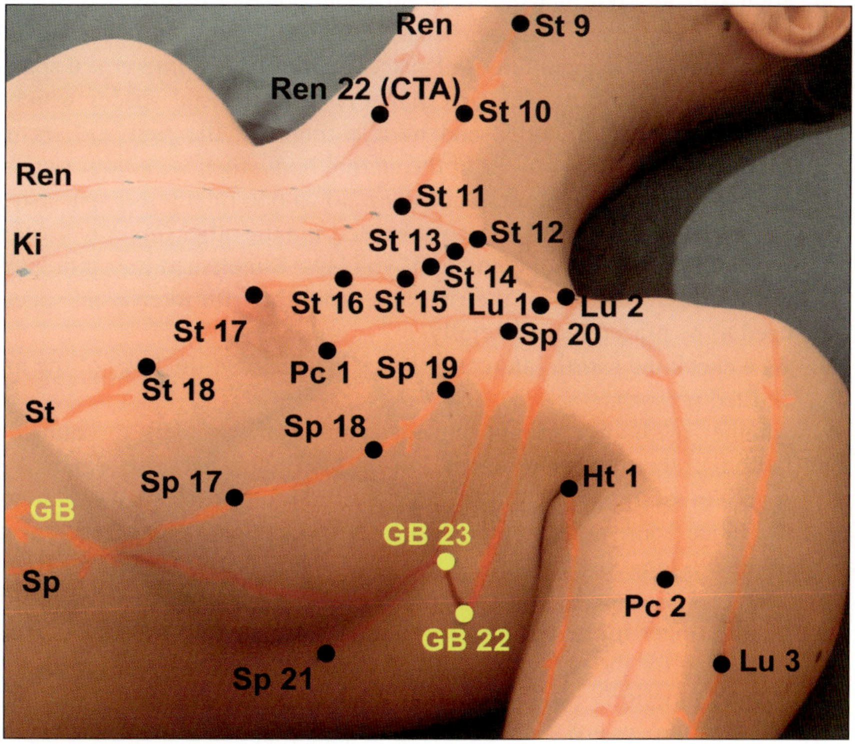

Tip:
a) GB 23 is located in the fourth intercostal space. As the fourth intercostal space cannot be palpated effectively due to muscle and breast tissue, the sixth intercostal space is easier to palpate and Sp 21 is used as a reference.
b) Locate the mid-axillary line which runs from the axilla (armpit) longitudinally along the most lateral aspect of the torso. To establish the mid-axillary line ask the patient to place their hands on their waist and locate the posterior border of the pectoralis major muscle (anterior border of the armpit), and the anterior border of the latissimus dorsi muscle (the posterior border of the armpit). Draw two parallel lines longitudinally along the lateral surface of the torso and the mid-axillary line is half way between these lines. Alternatively you can visualise where the mid-axillary line should be.
c) Draw a transverse line from the centre of the nipple laterally to the mid axillary line as in tip b) above.
d) Sp 21 is used as a reference for GB 22 and GB 23.
e) Sp 21 is located at the intersection of the mid-axillary line and the transverse line in the sixth intercostal space.
f) On a large breasted person you may need to ask them to lift their breast (left breast, right hand; right breast, left hand) to access the point. The nipple is usually in the fourth intercostal space on the anterior aspect of the chest.
g) As Sp 21 may be located in the seventh intercostal space, it is recommended that you use the lines of intersection to locate the sixth intercostal space.
h) Palpate from the sixth intercostal space on the mid-axillary line towards the axilla. As you palpate towards the axilla GB 22 is in the fourth intercostal space, approximately half way between Sp 21 and the apex of the axilla.
i) The pectoralis major muscle covers the surface of the ribs which can make it difficult to locate the intercostal spaces from the third intercostal space downwards.
j) If it is difficult locate the first and second intercostal spaces which are easier to palpate. Place your index and middle finger in the first and second intercostal spaces on the lateral border of the sternal body, then with your two fingers staying at the same distance apart, place them down one intercostal space so that you have one finger in the second intercostal space and the other finger in the third intercostal space. Repeating this method until you have established the sixth intercostal space.
k) Due to the formation of the rib cage, from the fifth intercostal space your fingers need to be placed more laterally.
l) As a check the fourth intercostal space is usually at the level of the nipple (in a flat chested person).
m) Another method of identifying the intercostal spaces is to count them from the bottom of the rib cage upwards. For the 9th intercostal space (there are 9 intercostal spaces in total) palpate for the inferior border of the rib cage which will be the 10th rib. Place your finger in the intercostal space superior to this rib. You will now be in the 9th intercostal space.
n) When the 9th intercostal space has been established, place the flat of your index or middle finger in the 9th intercostal space and palpate for the 8th intercostal space by feeling for the superior border of the 9th rib. Once you have located the 9th rib, palpate superiorly until you feel a softness, which will be the 8th intercostal space. Use this procedure to palpate and locate the other intercostal spaces. Sp 21 is located in the sixth intercostal space, on the mid axillary line.

o) GB 22 is used as a reference to locate GB 23. GB 22 is in the 4th intercostal space on the mid axillary line and GB 23 is 1 cun anterior it (1 cun anterior to the mid axillary line). On some people GB 23 may be located in the 5th intercostal space. Therefore if you cannot feel a *men* (depression) in 4th intercostal space, palpate in the 5th intercostal space.
p) Palpation will ensure accurate point location.
q) An alternative method is to use cun measurements to locate GB 22 and GB 23. When the arm is abducted the longitudinal distance between the axillary fold or apex of the axilla to the tip of the 11th rib is measured as 12 cun. Divide 12 cun in to 4 equal measurements of 3 cun.
r) GB 22 is located at approximately 3 cun inferior to the axillary fold and GB 23 is approximately 1 cun anterior to this. This point is located in the 4th (or sometimes 5th) intercostal space so palpation will take overall precedence over the cun measurements.
s) Many people may have more tissue in the area of the tip of the 11th rib. (To locate the tip of the 11th rib, please see Liv 13 tips section).

Note: Lawson-Wood (1973) and Worsley (1982) list this point as an ALARM/Front Collecting/Front Mu/Herald Point of Gall Bladder as well as VII (GB) 24. Lotan lists this point as a second GB front "Mu" point. Some Schools and texts also use this point as a RE-UNION/Crossing/Meeting Point of the Gall Bladder Channel with the Bladder Channel.- Foot Shao Yang Channel with the Foot Tai Yang Channel.

Note: Lawson-Wood (1973) locates VII 23 in the fifth intercostal space on the anterior paraxillary line of Weihe. Legge (1999) locates GB 23 at 1 cun anterior to GB 22 (in the fifth intercotal space), approximately level with the nipple. Lotan (2000) locates GB 23 in the fifth intercostal space, 1 cun anterior to the mid-axillary line; 1 cun anterior to GB 22. Lotan also includes the same location as our description but uses this as an alternative location. Voisin (1974) locates G 23 in relation to rib 5, upper border: 2 fb (finger breadth) medially to the anterior border of the axillary cavity.

Soulié (1994) locates GB 23 on the lateral part of the thorax: three FW (Finger Width) lateral to the vertical of the nipple; inferior edge of the fifth rib; in a hollow; three FW lateral to and under the nipple (men); five FW under and anterior to GB 22, passing through SP 21; one large FW under PC 1; two FW above and medial to GB 24; one large FW above and lateral to LR 14. Ellis (1991) locate GB 23 1" anterior to GB 22, approximately level with the nipple. Shanghai (1981) locates GB 23 at 1 unit anterior to GB 22 in the 5th intercostal space.

Cheng (1987) locates G 23 at 1 cin anterior to G 22, approximately level with the nipple. Eachou (1995) locates GB 23 in a lateral recumbent position, 3 inches inferior to the anterior axillary line and 1 inch anterior to GB 22, in the fifth intercostal space, approximately level with the nipple. Masayoshi (1975) locates GB 23 at 1 sun anterior to the midaxillary line, on the height of the papilla. Deadman (1998) locate GB 23 below the axilla in the fifth intercostal space, 1 cun anterior to GB 22, approximately level with the nipple. So (1985) locates GB 23 between the same rib bones as GB 22, in front of GB 22 1 and 1/4 divisions. Jayasuriya (1982) locates GB 23 at 1 cun anterior to GB 22, in the fifth intercostal space. Katsusuke (1983) locates GB 23 one sun behind SP 18; one sun in front of GB 22. Shandong (1982) locate Zhejin at 1 cun below Pt. Yuanye (GB 22).

GB 24 RI YUE – SUN AND MOON

⊥ ***0.3 TO 0.5 CUN*** ∆ ***5 TO 7***

- ALARM/Front Collecting/Front Mu/Herald Point of Gall Bladder
- RE-UNION/Crossing/Meeting Point of the Gall Bladder Channel with the Spleen Channel and the Yang Linking Vesse – Foot Shao Yang Channel with the Foot Tai Yin Channel and Yang Wei Mai

Pos: Position of patient: supine.

Loc: a) On the anterior aspect of the torso.
b) On the mid-abdomen (in the middle jiao).
c) Directly inferior to the nipple.
d) In the seventh intercostal space.
e) 4 cun lateral to the anterior median line.
f) Directly inferior to Liv 14 (which is in the sixth intercostal space)

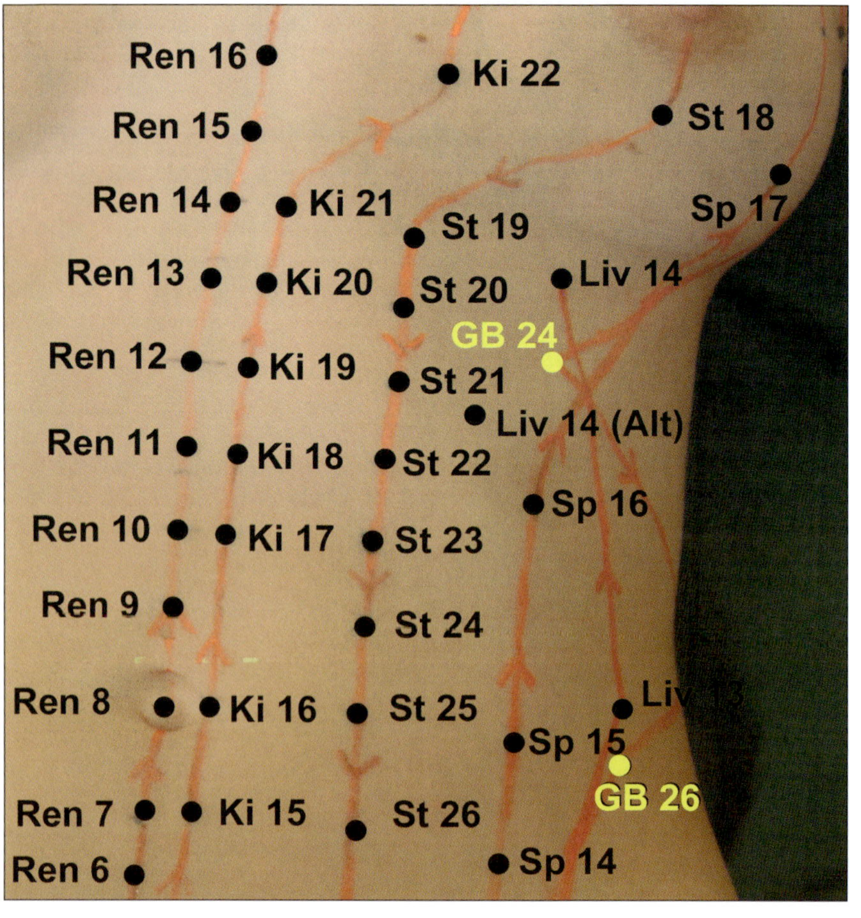

Cun: a) Draw a mark directly inferior to the nipple (4th intercostal space) towards the 6th intercostal space. On women you may need to ask them to lift their breast slightly (left breast, right hand; right breast, left hand) to allow you to visualise a "plumb" line inferior to the nipple. This may or not be 4 cun lateral to the nipple. As Liv 14 is on the middle jiao always measure 4 cun from the level of the umbilicus not from the clavicle (upper jiao). If you prefer to use the cun measurements to locate the point, see below, if not, advance to the tips section.

b) The transverse measurement for the middle and lower abdomen (middle and lower jiao) is 2 cun between the anterior median line (at the centre of the umbilicus) and the lateral border of the rectus abdominis muscle (at St 25).

c) The lateral border of the rectus abdominis muscle is not the actual edge of the muscle but the most prominent surface of the muscle before it begins to 'slope' in to the torso. By visualising the corner of an inverted 'L', the point is located on the antero-lateral edge of the muscle. To locate this muscle ask the patient to slightly raise their head. The lateral border of the rectus abdominis muscle is on the most lateral part of the palpable curve which is more medial than the actual edge of the muscle.

d) Another way to mark out the transverse cun measurements at the level of the umbilicus is to locate the medial border of the anterior superior iliac spine (part of the iliac crest). To locate the 4 cun line of the Spleen channel, place a pen longitudinally on the medial border of the anterior superior iliac spine approximately halfway between the centre of the umbilicus and the superior border of the symphysis pubis bone. For the Stomach channel divide the 4 cun measurement in half to get 2 cun. The edge of the rectus abdominis muscle is measured as 4 cun. Once established you can then divide the 4 cun into other cun measurements for use on the Stomach and Kidney and Spleen channels etc.

e) The transverse cun measurements for the middle and lower abdomen (middle and lower jiao) includes the Kidney, Stomach, Spleen, Gall Bladder and Liver channels (lateral to the anterior median line): Ki 11 to Ki 21 = 0.5 cun; St 19 to St 30 = 2 cun; Sp 12 = 3.5 cun; Sp 13 to Sp 16 = 4 cun; GB 24 = 4 cun; Liv 14 = 4 cun.

f) Ki 16, St 25 and Sp 15 are all transversely level with the centre of the umbilicus and used as reference points for marking their channels cun measurements.

g) The longitudinal measurement of the mid abdomen is 8 cun from the centre of the umbilicus to the xiphisternal joint (Ren 16).

Tip: a) Visualise and place a mark directly inferior to the nipple or mark in 4 cun lateral to the anterior median line (as explained in the cun measurements section).

b) Palpate and mark in the 6th intercostal space.

c) Palpate for the point which is directly inferior to the nipple, in the 6th intercostal space, (at 4 cun lateral to the anterior median line).

d) Place your finger in the seventh intercostal space between the seventh and eighth ribs and run laterally 4 cun. Ensure that your finger is in the deepest part of the intercostal space.

e) It may be difficult locating the third intercostal space onwards as the pectoralis major muscle covers the surface of the ribs. To assist with point location place a finger in both the first and second intercostal space.

f) Your fingers are now a "rib space" apart. If you place one finger in the second intercostal space, your other finger should then give you a good approximation of the position of the third intercostal space (intercostal spaces are approximately of equal width). You can continue with this method of locating the intercostal spaces. The spaces become more lateral at the level of the fourth intercostal space. At this level the costal cartilages of the lower ribs can merge together to attach to the sternum rather than having individual articulations with the sternum. The intercostal spaces are therefore only easily palpable more laterally.

g) Note that the nipples on men or 'flat chested' women are generally located at the fourth intercostal space.

h) Palpation in the area of 4 cun lateral to the anterior median line should reveal the accurate location for GB 24. Remember that the nipple lies in the 4th intercostal space, and the distance between the anterior median line to the nipple is 4 cun.

i) Another way of identifying the intercostal spaces is to count from the bottom of the rib cage upwards. For the 9th intercostal space (9 intercostal spaces in total) palpate for the inferior border of the rib cage which will be the 10th rib. Place your finger in the intercostal space superior to this rib. You will now be in the 9th intercostal space.

j) When the 9th intercostal space has been established, place the flat of your index or middle finger in the 9th intercostal space and palpate for the 8th intercostal space by feeling for the superior border of the 9th rib. Once you have located the 9th rib, palpate superiorly until you feel a softness, which will be the 8th intercostal space. Use this procedure to palpate and locate the seventh intercostal space.

k) Palpation gives ultimate accurately.

Note: Lawson-Wood (1973) locates VII 24 in the sixth intercostal space, on the anterior paraxillary line of Weihe. Wu (1973) locates GB 24 upon the thorax, on a line with the nipple, in the eighth intercostal space. Lavier (1974) in an illustration locates GB 24 medial to the rib cage at 4.5 pouce (4.5 cun) lateral to the anterior median line (which is the same lateral measurement for the his Spleen channel), and approximately one pouce (one cun) superior to Sp 16, transversely level with St 21, Ki 19 and VC 12 (Ren 12).

Voisin (1974) locates G 24 at rib 6, lower border: straight below the preceding point (which is 2 fb (finger breadth) medial to the anterior of the axillary cavity. Katsusuke (1983) locates GB 24 immediately below the lower edge of the ninth rib. Masayoshi (1975) locates GB 24 at 0.5 sun below LV 14. Huang (1993) locates GB 24 five fen below Cycle Gate (Liv 14). Worsley (1982) locates VII 24 in the seventh intercostal space, on the paramedian nipple line, approximately level with XIII 13 (Ren 13).

Soulié (1994) locates GB 24 on the lower part of the thorax: four large FW (Finger Width) lateral to the vertical of the nipple (and two FW below its level – men), inferior edge of the sixth rib (the nipple being on the superior edge of the fifth rib); in a hollow; two FW lateral and below GB 23; six FW above and anterior to GB 25.

GB 25 JING MEN – CAPITAL GATE

⊥ ***0.3 TO 0.5 CUN*** **Δ *5 TO 15***

- ALARM/Front Collecting/Front Mu/Herald Point of Kidney

Pos: Position of patient: supine or lateral recumbent (the person lying on their side with their legs bent).

Loc: a) On the lateral aspect of the torso.
b) Just inferior to the anterior tip of the twelfth rib (second floating rib).

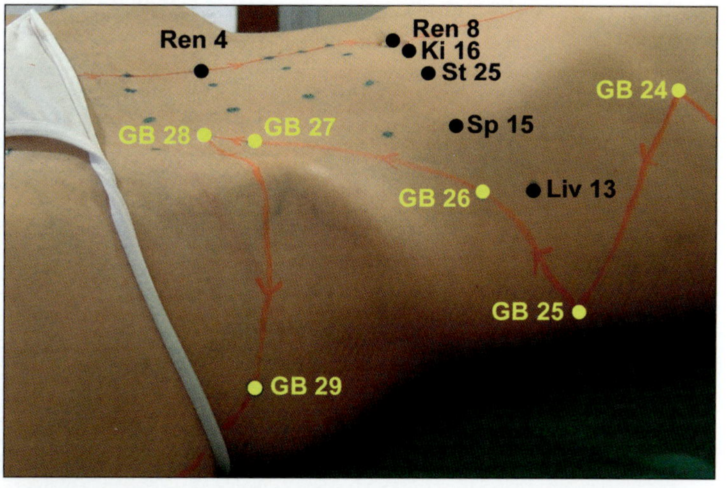

Tip: a) The length of the 12th rib varies from person to person. The point can be near to the mid axillary line either anterior or posterior. GB 25 may be located on the lateral aspect or on the posterior aspect of the torso
b) It may be difficult locating the 12th rib and its anterior tip.
c) If the person has alot of flesh in this area, ask them to turn on to their side (lateral recumbent position with their legs bent). This ensures that the rib cage is not as covered by flesh and the 12th rib would be more accessible. People who have alot of flesh covering their anatomy seem to have points that are easier to palpate.
d) With the person in the supine or lateral recumbent position, place two fingers on the rib cage on the back parallel to the ribs.
e) "Walk" your fingers inferiorly until you can only feel flesh, then go to the last place you were able to feel bone, which should be the inferior border of the 12th rib.
f) Palpate slightly anteriorly and superiorly until you locate the tip of the 12th rib which should be a sharp pointed structure. This should be near to the mid-axillary line.
g) Be careful with your finger pressure as this point can be sensitive. Always locate and needle the point with the person in the same position.

Note: Soulié (1994) locates GB 25 at the bottom of the lateral part of the thorax; at the angle between the inferior point of the twelfth and last rib and the anterior edge of the large vertical muscle (latissimus dorsi); in a hollow; about three FW (Finger Width) above GB 26; two large FW under and posterior to LR 13; two FW above and anterior to BL 51, lateral to BL 21. Huang (1993) locates GB 25 below the hip bone in the lumbar region lateral to the spine, one cun and eigth fen below the region of the free ribs.

GB 26 DAI MAI – GIRDLE VESSEL

⊥ ***0.5 TO 0.8 CUN*** Δ ***5 TO 15***
FORBIDDEN TO NEEDLE AND MOXA THIS POINT DURING PREGNANCY.

- 8 EXTRAORDINARY VESSEL/Coalescent Point of the Girdle Vessel (Dai Mai)
- RE-UNION/Crossing/Meeting Point of the Gall Bladder Channel with the Girdle Vessel – Foot Shao Yang Channel with the Dai Mai

Pos: Position of patient: supine.

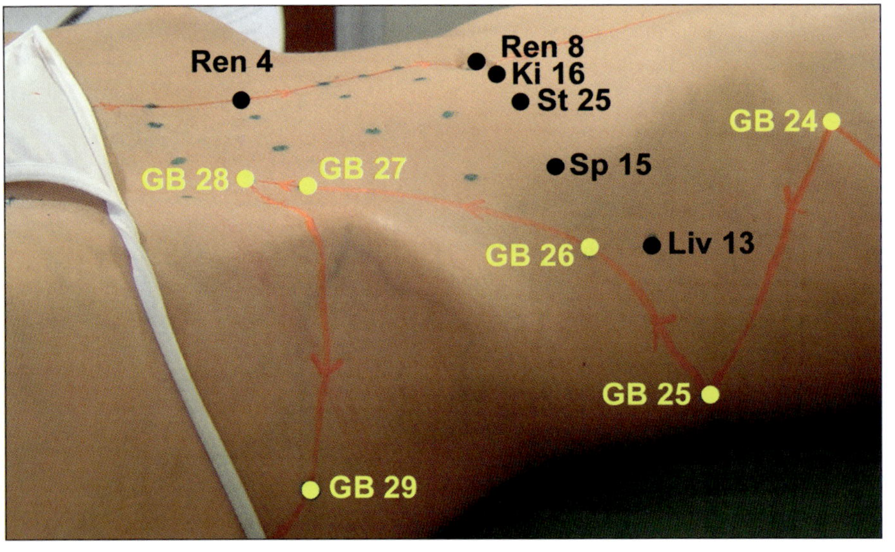

Loc:
a) On the anterior aspect of the torso.
b) In between the mid-abdomen and lower abdomen (in between the middle and lower jiao).
c) At the level of the umbilicus.
d) Inferior to the tip of the eleventh rib (where Liv 13 is located).
e) On a line from GB 25 to GB 27.

Tip:
a) Locate the tip of the 11th rib first.
b) Ask the patient to bend their elbow at 90 degrees with their upper arm at their side. The tip of their elbow should roughly be at the location of Liv 13 which will be just anterior to or on the mid-axillary line.
c) Press gently to locate the tip of the 11th rib (1st floating rib) and not the tip of the 12th rib (2nd floating rib) which is GB 25.
d) If your finger is palpating posterior to the mid-axillary line you will be near the tip of the 12th rib.
e) If you are having difficulties locating the tip of the 11th rib, first locate the tip of the 12th rib.

f) If the person has alot of flesh in this area, ask them to turn on to their side (lateralrecumbent position with their legs bent). This ensures that the rib cage is not as covered by flesh and the 11th rib would be more accessible. People who have alot of flesh covering their anatomy seem to have points that are easier to palpate.
g) With the person in the supine or lateral recumbent position, place two fingers on the rib cage on the back parallel to the ribs.
h) "Walk" your fingers inferiorly until you can only feel flesh, then go to the last place you were able to feel bone, which should be the inferior border of the 12th rib.
i) Then palpate the inferior border of the 12th rib anteriorly until you cannot feel anything.
j) From this area palpate superiorly until your fingers meet a resistence which is the inferior border of the 11th rib.
k) Palpate anteriorly again until there is no resistance.
l) Palpate slightly posteriorly and superiorly until you locate the tip of the 11th rib which should be a sharp pointed structure. This should be just anterior to the mid-axillary line.
m) From the 11th rib draw a longitudinal line inferior to the tip.
n) From the centre of the umbilicus, draw a transverse line towards the lateral aspect of the abdomen.
o) Where the longitudinal and transverse lines intersect this will give the approximate area of the point.
p) Palpation gives ultimate accurately.

Note: Jayasuriya (1982) locates GB 26 at the level of the umbilicus, on a vertical line drawn from the midpoint between the free ends of the 11th and 12th ribs. He goes on to say that according to some authoritirs it is directly below the free end of the 11th rib (Liv 13), at the level of the umbilicus. So (1985) locates GB 26 across from the umbilicus 8 divisions, at the same time level as the umbilicus, on the midaxillary line, at the top of the iliac crest. He notes that for fat or thin bodies, disregard the 8 divisions part of this measurement. Voisin (1974) locates G 26 on the flank: vertically below the anterior border of the axillary cavity, 1 fb (finger breadth) above the iliac crest. Masayoshi (1975) locates GB 26 in the centre on the side of the abdomen about 1.5 finger widths below the 11th intercostal; midway between the 11th rib and anterior superior iliac spine. Huang (1993) locates GB 26 at one cun and eight fen below the region of the free rib.

Soulié (1994) locates GB 26 at the mid-distance of the superior edge of the iliac crest (top of the hip) to the last rib, about vertical to the axilla; three FW (Finger Width) posterior to the anterior angle (of the ilium); on the anterior edge of the insertion on the hip of the large dorsal muscle (latissimus dorsi); in a large hollow (triangle of Petit); about three FW under GB 25; three FW above GB 27; about three large FW anterior to BL 25; four FW posterior to SP 14. Academy (1975) locates GB 26 midway between the free ends of the 11th and 12th ribs, level with the umbilicus.

The longitudinal measurements of the anterior torso are:

9 cun from the xiphisternal joint to the suprasternal fossa (with the space between 2 ribs measuring approximately 1.6 cun in the lower chest, and 1 cun in the upper chest)

8 cun from the centre of the umbilicus to the xiphisternal joint

For the descriptions relating to the channels in the middle jiao, the longitudinal cun measurements are given from the centre of the umbilicus superiorly or from the xiphisternal joint inferiorly, depending on the direction of the flow of the channel.

5 cun from the centre of the umbilicus to the superior border of the symphysis pubis bone

For the descriptions relating to the channels in the lower jiao, the longitudinal cun measurements are given from the centre of the umbilicus inferiorly or from the superior border of the symphysis pubis bone superiorly, depending on the direction of the flow of the channel.

GB 27 WU SHU – FIVE PIVOTS

⊥ ***0.5 TO 0.7 CUN*** ***∆ 3 TO 10***
FORBIDDEN TO NEEDLE AND MOXA THIS POINT DURING PREGNANCY.

- 8 EXTRAORDINARY VESSEL/Coalescent Point of the Girdle Vessel (Dai Mai)
- RE-UNION/Crossing/Meeting Point of the Gall Bladder Channel with the Girdle Vessel – Foot Shao Yang Channel with the Dai Mai

Pos: Position of patient: supine.

Loc: a) On the anterior aspect of the torso.
b) On the lower abdomen (lower jiao).
c) Just anterior to the border of the anterior superior iliac spine of the ilium.
d) 3 cun inferior to the level of the umbilicus.
e) Transversely level with Ren 4.

Tip: a) The longitudinal measurement of the lower abdomen is 5 cun from the centre of the umbilicus to the superior border of the symphysis pubis.
b) Mark out 5 equal cun measurements longitudinally from the superior border of the symphysis pubis to the centre of the umbilicus on the anterior median line.
c) If you cannot feel the superior border of the symphysis pubis, ask the patient to semi-flex their legs which will soften the abdominal muscles enough to palpate the superior border of the symphysis pubis.

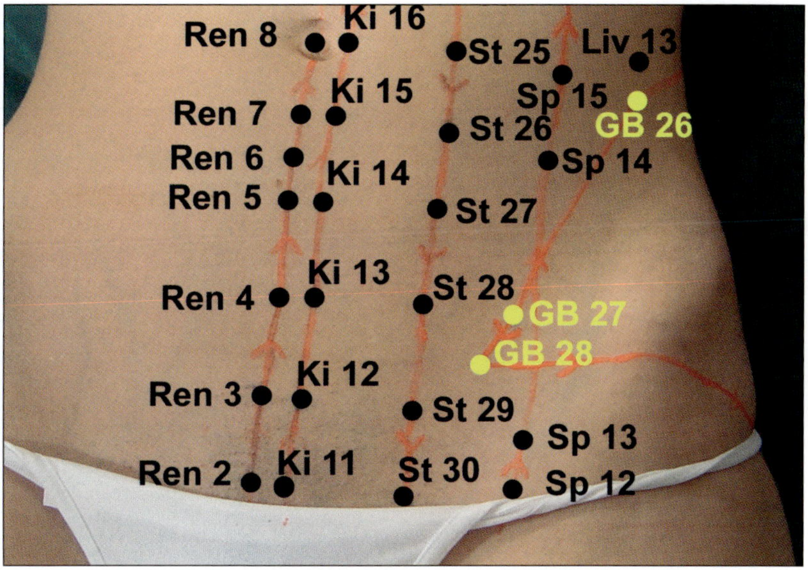

d) Place your finger on the anterior median line, (on Ren 4) at 3 cun inferior to the level of the centre of the umbilicus, and palpate laterally until you feel the border of the anterior superior iliac spine of the ilium.
e) GB 27 is located just anterior to the border of the anterior superior iliac spine of the ilium
f) Palpation gives ultimate accurately.

Note: Worsley (1982) locates VII 27 on the hip, inferior and slightly posterior to the anterior superior iliac spine, on a level with XIII 4 (Ren 4). Lavier (1974 in an illustration locates GB 27 in the same location as J.R.Worsley. Voisin (1974) locates G 27 on the pelvis: vertically below the preceding point, 1 fb (finger breadth) below the iliac crest. Wu (1973) locates GB 27 upon the hip, at three pouce below GB 26.

Lotan (2000) locates GB 27 medial to the ASIS, on the inguinal ligament superior (and medial) border, level with 3 cun inferior to the umbilicus. Academy (1975) locate GB 27 at 3 cun anterior and inferior to GB 26, level with Ren 4, in front of the anterior superior iliac spine. Soulié (1994) locates GB 27 on the lateral part of the hip: two FW (Finger Width) posterior to the vertical anterior part of the hip (iliac crest); two FW under the upper part; at the angle between the inferior edge of the large prominence of the crest and the anterior edge of the insertion of the muscle (gluteus medius); above the insertion of the gluteus minimus; in a hollow; three FW under GB 26; two FW above GB 29; two FW anterior to BL 53.

Huang (1993) locates GB 27 at three cun below Girdling Vessel (GB 26). It is also said to be one cun and five fen lateral to Water Way (St 28). Masayoshi (1975) locates GB 27 on the side of the abdomen along the edge of the ilium, slightly inside the anterior-superior-iliaca spine. Yang (1982) locates GB 27 at 0.5 cun in front of the anterior superior iliac spine. Qiu (1996) locates GB 27 on the lateral side of the abdomen, 0.5 cun anterior to the superior iliac spine, 3 cun below the level of the umbilicus. So (1985) locates GB 27 at 6 divisions lateral to CV 4 (Ren 4). Eachou (1995) locates GB 27 3 inches below GB 26, lateral to CV 4 (Ren 4) and 0.5 inches anterior to the anterior superior iliac crest.

GB 28 WEI DAO – BINDING PATH

⊥ ***0.5 TO 0.7 CUN*** ∆ ***3 TO 7***
FORBIDDEN TO NEEDLE AND MOXA THIS POINT DURING PREGNANCY.

- 8 EXTRAORDINARY VESSEL/Coalescent Point of the Girdle Vessel (Dai Mai)
- RE-UNION/Crossing/Meeting Point of the Gall Bladder Channel with the Girdle Vessel – Foot Shao Yang Channel with the Dai Mai

Pos: Position of patient: supine.

Loc: a) On the anterior aspect of the torso.
b) On the lower abdomen (lower jiao).
c) Anterior to the border of the anterior superior iliac spine of the ilium.
d) Inferior to GB 27.
e) Approximately 0.5 cun medial to the level of GB 27.

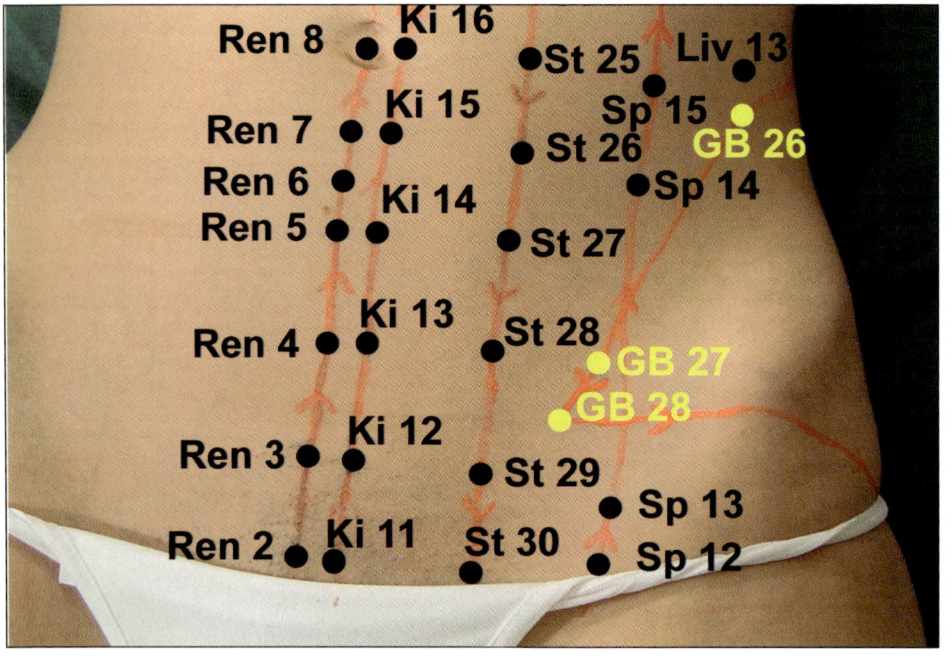

Tip: a) GB 27 is used as a reference point for GB 28.
b) The longitudinal measurement of the lower abdomen is 5 cun from the centre of the umbilicus to the superior border of the symphysis pubis.
c) Mark out 5 equal cun measurements longitudinally from the superior border of the symphysis pubis to the centre of the umbilicus on the anterior median line.
d) If you cannot feel the superior border of the symphysis pubis, ask the patient to semi-flex their legs which will soften the abdominal muscles enough to palpate the superior border of the symphysis pubis.

e) Place your finger on the anterior median line, (on Ren 4) at 3 cun inferior to the level of the centre of the umbilicus, and palpate laterally until you feel the border of the anterior superior iliac spine of the ilium.
f) GB 27 is located just anterior to the border of the anterior superior iliac spine of the ilium
g) From GB 27 palpate inferiorly and slightly medial until you can feel a *men* (depression).
h) How much you palpate inferiorly to GB 27 depends on the individual as the location of GB 28 can vary from person to person. Palpation is important as the point can be located between 0.5 and 2 cun.
i) When locating GB 28 ensure that you are still anterior to the anterior superior iliac spine of the ilium.

Note: Wu (1973) locates GB 28 at one pouce above the greater trochanter. Lavier (1974) in an illustration locates GB 28 on the lateral aspect of the hip, just superior to the greater trochanter of the femur. Voisin (1974) locates G 28 on the pelvis, below and slightly behind the anterior superior iliac spine. So (1985) locates GB 28 at 5 and 1/2 divisions lateral from between CV 4 (Ren 4) and CV 3 (Ren 3) and 1/2 division below GB 27. Shanghai (1981) locate GB 28 at 0.5 cun below GB 27, anterior to and slightly below the anterior superior iliac spine. Eachou (1995) locates GB 28 in the medial inferior margin of the anterior superior iliac crest, and 0.5 inch anterior and inferior to GB 27.

Worsley (1982) locates VII 28 on the hip, mid-way between VII 27 and VII 29. Shandong (1982) locate Weidao anterior and inferior to the spina iliac anterior superior, 0.5 cun anterior and inferior to Pt. Wushu (GB 27). Lotan (2000) locates GB 28 superior to the inguinal ligament, about 0.5 cun medial (and inferior) to the ASIS, about 0.5 cun medial (and inferior) to GB 27. Academy (1975) locate GB 28 anterior and inferior to the anterior superior iliac spine, 0.5 cun anterior and inferior to GB 27.

Soulié (1994) his GB 30 is our GB 28. He locates this on the lateral, superior part of the thigh, hip: anterior edge of the large bulge of the thigh (greater trochanter), angle of the deep anterior edge of the femur; posterior edge of the large muscle (tensor fascia lata); in a hollow; three FW (Finger Width) below GB 30; five FW above GB 31. Masayoshi (1975) locates GB 28 at the inner lower part of the anterior-superior iliaca spine. Huang (1993) locates GB 28 at five cun and three fen below Camphorwood Gate (Liv 13).

GB 29-30 on the lateral aspect of the hip.

GB 29 JU LIAO – DWELLING IN THE BONE

⊥ ***0.5 TO 0.8 CUN*** Δ ***3 TO 7***

- 8 EXTRAORDINARY VESSEL/Coalescent Point of Yang Heel/Yang Motility Vessel (Yang Qiao Mai)
- RE-UNION/Crossing/Meeting Point of the Gall Bladder Channel with the Yang Heel/Yang Motility Vessel – Foot Shao Yang Channel with the Yang Qiao Mai

Pos: Position of patient: supine or lateral recumbent.

Loc: a) On the lateral aspect of the torso.
b) On the lateral aspect of the hip.
c) Midway between the anterior superior iliac spine of the ilium and the prominence of the greater trochanter of the femur.
d) Approximately 3 cun posterior to GB 28.
e) Traditionally described in the anterior fossa of the greater trochanter of the femur.

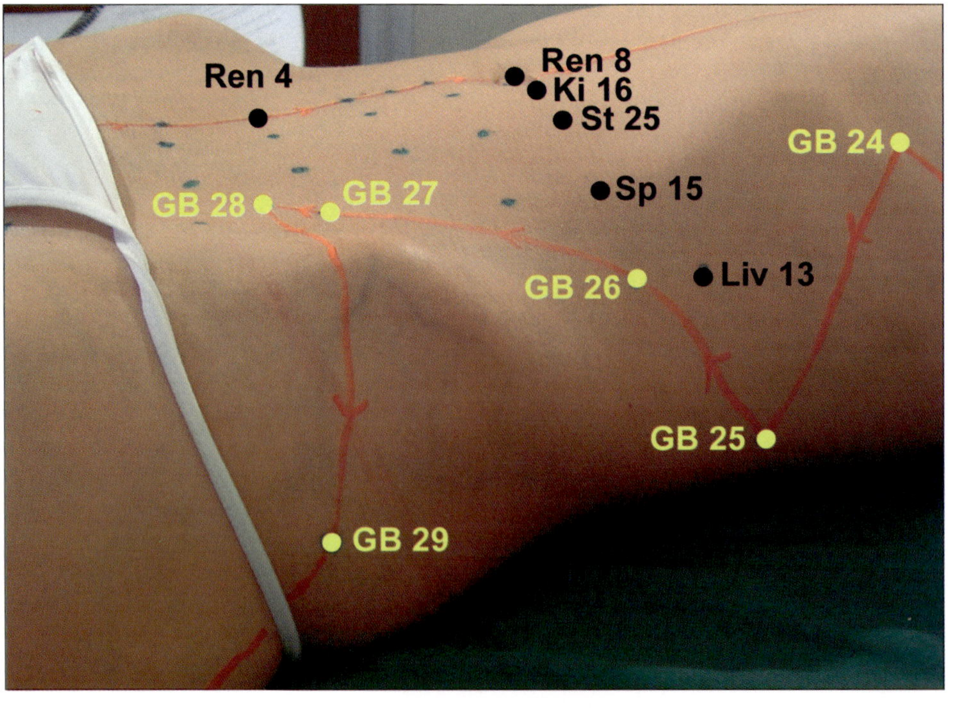

Tip:
a) By vision and by palpation, place a mark on the anterior superior iliac spine of the ilium.
b) Palpate for the prominence of the greater trochanter of the femur. The prominence is usually visible, if not, palpate towards the hip from the knee on the lateral aspect of the thigh to the part of the bone that is most prominent. Place a mark on the prominence.
c) Palpate for GB 29 which is approximately midway between these two marks.
d) An alternative method for locating GB 29 is to locate GB 27 and GB 28.
e) GB 27 is used as a reference point for GB 28.
f) The longitudinal measurement of the lower abdomen is 5 cun from the centre of the umbilicus to the superior border of the symphysis pubis.
g) Mark out 5 equal cun measurements longitudinally from the superior border of the symphysis pubis to the centre of the umbilicus on the anterior median line.
h) If you cannot feel the superior border of the symphysis pubis, ask the patient to semi-flex their legs to relax the abdominal muscles enabling palpation of the superior border of the symphysis pubis.
i) Place your finger on the anterior median line, (on Ren 4) at 3 cun inferior to the level of thecentre of the umbilicus, and palpate laterally until you feel the border of the anterior superior iliac spine of the ilium (ASIS).
j) GB 27 is located just anterior to the border of the anterior superior iliac spine of the ilium
k) From GB 27 palpate inferiorly and slightly medially until you feel a *men* (depression).
l) Palpation of GB 28 inferior to GB 27 is important as the point can be located between 0.5 and 2 cun.
m) When locating GB 28 ensure that you are still anterior to the anterior superior iliac spine.
n) GB 29 is 3 cun posterior to GB 28.
o) The anterior fossa of the greater trochanter of the femur is often visible as a depression, but on some people there can be more flesh covering the fossa. GB 29 is located in the anterior fossa of the greater trochanter. The fossa is anterior to your mark made on the prominence of the greater trochanter of the femur. Palpation will locate the fossa and the point.

Note: Soulié (1994), his GB 28 is our GB 29. He locates this point on the lateral part of the hip: one small FW (Finger Width) above the large bulge of the femur (greater trochanter); upper part of a large hollow; inferior angle between two muscles in front of the gluteus minimus (behind the gluteus medius); two FW under GB 27; three FW above GB 28. Voisin (1974) locates G 29 on the pelvis: 1.5 fb (finger breadth) above and in front of the summit of the greater trochanter. Lavier (1974) in an illustration locates GB 29 on the region of the hip, anterior to the prominence of the greater trochanter of the femur. Huang (1993) locates GB 29 at eight cun and three fen below Camphorwood Gate (Liv 13) in a depression on the hip bone. Wu (1973) locates GB 29 upon the hip, at one and one half pouce below GB 27 (which is three pouce below GB 26). So (1985) locates GB 29 with the leg bent at a 90 degree angle, on the iliac side of the greater trochanter of the femur, opposite GB 30. Masayoshi (1975) locates GB 29 at the lower part of the front edge of the anterior-superior iliaca spine.

To locate GB 30 on one side, have the patient in a lateral recumbent position, with that lower leg extended and the thigh flexed.

GB 30 HUAN TIAO – JUMPING CIRCLE

⊥ *1.0 TO 1.5 CUN* Δ *7 TO 20*

- RE-UNION/Crossing/Meeting Point of the Gall Bladder Channel with the Bladder Channel – Foot Shao Yang Channel with the Foot Tai Yang Channel

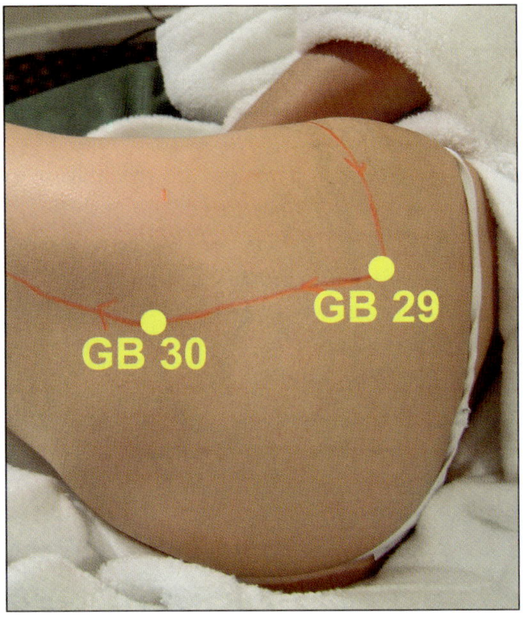

Pos: Position of patient: in a lateral recumbent position, with the lower leg extended and the thigh flexed, with the knee near to the abdomen.

Loc: a) On the lateral aspect of the upper thigh.
b) Posterior to the prominence of the greater trochanter of the femur.
c) One third of the distance between the prominence of the greater trochanter of the femur and the sacral hiatus of the sacrum (Du 2).
d) In the middle of a triangle formed by the greater trochanter of the femur, the posterior superior iliac spine of the ilium and the ischial tuberosity of the ischium.

Tip: a) Place a mark on the prominence of the greater trochanter of the femur.
b) Place a mark on the posterior median line of the sacral hiatus of the sacrum. The sacral hiatus is located at the base of the sacrum. Inferior to the sacral hiatus of the sacrum is the superior border of the coccyx. Du 2 is located between these two structures (on the posterior median line in the sacro-coccygeal articulation).
c) Divide the distance between the two marks in to three.
d) GB 30 is one third of the distance between the prominence of the greater trochanter of the femur and the sacral hiatus of the sacrum, therefore nearer the greater trochanter than the sacral hiatus.
e) Palpation will give overall accuracy, although you may see a large depression, if so, palpate in the depression.
f) An alternative way of locating GB 30 is to locate the greater trochanter of the femur, the posterior superior iliac spine (PSIS) of the ilium and the ischial tuberosity of the ischium.

g) Place a mark on the prominence of the greater trochanter of the femur and on the posterior superior iliac spine of the ilium, (the bony protruberance on the posterior aspect of the lower torso, in the sacral region).

h) If you are having difficulty locating the posterior superior iliac spine, locate the second sacral foramen on the sacral body, which has a large *men* (depression) and is the easiest of the four sacral foramen to palpate. On a level with the second sacral foramen palpate laterally to the sacroiliac joint until you can palpate a bony protruberance which is the posterior superior iliac spine of the ilium. When located, place a mark on the bony protruberance.

i) To locate the ischial tuberosity of the ilium visualise the location of the anus. Lateral to the anus there is a a sharp bony structure, which is the ischial tuberosity of the ischium (the bone you sit on).

j) Once the three structures have been located (g, h and i), draw in a triangle from the three marks. Palpate for GB 30 which is in the middle of the triangle.

k) The outer line of the Bladder channel connects to GB 30 before it travels down the leg and connects to the Bladder channel again at Bl 40 (Bl 54 in some references).

Note: Soulié (1994) his GB 29 is our GB 30. located on the superior lateral part of the thigh: superior and anterior to the large bulge of the femur (greater trochanter): deep; the superior edge of the lower spine; between the anterior edge of the bone and the posterior edge of the large muscle (tensor fascia lata muscle) and of the insertion of the gluteus medius; one FW (Finger Width) above GB 28; eight FW above GB 31. Voisin (1974) locates G 30 on the greater trochanter, summit: posterior border if standing, touching the summit if sitting. Wu (1973) locates GB 30 upon the hip, behind the greater trochanter, at the bottom of the gluteal fold which is formed in a standing position.

So (1985) locates the point with the patient laying to one side, with the top leg bent so that the thigh is close to the abdomen. The point is at the edge of the round shaped bone (greater trochanter) which faces the tip of the butt. Li (1991) locates GB 30 at the junction of the middle and lateral third of the distance along a line connecting the anterosuperior border of the greater trochanter with the hiatus of the sacrum. When the point is being located, have the patient assume a lateral recumbent position, with the leg extended and the thigh flexed about 90 degrees. Place the transverse crease of the interphalangeal joint of the thumb on the highrest point of the greater trochanter, with the tip of the thumb directed towards the spinal columb. The point is where the tip of the thumb touches.

Worsley (1982) locates VII 30 on the lateral surface of the hip, posterior to the prominence of the greater trochanter. Yang (1982) locates GB 30 midway between the anterior superior border of the greater trochanter and the hiatus of the sacrum. Masayoshi (1975) locates GB 30 on the outer part of the hip joint, anterior superior. in the greater trochanter. Huang (1993) locates GB 30 in the hip joint.

Cun Measurements of the Upper Leg

GB 31-33 lie on the lateral aspect of the thigh, GB 34-44 on the lateral aspect of the lower leg and the dorsal surface of the foot.

The distance from a line drawn transversely between the gluteal groove and the medial root of the lower limb (at the level of the lower border of the pubic symphysis where the medial side of the upper leg joins the torso), to the medial popliteal crease (flexure of the knee) is 14 cun.

The distance between the popliteal crease (flexure of the knee) to the superior border of the greater trochanter of the femur, when the leg is abducted, is measured as 19 cun. There seems to be great discrepancies with other descriptions of the anatomy that have used the 19 cun measurement, eg. 19 cun from the popliteal crease to the superior and inferior borders of the pubic symphysis and 19 cun from the popliteal crease to the prominence or inferior border of the greater trochanter of the femur.

14 cun is the accepted bone proportional measurement of the thigh.

Note: Wu (1973) gives St 31/St 32 as "13 and 7 pouce above the flexure", whereas St 33 is "3 pouce above the upper edge of the patella" and St 34 is "1 pouce below St 33". Lavier (1974) shows the total longitudinal measurement of the thigh to be 13 pouce, with St 31/32/33/34 at 13/7/5/4 pouce respectively. Worsley (1982) uses 13 ACI from the medial extremity of the knee crease to the medial extremity of the groin and locates St 31/32/33/34 at 13/7/5/4 ACI proximal to the flexure of the knee. Shanghai (1993) locates ST 30 lateral and superior to the pubis tubercle, 2 cun lateral to the anterior midline, above the inguinal groove and on the medial side of the artery. Shandong (1982) locates Qichong (St 30) laterao-superior to the tuberculum pubicum, 2 cun lateral to the midline, upper portion of inguinal region, medial to the artery.

GB 31, GB 32 and GB 33 are located on the lateral aspect of the thigh.

GB 31 FENG SHI – WIND MARKET

⊥ ***0.5 TO 0.7 CUN*** ***Δ 5***

Pos: Position of patient: supine or standing.

Loc: a) On the midline of the lateral aspect of the thigh.
b) Distal to the greater trochanter of the femur.
c) In a seam between the vastus lateralis and biceps femoris muscles.
d) 7 cun proximal to the popliteal crease (flexure of the knee).
e) Traditionally located with the person standing with their hands at their sides, where the tip of their middle finger touches the lateral aspect of the thigh.

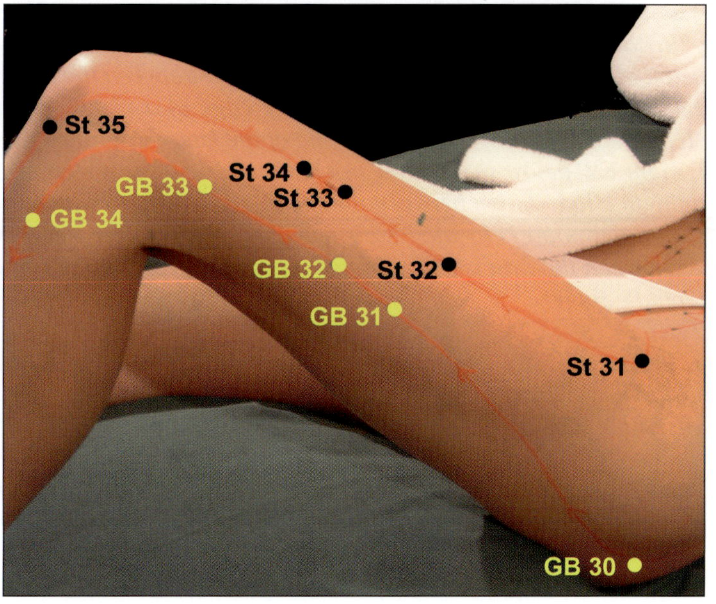

Tip: a) Mark out the level of the inferior border of the symphysis pubis bone (where the medial side of the upper leg joins the torso).

b) Measure 14 cun from the inferior border of the symphysis pubis bone (where the medial side of the upper leg joins the torso) to the medial popliteal crease (flexure of the knee).

c) Draw a transverse line between the two marks laterally to the lateral aspect of the thigh. The measurement between these two marks is 14 cun.

d) GB 31 is located approximately 7 cun proximal to the lateral popliteal crease on the lateral thigh, and distal to the greater trochanter of the femur.

e) Palpate for the seam between the vastus lateralis and biceps femoris muscles with the flow of the Gall Bladder channel from GB 30 down the lateral aspect of the leg to 7 cun measurement, then palpate for a *men* (depression).

f) The point lies approximately where the person's finger tips touch the lateral aspect of the thigh when their hands are at their sides. The traditional location states that the point with the patient in the standing position, but if supine there should be little difference.

g) There are few anatomical structures to locate GB 31 therefore palpate with the flow of the channel from GB 30 down the midline of the lateral aspect of the leg to the until the 7 cun measurement, then palpate to locate a *men* (depression).

Note: Lavier (1974) in an illustration locates GB 31 on the lateral side of the thigh, at 6 pouce proximal to the popliteal crease (knee crease). Note that he uses 13 pouce from the popliteal crease to the prominence of the greater trochanter of the femur. Jayasuriya (1982) locates GB 31 on the lateral aspect of the thigh, 7 cun proximal to the transverse popliteal crease, on the groove between the vastus lateralis and biceps femoris muscles. Wu (1973) locates GB 31 upon the external surface of the thigh, at six pouce above the flexure of the knee. He uses 13 pouce between the crease of the groin at the femoral artery and the interior edge of the popliteal crease.

Soulié (1994) locates GB 31 on the lateral part of the thigh, about mid-height; five FW (Finger Width) below the large, upper protrusion of the femur (greater trochanter). Ten FW above the lateral protrusion of the knee (lateral condyle); the angle between the posterior edge of a large flat tendon (band of the fascia lata) and the lower edge of a transverse mass; on the biceps femoris muscle; eight FW above the lateral bone of the knee (lateral condyle), GB 33; two FW above GB 32; eight FW below the greater trochanter, GB 30. Eachou (1995) locates GB 31 on the lateral thigh, on a line drawn between the greater trochanter of the the femur and the head of the fibula, the point point is located 7 inches above the skin crease of the knee, or 2 inches above GB 32. Or when the arm is straightened against the lateral thigh the point is located at the tip of the middle finger.

Worsley (1982) locates VII 31 on the lateral surface of the thigh, 6 ACI (Anatomical Chinese Inch) proximal to the flexure of the knee, between the vastus lateralis and the biceps femoris. J.R. Worsley uses 13 ACI for the thigh measurement from the medial extremity of the groin to the popliteal crease. Academy (1975) locates GB 31 at the lateral side of the thigh, 7 cun above the transverse popliteal crease, between the m. vastus lateralis and m. biceps femoris. With the patient standing erect, hands close to thighs, the point is at the tip of the middle finger.

Masayoshi (1975) locates GB 31 at 2 to 3 cm above the centre of the outer side of the thigh; at the point of the middle finger when standing straight and touching on the outer side of the thigh with the palm. Katsusuke (1983) locates GB 31 at seven sun above the knees on the outersides of the thighs, at a point where there are two muscles.

GB 32 ZHONG DU – MIDDLE DITCH

⊥ ***0.5 TO 0.7 CUN*** **Δ** ***5 TO 7***

Pos: Position of patient: supine or standing.

Loc: a) On the lateral aspect of the thigh.
b) Distal to the greater trochanter of the femur.
c) In a seam between the vastus lateralis and biceps femoris muscles.
d) 5 cun proximal to the popliteal crease (flexure of the knee).
e) 2 cun inferior to GB 31.

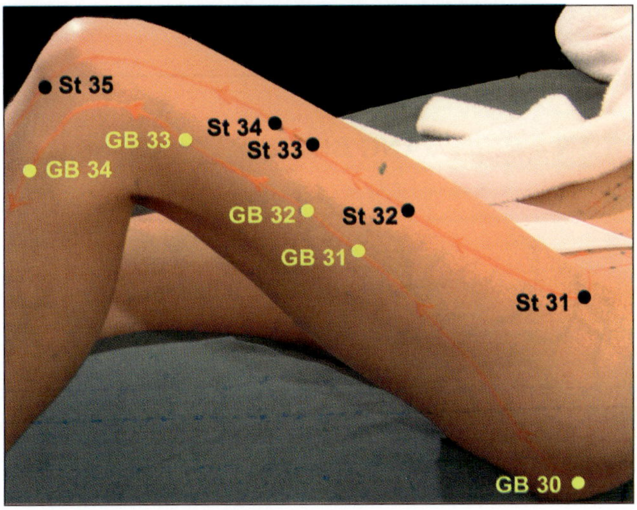

Tip: a) Mark out the level of the inferior border of the symphysis pubis bone (where the medial side of the upper leg joins the torso).
b) Measure 14 cun from the inferior border of the symphysis pubis bone (where the medial side of the upper leg joins the torso) to the medial popliteal crease (flexure of the knee).
c) Draw a transverse line between the two markslaterally to the lateral aspect of the thigh. The measurement between these two marks is 14 cun.
d) GB 32 is located approximately 5 cun proximal to the lateral popliteal crease on the lateral thigh, and distal to the greater trochanter of the femur.
e) Palpate for the seam between the vastus lateralis and biceps femoris muscles with the flow of the Gall Bladder channel from GB 30 down the lateral aspect of the leg to 5 cun proximal to the popliteal crease, then palpate for a *men* (depression).

Note: Lavier (1974) in an illustration locates GB 32 on the lateral side of the thigh, at 5 pouce proximal to the popliteal crease (knee crease). Note that he uses 13 pouce from the popliteal crease to the prominence of the greater trochanter of the femur. Wu (1973) locates GB 32 upon the external surface of the thigh, at five pouce above the flexure of the knee. He uses 13 pouce between the crease of the groin at the femoral artery and the interior edge of the popliteal crease.

Worsley (1982) locates VII 32 on the lateral surface of the thigh, 5 ACI (Anatomical Chinese Inch) proximal to the flexure of the knee, between the vastus lateralis and the biceps femoris. J.R. Worsley uses 13 ACI for the thigh measurement from the medial extremity of the groin to the popliteal crease. Soulié (1994) locates GB 32 on the lateral thigh, about at the lower third; six FW (Finger Width) above the lateral protruding bone of the knee (lateral condyle of the femur); at the angle between the posterior edge of a flat ligament (band of tensor fascia lata) and the lower edge of a transverse mass, on the vastus intermedius muscle; in a hollow; two FW (Finger Width) below GB 31; four FW above GB 33; at the level and lateral to ST 32.

Voisin (1974) locates G 32 on the thigh, lateral aspect: 2 fb (finger breadth) below preceding point. So (1985) locates GB 32 at 5 divisions above GB 33 (from the posterior knee crease on the middle of the thigh. Masayoshi (1975) locates GB 32 at the centre of the outer side of the thigh at the edge of the iliofemoral tendon. Katsusuke (1983) locates GB 31 at seven sun above the knees on the outersides of the thighs, at a point where there are two muscles.

GB 33 XI YANG GUAN – KNEE YANG BORDER

⊥ ***0.5 CUN*** ***Δ FORBIDDEN TO USE MOXA***

Pos: Position of patient: supine with the leg flexed.

Loc:
a) On the lateral aspect of the lower thigh.
b) In a fossa between the tendon of the biceps femoris muscle and the femur.
c) Just proximal to the flare of the lateral epicondyle of the femur.
d) Approximately 3 cun proximal to GB 34.

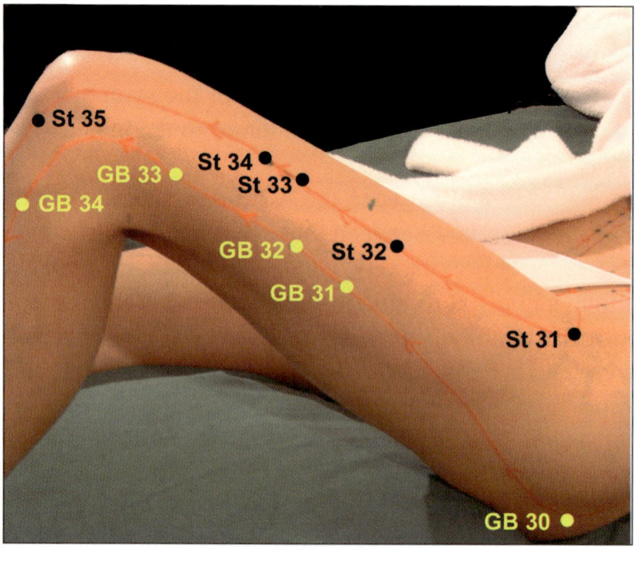

Tip: a) With the patient supine, feel for the anterior border of the biceps femoris muscle on the lateral aspect of the popliteal crease. Usually you can see a dimple at the lateral end of the posterior aspect of the popliteal crease which is formed by the medial border of the biceps femoris muscle.

b) Palpate and run the flat of your finger with the flow of the Gall Bladder channel on the lateral aspect of the thigh in the seam between the anterior border of the tendon of the biceps femoris muscle and the femur.

c) You will feel some resistance in the seam proximal to the lateral popliteal crease, which is the flare of the lateral epicondyle of the femur.

d) The point is located just proximal to the flare of the lateral epicondyle of the femur. Palpation will give overall accuracy for GB 33.

e) If you are having difficulty locating the lateral aspect of the popliteal crease ask the patient to flex their leg, and then mark in the popliteal crease.

Note: Worsley (1982) locates VII 33 on the lateral surface of the leg, between the lateral condyle of the femur and the lateral condyle of the tibia, J.R. Worsley uses 13 ACI for the thigh measurement from the medial extremity of the groin to the popliteal crease. Wu (1973) locates GB 33 upon the external surface of the thigh, in a depression above the head of the femur. He uses 13 pouce between the crease of the groin at the femoral artery and the interior edge of the popliteal crease. Voisin (1974) locates G 33 on the thigh, lateral aspect: 3 fb (finger breadth) above the lateral condyle. Lavier (1974) in an illustration locates GB 33 on the lateral surface of the leg, approximately one pouce proximal to the popliteal crease of the knee. Note that he uses 13 pouce from the popliteal crease to the prominence of the greater trochanter of the femur.

Legge (1999) locates GB 33 in the depression above the lateral condyle of the femur between the tendon of the biceps femoris and the ilio-tibial tract. Jayasuriya (1982) locates GB 33 lateral to the knee joint, in the depression above the lateral epicondyle of the femur, between the bone and the biceps femoris tendon. This point is located with the knee flexed. So (1985) locates GB 33 from the outer eye of the knee, lateral two divisions, between the femur and the tibia. To locate and treat this point, bend the leg so that the calf touches the thigh; the point is at the hollow between and behind the two bones. Ellis (1991) locates GB 33 at 3.0" above GB 34, in the depression between the tendon of the biceps muscle of the femur (m. biceps femoris) and the lateral condyle of the femur. This point is located posterior to the joint when the knee is bent.

Lotan (2000) locates GB 33 with the knee flexed, it is between the femur lateral epicondyle and the biceps femoris, proximal to the knee joint, level with the patella inferior border. Eachou (1995) locates GB 33 on the lateral thigh between the iliotibial tract and the tendon of the biceps femoris 3 inches above GB 34 and lateral to ST 35; or at the same point of the superior margin of the patella, the point is located in the fossa of the lateral epicondyle of the femur. Soulié (1994) locates GB 33 on the upper, lateral part of the knee: two FW (Finger Width) above the round head of the fibula; anterior to the posterior opening of the tibial-femural articulation; at the angle between the upper edge of the head of the femur and the body of the bone; on the anterior edge of a large tendon (biceps femoris); in a hollow; four FW below GB 32; three FW above GB 34. At the level of and lateral to ST 34; three FW anterior to BL 39. Huang (1993) locates GB33 at three cun above Yang Mound Spring (GB 34) in a depression lateral to Calf's Nose (St 35). Masayoshi (1975) locates GB 33 on the lower 1/4th of the outer side of the thigh, in a depression directly above the lateral condyle of the femur.

The distance between the popliteal crease to the prominence of the lateral malleolus is measured as 16 cun.

GB 34 YANG LING QUAN – YANG MOUND SPRING

⊥ ***0.5 TO 0.7 CUN*** **Δ** ***3 TO 10***

- EARTH
- HE – SEA/Shu – Transporting/Antique
- LOWER HE-SEA point of the Gall Bladder
- INFLUENTIAL/Hui – Meeting/Gathering/Assembling Point of Tendons (Sinews)
- COUSIN in association with Sp 9
- ONE OF THE HEAVENLY STAR POINTS OF MA DAN-YANG (the others are: Lu 7, LI 4, LI 11, St 36, St 44, Bl 40, Bl 57, Bl 60, Ht 5, GB 39 and Liv 3)

Pos: Position of patient: supine with the leg semi flexed.

Loc: a) On the lateral aspect of the lower leg.
b) Inferior and anterior to the head of the fibula.
c) Approximately 14 cun proximal to the prominence of the lateral malleolus.
d) Aproximately on a level with Sp 9 (which is on the inferior border of the medial condyle of the tibia).

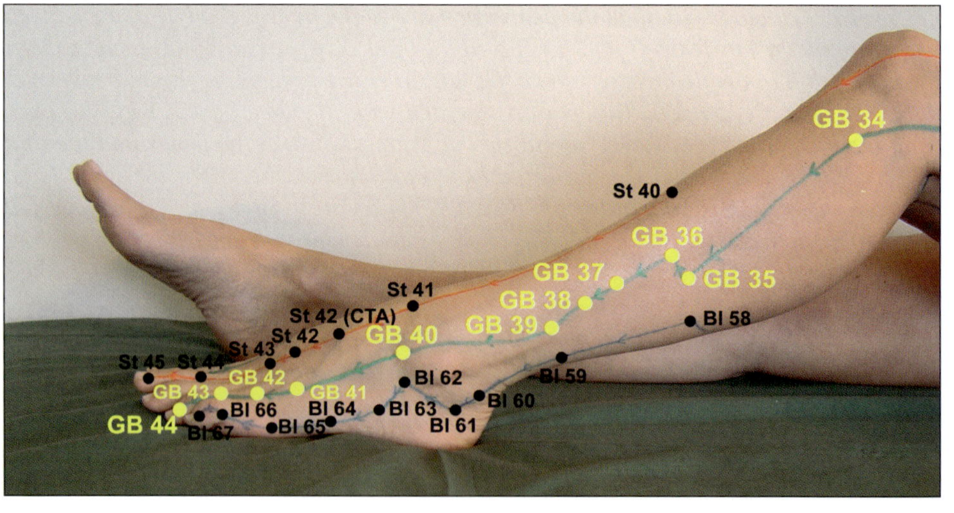

Tip: a) When locating GB 34 the emphasis should be placed on the anatomical description rather than the cun measurement, which is not always accurate due to the size of the head of the fibula.
b) Palpation of the anterior and inferior borders of the head of the fibula takes overall precedence when locating this point.

c) Palpate with the flow of the Gall Bladder channel from the lower thigh towards the knee in the seam between the anterior border of the tendon of the biceps femoris muscle and the femur. Begin palpating from the level of the flare that is proximal to the lateral condyle of the femur (GB 33 location).
d) Continue to palpate the lower leg past the lateral popliteal crease until the lateral border of the biceps femoris muscle can no longer be palpated.
e) Still with the flow of the Gall Bladder channel your finger should then be able to palpate the anterior border of the head of the fibula (on the lateral aspect of the lower leg).
f) Palpate around the border until you are inferior and anterior (the corner) to the head of the fibula.
g) Palpation for accurate point location as the cun measurement should only be used as a guide.
h) If you prefer to use the 14 cun measurement, mark 16 cun from the popliteal crease on the lateral side of the knee flexure to the prominence of the lateral malleolus and then palpate at 14 cun proximal to the prominence of the lateral malleolus.
i) Anatomy takes precedence with point location. Palpating at 14 cun may not accurately locate GB 34, therefore you need to locate the inferior and anterior border of the fibula which may or may not be at 14 cun.
j) Also as a guide, GB 34 is approximately on a level with the inferior border of the medial condyle of the tibia (location of Sp 9). Imagine a bolt going through GB 34, it should meet Sp 9.

Note: Wu (1973) locates GB 34 upon the external surface of the leg, below the head of the fibula, between the two muscles. Lavier (1974) in an illustration locates GB 34 inferior and posterior to the head of the fibula. Lotan (2000) locates GB 34 on the knee, lateral aspect, anterior and distal to the fibula's head, about 1 cun distal (and anterior) to the fibula's head peak, approximately level with 2 cun inferior to the popliteal joint and crease. so (1985) locates GB 34 at the cleft between the proximal ends of the tibia and fibula. Deadman (1998) locates GB 34 below the lateral aspect of the knee; in the tender depression approximately 1 cun anterior and inferior to the head of the fibula. Huang (1993) locates GB 34 one cun below the knee in a depression at the lateral aspect of the leg.

Soulié (1994) locates GB 34 on the lateral, upper part of the lower leg, just at the anterior edge of the round head of the fibula. In the angle between the lower edge of the head of the tibia and the posterior edge of the insertion of the extensor digitorum longus muscle; in a hollow; three FW (Finger Width) below GB 33; six FW above GB 35; one large FW posterior and slightly below ST 36. Masayoshi (1975) locates GB 34 on the upper extremity of the exterior region of the lower leg, medial and inferior to the capitulum. Katsusuke (1983) locates GB 34 on the little toe side of the calf about one sun below the knee. On the little toe side directly below and in front of the head of the fibula.

GB 35 YANG JIAO – YANG CROSSING

⊥ ***0.5 TO 0.7 CUN*** Δ ***3 TO 7***

- ACCUMULATION/Xi Cleft/Gueki Point of the Yang Linking Vessel (Yang Wei Mai)
- 8 EXTRAORDINARY VESSEL/Coalescent Point of Yang Linking Vessel (Yang Wei Mai)

Pos: Position of patient: supine with the leg semi flexed.

Loc: a) On the lateral aspect of the lower leg.
b) Posterior to the posterior border of the fibula.
c) Posterior to and on a level with GB 36.
d) 7 cun proximal to the prominence of the lateral malleolus.

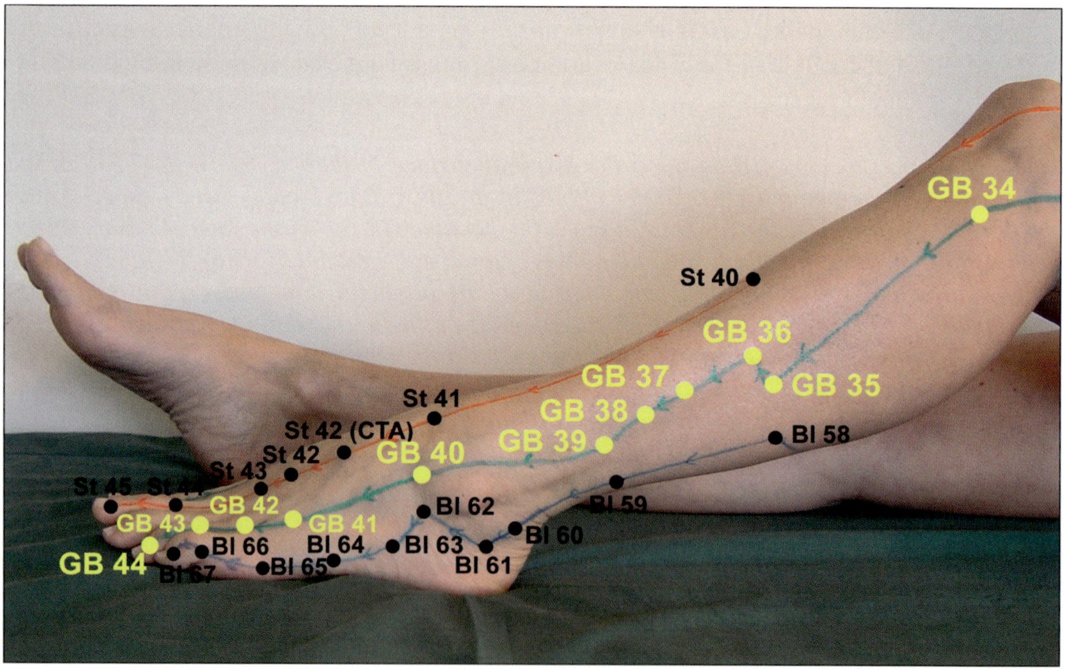

Tip: a) Mark out 7 cun proximal to the prominence of the lateral malleolus. There are 16 cun from the lateral popliteal crease to the prominence of the lateral malleolus.

b) Palpate the anterior border of the fibula either from the knee (from GB 34 – see separate description) or from the anterior border of the lateral malleolus to 7 cun. Make sure the leg is semi flexed to allow the peroneus brevis (fibularis brevis) and peroneus longus (fibularis longus) muscles to become flacid to facilitate palpation.

c) Palpate for GB 36, approximately 7 cun proximal to the prominence of the lateral malleolus, which is anterior to the anterior border of the fibula.

d) At the level of GB 36, palpate posteriorly until you locate the posterior border of the fibula. GB 35 is located posterior to the posterior border of the fibula at 7 cun proximal to the prominence of the lateral malleolus. You should be able to palpate a *men* (depression).

Note: Soulié (1994) locates GB 35 on the lateral part of the lower leg: six large FW (Finger Width) below the round head of the fibula; angle between the anterior edge of the fibula (with the peroneus longus muscle) and the upper edge of a transverse mass, posterior edge of the extensor digitorum longus; in a hollow; six FW below GB 34; two above and posteror to GB 36; two posterior (lateral) to ST 38; at the level of BL 57, between the gastrocnemius muscle. Voisin (1974) locates G 35 on the leg, lateral aspect; 8 fb (finger breadth) above the lateral malleolus, anterior to the border of the fibula.

Wu (1973) locates GB 35 upon the external face of the leg, at seven pouce above the external malleus. Academy (1975) locate GB 35 at 7 cun above the tip of the external malleolus, in the anterior border of the fibula, on the line connecting the tip of the external malleolus with GB 34. Shandong (1982) locate GB 35 at 7 cun above the malleolus lateralis, on the anterior border of the fibula. Worsley (1982) locates VII 35 on the lateral surface of the leg, 7 ACI (Anatomical Chinese Inch) proximal to the prominence of the lateral malleolus, posterior to the edge of the fibula, 0.5 ACI posterior to VII 36.

Lavier (1974) in an illustration has GB 35 located on the Bladder channel at one pouce inferior to Bl 58, between the lateral border of the soleus/gastrocnemius and the posterior border of the peroneus longus muscle, posterior to GB 36, seven pouce proximal to the prominence of the external malleolus. Ellis (1991) locate GB 35 at 7" above the tip of the external malleolus, on the posterior border of the fibula, level with GB 36 and BL 58. So (1985) locates GB 35 at 7 divisions directly above the upper edge of the lateral malleolus in front of the fibula. Masayoshi (1975) locates GB 35 at the centre of the external region of the lower leg, slightly in front of GB 36, between the extensor digitorum longus and the peroneus longus.

GB 36 WAI QIU – OUTER MOUND

⊥ ***0.3 TO 0.5 CUN*** Δ ***3***

- ACCUMULATION/Xi Cleft/Gueki Point

Pos: Position of patient: supine with the leg semi flexed.

Loc:
a) On the lateral aspect of the lower leg.
b) Anterior to the anterior border of the fibula.
c) 7 cun proximal to the prominence of the lateral malleolus.
d) Between the peroneus longus (fibularis longus) and extensor digitorum longus muscles.
e) Anterior to and on a level with GB 35.

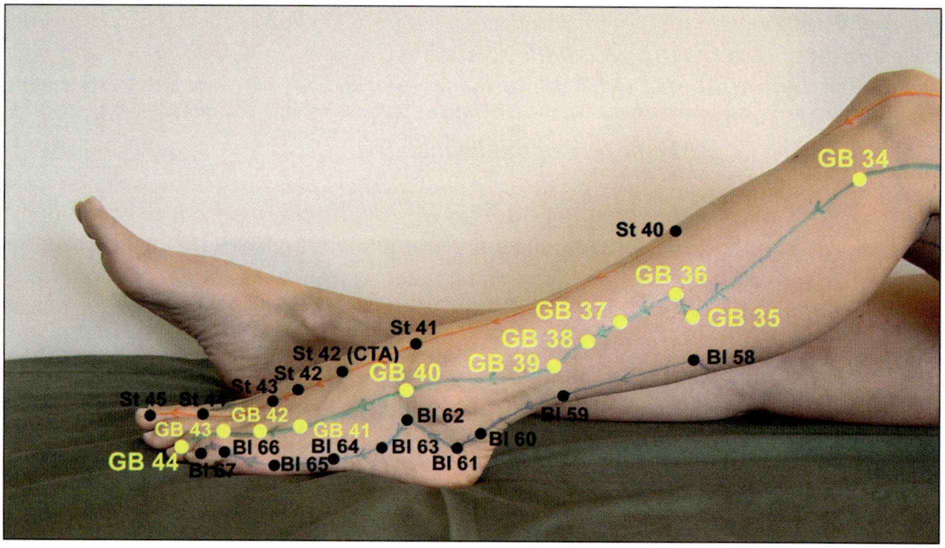

Tip:
a) Mark out 7 cun proximal to the prominence of the lateral malleolus. There are 16 cun from the lateral popliteal crease to the prominence of the lateral malleolus.
b) Palpate the anterior border of the fibula either from the knee (from GB 34 – see separate description) or from the anterior border of the lateral malleolus to the 7 cun measurement.
c) Make sure the leg is semi flexed to allow the peroneus longus (fibularis longus) and extensor digitorum longus muscles to become flacid to facilitate palpation.
d) Everting the foot (raising the lateral side of the foot off the couch) can demonstrate the peroneus longus muscles. To expose the extensor digitorum longus muscle, dorsiflex the foot (so that the heel is the only part of the foot making contact with the couch). The point lies in between the peroneus longus and the extensor digitorum longus muscles.
e) Palpate for GB 36, approximately 7 cun proximal to the prominence of the lateral malleolus, anterior to the anterior border of the fibula.
f) You should be able to palpate a *men* (depression).

Note: Soulié (1994) locates GB 36 on the lateral lower leg: six FW (Finger Width) above the bone of the ankle (external malleolus), at the angle between the anterior edge of the fibula and the upper edge of a bulge curving backwards (groove of the peroneus muscle); on the inferior and anterior edge of the peroneus longus muscle; in a hollow; two FW below and posterior to GB 35; one large FW posterior to and above GB 37; two FW in front of BL 58; three FW posterior and slightly above ST 39. Wu (1973) locates GB 36 upon the anterio-external surface of the leg, before GB 35 at the opposite side of the muscle.

Voisin (1974) locates G 36 on the leg, lateral aspect: same level as G 35 but just behind the posterior border of the fibula. Shanghai (1993) locates GB 36 on the lateral aspect of the leg, 7 cun above the tip of the lateral malleolus, anterior to the fibula, at the level with GB 35, (1 cun anterior to GB 35). Lavier (1974) in an illustration locates GB 36 on the lateral aspect of the lower leg, at seven pouce proximal to the prominence of the lateral malleolus, on the anterior border of the peroneus longus muscle, on a level with and anterior to GB 35. So (1985) locates GB 36 one finger division directly behind GB 35 on the fibula.

Academy (1975) locate GB 36 level and 1 cun posterior to GB 35 and posterior to the border of the fibula. Ellis (1991) locate GB 36 at 7" above the tip of the external malleolus, on the anterior border of the fibula, level with GB 35 and ST 39, between the m. peroneus longus and the m. flexor digitorum longus. Shanghai (1981) locate GB 36 midway between GB 34 and the lateral malleolus, in front of GB 35, at the anterior margin of the fibula. Masayoshi (1975) locates GB 36 on the centre of the exterior region of the lower leg, on the posterior edge of the peroneus longus. Shandong (1982) locate Waiqiu at 7 cun above the malleolus lateralis in the posterior border of the fibula

---

GB 37 GUANG MING – BRIGHT AND CLEAR

⊥ ***0.5 TO 0.7 CUN*** Δ ***5 TO 7***

- JUNCTION/Luo/Connecting/Passage/Lo/Lê
- RE-UNION/Crossing/Meeting Point of the Gall Bladder Channel with the Liver Channel.- Foot Shao Yang Channel with the Foot Jue Yin Channel
- HOST/GUEST COMBINATION – Source Point with the Junction Point of its Paired Official/Organ Therefore GB 37 is combined with Liv 3

Pos: Position of patient: supine with the leg semi flexed.

Loc: a) On the lateral aspect of the lower leg.
b) Anterior to the anterior border of the fibula.
c) 5 cun proximal to the prominence of the lateral malleolus.
d) Between the peroneus brevis (fibularis brevis) and extensor digitorum longus muscles.

Tip:
a) Mark out 5 cun proximal to the prominence of the lateral malleolus. There are 16 cun from the lateral popliteal crease to the prominence of the lateral malleolus.
b) Palpate the anterior border of the fibula either from the knee (from GB 34 – see separate description) or from the anterior border of the lateral malleolus to the 5 cun measurement.
c) Palpate the anterior border of the fibula either from the knee (from GB 34 – see separate description) or from the anterior border of the lateral malleolus to 7 cun. Make sure the leg is semi flexed to allow the peroneus brevis (fibularis brevis) and extensor digitorum longus muscles to become flacid to facilitate palpation.
d) Everting the foot (raising the lateral side of the foot off the couch) can demonstrate the peroneus longus muscles. To expose the extensor digitorum longus muscle, dorsiflex the foot (so that the heel is the only part of the foot making contact with the couch). The point lies in between the peroneus longus and the extensor digitorum longus muscles.
e) Palpate for GB 37, approximately 5 cun proximal to the prominence of the lateral malleolus, anterior to the anterior border of the fibula.
f) You should be able to palpate a *men* (depression).

Note: Wu (1973) locates GB 37 upon the external surface of the leg, at five pouce above the external malleus. Lavier (1974) in an illustration locates GB 37 on the lateral aspect of the lower leg, at five pouce proximal to the prominence of the lateral malleolus, on the anterior border of the peroneus longus muscle. Voisin (1974) locates G 37 on the leg, lateral aspect: 6 fb (finger breadth) above the lateral malleolus, on the anterior border of the fibula.

Soulié (1994) locates GB 37 on the lateral lower leg: five FW (Finger Width) above the ankle bone (lateral malleolus); in the angle between the anterior edge of the fibula (with peroneus longus muscle), just at a small bony eminence, and the upper edge of a transverse mass (insertion of the peroneus anterior muscle); on the posterior edge of the extensor digitoum longus muscle; one large FW under GB 36; one FW above GB 38; two FW posterior to ST 40; one large FW anterior to BL 59. Ellis (1991) locate GB 37 at 5.0" above the tip of the external malleolus, on the anterior border of the fibula; between the m. peroneus longus and the m. flexor digitorum longus.

Lawson-Wood (1973) locates VII 37 on the antero-external aspect of the leg, 6cm below the middle of a line drawn from the anterior tuberosity of the tibial plateau to the external malleolus. Eachou (1995) locates GB 37 on the lateral side of the leg, on the anterior margin of the fibula 5 inches above the lateral malleolus of the fibula and 2 inches below GB 36. Yang (1982) locates GB 37 at 5 cun above the tip of the external malleolus, on the posterior border of the fibula. Masayoshi (1975) locates GB 37 at 5 sun above the lateral malleolus.

GB 38 YNG FU – YANG SUPPORT

⊥ ***0.5 TO 0.7 CUN*** **Δ** ***3 TO 15***

- FIRE
- SEDATION/Reducing/Dispersing
- CHILD
- JING – RIVER/Shu – Transporting/Antique

Pos: Position of patient: supine with the leg semi flexed.

Loc: a) On the lateral aspect of the lower leg.
b) Anterior to the anterior border of the fibula.
c) 4 cun proximal to the prominence of the lateral malleolus.
d) Between the peroneus brevis (fibularis brevis) and extensor digitorum longus muscles.

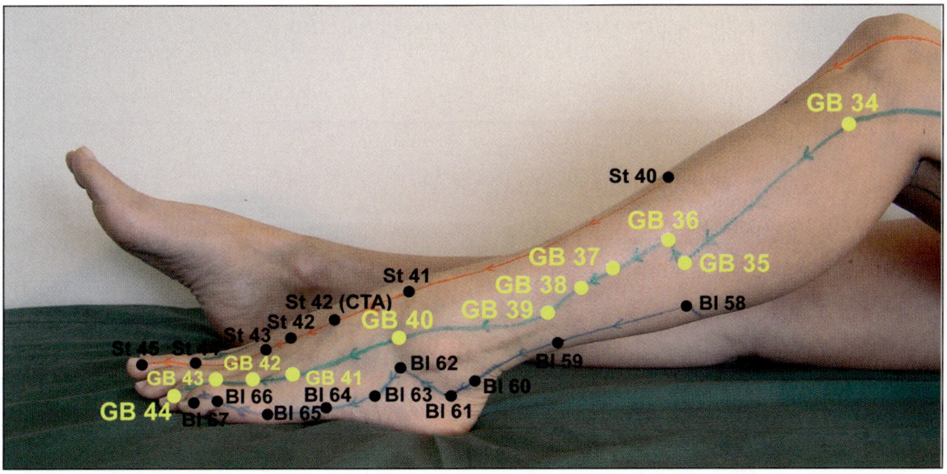

Tip: a) Mark out 4 cun proximal to the prominence of the lateral malleolus. There are 16 cun from the lateral popliteal crease to the prominence of the lateral malleolus.
b) Palpate the anterior border of the fibula either from the knee (from GB 34 – see separate description) or from the anterior border of the lateral malleolus to the 4 cun measurement. c) Palpate the anterior border of the fibula either from the knee (from GB 34 – see separate description) or from the anterior border of the lateral malleolus to 4 cun. Make sure the leg is semi flexed to allow the peroneus brevis (fibularis brevis) and extensor digitorum longus muscles to become flacid to facilitate palpation.
d) Everting the foot (raising the lateral side of the foot off the couch) can demonstrate the peroneus longus muscles. To expose the extensor digitorum longus muscle, dorsiflex the foot (so that the heel is the only part of the foot making contact with the couch). The point lies in between the peroneus longus and the extensor digitorum longus muscles.
e) Palpate for GB 38, approximately 4 cun proximal to the prominence of the lateral malleolus, anterior to the anterior border of the fibula.
f) You should be able to palpate a *men* (depression).

Note: Soulié (1994) locates GB 38 on the lateral part of the lower leg: four FW (Finger Width) above the ankle bone (external malleolus); just at the anterior edge of the fibula; in the angle between the anterior edge of the upper prominence of a notch in the bone (the groove of the peroneus muscle) and the upper edge of a transverse mass; posterior to the extensor digitorum longus and the peroneus anterior; one FW below GB 37; two FW above GB 39. Voisin (1974) locates G 38 on the leg, lateral aspect: 5 fb (finger breadth) above the lateral malleolus, on the anterior border of the fibula. Lavier (1974) in an illustration locates GB 38 on the lateral aspect of the lower leg, at four pouce proximal to the prominence of the lateral malleolus, on the anterior border of the peroneus longus muscle.

Wu (1973) locates GB 38 upon the external surface of the leg, at four pouce above the external malleus. Lawson-Wood (1973) locates VII 38 on the antero-external aspect of the leg, 10cm above the external malleolus, on the line drawn from the external malleolus to the external border of the anterior tuberosity of the tibia. So (1985) locates GB 38 at four divisions proximal to the upper edge of the lateral malleolus, between the tibia and fibula. Huang (1993) locates GB 38 at four cun above the lateral malleolus, at the end of the severed bone, three fen anterior to the assisting bone, seven cun proximal to Hill Ruins (GB 40). Masayoshi (1975) locates GB 38 on the exterior region of the lower leg, directly on the peroneum, 4 sun above the lateral malleolus.

GB 39 XUAN ZHONG – HANGING CUP

⊥ ***0.3 TO 0.5 CUN*** Δ ***3 TO 5***

- INFLUENTIAL/Hui – Meeting/Gathering/Assembling Point of Marrow
- RE-UNION/Crossing/Meeting Point of the Three Yang (Leg) Channels: Gall Bladder, Bladder and Stomach Channels – Foot Shao Yang, Foot Tai Yang and Foot Yang Ming Channels
- ONE OF THE HEAVENLY STAR POINTS OF MA DAN-YANG (the others are: Lu 7, LI 4, LI 11, St 36, St 44, Bl 40, Bl 57, Bl 60, Ht 5, GB 34, and Liv 3)

Pos: Position of patient: supine with the leg semi flexed.

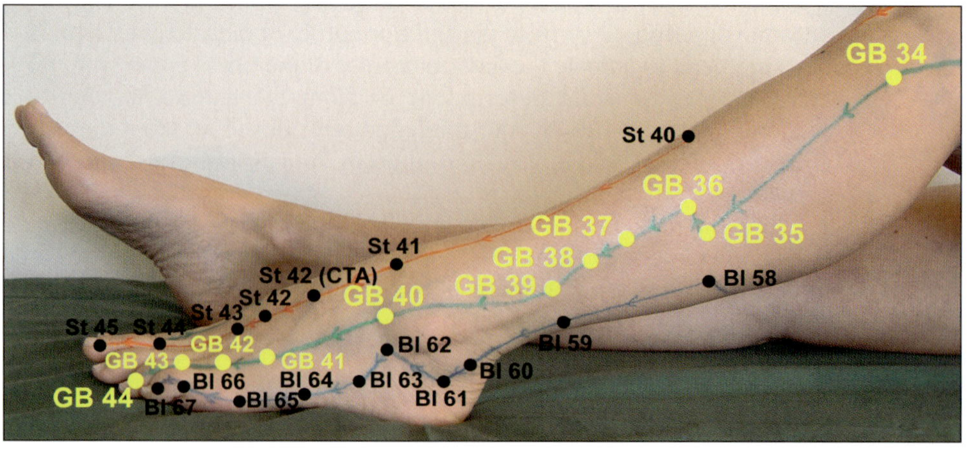

Loc: a) On the lateral aspect of the lower leg.
b) On the posterior border of the fibula.
c) Between the posterior border of the fibula and the anterior border of the tendons of the peroneus brevis (fibularis brevis) and peroneus longus (fibularis longus) muscle.
c) 3 cun proximal to the prominence of the lateral malleolus.

Tip: a) Mark out 3 cun proximal to the prominence of the lateral malleolus. There are 16 cun from the lateral popliteal crease to the prominence of the lateral malleolus.
b) Palpate tightly against the posterior border of the fibula from the posterior border of the lateral malleolus to 3 cun.
c) Make sure the leg is semi flexed to allow the tendons of the peroneus longus and peroneus brevis muscles to become flacid, facilitating palpation of the posterior border of the fibula. Everting the foot (raising the lateral side of the foot off the couch) can demonstrate the peroneus longus (fibularis longus) and peroneus brevis (fibularis brveis) muscles. The point lies in between the tendons of the peroneus brevis and peroneus longus muscle and the posterior border of the fibula.
d) GB 39 is located on the bone as the tendons of the peroneus longus and peroneus brevis muscles begin to cover the fibula, hence making the point move anteriorly on to the bone. As you palpate anteriorly it can be difficult palpating for the fibula as it is covered by these two muscles.
e) The identification of the tendons of the peroneus brevis and peroneus longus muscles can cause difficulties. The tendon of the peroneus brevis muscle is more anterior and closer to the fibula than the tendon of the peroneus longus muscle, although this may vary on people.
f) The description may state that the point lies between the anterior border of the tendon of the peroneus brevis muscle and the posterior border of the fibula.
g) Palpate for GB 39, approximately 3 cun proximal to the prominence of the lateral malleolus.

Note: Wu (1973) locates GB 39 upon the external surface of the leg, at three pouce above the external malleus. Lavier (1974) in an illustration locates GB 39 on the lateral aspect of the lower leg, at three pouce proximal to the prominence of the lateral malleolus, on the anterior border of the peroneus longus muscle. Voisin (1974) locates G 39 on the leg, lateral aspect: 4 fb (finger breadth) above the lateral malleolus, on the anterior border of the fibula.

Shanghai (1993) locate GB 39 on the lateral aspect of the leg,3 cun above the tip of the lateral malleolus, anterior to the fibula. Worsley (1982) locates VII 39 on the lateral surface of the leg, 3 ACI proximal to the prominence of the lateral malleolus. With the body supine and the knee semiflexed, the point lies anterior to the fibula. Shandong (1982) locate Xuanzhong at 3 cun above the top of the malleolus lateralis, on the anterior border of the fibula.

Soulié (1994) locates GB 39 on the lateral part of the leg: two FW (Finger Width) above the ankle bone (external malleolus); in the angle between the anterior edge of the peroneus muscle and the inferior edge of a transverse mass. Between the bone and the peroneus brevis muscle, which is just posterior to the extensor digitorum longus; in a hollow; two FW under GB 38; three large FW above GB 40. So (1985) locates GB 39 at three divisions proximal to the lateral malleolus; 1/4 division lateral from the vertical line drawn through GB 38. Masayoshi (1975) locates GB 39 about 3 sun above the lateral malleolus directly on the peroneum.

GB 40 is on the anterior aspect of the flexure of the ankle.

GB 40 QIU XU – WILDERNESS MOUND

⊥ ***0.3 TO 0.5 CUN*** Δ ***3 TO 5***

- SOURCE/Yuan/Regulator/Primary
- ORIGINAL (for specific symptoms)
- HOST/GUEST COMBINATION – Source Point with the Junction Point of its Paired Official/Organ Therefore GB 40 is combined with Liv 5

Pos: Position of patient: supine.

Loc: a) On the lateral aspect of the ankle.
b) Anterior and inferior to the lateral malleolus.
c) Lateral to the extensor digitorum longus muscle.
d) In a hollow between the lateral malleolus and the tendon of the extensor digitorum longus muscle.

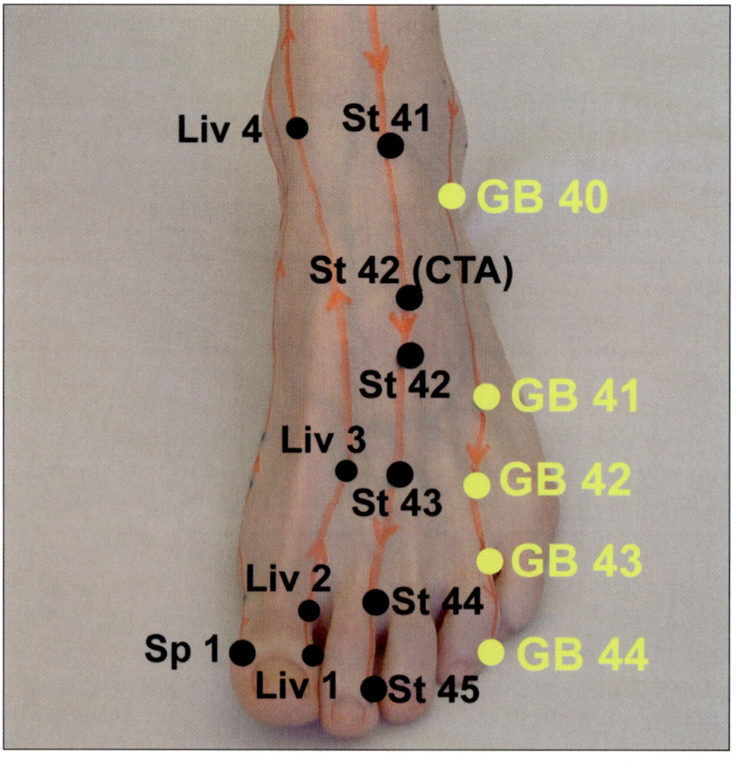

Tip: a) The point lies in the deepest part of a hollow formed by the lateral malleolus and the lateral border of the tendon of the extensor digitorum longus muscle.

b) To demonstrate the tendon of the extensor digitorum longus muscle, dorsiflex the foot (so that the heel is the only part of the foot making contact with the couch) and evert the foot (raising the lateral side of the foot off the couch). The tendon can be on or slightly posterior to the prominence of the lateral malleolus.

c) With your finger on the anterior border of the lateral malleolus approximately level with the prominence of the malleolus, palpate along the border towards the foot until you feel a resistance and you cannot palpate further around the malleolus. You should be approximately anterior and inferior to the lateral malleolus.

d) Palpate for the deepest part of the hollow where your finger met with resistance. The point should be in the deepest part, in the ankle joint (the gap between the bones of the foot and the fibula).

e) Have the foot in a relaxed position and place your two index fingers anterior and inferior to the lateral and medial malleoli respectively. Wiggle the foot from side to side and the fingers should fall in to two hollows. Your fingers would look like a bolt going straight through from one side to the other. The medial side is more proximal than the lateral side The two points in these hollows are GB 40 (lateral surface hollow) and Sp 5 (medial surface hollow).

Note: Wu (1973) locates GB 40 upon the foot, at one pouce before and below the external malleus. Voisin (1974) locates G 40 on the foot: 1 fb (finger breadth) in front and below the lateral malleolus, centre of the calcaneocuboid joint. Shandong (1982) locate Qiuxu anterior and inferior to the malleolus lateralis, in the depression on the tendon of the m. extensor digitorum longus. Eachou (1995) locates GB 40 on the dorsum of the foot, in the fossa anterior and inferior to the lateral malleolus of the fibula, and at the midpoint between ST 41 and the trochlear tubercle of the calcaneus.

Lawson-Wood (1973) locates VII 40 on the antero-external aspect of the foot (instep) in the centre of the calcaneo-cuboid articulation. So (1985) locates GB 40 at 1/2 division anterior to the anterior edge of the lateral malleolus, in the hollow posterior to the tendon. Masayoshi (1975) locates GB 40 on the talofibular joint, on lower anterior part of the lateral malleolus. Huang (1993) locates GB 40 inferior and a little anterior to the lateral malleolus in a depression three cun proximal to Overlooking Tears (GB 41).

GB 41 ZU LIN QI – FOOT ABOVE TEARS

⊥ ***0.3 CUN*** Δ ***3***

- WOOD
- EXIT
- HORARY from 11 p.m. to 1 a.m.
- SEASONAL HORARY – Spring
- SHU – STREAM/Shu – Transporting/Antique
- 8 EXTRAORDINARY CHANNELS CONFLUENT/8 Extraordinary Meridians Confluent/8 Extraordinary Vessels Opening/Master Point of the Girdle Vessel (Dai Mai)
- 8 EXTRAORDINARY VESSEL/Coupled Point of the Yang Linking Vessel (Yang Wei Mai)
- RE-UNION/Crossing/Meeting Point of the Gall Bladder Channel with the Liver Channel – Foot Shao Yang Channel with the Foot Jue Yin Channel

Pos: Position of patient: supine.

Loc: a) On the dorsum of the foot.
b) In the angle just distal to the junction of the fourth and fifth metatarsal bones.
c) Just distal and lateral to the flare of the base of the fourth metatarsal bone.
d) Lateral to the border of the fourth slip of the tendon of the extensor digitorum longus muscle.

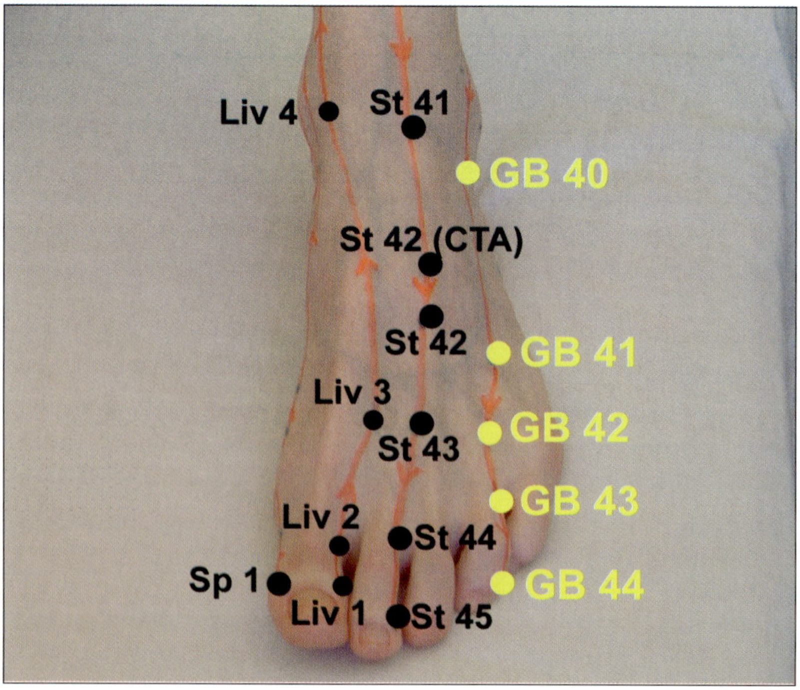

Tip: a) Run your finger with the flow of the channel from GB 40, towards the lateral aspect of the base of the fourth metatarsal bone until you can palpate a soft area just distal to the junction of the flares of the bases between the fourth and fifth metatarsals.

b) If you tried to palpate too distally you will feel resistance from the medial border of the fifth metatarsal and the lateral border of the fourth slip of the tendon of the extensor digitorum longus muscle. The fourth slip crosses over the space between the fourth and fifth metatarsals and attaches to the fifth digit.

c) To demonstrate the tendon of the extensor digitorum longus muscle, dorsiflex the foot, especially the fifth digit (so that the heel is the only part of the foot making contact with the couch).

d) The point can be palpated in a *men* (depression) in the angle just distal to the bases of the fourth and fifth metatarsals and just lateral to the tendon of the extensor digitorum longus muscle.

e) Another method to locate GB 41 is to palpate proximally from the web margin between the fourth and fifth metatarsal bones towards the flares of their bases. Locate the fourth slip of the tendon of the extensor digitorum longus muscle and palpate laterally until you feel a soft area between the two metatarsals.

f) Palpate for the point in the angle just distal to the junction of the fourth and fifth metatarsals and just distal to the base of the fourth metatarsal.

g) If you cannot feel the angle at the junction of the fourth and fifth metatarsals, palpate against the channel by feeling for the anatomy of the fourth and fifth metatarsophalangeal joints. To identify these, press your fingers against the plantar surface of the foot level with the metatarsophalangeal joints, to visualise the fourth and fifth metatarsal bones on the dorsum surface of the foot.

h) Run your fingers proximally from the metatarsophalangeal joints palpating over the fourth slip of the tendon until you feel the flare at the bases of the fourth and fifth metatarsals. The point lies in a hollow just distal to the flare at the base of the fourth metatarsal.

i) Another method to locate the point is to visualise the lateral aspect of the foot. You should see and feel a bony prominence which is the tuberosity of the fifth metatarsal (the tuberosity is the base of the fifth metatarsal).

j) Run your finger medially from the tuberosity of the fifth metatarsal until you feel a small space between the fourth and fifth metatarsal. GB 41 is located in this space just distal to flare of the 4th metatarsal.

Note: Gray's (1978) The tendon of the extensor digitorum longus divides in to four slips which run forward on the dorsum of the foot; Soulié (1994) locates GB 41 on the dorsum of the foot, between the fourth and fifth metatarsal bones (long bones of the fourth and fifth toes); at the mid-length of the bones; on the lateral edge of the tendon coming obliquely from the fifth toe (extensor digitorum longus muscle); on the medial edge (towards the toe) of the fourth metatarsal with the dorsal tendon (extensor digitorum brevis; in a hollow; on the edge of a transverse mass; four FW (Finger Width) under GB 40; one FW posterior to GB 42; one FW lateral to ST 42; three FW medial to BL 63. Shandong (1982) locate Foot-Linqi in the depression anterior to the junction of the ossa metatarsalia IV and V.

Li (1991) locates GB 41 in the depression distal to the junction of the 4th and 5th metatarsal bones, 1.5 cun above GB 43, lateral to the tendon of the m. extensor distorum. Cheng (1987) locates G 41 in the depression distal to the junction of the fourth and fifth metatarsal bones, on the lateral side of the tendon of m. extensor digiti minimi of the foot. Shanghai (1993) locate GB 41 on the lateral aspect of the dorsum of the foot, posterior to the 4th metatarsophalageal joint, in the depression lateral to the tendon of the extensor muscle of the little toe. Qiu 91996) locates GB 41 in the depression distal to the junction of the 4th and 5th metatarsal bones, on the lateral side of the tendon of the m. extensor digiti minimi of the foot.

Legge (1999) locates GB 41 in the depression just distal to the 4th and 5th tarso-metatarsal joints. So (1985) locates GB 41 one division proximal to the joint, between the 4th and 5th metatarsal bones. Yang (1982) locates GB 41 posterior to the tendon of the m. extensor digiti minimi pedis, in front of the junction of the 4th and 5th metatarsal bones. Ellis (1991) locate GB 41 in the depression distal to the junction of the 4th and 5th metatarsal bones, on the lateral side of the tendon of the short extensor muscle of the small toe (m. extensor digitorum brevis). Huang (1993) locates GB 41 proximal to the base joint of the phalanx in a depression one cun and five fen from Pinched Ravine (GB 43)

GB 42 DI WU HUI – EARTH FIVE MEETINGS

⊥ ***0.3 CUN*** Δ ***1 TO 3***

Pos: Position of patient: supine.

Loc: a) On the dorsum of the foot.
b) Between the fourth and fifth metatarsal bones.
c) Proximal to the fourth metatarso-phalangeal joint.
d) Just proximal to the flare of the head of the fourth metatarsal bone.
e) Medial to the fourth slip of the tendon of the extensor digitorum longus muscle.

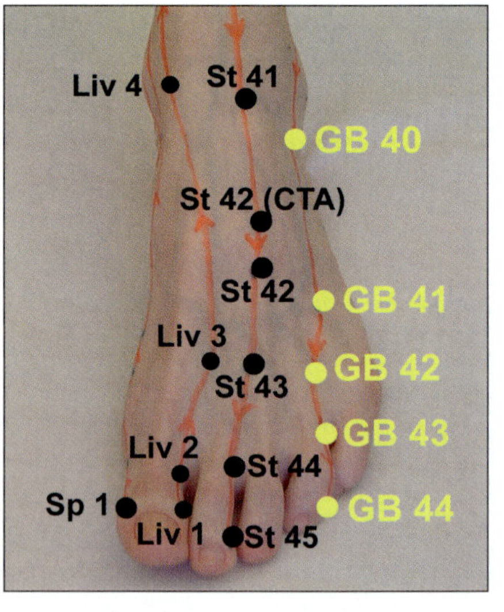

Tip: a) The point can be palpated in a *men* (depression) just proximal to the flare of the head of the fourth metatarsal and medial to the tendon of the extensor digitorum longus muscle.
b) Palpate proximally from the web margin between the fourth and fifth metatarsals towards the flare of the heads of the fourth and fifth metatarsals.
c) You should be able to feel the tendon of the extensor digitorum longus muscle, but if you palpate over this you have palpated too proximally. Before the tendon you should be able to feel a soft area between the heads of the two metatarsals. In the soft area, palpate for the point which is proximal to the flare of the head of the fourth metatarsal and medial to the fourth slip of the tendon of the extensor digitorum longus muscle, which attaches to the fifth digit.

d) If you cannot feel the metatarsophalangeal joint of the fourth metatarsal, press your fingers against the plantar surface of the foot level with the metatarsophalangeal joints, to visualise the fourth and fifth metatarsals on the dorsum surface of the foot.
e) Run your finger proximally from the fourth metatarsophalangeal joint until you feel the bone flare just proximal to the head of the fourth metatarsal.
f) Palpate to accurately locate GB 42.

Note: Gray's (1978) The tendon of the extensor digitorum longus divides in to four slips which run forward on the dorsum of the foot; Eachou (1995) locates GB 42 1.5 inches proximal to the toe web, in the fossa between the fourth and fifth metatarsals, on the medial side of the tendon of the extensor digitorum brevis. Soulié (1994) locates GB 42 on the dorsal and lateral part of the foot: one FW (Finger Width) posterior to the joint of the fourth toe (metatarsophalangeal joint); in the angle between the lateral edge of the body of the fourth metatarsal and the anterior edge of the oblique tendon (extensor of the fifth toe); in a hollow; one FW in front of GB 41; one FW posterior to GB 43; two FW medial to BL 66; two FW lateral to ST 44.

Cheng (1987) locates GB 42 between the fourth and fifth metatarsal bones, on the medial side of the tendon of the m. extensor digiti minimi of the foot. Shanghai (1993) locate GB 42 on the lateral aspect of the dorsum of the foot, between the 4th and 5th metatarsal bones, on the medial side of the tendon of the extensor muscle of the little toe, 0.5 cun below GB 41 and 1 cun above GB 43. Wu (1973) locates GB 42 upon the dorsal surface of the foot, behind the metatarsal-phalangeal articulation of the fourth toe, on the side toward the fifth toe. Qiu (1996) locates GB 42 between the 4th and 5th metatarsal bones, on the medial side of the tendon of the m. extensor digiti minimi of the foot.

Legge (1999) locates GB 42 between the 4th and 5th metatarsal bones, proximal to the metatarso-phalangeal joints, on the medial side of the tendon of the m. extensor digiti minimi of the foot. So (1985) locates GB 42 at 1/2 division proximal to the joint between the 4th and 5th metatarsals. Ellis (1991) locate GB 42 between the 4th and 5th metatarsal bones, on the medial side of the tendon of the short extensor muscle of the small toe (m. extensor digitorum brevis). Academy (1975) locate GB 42 on the cleft between the 4th and 5th metatarsal bones, 0.5 cun anterior to GB 41.

Jayasuriya (1982) locates GB 42 at 1.0 cun proximal to GB 43. Shanghai (1981) locate GB 42 between the 4th and 5th metatarsal bones, 1 unit above GB 43. Shandong (1982) locate Diwuhui between the ossa metatarsalia IV and V, 0.5 cun anterior to Pt. Foot-linqi (GB 41). Li (1991) locates GB 42 between the 4th and the 5th metatarsal bones, posterior to the metatarsodigital joints and 1 cun above GB 43.

GB 43 XIA XI – VALIANT STREAM

⊥ ***0.3 CUN*** Δ ***3***

- WATER
- TONIFICATION/Reinforcing
- MOTHER
- YING – SPRING/Shu – Transporting/Antique

Pos: Position of patient: supine.

Loc: a) On the dorsum of the foot.
b) Between the fourth and fifth digits.
c) Distal to the metatarso-phalangeal joint of the fourth digit.
d) Just distal to the flare of the base of the proximal phalanx of the fourth digit.
e) Proximal to the web margin (between the fourth and fifth digits).

Tip: a) To help demonstrate the metatarsophalangeal joint, push the pads of your fingers gently in to the plantar surface of the foot directly underneath the base of the fourth digit. You should be able to feel the metatarsophalangeal (knuckle) joint on the dorsal surface of the foot as the bones have been pushed upwards and the tendons are more relaxed.
b) Run your finger from the proximal lateral border of the fourth metatarsophalangeal joint with the flow of the channel (GB 42) towards the proximal phalanx of the fourth digit.
c) Palpate distally over the fourth metatarsophalangeal joint to the distal edge of the flare (distal to the base of the proximal phalanx of the fourth digit).
d) Palpation will accurately locate GB 43.

Note: Lawson-Wood (1973) locates VII 43 on the dorsum of the foot, lateral to the base of the fourth toe. Voisin (1974) locates G 43 on the MTP joint 4: lateral to it. Wu (1973) locates GB 43 upon the dorsal surface of the foot, in front of the metatarsal-phalangeal articulation of the fourth toe; on the side toward the fifth toe. Academy (1975) locate GB 43 on the cleft between the 4th and 5th metatarsal bones, 0.5 cun proximal to the margin of the web.

Eachou (1995) locates GB 43 on the dorsum of the foot, in the fossa between the fourth and fifth proximal phalanges at the midpoint of the toe web. Soulié (1994) locates GB 43 on the dorsum of the foot, just behind the joint at the base of the fourth and fifth toes; at the lateral angle of the head and body of the fourth metatarsal bone of the fourth toe; between the bone and artery, vein and nerve; in a hollow; one FW (Finger Width) in front of GB 42. So (1985) locates GB 43 between the 4th and 5th metatarsals between the joint and the web. Shanghai (1981) locate GB 43 at 0.5 unit posterior to the web between the 4th and 5th toes. Lotan (2000) locates GB 43 between the 4th and 5th toes, midway between the web margin and the metatarsophalangeal joint.

GB 44 ZU QIAO YIN – FOOT HOLE YIN

⊥ ***0.1 CUN*** Δ ***3 TO 5***

- METAL
- JING – WELL/Shu – Transporting/Antique

Pos: Position of patient: supine.

Loc: a) On the foot.
b) The lateral nail point of the fourth digit.
c) Approximately 0.1 cun proximal to the corner of the nail.
d) Just distal to the flare of the distal phalanx.

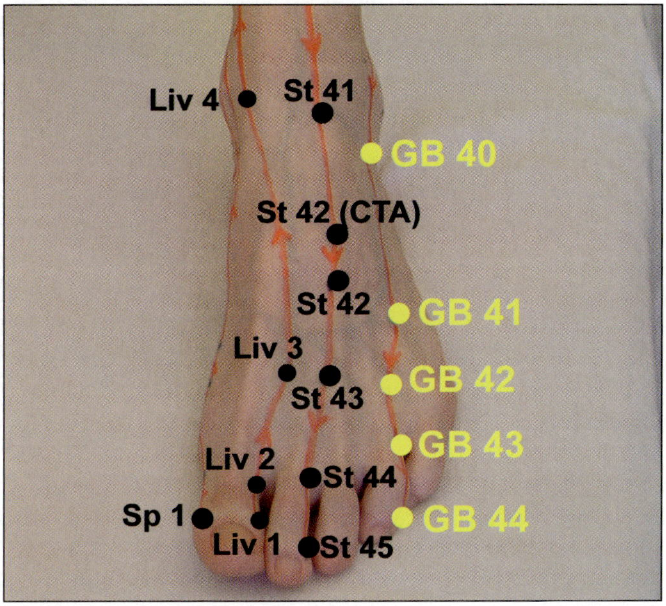

Tip: a) The point is level with the nail bed (where the nail attaches to the skin) rather than the cuticle.
b) Draw a horizontal line across the nail bed.
c) Draw a vertical line from the lateral border of the nail towards the nail bed.
d) The lines drawn from b) and c) (vertical and horizontal) form an intersection. This is approximately where the point is located.

Note: Ellis (1991) in a Classical description locates GB 44 on the outer side of the toe next to the little toe, the width of a Chinese leek leaf away from the corner of the nail (The Great Compendium). Huang (1993) locates GB 44 at the tip of the toe next to the small one, the distance of a leek leaf from the corner of the nail.

REFERENCES FOR THE GALL BLADDER CHANNEL

Note that the following numbers in brackets are the individual author's numbering, eg. Soulié (1994) GB 15 (GB 11), GB 11 is Soulié's numbering for our GB 15.

Soulié De Morant, George. 1994 Chinese Acupuncture – GB 1: 477; GB 2: 478; GB 3: 478; GB 4: 479; GB 5: 479; GB 6: 480; GB 7: 480; GB 8: 481; GB 9 (GB 15): 484; GB 10 (GB 16): 484; GB 11 (GB 18): 485; GB 12 (GB 17): 484; GB 13 (GB 9): 481; GB 14 (GB 10): 482; GB 15 (GB 11): 482; GB 16 (GB12): 482; GB 17 (GB 13): 483; GB 18 (GB 14): 483; GB 19: 485/486; GB 20: 486; GB 21: 487; GB 22: 487; GB 23: 488; GB 24: 488; GB 25: 489; GB 26: 489; GB 27: 490; GB 28 (GB 30): 491; GB 29 (GB 28): 490: 490; GB 30 (GB 29): 491; GB 31: 491/492; GB 32: 492; GB 33: 492; GB 34: 493; GB 35: 493; GB 36: 494; GB 37: 494; GB 38: 495; GB 39: 495; GB 41: 496/497

Voisin, Dr. H 1974 Essentials of Acupuncture – G 1: 60; G 2: 60; G 3: 60; G 4: 60; G 5: 60; G 6: 60; G 7: 60; G 8: 60; G 9: 60; GB 10 (G 15): 60; GB 11 (G 16): 60; GB 12 (G 18): 60; GB 13: (G 11): 60; GB 14 (G 10): 60; GB 15 (Illustration of the Gall Bladder Channel): 61; GB 16 (G 12): 60; GB 17: (G 13): 60; GB 18 (G 14): 60; G 19: 60; G 20: 60; G 21: 60; G 22: 62; G 23: 62; GB 24: 62; GB 26: 62; G 27: 62; G 28: 62; G 29: 62; G 30: 62; G 32: 62; G 33: 62; G 35: 62; G 36: 62; G 37: 62; G 38: 62; G 39: 62; G 43: 64

Worsley, J R 1982 Traditional Chinese Acupuncture Volume 1 – Meridians and Points – VII 2: 147; VII 4: 147; VII 5: 147; VII 6: 147; VII 7: 149; VII 10: 149; VII 11: 149; VII 12: 151; VII 14: 151; VII 15: 151; VII 17: 153; VII 18: 153; VII 20: 153; VII 21: 153; VII 23: 155; VII 24: 155; VII 27: 157; VII 28: 157; VII 30: 157; VII 31: 159; VII 32: 159; VII 33: 159; VII 35: 159; VII 39: 161

So, James Tin Yau (Dr) 1985 The Book of Acupuncture Points – GB 2: 21; GB 3: 224; GB 4: 224; GB 5: 225; GB 6: 225; GB 7: 226; GB 8: 226; GB 10: 227; GB 11: 227; GB 12: 228; GB 13: 16; GB 14: 25; GB 19: 229; GB 20: 19; GB 21: 71; GB 22: 229; GB 23: 230; GB 26: 49; GB 27: 231; GB 28: 232; GB 29: 232; GB 30: 161; GB 32: 232; GB 33: 162; GB 34: 163; GB 35: 233; GB 36: 233; GB 38: 163; GB 39: 164; GB 40: 164; GB 41: 234; GB 42: 235; GB 43: 235

Masayoshi Hyodo 1975 Ryodoraku Acupuncture – GB 2: 60; GB 4: 59; GB 5: 59; GB 6: 59; GB 7: 59; GB 10: 59; GB 11: 59; GB 12: 59; GB 13: 60; GB 16: 59; GB 17: 59; GB 18: 59; GB 19: 59; GB 23: 60; GB 24: 60; GB 26: 60; GB 27: 60; GB 28: 60; GB 29: 60; GB 30: 61; GB 31: 61; GB 32: 61; GB 33: 61; GB 34: 61; GB 35: 61; GB 36: 61; GB 37: 62; GB 38: 62; GB 39: 62; GB 40: 62

Wu, Wei-P'ing 1973 Chinese Acupuncture – GB 2: 110; GB 3: 110; GB 4: 110; GB 5: 111; GB 6: 111; GB 7: 111; GB 9: 111; GB 10: 111; GB 11: 112; GB 12: 112; GB 13: 112; GB 15: 112; GB 16: 113; GB 17: 113; GB 18: 113; GB 19: 113; GB 20: 113; GB 21: 113; GB 24: 114; GB 27: 114; GB 28: 115; GB 29: 115; GB 30: 115; GB 31: 115; GB 32: 115; GB 33: 115; GB 34: 116; GB 35: 116; GB 36: 116; GB 37: 116; GB 38: 116; GB 39: 116; GB 40: 117; GB 42: 117; GB 43: 117

Lotan, Alon 2000 Acupoint Location Guide – GB 3: 129; GB 7: 131; GB 14: 133; GB 21: 137; GB 22: 139; GB 23: 139; GB 27: 141; GB 28: 141; GB 33: 145; GB 34: 147; GB 43: 149

Academy of Traditional Chinese Medicine, The. 1975 – Outline of Chinese Acupuncture, An. – GB 4: 172; GB 5: 172; GB 6: 175; GB 7: 175; GB 10: 175; GB 11: 175; GB 13: 176; GB 16: 176; GB 17: 176; GB 18: 176; GB 26: 179; GB 27: 179; GB 28: 179; GB 31: 181; GB 35: 182; GB 36: 162; GB 42: 184; GB 43: 184

Eachou Chen 1995 Cross-sectional Anatomy of Acupoints – GB 4: 108; GB 7: 128; GB 9: 109; GB 10: 111; GB 11: 112; GB 12: 113; GB 19: 111; GB 20: 221; GB 22: 206; GB 23: 206; GB 27: 208; GB 28: 208; GB 31: 56; GB 33: 58; GB 37: 79; GB 40: 89; GB 42: 94; GB 43: 95

Lavier, Dr. J 1974 Points of Chinese Acupuncture – GB 4: 73; GB 5: 73; GB 6: 73; GB 7: 73 & 75; GB 8: 75; GB 9: 75; GB 10: 75; GB 11: 75; GB 21: 65; GB 24: 51; GB 27: 55; GB 28: 55; GB 29: 55; GB 31: 29; GB 32: 29; GB 33: 29; GB 34: 37; GB 35: 37; GB 36: 37; GB 37: 37; GB 38: 37; GB 39: 37

Shandong Medical College and Shandong College of Traditional Chinese Medicine 1982 Anatomical Atlas of Chinese Acupuncture Point – Hanyan (GB 4): 50; Xuanli (GB 6): 50; Head-Qiaoyin (GB 11): 51; Muchuang (GB 16): 51; Zhengying (GB 17): 51; Chengling (GB 18): 51; Naokong (GB 19): 51; Zhejin (GB 23): 51; Weidao (GB 28): 52; Yangjiao(GB 35): 52; Waiqiu (GB 36): 52; Xuanzhong (GB 39): 53; Qiuxu (GB 40): 53l; Foot-Linqi (GB 41): 53; Diwuhui (GB 42): 53

Legge, David 1999 Acupuncture Points and Meridians – GB 6: 79; GB 12: 80; GB 20: 80; GB 21: 80; GB 22: 80; GB 23: 81; GB 33: 82; GB 41: 82; GB 42: 83

Jayasuriya, Anton 1982 Clinical Acupuncture – GB 6: 402; GB 10: 402; GB 11: 402; GB 12: 402; GB 20: 403; GB 21: 403; GB 22: 403; GB 23: 403; GB 26: 403; GB 31: 403; GB 33: 404; GB 42: 404; GB 43: 404

Ellis, Wiseman and Boss. 1991 Fundamentals of Chinese Acupuncture – GB 6: 303; GB 21: 312; GB 23: 313; GB 33: 319; GB 35: 320; GB 36: 321; GB 37: 321; GB 41: 324; GB 42: 325; GB 44: 326

Cheng Xinnong (Editor) 1987 Chinese Acupuncture and Moxibustion – GB 7: 200; GB 20: 203; GB 23: 204; GB 41: 210; GB 42: 210

Shanghai College of Traditional Chinese Medicine. 1993 Applied Anatomical Charts of Acupuncture and Moxibustion – GB 7: 134; GB 10: 136; GB 11: 136; GB 16: 138; GB 17: 140; GB 18: 140; GB 21: 142; GB 36: 150; GB 39: 150; GB 41: 152; GB 42: 152

Qiu Mao-Liang 1996 – Chinese Acupuncture and Moxibustion – GB 7: 138; GB 16: 139; GB 17: 139; GB 18: 140; GB 27: 142; GB 41: 144; GB 42: 145

Katsusuke Serizawa 1983 Tsubo – Vital Points for Oriental Therapy – GB 7: 239; GB 11: 180; GB 12: 179;

GB 20: 180; GB 23: 246; GB 24: 113; GB 31: 120; GB 34: 161

Li Ding (Prof.). 1991. Acupuncture, Meridian Theory and Acupuncture Points – GB 9: 260; GB 10: 261; GB 11: 261; GB 16: 263; GB 17: 263; GB 18: 264; GB 19: 264; GB 21: 265; GB 30: 270; GB 41: 278; GB 42: 279

Yang Jiasan (Prof) 1982 The Way to Locate Acu-Points – GB 9: 45; GB 10: 45; GB 19: 46; GB 20: 46; GB 21: 46; GB 27: 46; GB 30: 46; GB 37: 47

Shanghai College of Traditional Medicine 1981 Acupuncture – A Comprehensive Text – GB 10: 320; GB 11 320; GB 12: 320; GB 20: 168; GB 21: 194; GB 22: 321; GB 28: 322; GB 36: 322; GB 42: 323; GB 43: 323

Deadman, Peter; Al-Khafaji, Mazin; Baker, Kevin 1998 Manual of Acupuncture, An – GB 11: 429; GB 20: 436; GB 21: 438; GB 22: 440; GB 23: 440; GB 34: 450

Lawson-Wood 1973 Acupuncture Handbook – VII 23: 18; VII 24: 19; VII 37: 50; VII 38: 34; VII 40: 42; VII 43: 26

Huang-fu Mi. Trans: Yang Shou-zhong and Charles Chace 1993 The Systematic Classic of Acupuncture & Moxibustion – GB 20: 136; GB 24: 168; GB 25: 170; GB 26: 169; GB 27: 169; GB 28: 170; GB 29: 170; GB 30: 194; GB 33: 194; GB 34: 194; GB 38: 193; GB 40: 193; GB 41: 193; GB 44: 192

Gray, H; Warwick, Roger; Williams, Peter L 1978 Gray's Anatomy 35th Edition. (GB 2) Intertragic Incisure: ; (GB 16) Coronal Suture: 261; (GB 41 & GB 42) Extensor Digitorum Longus: 572

THE LIVER CHANNEL OF THE FOOT (JUE YIN)

Primary Channel

The Liver channel starts superficially at Liv 1 on the lateral aspect of the first digit, and runs up the medial aspect of the lower leg (meeting with Sp 6) and thigh to Liv 11. Here the channel connects with the spleen at Sp 12 and Sp 13. It loops round the genital area, round the reproductive organs, and goes up through Ren 2, 3 and 4 to the stomach and to Liv 13/14, connecting with the liver and Gallbladder organs and the side of the abdominal wall.

One deep channel arises in the liver, and passes through the diaphragm to flow into the lungs, to link with the Lung channel. The main channel runs up through the diaphragm, crosses by the ribs, goes behind the trachea, larynx and pharynx and up onto the face. It passes through the nasal cavities to the lachrymal canal where it connects with the eye, then travels up the forehead and over the frontal bone to Du 20. Another deep branch travels down from the eye, down the mandible and encircles the lips.

Divergent Channel

This leaves the primary channel on the foot and continues up to the pubic region, where it joins the Gallbladder primary channel.

Connecting Channel

This leaves the primary channel at Liv 5 on the medial aspect of the lower leg and connects with the Gallbladder channel. A branch passes up the leg to the genitals.

Muscle Channel

This begins on the dorsal aspect of the first digit, binds anterior to the medial malleolus, and passes up the medial aspect of the tibia binding at the medial aspect of the knee. It traverses the medial aspect of the thigh, binding with the hip then joining the reproductive organs (and other muscle channels). It crosses the abdomen binding with the umbilicus, then enters the abdominal cavity, binds with the ribs and disperses through the chest. An internal branch adheres to the spine.

THE LIVER CHANNEL OF THE FOOT

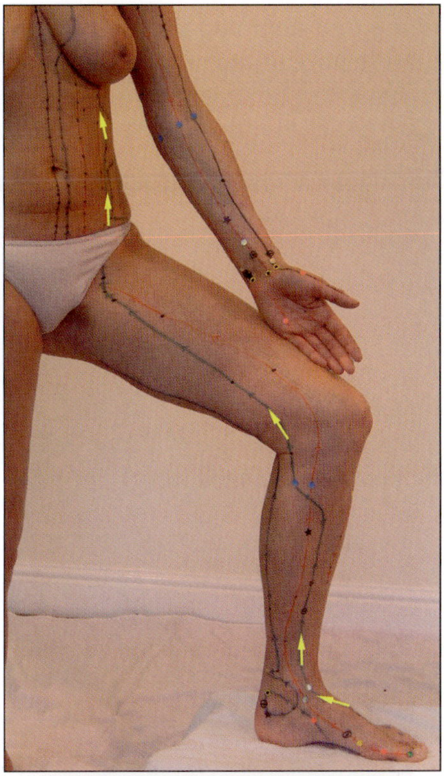

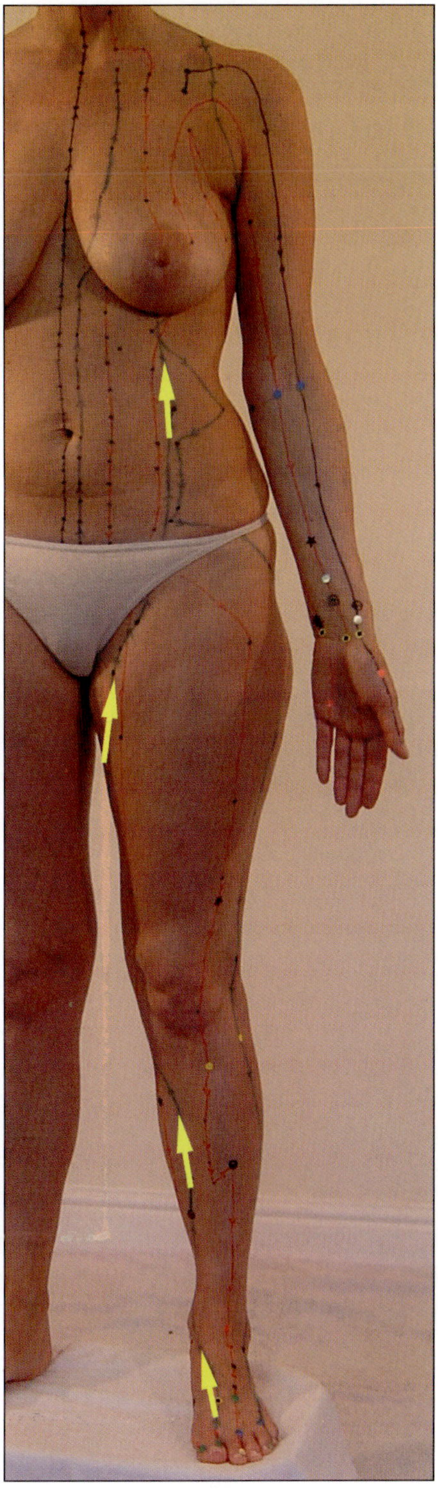

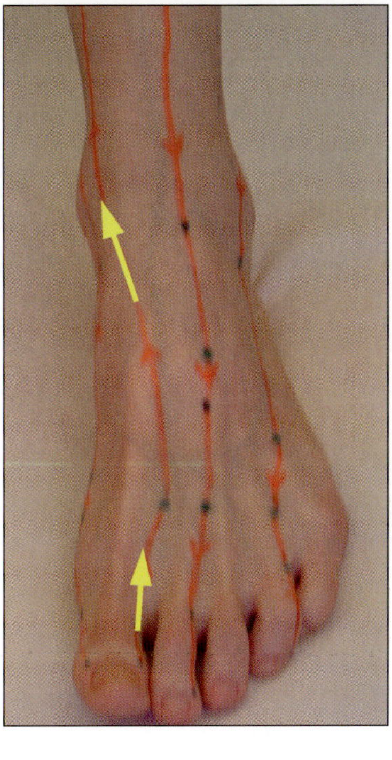

Points of the Liver Channel – Foot Jue Yin (Liv/Li/LIV/LV/LR/VIII)

Liv 1-3 are on the dorsal surface of the first digit and the foot, Liv 4 on the anterior aspect of the flexure of the ankle.

Liv 1 DA DUN – GREAT ESTEEM

⊥ ***0.1 TO 0.2 CUN*** ∆ ***3 TO 7***

- WOOD
- ENTRY
- HORARY from 1 a.m. to 3 a.m.
- SEASONAL HORARY – Spring
- JING – WELL/Shu – Transporting/Antique
- RE-UNION/Crossing/Meeting Point of the Liver Channel with the Gall Bladder Channel.- Foot Jue Yin Channel with the Foot Shao Yang Channel

Pos: Position of patient: supine.

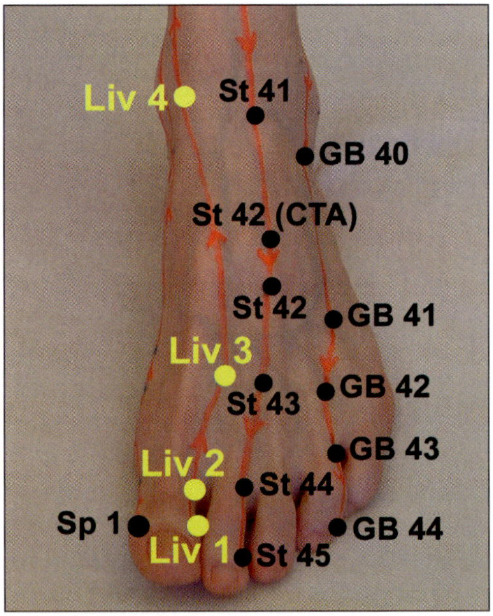

Loc: a) On the foot.
b) On the dorsal aspect of the first digit (big toe).
c) The lateral nail point of the first digit.
d) Approximately 0.1 cun proximal to the corner of the nail.
e) Just distal to the flare of the distal phalanx.
f) Between the lateral corner of the nail and the interphalangeal joint.

Tip: a) The point is level with the nail bed (where the nail attaches to the skin) rather than the cuticle.
b) Draw a horizontal line across the nail bed.
c) Draw a vertical line from the lateral border of the nail towards the nail bed.
d) The lines drawn from b) and c) (vertical and horizontal) form an intersection. This is approximately where the point is located.
e) The point may lie approximately halfway between the corner of the nail and the interphalangeal joint (the joint between the distal and proximal phalanges of the big toe).

Note: Ellis (1991) in a Classical description locates LV 1 on the lateral side of the great toe, about the width of a Chinese leek leaf away from the nail, on the lateral side amid the "three hairs" (The Golden Mirror). Huang (1993) locates Liv 1 at the tip of the big toe, the distance of a leek leaf from the corner of the nail in the three hair region.

Liv 2 XING JIAN – WALK BETWEEN

⊥ ***0.3 TO 0.5 CUN*** **Δ *3 TO 7***

- FIRE
- SEDATION/Reducing/Dispersing
- CHILD
- YING – SPRING/Shu – Transporting/Antique

Pos: Position of patient: supine.

Loc:
a) On the dorsal surface of the foot.
b) Between the first and second digits.
c) On the dorsal surface the first digit (big toe)
d) Distal to the metatarsophalangeal joint of the first digit.
e) Just distal to the flare of the base of the proximal phalanx.
f) Proximal to the web margin.

Tip:
a) From the lateral nail point (Liv 1) of the big toe, palpate along the Liver channel, with the flow until you can feel a flare arise at the distal end of the base of the first proximal phalanx.
b) The metatarsophalangeal joint of the first digit (knuckle of the big toe) is formed by the base of the proximal phalanx and the head of the the first metatarsal bone.
c) Palpation should be proximal to the web margin, between the first and second toes.
d) It is important that you do not palpate too proximal (no more than 0.5 cun proximal to the web margin) otherwise you will end up on the flare itself. Even though the description of the point locates Liv 2 on the dorsal surface of the first digit, the channel can often flow towards the dorsal and lateral corners of the first digit, therefore to accurately locate Liv 2 palpation is vital.

Note: Shanghai (1993) locates LR 2 on the dorsum of the foot, on the web margin between the 1st and 2nd toes. Shandong (1982) locate Xingjian on the web margin between the 1st and 2nd toes. Huang (1993) locates Liv 2 in the web of the big toe, where a pulsating vessel is palpable. Eachou (1995) locates LIV 2 on the dorsum of the foot, in the fossa between the first and second proximal phalanges, and proximal to the margin of the toe web. Lotan (2000) locates Liv 2 between the big and 2nd toes, midway between the web margin and the metatarsophalangeal joint.

So (1985) locates LV 2 in between the big and second toe, half-way between the web and the joint. Soulié (1994) locates LR 2 on the dorsum of the foot: at the metatarsophalangeal joint at the base of the big toe, facing the second toe; in the angle between the body and the head of the first metatarsal and the posterior edge of a transverse ligament; in a hollow. Wu (1973) locates LI 2 upon the dorsal surface of the foot, in the interdigital space between the first and second toe, on the median side, toward the first toe. Voisin (1974) locates Liv 2 on the dorsum of the foot, slightly behind the junction of toes 1 and 2. Masayoshi (1975) locates LV 2 in front of the first metatarsophalangeal joint.

Liv 3 TAI CHONG – SUPREME RUSHING

⊥ *0.3 TO 0.5 CUN* Δ *3 TO 7*

- SOURCE/Yuan/Regulator/Primary
- EARTH
- SHU – STREAM/Shu – Transporting/Antique
- HOST/GUEST COMBINATION – Source Point with the Junction Point of its Paired Official/Organ Therefore Liv 3 is combined with GB 37
- ONE OF THE HEAVENLY STAR POINTS OF MA DAN-YANG (the others are: Lu 7, LI 4, LI 11, St 36, St 44, Bl 40, Bl 57, Bl 60, Ht 5, GB 34 and GB 39)

Pos: Position: supine.

Loc:
a) On the dorsal surface of the foot.
b) Distal to the junction of the first and second metatarsal bones.
c) Just distal to the flare of the bases of the metatarsal bones.
d) Lateral to the tendon of the extensor hallucis longus.

Tip:
a) Palpate proximally from the web margin between the first and second toes until you feel some resistance. This resistance is where the bases of the first and second metatarsal bones meet i.e. the junction of the first and second metatarsal bones.
b) If you cannot feel the junction then you may need to feel for the anatomy of the first and second metatarsophalangeal joints. To do this, press your fingers in to the plantar surface of the foot at the level of the first and second metatarsophalangeal joints, which will make the first and second metatarsal bones on the dorsum surface of the foot more clearly visible.
c) The point lies just distal to the flare at the base of the first and second metatarsal bones (which is also just distal to the junction of the first and second metatarsal bones).
d) The point lies lateral to the tendon of the hallucis longus, which inserts into the phalanges of the first digit.
e) Liv 3 is located in the hollow just distal to the resistance formed by the junction of the bases of the first and second metatarsal bones.

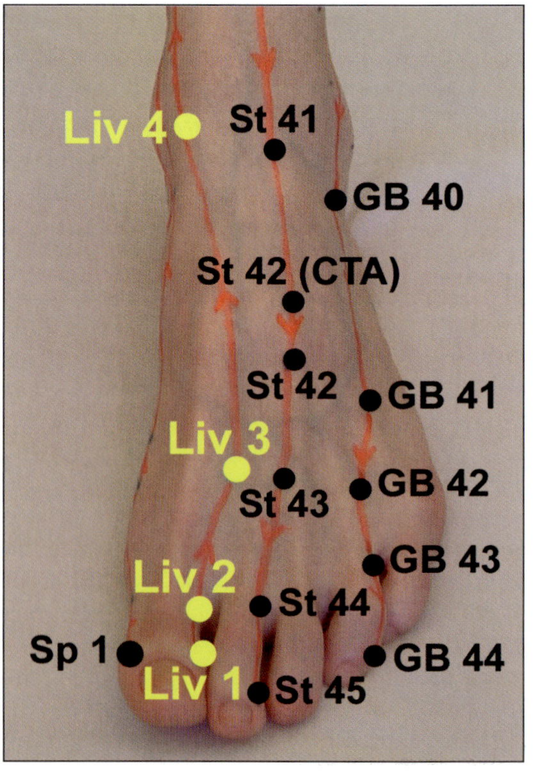

Note: Shanghai (1981) locates Li 2 on the foot, 1.5 – 2 units above the web betweenthe first and second toes. Eachou (1995) locates LIV 3 on the dorsum of the foot in the fossa distal to the junction of the first and second metatarsal bones, 2 inches above the web of the toe. Lotan (2000) locates Liv 3 between the 1st and 2nd metatarsals, proximal to the bone heads. Jayasuirya (1982) locates Liv 3 at 2 cun proximal to the margin of the web between the 1st and 2nd toes.

So (1985) locates LV 3 at 1.5 divisions proximal to the metatarsophalangeal joints, between the first and second metatarsal. Academy (1975) locate Liv 3 between the 1st and 2nd toe, 2 cun proximal to the margin of the web. Huang (1993) locates Liv 3 either at 2 cun or at one and five fen proximal to the base joint of the phalanx of the big toe. Lawson-Wood (1973) locates VIII 3 on the anterior of the instep, between the first and second metatarsals, a little in front of their articulation with the first cuneiform.

Liv 4 ZHONG FENG – MIDDLE SEAL

⊥ ***0.3 TO 0.5 CUN*** Δ ***3 TO 5***

- METAL
- JING – RIVER/Shu – Transporting/Antique

Pos: Position of patient: supine.

Loc: a) On the anterior aspect of the flexure of the ankle.
b) Between the medial malleolus and the tendon of the tibialis anterior muscle.
c) Level with the prominence of the medial malleolus when the foot is dorsiflexed.
d) 1 cun anterior to the level of the prominence of the medial malleolus.

Tip: a) Draw a transverse line across the prominence of the medial malleolus to the tendon of the tibialis anterior muscle.
b) Palpate on this line between the anterior aspect of the medial malleolus and the tendon of the tibialis anterior muscle.
c) You should be able to feel a good *men* (depression) in between the medial malleolus and the tendon, if not ask the patient to dorsiflex (so that the heel is the only part of the foot making contact with the ground) and invert their foot (turning inwards) to expose the tendon of the tibialis anterior muscle. The point is located in between the medial side of the tendon and the anterior aspect of the medial malleolus level with the prominence of the medial malleolus.
d) Remember that you need to locate and needle the patient in the same position, therefore after asking the patient to dorsiflex and extend their foot, you need to get them to relax and then palpate for Liv 4.

Note: Wu (1973) locates LI 4 upon the foot, at one pouce before the internal malleus. Voisin (1974) locates Liv 4 on the dorsum of the foot, in the centre of the talonavicular joint. So (1985) locates LV 4 at approximately one division anterior to the medial malleolus in between the two tendons. Jayasuriya (1982) locates Liv 4 in the medial aspect of the ankle, in the depression on the medial side of the tendon of the tibialis anterior muscle, midway between Sp 5 and St 41. Legge (1999) locates Liv 4 on the medial side of the tendon of the tibialis anterior, 1 cun anterior to the medial malleolus, midway between Sp 5 and St 41.

Shandong (1982) locates Zhongfeng anteior to the medial malleolus, between the tendons of the m. tibialis anterior and the m. extensor hallucis longus. Cheng (1987) locates Liv 4 at 1 cun anterior to the medial malleolus, midway between Sp 5 and St 41, in the depression on the medial side of the tendon of m. tibialis anterior. Li (1991) locates Liv 4 at 1 cun anterior to the tip of the medial malleolus, in the depression between the tendons of m. tibialis anterior and the m. extensor hallucis longus. It lies between the borders of these two tendons. Note that the illustration differs to the description in that it shows the point medial to the border of the m. tibialis anterior and not not in between these two tendons.

Worsley (1982) locates VIII 4 at the anterior flexure of the ankle, between the tendons of the tibialis anterior and the extensor hallucis longus. Soulié (1994) locates LR 4 at the arch, medial side (facing the big toe): about three FW (Finger Width) anterior to and lateral to the medial malleolus; in the angle between the anterior edge of a transverse bone (scaphoid) and the medial edge of the extensor hallucis longus muscle; lateral to the flat tendon of the tibialis anterior; in a hollow; about three FW posterior to LR 3; about six FW in front of LR 5; separated by the extensor hallucis longus muscle from ST 42, by the tibialis anterior from SP 4.

Shanghai (1993) locates LR 4 anterior to the medial malleolus, on the midway of the line connecting SP 5 and ST 41, in the depression medial to the tendon of the anterior tibial muscle. Eachou (1995) locates LIV 4 on the medial side of the foot 1 inch anterior to the medial malleolus of the tibia, and between the tendons of the tibialis anterior and extensor hallucis longus muscles. Shanghai (1981) locates Li 4 one unit anterior to the inferior margin of the medial malleolus of the ankle, midway between S 41 and Sp 5. Ellis (1991) locates LV 4 at 1 inch anterior to the medial malleolus, midway between SP 5 and ST 41, in the depression on the medial side of the tendon of the anterior tibial muscle (m. tibialis anterior).

Deadman (1998) locates LIV 4 on the ankle, anterior to the prominence of the medial malleolus, just medial to the tendon of the tibialis anterior when the ankle is extended (dorsiflexed). Academy (1975) locates Liv 4 at 1 cun anterior to the medial malleolus, in the depression medial to the tendon of the m. tibialis anticus.

Cun Measurements of the Medial Aspect of the Leg

The distance from the prominence of the medial malleolus (ankle) bone to the popliteal crease on the medial side of the knee flexure is measured as 15 cun. This is measured with the patient in a supine position with the leg flat. This method may seem more user friendly than using the 13 cun measurement as it should be easier to divide your 15 cun measurement in to 3 sections of 5 and then to divide the 5 in to 1 cun measurements.

The distance from the prominence of the medial malleolus to the inferior border of the medial condyle of the tibia bone (Sp 9) is measured as 13 cun. This is measured with the patient in a seated position with the knee bent at 90 degrees. The difficulty of measuring 13 cun is not just dividing your 13 cun in to equal 1 cun measurements but to accurately mark the inferior border of the medial condyle of the tibia where Sp 9 is located can be difficult.

Note: There are approximately 2 cun between the inferior border of the medial condyle of the tibia bone and the popliteal crease on the medial flexure of the knee, hence 15 cun, but this is only accurate in the seated position. If you were to measure 13 cun and then measure 2 cun to the popliteal crease of the medial flexure of the knee from the 13 cun with the person in a supine position, the 2 cun measurement will seem greater compared to the 13 equal cun measurements as the leg will be in a flat position as opposed to a seated position. The seated position allows the 2 cun measurement to be more accurate as the leg is bent at 90 degrees.

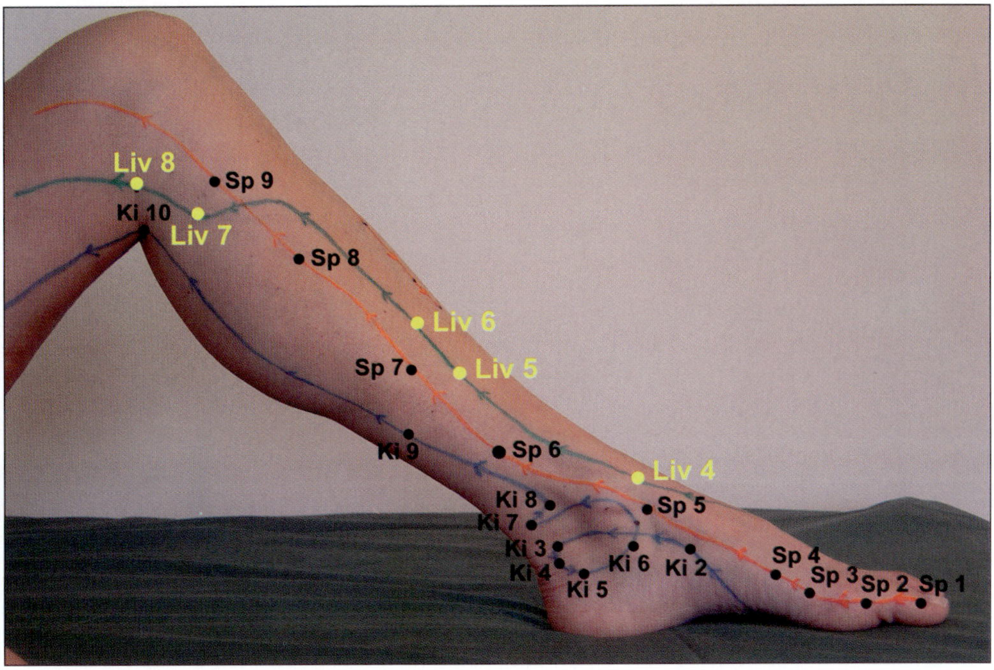

Liv 5-7 are on the medial aspect of the lower leg.

Liv 5 LI GOU – INSECT DITCH

⊥ ***0.3 TO 0.5 CUN*** Δ ***3 TO 7***

- JUNCTION/Luo/Connecting/Passage/Lo/Lê
- RE-UNION/Crossing/Meeting Point of the Liver Channel with the Gall Bladder Channel – Foot Jue Yin Channel with the Foot Shao Yang Channel
- HOST/GUEST COMBINATION – Source Point with the Junction Point of its Paired Official/Organ Therefore Liv 5 is combined with GB 40

Pos: Position of patient: supine (at 15 cun) with the leg flat, or in a seated position with the leg bent at 90 degrees (at 13 cun).

Loc: a) On the lower leg.
b) On the medial aspect of the lower leg.
c) On the medial surface of the tibia.
d) Near to the medial border of the tibia.
e) On the medial border of the soleus/gastrocnemius muscle.
f) 5 cun proximal to the prominence of the medial malleolus.

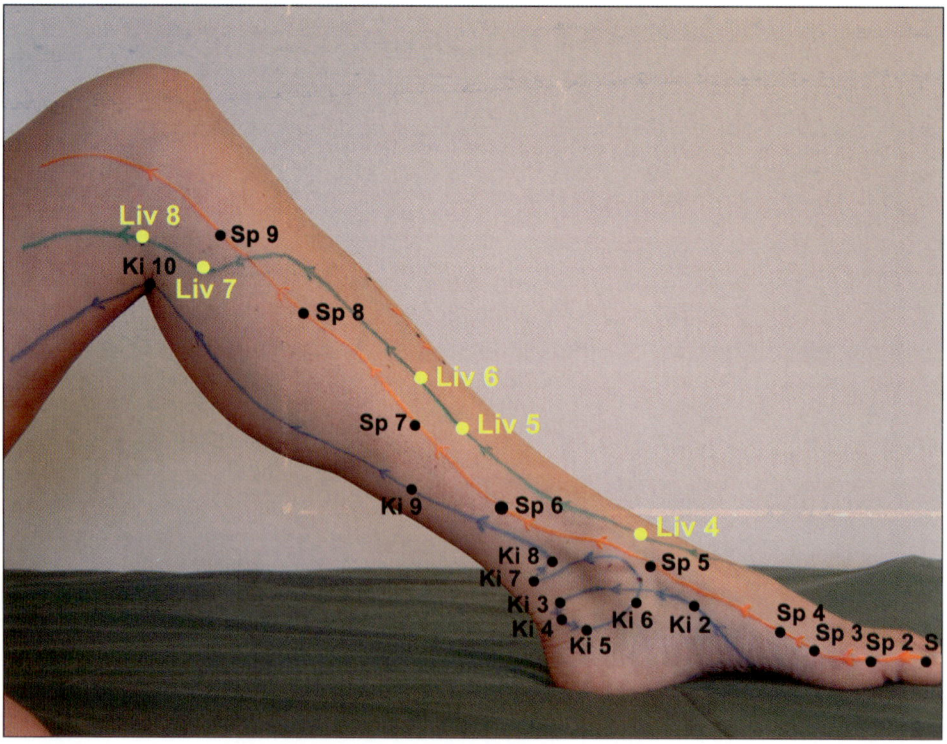

Cun: a) The distance from the prominence of the medial malleolus (ankle) bone to the popliteal crease on the medial side of the knee flexure is measured as 15 cun.

b) 15 cun is measured with the patient in a supine position with the leg flat.

c) This method may seem more user friendly than using the 13 cun measurement as it should be easier to divide 15 cun in to 3 sections of 5 and then to divide the 5 in to 1 cun measurements.

d) 13 cun is measured with the patient's leg bent at 90 degrees. It is measured from the prominence of the medial malleolus to the inferior border of the medial condyle of the tibia bone, please refer to Sp 9 cun measurements sections c) to g).

Tip: a) Liv 5 is in a seam formed when you lift and slightly turn the body of the gastrocnemius and soleus muscless medially and anteriorly.

b) Placing a rolled towel under the leg at the level of the middle of the shin will highlight the borders of the gastrocnemius and soleus muscles as they are moved medially and anteriorly. You should then be able to palpate a seam near to the medial border of the tibia.

c) Run the flat of your finger with the flow of the Liver channel from the flexure of the ankle along the seam towards the popliteal crease.

d) Palpating approximately 5 cunproximal to the medial malleolus should reveal the accurate location of Liv 5.

e) At the level of 5 cun the soleus can be more prominent than the gastrocnemius and conversely the gastrocnemius can be more prominent than the soleus.

Note: Grays (1978) The tendo calcaneus is about 15 cm in length and begins near the middle of the leg, but its anterior surface receives muscle fibres from the soleus. It gradually becomes more rounded towards a level of approximately 4 cm above the calcaneus.

Note: There are some Schools and texts that locate the Liver and Spleen channels in the same position on the medial side of the lower leg, posterior to the edge of the tibia. Worsley (1982) has the Liver and Spleen sharing the same channel, although an explanation for this could be that the Liver and Spleen channels flow more superficially at their points and therefore they do not flow into each other, they only share the same anatomical features instead. He locates VIII 5 on the medial surface of the leg, 6 ACI (Anatomical Chinese Inch) proximal to the prominence of the medial malleolus, posterior to the edge of the tibia. Wu (1973) locates LI 5 upon the internal surface of the leg, posterior to the edge of the tibia, at six pouce above the internal malleus. Legge (1999) locates Liv 5 at 5 cun above the tip of the medial malleolus, just posterior to the medial border of the tibia. Lotan (2000) locates Liv 5 on the medial aspect of the leg, 5 cun proximal to the medial malleolus peak, posterior to the tibia.

Jayasuriya (1982) locates Liv 5 at 5 cun superior to the tip of the medial malleolus, one fingerbreadth anterior to the medial border of the tibia. Soulié (1994) locates LR 5 on the anterior side of the lower limb; lateral edge of tibia. Three FW (Finger Width) above the lower edge of the tibia; at the edge of an anterior notch of the bone. In the angle of the upper edge of a transverse mass; in a hollow; approximately six FW above LR 4; five FW inferior to LR 6; one and a half FW in front of and a little below SP 6; four FW below and in front of GB 37; three FW anterior and above KI 4.

Voisin (1974) locates Liv 5 on the tibia, midwidth: 1 handbreadth above the medial malleolus. Lawson-Wood (1973) uses VIII 6 (Liv 6) as the Junction (Passage) point. He locates this point on the antero-internal aspect of the leg on the centre line of the tibia, about 4cm below the midpoint of a line drawn from the internal malleolus to the antero-intern of the tibio-femoral articulation. This location is closer to our Liv 5 than our Liv 6. Lavier (1974) in an illustration clear shows the Spleen and Liver channels share the same line at the posterior border of the tibia. LI 5 is illustrated as being located on the medial side of the lower, on the posterior border of the tibia, at 6 pouce proximal to the prominence of the medial malleolus.

So (1985) locates LV 5 at 5 divisions above the upper edge of the medial malleolus, behind the border of the tibia. Academy (1975) locate Liv 5 at 5 cun superior to the medial malleolus, on the posterior border of the tibia. Their illustration shows the Liver channel in the same location as our Liver channel.

Liv 6 ZHONG DU – MIDDLE CAPITAL

⊥ ***0.3 TO 0.5 CUN*** Δ ***3 TO 5***

- ACCUMULATION/Xi Cleft/Gueki Point

Pos: Position of patient: supine (at 15 cun) with the leg flat, or in a seated position with the leg bent at 90 degrees (at 13 cun).

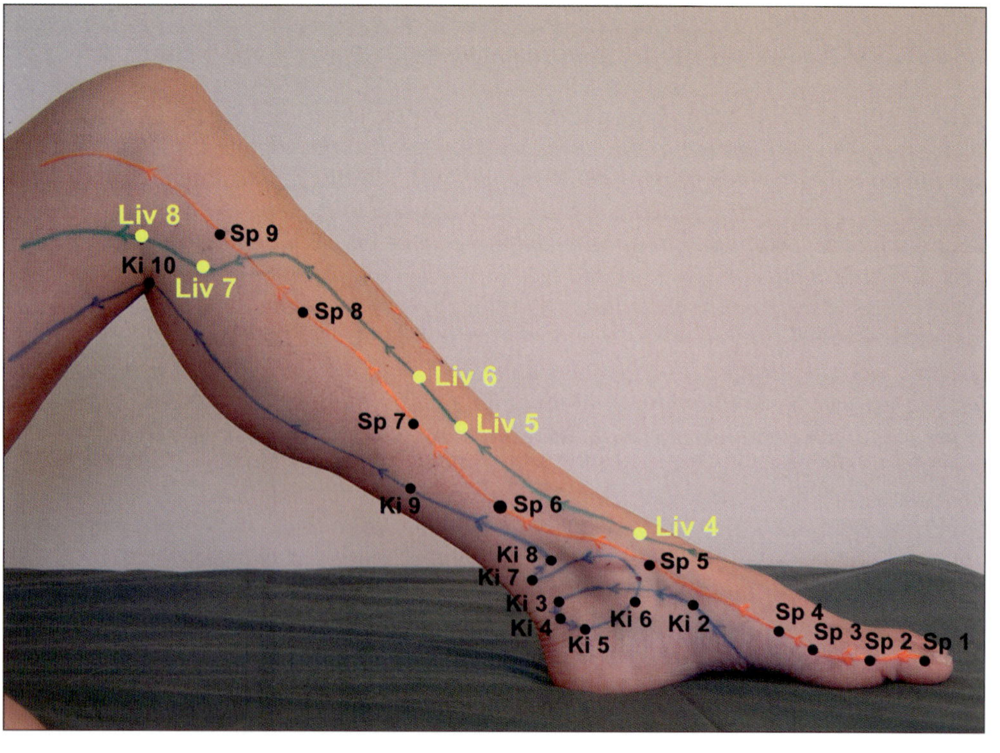

Loc: a) On the lower leg.
b) On the medial aspect of the lower leg.
c) On the medial surface of the tibia.
d) Near the medial border of the tibia.
e) Between the medial border of the tibia and the gastrocnemius muscle.
f) 7 cun proximal to the prominence of the medial malleolus.

Cun: a) The distance from the prominence of the medial malleolus (ankle) bone to the popliteal crease on the medial side of the knee flexure is measured as 15 cun.
b) 15 cun is measured with the patient in a supine position with the leg flat.
c) This method may seem more user friendly than using the 13 cun measurement as it should be easier to divide 15 cun in to 3 sections of 5 and then to divide the 5 in to 1 cun measurements.
d) 13 cun is measured with the patient's leg bent at 90 degrees. It is measured from the prominence of the medial malleolus to the inferior border of the medial condyle of the tibia bone, please refer to Sp 9 cun measurements sections c) to g).

Tip: a) Liv 6 is in a seam formed when you lift and slightly turn the body of the gastrocnemius and soleus muscless medially and anteriorly.
b) Placing a rolled towel under the leg at the level of the middle of the shin will highlight the borders of the gastrocnemius and soleus muscles as they are moved medially and anteriorly. You should then be able to palpate a seam near to the medial border of the tibia.
c) Run the flat of your finger with the flow of the Liver channel from the flexure of the ankle along the seam towards the popliteal crease.
d) Palpating approximately 7 cun proximal to the medial malleolus should reveal the accurate location of Liv 6.
e) At the level of 7 cun the soleus can be more prominent than the gastrocnemius and conversely the gastrocnemius can be more prominent than the soleus.

Note: There are some Schools and texts that locate the Liver and Spleen channels in the same position on the medial side of the lower leg, posterior to the edge of the tibia. Worsley (1982) has the Liver and Spleen sharing the same channel, although an explanation for this could be that the Liver and Spleen channels flow superficially at their points and therefore they do not flow into each other, they only share the same anatomical features instead. He locates VIII 6 on the medial surface of the leg, 8 ACI (Anatomical Chinese Inch) proximal to the prominence of the medial malleolus, posterior to the edge of the tibia. Wu (1973) locates LI 6 upon the internal surface of the leg, at eight pouce above the internal malleus, posterior to the edge of the tibia.

Legge (1999) locates Liv 6 at 7 cun above the tip of the medial malleolus, just posterior to the medial border of the tibia. Lotan (2000) locates Liv 6 on the medial aspect of the leg, 7 cun proximal to the medial malleolus peak, posterior to the tibia. Voisin (1974) locates Liv 6 on the tibia, midwidth and midlength. Lavier (1974) in an illustration clear shows the Spleen and Liver channels share the same line at the posterior border of the tibia. LI 6 is illustrated as being located on the medial side of the lower, on the posterior border of the tibia, at 8 pouce proximal to the prominence of the medial malleolus.

Lawson-Wood (1973) uses VIII 6 (Liv 6) as the Junction (Passage) point. He locates this point on the antero-internal aspect of the leg on the centre line of the tibia, about 4cm below the midpoint of a line drawn from the internal malleolus to the antero-intern of the tibio-femoral articulation. This location is closer to our Liv 5 than our Liv 6.

Soulié (1994) locates LR 6 on the anterior lower leg, just on the anterior edge of the tibia; between it and a large muscle (tibialis anterior muscle); in a hollow; in the angle on the upper edge of a transverse mass; five FW (Finger Width) above LR 5; seven large FW below LR 7; a little below the level of SP 7 and anterior to it. Jayasuriya (1982) locates Liv 6 at 7 cun superior to the tip of the medial malleolus, one finger breadth anterior to the medial border of the tibia. Academy (1975) locate Liv 6 at 7 cun superior to the tip of the medial malleolus, on the posterior border of the tibia.

Liv 7 XI GUAN – KNEE BORDER

⊥ ***0.5 TO 0.8 CUN*** Δ ***3***

Pos: Position of patient: supine with the leg flat (at 15 cun), or in a seated position with the leg bent at 90 degrees (at 13 cun).

Loc:
a) On the lower leg.
b) On the medial aspect of the lower leg.
c) In the medial head of the gastrocnemius muscle.
d) Approximately 13 cun proximal to the prominence of the medial malleolus.
e) 1 cun posterior to Sp 9.

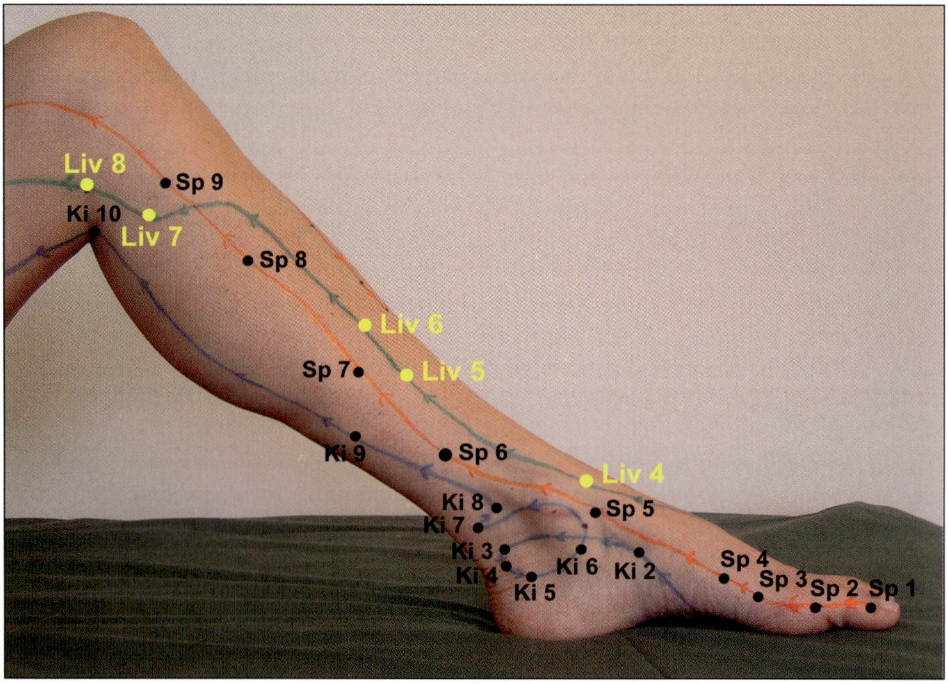

Cun: a) The distance from the prominence of the medial malleolus (ankle) bone to the popliteal crease on the medial side of the knee flexure is measured as 15 cun.
b) 15 cun is measured with the patient in a supine position with the leg flat.
c) This method may seem more user friendly than using the 13 cun measurement as it should be easier to divide 15 cun in to 3 sections of 5 and then to divide the 5 in to 1 cun measurements.
d) 13 cun is measured with the patient's leg bent at 90 degrees. It is measured from the prominence of the medial malleolus to the inferior border of the medial condyle of the tibia bone, please refer to Sp 9 cun measurements sections c) to g).

Tip: a) Locate Sp 9 first as this point is used to locate Liv 7.
b) Sp 9 is located on the posterior border of the medial aspect of the tibia bone, on the inferior border of the medial condyle of the tibia, between the tibia bone and the gastrocnemius muscle, 13 cun proximal to the prominence of the medial malleolus. A detailed guide for the location of Sp 9 can be referenced in the tips section for Sp 9.
c) When you have located Sp 9, Liv 7 is approximately 1 cun posterior to it, in the medial head of the gastrocnemius muscle.
d) Alternatively, palpate posteriorly from the inferior border of the medial condyle of the tibia on to the medial head of the gastrocnemius muscle and you should be able to feel a *men* (depression). This is approximately 13 cun proximal to the prominence of the medial malleolus.
e) If you are unable to locate the inferior border of the medial condyle of the tibia, run the flat of your finger from the flexure of the ankle towards the popliteal crease along the posterior border of the medial aspect of the tibia (along the Spleen channel). Your finger should begin to curve with the contour, which is the inferior border of the medial condyle of the tibia.

Note: Wu (1973) Liv 7 upon the internal surface of the leg, posterior to the tibia. He also locates this point at three pouce below the crease formed by the articulation of the knee. Lavier (1974) clearly illustrates the Liver and Spleen channels sharing the same channel between Sp 6 and Sp 8 on the posterior border of the medial aspect of the tibia, with Liv 5/6/7 at 6/8/12 pouce, and Sp 6/7/8/9 at 4/7/9/13 pouce.

Worsley (1982) has the Liver and Spleen sharing the same channel, although an explanation for this could be that the Liver and Spleen channels flow superficially at their points and therefore they do not flow into each other, they only share the same anatomical features instead. The location of VIII 7 is on the medial surface of the leg, 12 ACI (Anatomical Chinese Inch) proximal to the prominence of the medial malleolus, posterior to the edge of the tibia.

Soulié (1994) locates LR 7 on the upper medial side of the lower leg. On the tibia, just at the lower and medial edge of the anterior bulge of the anterior tibial tuberosity, on the lower edge of a transverse mass; in a hollow; four FW (Finger Width) inferior and anterior to LR 8; seven large FW above LR 6. Lotan (2000) locates Liv 7 on the medial aspect of the leg, 1 cun posterior to the tibial neck, level with the tibial tuberosity inferior border. Masayoshi (1975) locates LV 7 at the lower edge of the medial condyle of the tibia; posterior to the semitendinosus. Voisin (1974) locates Liv 7 on the knee, just below the tibial tuberosity. Shandong (1982) locate Xiguan in the posterior and inferior aspect of the condylus medialis of the tibia, 1 cun posterior to Pt. Yinglingquan (Sp 9).

Liv 8 is on the medial aspect of the flexure of the knee.

Liv 8 QU QUAN – CROOKED SPRING

⊥ *0.3 TO 0.7 CUN* Δ *3 TO 5*

- WATER
- TONIFICATION/Reinforcing
- MOTHER
- HE – SEA/Shu – Transporting/Antique

Pos: Position of patient: supine with the knee flexed, or seated with the leg bent at 90 degrees.

Loc:
a) On the medial aspect of the knee.
b) On the medial border of the joint of the knee.
c) Superior to the medial end of the popliteal crease when the knee is flexed
d) Posterior to the medial condyle of the tibia.
e) Medial and anterior to the tendon of the semimembranosus muscle.

Tip:
a) With the patients' knee flexed, place a mark at the superior end of the medial popliteal crease.
b) From the centre of the patella palpate medially along the knee joint until you can no longer feel the medial condyle of the tibia. Place a mark at this location.

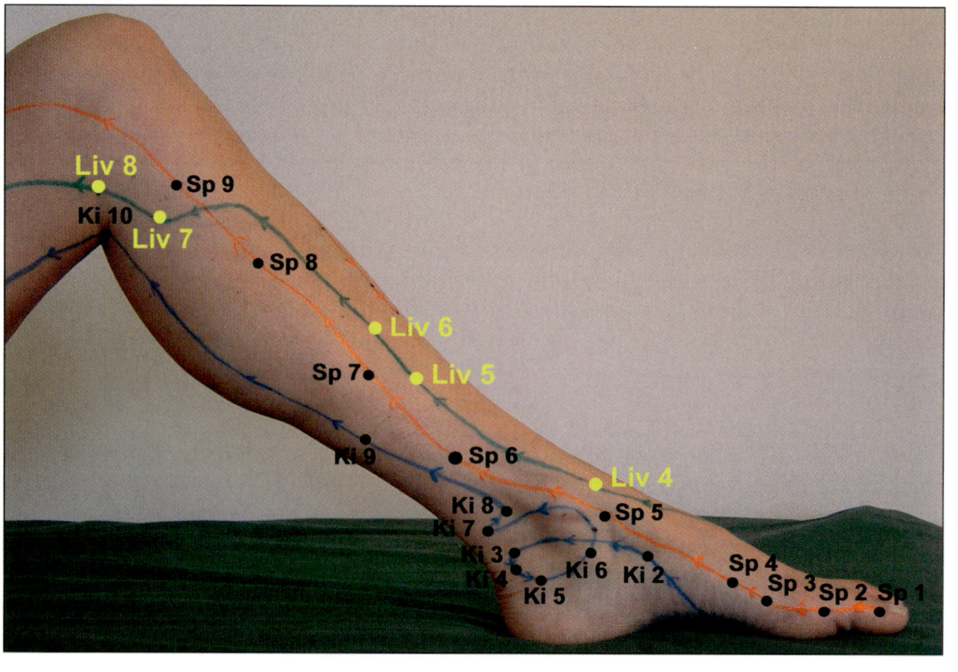

c) The point can be palpated in between the superior end of the popliteal crease and the mark drawn in b).
d) The point may not always be at the superior end of the medial popliteal crease. Liv 8 is located medial and anterior to the tendon of the semimembranosus muscle. To identify this ask the patient to push their heel against your hand. Once identified ask the patient to slowly relax their foot and then mark the tendon of the semimembranosus muscle.
e) The tendon and the posterior aspect of the medial condyle of the tibia can be used as landmarks. Palpate for the point in between these two landmarks in the joint of the knee.
f) A common error when locating Liv 8 is to mark it too close to the tendon. Use the superior end of the popliteal crease as a guide.

Note: All of the following references have the knee in a flexed position. Some mention the bones of the knee while others omit them. Worsley (1982) locates VIII 8 on the medial surface of the knee, posterior to the medial condyle of the tibia, close to the extremity of the crease formed when the knee is flexed, This seems to be a Japanese location (see Shudo (1979)). Deadman (1998) locates it just superior to the medial end of the popliteal crease, anterior to the tendons of the m. semitendinosus and m. semimembranosus, about 1 cun anterior to KID 10.

Lawson-Wood (1973) locates VIII 9 where we locate Liv 8. He also lists VIII 9 as the Toning point where we use Liv 8 as the Tonification point. He locates it on the internal aspect of the flexed knee, at the extremity of the transverse fold. Voisin (1974) locates Liv 8 on the knee, medial aspect: in front of the flexion fold. Wu (1973) locates LI 8 at the internal extremity of the flexure of the knee, posterior to the protruberance of the tibia. Lavier (1974) in an illustration locates LI 8 on the medial aspect of the knee, medial to the tendons of the semimembranosus and semitendinosus, at 15 pouce proximal to the tip of the internal malleolus and posterior to KI 10. Li (1991) locates LIV 8 on the medial side of the knee joint. When the knee is flexed, the point lies in the depression posterior and superior to the medial end of the transverse popliteal crease, on the anterior border of the m. semimembranosus and posterior to the medial condyle of the tibia. Yang (1982) locates Liv 8 in the depression between the upper border. Cheng (1987) locates Liv 8 above the medial end of the transverse popliteal crease, posterior to the medial epicondyle of the femur, on the anterior part of the insertion of m. semimembranosus and m. semitendinosus.

Eachou (1995) locates LIV 8 on the medial aspect of the thigh in the fossa on the medial side of the popliteal skin crease, between the medial epicondyle of the femur and the tendon of the semimembranosus. Shanghai (1993) locates LR 8 on the medial aspect of the thigh, when the knee is flexed, at the medial end of the transverse popliteal crease, on the medial border of the knee joint, posterior to the medial epicondyle of the tibia, in the depression anterior to the insertion of the semitendinous and the semimembranous muscles. Shanghai (1981) locates Li 8 in the depression at the medial end of the transverse crease on the posterior aspect of the knee. So (1985) locates LV 8 on the inner side of the knee; the point is found by pressing down from the meeting of the two bones, to the hollow. The point is not necessarily at the end of the knee crease.

Shandong (1982) locates Ququan in the depression at the medial end of the transverse crease of the art. genus with the knee flexed. Legge (1999) locates Liv 8 in the depression at the medial end of the cubital (knee) crease just anterior to the tendinous insertions of the medial hamstrings. Academy (1975) locate Liv 8 at the medial end of the transverse crease of the knee joint, in a depression at the anterior border of m. semimembranosus and m. semitendinosus. Jayasuriya (1982) locates Liv 8 in the transverse crease of the knee joint, at the medial border of the semimembranosus tendon. The point is better located at the medial end of the popliteal crease when the knee is fully flexed.

Masayoshi (1975) locates LV 8 on the popliteus between the semitendinous and sartorius m. Qiu (1996) locates LIV 8 in the depression above the medial end of the transverse popliteal crease. Ellis (1991) locates LV 8 on the medial side of the knee joint. When the knee is bent, the point is posterior to the medial condyle of the tibia and superior to the border of the tendons of those muscles attaching at the medial side of the knee. Lotan (2000) locates Liv 8 on the medial aspect of the leg. between the semimembranosus tendon and gracilis muscle, proximal to the knee joint. Posterior to the femur medial epicondyle.

Soulié (1994) locates LR 8 on the knee: medial side and lower part; in the posterior angle between the heads of the femur and tibia; in the angle between the head of the tibia and the posterior edge of the tibiofemoral ligament; in a hollow; four FW (Finger Width) above and medial to LR 7; eight FW below LR 9; two FW above SP 9; four FW above SP 8. Huang (1993) locates Liv 8 on the inside of the knee below the inner assisting bone in a depression above the major sinew and beneath the lesser one. Katsusuke (1983) locates LV 8 on the inner side of the knee joint. The extremity of the groove formed when the knee is bent.

Cun Measurements of the Upper Leg

The distance from a line drawn transversely between the gluteal groove and the medial root of the lower limb (at the level of the lower border of the pubic symphysis where the medial side of the upper leg joins the torso), to the medial popliteal crease (flexure of the knee) is 14 cun.

The distance between the popliteal crease (flexure of the knee) to the superior border of the greater trochanter of the femur, when the leg is abducted, is measured as 19 cun. There seems to be great discrepancies with other descriptions of the anatomy that have used the 19 cun measurement, eg. 19 cun from the popliteal crease to the superior and inferior borders of the pubic symphysis and 19 cun from the popliteal crease to the prominence or inferior border of the greater trochanter of the femur.

14 cun is the accepted bone proportional measurement of the thigh.

Liv 9-11 on the medial aspect of the thigh.

Liv 9 YIN BAO – YIN WRAPPING

⊥ *0.5 TO 0.7 CUN* Δ *3*

Pos: Position of patient: supine.

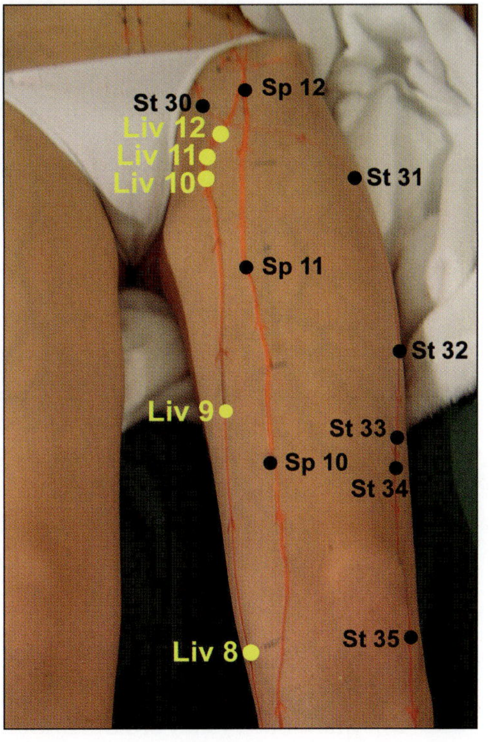

Loc:
a) On the medial aspect of the upper thigh.
b) In a seam between the vastus medialis and sartorius muscles.
c) 6 cun proximal to the medial popliteal crease (flexure of the knee).
d) 4 cun proximal to the medial epicondyle of the femur.

Cun:
a) Mark out the level of the inferior border of the symphysis pubis bone (where the medial side of the upper leg joins the torso) and the medial popliteal crease (flexure of the knee).
b) There are 14 cun between these two marks.
c) There are four ways of checking the cun measurements: see f), g), h) and i).
d) Mark out 14 cun proximal to the medial popliteal crease, as explained in a) and b) and mark 4 cun proximal to the popliteal crease.
e) The longitudinal measurement of the patella is 2 cun, therefore double this to give 4 cun. Use this measurement from the popliteal crease or the inferior border of the patella bone to get the approximate location on the prominence of the vastus medialis muscle.
f) Use the following method if you don't want to mark out 14 cun from the inferior border of the symphysis pubis to the medial popliteal crease. The superior border of the patella to the inferior border of the symphysis pubis measures 12 cun, which can be divided in to equal cun measurements by using the width of 4 fingers held close together which measures 3 cun. You will need the patient's own fingers to give guidance as to the width used as their fingers may be a different size than your own. The measurement for the width of the fingers are taken from the joint that is formed by the proximal and intermediate (middle) phalanges.

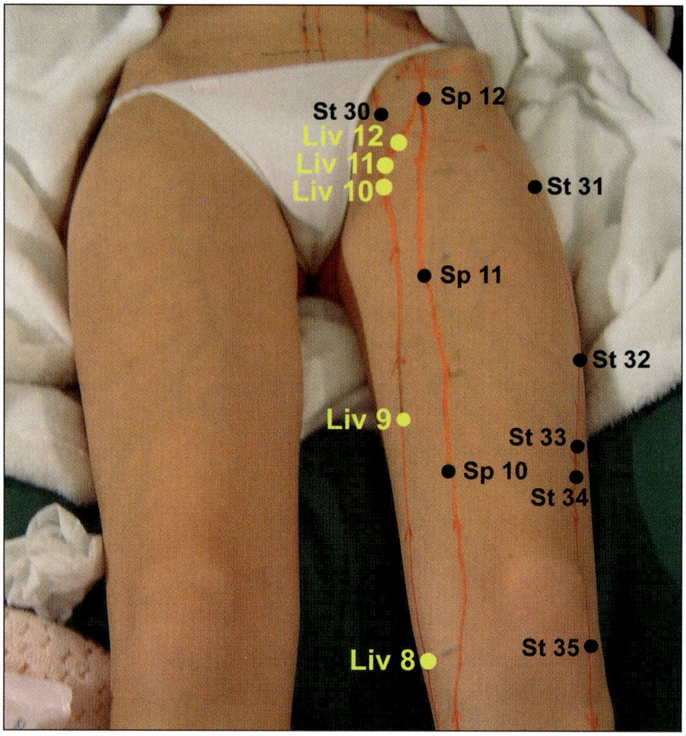

Tip:

a) Flex and extend the knee to expose the vastus medialis muscle. To locate the point the patient must have their leg in a relaxed position.

b) The point is located in a seam formed by the lateral border of the vastus medialis and the lateral border of the sartorius muscles.

c) The point is located approximately 6 cun proximal to the medial popliteal crease or 4 cun proximal to the medial epicondyle of the femur. (The distance between the medial popliteal crease and the medial epicondyle of the femur is approximately 2 cun).

d) Mark out 14 cun proximal to the medial popliteal crease, as explained in a) and b) and mark 6 cun measurement proximal to the popliteal crease.

e) The longitudinal measurement of the patella is 2 cun. If you treble this to 6 cun by taking this measurement from the popliteal crease or the inferior border of the patella bone, it will give the approximate cun where to locate the point, between the medial border of the vastus medialis and the sartorius muscles.

f) Use the following method if you don't want to mark out 14 cun from the inferior border of the symphysis pubis to the medial popliteal crease. The width of 4 fingers measures as 3 cun. You will need to look at the patient's own fingers to give you some guidance as to the width you should use as their fingers may be wider or narrower than yours. The measurement for the width of the fingers are taken from the joint that is formed by the proximal and intermediate (middle) phalanges. Once the width of the fingers is established, place the edge of the joint of your little finger on the popliteal crease. Place the edge of the index finger on the thigh and mark to give 3 cun From this mark place repeat the first step again along the thigh to give another 3 cun,therefore 6 cun proximal to the medial popliteal crease. Divide these measurements to give 4 cun proximal to the popliteal crease.

g) Palpation with the flow of the channel from the posterior border of the medial condyle of the tibia to the vastus medialis muscle (4 cun proximal to the popliteal crease) should give you accurate point location.

Note: Lotan (2000) locates Liv 9 level with 4 cun superior to the medial epicondyle superior border, anterior to the sartorius muscle. Qiu (1996) locates LIV 9 at 4 cun above the medial epicondyle of the femur, at the posterior border of the m. sartorius. Masayoshi (1975) locates LV 9 on the lower third, on the inner side of the thigh, between the sartorius m. and the gracilis m. Shandong (1982) locates Yinbao at 4 cun above the epicondylus medialis of the femur, between the m. gracilis and the m. sartorius.

Shanghai (1993) locate LR 9 on the medial aspect of the thigh, 4 cun above the medial epicondyle of the femur, posterior to the sartorius muscle. Soulié (1994) locates LR 9 on the thigh, inferior third, medial surface; three FW (Finger Width) above the condyle (lower head) of the femur, mid-width on the medial face of the femur; in the angle between the posterior (medial) edge of the longitudinal tendon and the lower edge (towards the patella) of a transverse mass; in a hollow; three FW above LR 8; three FW below LR 10; three FW anterior and below SP 11; three FW medial to ST 33; Lavier (1974) in an illustration locates LI 9 on the medial side of the upper leg, at 5 pouce proximal to the popliteal crease of the knee, and between two muscles. Eachou (1995) locates LIV 9 on the medial thigh, 4 inches above the medial epicondyle of the femur, and in the fossa between the posterior margin of the sartorius muscle and the gracilis muscle. Yang (1982) locates Liv 9 at 4 cun above Liv 8, on the border of the m. vastus medialis.

Li (1991) locates LIV 9 on the medial aspect of the thigh between the kidney and spleen meridians, 4 cun above LIV 8, on the border of the m. vastus medialis. Worsley (1982) locates VIII 9 on the medial surface of the thigh, 5 ACI (Anatomical Chinese Inch) proximal to the flexure of the knee, between the sartorius and the vastus medialis. Wu (1973) locates LI 9 upon the internal surface of the thigh, at five pouce above the popliteal area. Voisin (1974) locates Liv 9 on the thigh, medial aspect: 5fb (finger breadth) above the knee joint, on the posterior border of the sartorius. Lawson-Wood (1973) locates VIII 9 where we locate Liv 8. He also lists VIII 9 as the Toning point where we use Liv 8 as the Tonification point. He locates it on the internal aspect of the flexed knee, at the extremity of the transverse fold.

Liv 10 ZU WU LI – FIVE MILES

⊥ ***0.5 TO 0.8 CUN*** Δ ***3 TO 5***

Pos: Position of patient: supine.

Loc:
a) On the medial aspect of the upper thigh.
b) On the lateral border of the adductor longus muscle.
c) Medial and superior to the sartorius muscle.
d) At the medial margin of the femoral artery.
e) Inferior to the pubic tubercle.
f) 2 cun lateral to the anterior median line (of the lower abdomen).
g) Directly inferior to St 30.
h) 2 cun below Liv 12 (inguinal groove).
i) 1 cun below Liv 11.

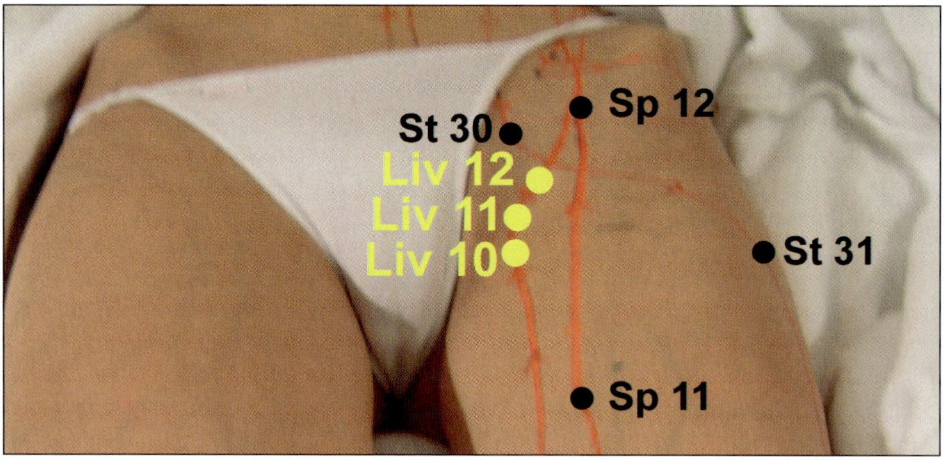

Tip:
a) Adduct (towards the median line) the leg against resistance to expose the adductor longus. This muscle is particularly noticeable with horseriders as they have to adduct their legs (grip them) against the horse.
b) The adductor longus muscle is triangular in shape and is attached by its tendon to the anterior part of the pubis, in the angle between the crest and the symphysis (Gray 1978). The tendon of the adductor longus muscle is the most prominent tendon in the region of the groin. It can be palpated just lateral to where the medial upper leg attaches to the torso.
d) Locate St 30 which is on the anterior aspect of the torso, on the lower abdomen, 2 cun lateral to the anterior median line, level with the superior border of the symphysis pubis (level with Ren 2).
e) Draw a line directly inferior to St 30 on to the thigh.
f) Locate Liv 12 on the inguinal groove, 0.5 cun lateral and inferior to St 30. Liv 12 lies on the femoral artery, where you should be able to palpate a pulse.
g) At 2 cun below Liv 12 palpate for Liv 10 on the line previously drawn.
e) The longitudinal measurement of the patella is 2 cun. You can use this to measure the distance from Liv 12 (inguinal groove) to locate Liv 10.

Note: Qiu (1996) locates LIV 10 in the same location but uses a different description. He locates the point at 2 cun lateral to Ren 2 and then 3 cun below. Soulié (1994) locates LR 10 on the anteromedial surface of the thigh: five large FW (Finger Width) above a large protrusion of the femur of the knee (the medial condyle). About mid-width of the femur; in the angle between the posterior (medial) edge of a longitudinal tendon and the lower edge of a transverse mass; in a hollow; three FW above LR 9; three FW below LR 11; two FW above and anterior to SP 11.

Worsley (1982) locates VIII 10 on the anterior surface of the thigh, lateral to the adductor longus, just medial to the femoral artery. 1 ACI (Anatomical Chinese Inch) distal to the flexure of the groin. Li (1991) locates LIV 10 at 2 cun lateral and 3 cun directly below Ren 2 and 5 cun above Sp 11.

Masayoshi (1975) locates LV 10 at 3 cun below SP 12. Lavier (1974) in an illustration locates LI 10 on the adductor longus muscle, one pouce below and medial to LI 11. Voisin (1974) locates Liv 10 on the medial aspect of the thigh: 3 fb (finger breadth) above and slightly lateral to Liv 9. Wu (1973) locates LI 10 upon the anterior surface of the thigh at one pouce below the flexure of the groin, upon the femoral artery. Shandong (1982) locate Femur-Wuli at 3 cun below Pt. Qichong (St 30) lateral to the m. adductor longus.

Liv 11 YIN LIAN – YIN ANGLE

⊥ ***0.3 TO 0.5 CUN*** **Δ 3**

Pos: Position of patient: supine.

Loc:
a) On the medial aspect of the upper thigh.
b) On the lateral border of the adductor longus muscle.
c) Medial to the femoral artery.
d) Inferior to the pubic tubercle.
e) 2 cun lateral to the anterior median line (of the lower abdomen).
f) Inferior to St 30.
g) 1 cun below Liv 12.

Tip:
a) Adduct (towards the median line) the leg against resistance to expose the adductor longus. This muscle is particularly noticeable with horseriders as they have to adduct their legs (grip them) against the horse.
b) The adductor longus muscle is triangular in shape and is attached by its tendon to the anterior part of the pubis, in the angle between the crest and the symphysis (Gray 1978). The tendon of the adductor longus muscle is the most prominent tendon in the region of the groin. It can be palpated just lateral to where the medial upper leg attaches to the torso.
c) Locate St 30 which is on the anterior aspect of the torso, on the lower abdomen, 2 cun lateral to the anterior median line, level with the superior border of the symphysis pubis (level with Ren 2).

d) Draw a line directly inferior to St 30 on to the thigh.
e) Locate Liv 12 on the inguinal groove, 0.5 cun lateral and inferior to St 30. Liv 12 lies on the femoral artery, where you should be able to palpate a pulse.
f) At 1 cun below Liv 12 palpate for Liv 11 on the line previously drawn.
g) The longitudinal measurement of the patella is 2 cun. You can use this to measure the distance from Liv 12 (inguinal groove) to locate Liv 11 by halving the cun to give 1 cun below Liv 12.

Note: Worsley (1982) locates VIII 11 on the flexure of the groin, just lateral to the femoral artery. Eachou (1995) locates this point as in the main location above. He also locates LIV 11 at 2 inches lateral and 2 inches inferior to CV 2 (Ren 2), and lateral to the adductor muscle and medial to the femoral artery. So (1985) locates LV 11 at two divisions below ST 30 in the crease between the lower abdomen and the top of the thigh, in the hollow at the upper side of the big tendon.

Qiu (1996) locates LIV at 2 cun lateral to Ren 2 and then 2 cun below. Shanghai (1993) locate LR 11 on the medial aspect of the thigh, 2 cun directly below ST 30, at the end of the thigh, below the pubic tubercle. Soulié (1994) locates LR 11 on the thigh, medial face; eight large FW (Finger Width) above the protrusion of the lower head of the femur (medial condyle); at the mid-width of the femur; on the anterior edge of the gracilis and posterior edge of the rectus femoris; in a marked hollow; three FW above LR 10; four FW below LR 12. Academy (1975) locates Liv 11 at 1 cun inferior to the lateral aspect of the femoral artery in the inguinal groove.

Masayoshi (1975) locates LV 11 at 2 cun below SP 12. Lavier (1974) in an illustration locates LV 11 on the inguinal fold, medial to LR 12 which is also in the inguinal fold, directly inferior to KI 11. In this case the Ki channel is1.5 pouce lateral to the anterior median line (Ren channel). Wu (1973) locates LI 11 upon the flexure of the groin, upon the femoral artery. Voisin (1974) locates Liv 11 on the thigh, anterior aspect: 1.5 fb (finger breadth) below and medial to the centre of the inguinal fold, behind the medial border of the sartorius. Li (1991) locates LIV 11 at 2 cun lateral to and 2 cun below Ren 2. Shandong (1982) locate Yinlian at 2 cun below Pt. Qichong (St 30).

Liv 12 in the inguinal groove on the anterior torso.

Liv 12 JI MAI – HASTY PULSE

⊥ *FORBIDDEN TO NEEDLE* Δ *3*

Pos: Position of patient: supine.

Loc: a) On the anterior torso.
b) In the inguinal groove of the groin.
c) On the femoral artery.
d) On the inferolateral corner of the pubic crest.
e) 2.5 cun lateral to the anterior median line (of the lower abdomen).
f) Lateral and inferior to St 30.

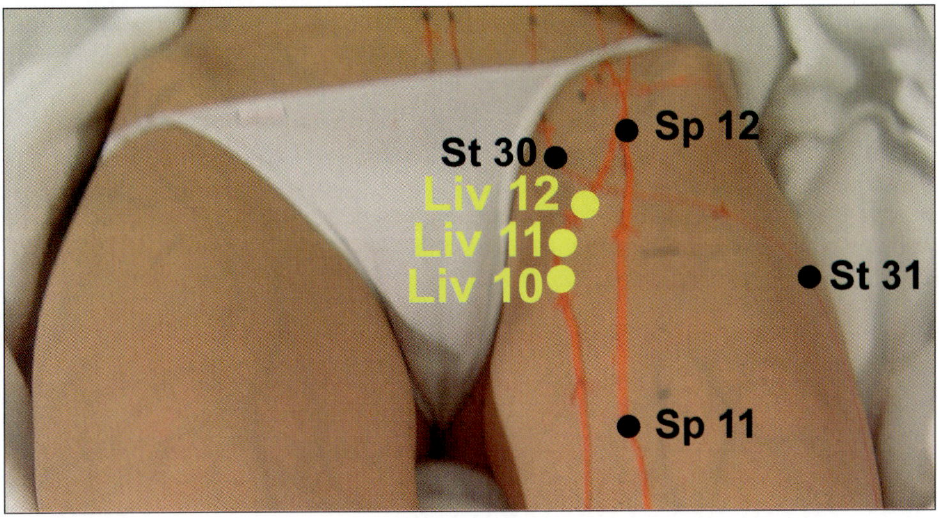

Tip: a) Adduct (towards the median line) the leg against resistance to expose the adductor longus. This muscle is particularly noticeable with horseriders as they have to adduct their legs (grip them) against the horse.
b) The adductor longus muscle is triangular in shape and is attached by its tendon to the anterior part of the pubis, in the angle between the crest and the symphysis (Gray 1978). The tendon of the adductor longus muscle is the most prominent tendon in the region of the groin. It can be palpated just lateral to where the medial upper leg attaches to the torso.
c) Locate St 30 which is on the anterior aspect of the torso, on the lower abdomen, 2 cun lateral to the anterior median line, level with the superior border of the symphysis pubis (level with Ren 2).
d) Draw a line directly inferior to St 30 on to the thigh.
e) Locate Liv 12 on the inguinal groove, 0.5 cun lateral and inferior to St 30. Liv 12 lies on to the femoral artery, where you should be able to palpate a pulse.

Note: Worsley (1982) locates VIII 12 on the flexure of the groin, 2 ACI (Anatomical Chinese Inch) lateral to the mid-line of the pubic symphysis. Voisin (1974) locates Liv 12 in the inguinal fold: superficial to the femoral artery. Lavier (1974) locates LI 12 in an illustration in the inguinal fold, approximately 2 pouce lateral to LI 11 (which is also in the inguinal fold, approximately 3.5 pouce lateral to the anterior median line (Ren channel). He also locates LI 12 inferior to and approximately halfway between ST 30 (at 3 pouce lateral to the anterior median line) and SP 12 (at 4.5 pouce lateral to the anterior median line). Wu (1973) locates LI 12 within the flexure of the groin, at two pouce lateral to the root of the penis.

Jayasuriya (1982) locates Liv 12 at 2.5 cun lateral to the centre of the pubic symphysis. Academy (1975) locate Liv 12 at 2.5 cun lateral to and 1 cun inferior to the superior border of the pubic symphysis, at the lower portion of the inguinal groove. Soulié (1994) locates LR 12 on the upper medial surface of the thigh: just at the lower edge of the apparent extremity of the pubis; in the angle between the bone and the lateral edge of the muscle passing over the pubis (psoas major muscle); just medial to the artery; four FW (Finger Width) above LR 11. Li (1991) locates LIV 12 at2.5 cun lateral to the mid-point of the lower border of the symphysis pubis, at the inguinal groove. The pulse of the arteria femoralis passes the point, and can be palpated.

Eachou (1995) locates LIV 12 at 2,5 inches lateral to the anterior midline level with the inferior margin of the pubic symphysis; or in the inguinal groove lateral and inferior to ST 30. Shanghai (1981) locates Li 12 below the pubic symphysis and lateral to the median line 2.5 units. Deadman (1998) locates LIV 12 at 1 cun inferior and 2.5 cun lateral to Ren 2, in the crease of the groin, medial to the femoral vein. So (1985) locates LV 12 at 1 division directly below ST 30 on top of the pubic bone.

LIV 13-14 are on the anterior torso.

Liv 13 ZHANG MEN – CHAPTER GATE

⊥ ***0.5 TO 0.8 CUN*** ***Δ 3 TO 20***
FORBIDDEN TO NEEDLE AND MOXA THIS POINT DURING PREGNANCY.

- ALARM/Front Collecting/Front Mu/Herald Point of Spleen
- INFLUENTIAL/Hui – Meeting/Gathering/Assembling Point of the Yin or Zang(Solid) Organs: Liver, Heart, Pericardium, Spleen, Kidney and Lŭng – Foot Jue Yin, Hand Shao Yin, Hand Jue Yin, Foot Tai Yin, Foot Shao Yin and Hand Tai Yin
- RE-UNION/Crossing/Meeting Point of the the Yin Channels: Liver, Heart, Pericardium, Spleen, Kidney and Lung – Foot Jue Yin, Hand Shao Yin, Hand Jue Yin, Foot Tai Yin, Foot Shao Yin and Hand Tai Yin Channels
- RE-UNION/Crossing/Meeting Point of the Liver Channel with the Gall Bladder Channel and the Girdle Vessel – Foot Jue Yin Channel with the Foot Shao Yang Channel and Dai Mai (Dai Mai originates from this location)

Pos: Position of patient: supine or lateral recumbent (the person lying on their side with their legs bent).

Loc:
a) On the anterior aspect of the torso.
b) On the mid-abdomen (the middle jiao).
c) Just inferior and anterior to the tip of the eleventh rib (1st of two floating ribs).
d) Just anterior to or on the mid-axillary line.

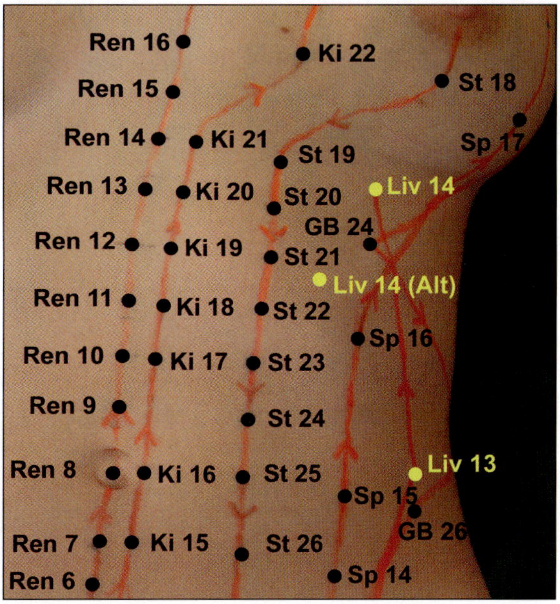

Tip:
a) Ask the patient to bend their elbow at 90 degrees with their upper arm at their side. The tip of their elbow should roughly be at the location of Liv 13 which will be just anterior to or on the mid-axillary line.
b) Press gently to locate the tip of the 11th rib (1st floating rib) and not the tip of the 12th rib (2nd floating rib) which is GB 25.
c) If your finger is palpating posterior to the mid-axillary line you will be near the tip of the 12th rib.
d) If you are having difficulties locating the tip of the 11th rib, first locate the tip of the 12th rib.
e) If the person has alot of flesh in this area, ask them to turn on to their side (lateral recumbent position with their legs bent). This ensures that the rib cage is not as covered by flesh and the 11th rib would be more accessible. People who have alot of flesh covering their anatomy seem to have points that are easier to palpate.
f) With the person in the supine or lateral recumbent position, place two fingers on the rib cage on the back parallel to the ribs.
g) "Walk" your fingers inferiorly until you can only feel flesh, then go to the last place you were able to feel bone, which should be the inferior border of the 12th rib.
h) Then palpate the inferior border of the 12th rib anteriorly until you cannot feel anything.
i) From this area palpate superiorly until your fingers meet a resistence which is the inferior border of the 11th rib.
j) Palpate anteriorly again until there is no resistance.
k) Palpate slightly posteriorly and superiorly until you locate the tip of the 11th rib which should be a sharp pointed structure. This should be just anterior to or on the mid-axillary line
l) From the tip of the 11th rib, palpate for the point. Be careful with your finger pressure as this point can be sensitive. Always locate and needle the point with the person in the same position.

Note: Soulié (1994) locates LR 13 on the lateral part of the lower thorax: above the floating point of the eleventh rib, between the ninth and tenth rib; in the angle between the lower edge of the ninth rib and the anterior edge of a vertical ligament (intercostal). About two FW (Finger Width) lateral to the lateral angle between the ninth and tenth ribs; in a hollow; four FW below LR 14; two FW anterior (medial) to SP 16; two FW posterolateral to ST 23.

So (1985) locates LV 13 up two divisions from the umbilicus, across 6 divisions, just below the end of the 11th rib. Legge (1999) locates Liv 13 just below the free end of the 11th floating rib, close to the mid-axillary line. Li (1991) locates LIV 13 on the lateral side of the abdomen, below the free end of the 11th floating rib. When the elbow is flexed and the arm abducted, the point is located at where the tip of the elbow touches.

Shanghai (1981) locate Li 13 at the anterior end of the eleventh rib on the mid-axillary line. (when the arm is bent at the elbow and held against the side, the tip of the elbow roughly corresponds to the position of the point). Voisin (1974) locates Liv 13 at the upper border of the 11th rib, anterior extremity.

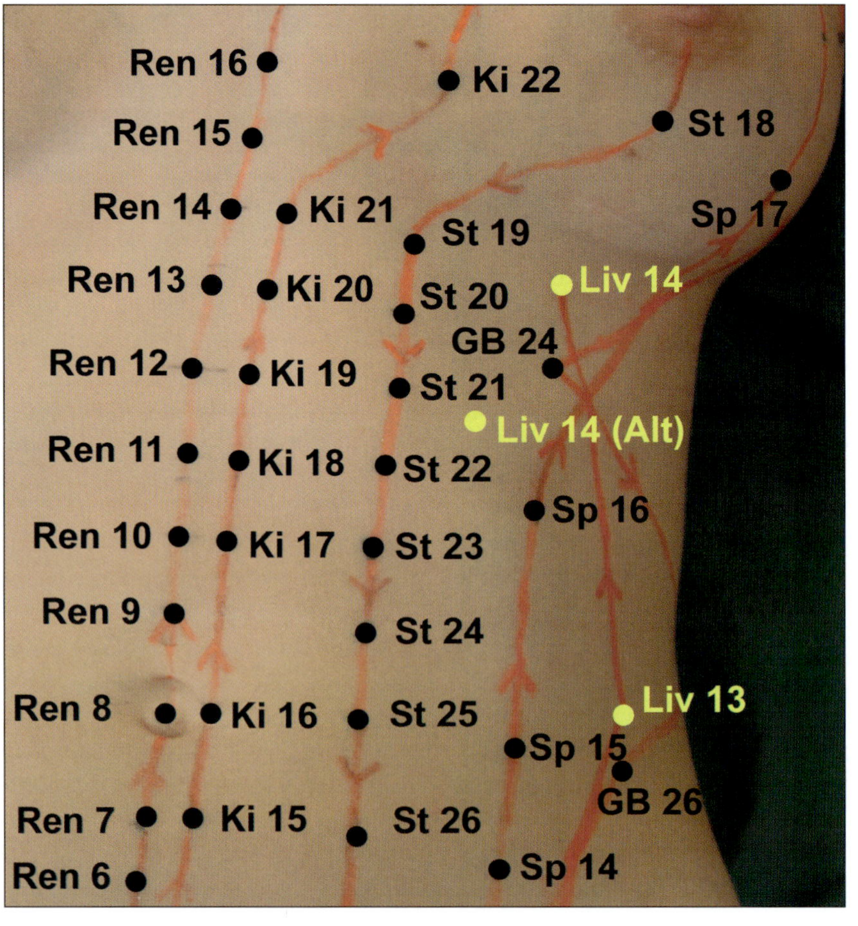

Liv 14 QI MEN – GATE OF HOPE

⊥ ***0.3 TO 0.5 CUN*** Δ ***5 TO 7***

- EXIT
- ALARM/Front Collecting/ Front Mu/Herald Point of Liver
- 8 EXTRAORDINARY VESSEL/Coalescent Point of the Yin Linking Vessel (Yin Wei Mai)
- RE-UNION/Crossing/Meeting Point of the Liver Channel with the Gall Bladder Channel and the Yin Linking Vessel – Foot Jue Yin Channel with the Foot Shao Yang Channel and Yin Wei Mai

NOTE: AN ALTERNATIVE LOCATION IS USED BY SOME TRADITIONAL PRACTITIONERS.

Pos: Position of patient: supine.

Loc: a) On the anterior aspect of the torso.
b) On the mid-abdomen (in the middle jiao).
c) Directly inferior to the nipple.
d) In the sixth intercostal space.
e) 4 cun lateral to the anterior median line.
f) Directly superior to GB 24 (which is in the seventh intercostal space).

Cun: a) Draw a mark directly inferior to the nipple (4th intercostal space) towards the 6th intercostal space. On women you may need to ask them to lift their breast slightly (left breast, right hand; right breast, left hand) to allow you to visualise a "plumb" line inferior to the nipple. This may or not be 4 cun lateral to the nipple. As Liv 14 is on the middle jiao always measure 4 cun from the level of the umbilicus not from the clavicle (upper jiao). If you prefer to use the cun measurements to locate the point, see below, if not, advance to the tips section.
b) The transverse measurement for the middle and lower abdomen (middle and lower jiao) is 2 cun between the anterior median line (at the centre of the umbilicus) and the lateral border of the rectus abdominis muscle (at St 25).
c) The lateral border of the rectus abdominis muscle is not the actual edge of the muscle but the most prominent surface of the muscle before it begins to 'slope' in to the torso. By visualising the corner of an inverted 'L', the point is located on the antero-lateral edge of the muscle. To locate this muscle ask the patient to slightly raise their head. The lateral border of the rectus abdominis muscle is on the most lateral part of the palpable curve which is more medial than the actual edge of the muscle.
d) Another way to mark out the transverse cun measurements at the level of the umbilicus is to locate the medial border of the anterior superior iliac spine (part of the iliac crest). To locate the 4 cun line of the Spleen channel, place a pen longitudinally on the medial border of the anterior superior iliac spine approximately halfway between the centre of the umbilicus and the superior border

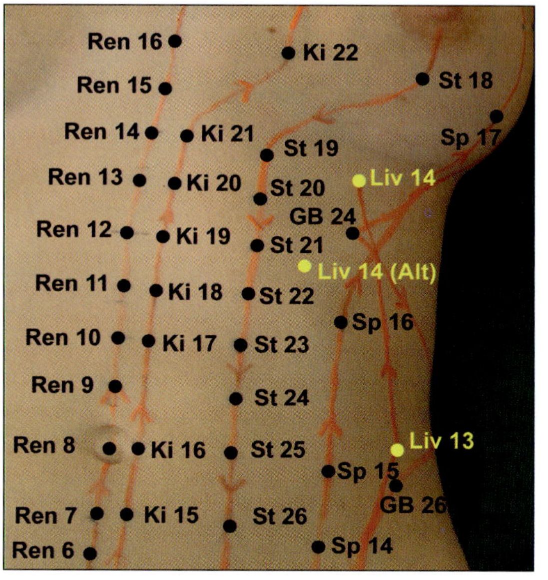

of the symphysis pubis bone. For the Stomach channel divide the 4 cun measurement in half to get 2 cun. The edge of the rectus abdominis muscle is measured as 4 cun. Once established you can then divide the 4 cun into other cun measurements for use on the Stomach and Kidney and Spleen channels etc.

e) The transverse cun measurements for the middle and lower abdomen (middle and lower jiao) includes the Kidney, Stomach, Spleen, Gall Bladder and Liver channels (lateral to the anterior median line): Ki 11 to Ki 21 = 0.5 cun; St 19 to St 30 = 2 cun; Sp 12 = 3.5 cun; Sp 13 to Sp 16 = 4 cun; GB 24 = 4 cun; Liv 14 = 4 cun.

f) Ki 16, St 25 and Sp 15 are all transversely level with the centre of the umbilicus and used as reference points for marking their channels cun measurements.

g) The longitudinal measurement of the mid abdomen is 8 cun from the centre of the umbilicus to the xiphisternal joint (Ren 16).

Tip: a) Visualise and place a mark directly inferior to the nipple or mark in 4 cun lateral to the anterior median line (as explained in the cun measurements section).

b) Palpate and mark in the 6th intercostal space.

c) Palpate for the point which is directly inferior to the nipple, in the 6th intercostal space, (at 4 cun lateral to the anterior median line).

e) Place your finger in the sixth intercostal space between the sixth and seventh ribs and run laterally 4 cun. Ensure that your finger is in the deepest part of the intercostal space.

f) It may be difficult locating the third intercostal space onwards as the pectoralis major muscle covers the surface of the ribs. To assist with point location place a finger in both the first and second intercostal space.

g) Your fingers are now a "rib space" apart. If you place one finger in the second intercostal space, your other finger should then give you a good approximation of the position of the third intercostal space (intercostal spaces are approximately of equal width). You can continue with this method of locating the intercostal spaces. The spaces become more lateral at the level of the fourth intercostal space. At this level the costal cartilages of the lower ribs can merge together to attach to the sternum rather than having individual articulations with the sternum. The intercostal spaces are therefore only easily palpable more laterally.

h) Note that the nipples on men or 'flat chested' women are generally located at the fourth intercostal space.

i) Palpation in the area of 4 cun lateral to the anterior median line should reveal the accurate location for Liv 14. Remember that the nipple lies in the 4th intercostal space, and the distance between the anterior median line to the nipple is 4 cun.
j) Another way of identifying the intercostal spaces is to count from the bottom of the rib cage upwards. For the 9th intercostal space (9 intercostal spaces in total) palpate for the inferior border of the rib cage which will be the 10th rib. Place your finger in the intercostal space superior to this rib. You will now be in the 9th intercostal space.
k) When the 9th intercostal space has been established, place the flat of your index or middle finger in the 9th intercostal space and palpate for the 8th intercostal space by feeling for the superior border of the 9th rib. Once you have located the 9th rib, palpate superiorly until you feel a softness, which will be the 8th intercostal space. Use this procedure to palpate and locate the sixth intercostal space.
l) Palpation gives ultimate accurately.

Note: Shanghai (1981) locate Li 14 at 6 units above the navel and 3 units lateral to Co 14 (Ren 14), in the sixth intercostal space. Lotan (2000) locates Liv 14 in the 6th intercostal, 4 cun lateral to the front midline. Shandong (1982) locates Qimen directly below the nipple in the 6th intercostal space. Academy (1975) locate Liv 14 on the mamillary line, directly below the nipple, in the intercostal space of the 6th and 7th ribs. Eachou (1995) locates LIV 14 in the sixth intercostal space, and on the mid-clavicular line.

Deadman (1998) locate LIV 14 on the mamillary line, in the sixth intercostal space, 4 cun lateral to the midline. Li (1991) locates LIV 14 two ribs below the nipple, in the depression of the 6th intercostal space. So (1985) locates LV 14 up from the umbilicus six divisions and across from the midline four divisions; in between two ribs, between the sixth and seventh rib bones. Soulié (1994) locates LR 14 on the anterolateral thorax: five FW (Finger Width) above the tip of the eleventh rib. Between the sixth and seventh ribs; two FW lateral to and below the nipple (men). In the angle between the lower edge of the sixth rib and the lateral edge of a vertical ligament (interosseous); in a hollow; four FW above and slightly lateral to LR 13; four FW lateral to ST 19; two FW below and lateral to SP 18; two FW anterior to GB 24.

Lawson-Wood (1973) locates VIII 14 below the nipple in the fifth intercostal space. Masayoshi (1975) locates LV 14 on the papillary line below the adhesive part of the costal cartilage. Huang (1993) locates Liv 14 at the tip of the angle of the second rib (this could be a printing error), one cun and five fen lateral to Not Contained (St 19), directly inferior to the breast. Located with the patient's arm raised. Voisin (1974) locates Liv 14 on the lower border of the eighth rib: 1 fb (finger breadth) lateral to the mammary line.

Worsley (1982) locates VIII 14 on the inferior edge of the thoracic cage, on the paramedian nipple line. The point lies at the level half-way between XIII 11 (Ren/CV 11) and XIII 12 (Ren/CV 12). Wu (1973) locates LI 14 upon a line vertical to the nipple at the lower edge of the thoracic cage . Lavier (1974) in an illustration locates LI 14 in the same location as Wu. Katsusuke (1983) locates LV 14 on the extremities of the ninth ribs. Or a place located at the boundary between the rib and the abdomen, directly below the nipple of the breast. The zone between the edge of the rib and the diaphragm.

THIS LOCATION IS SOMETIMES USED BY TRADITIONAL PRACTITIONERS USING FIVE ELEMENTS ACUPUNCTURE.

Liv 14 (Alt) QI MEN – GATE OF HOPE

⊥ ***0.3 TO 0.5 CUN*** ***∆ 5 TO 7***

- EXIT
- ALARM/Front Collecting/Front Mu/Herald Point of Liver
- 8 EXTRAORDINARY VESSEL/Coalescent Point of the Yin Linking Vessel (Yin Wei Mai)
- RE-UNION/Crossing/Meeting Point of the Liver Channel with the Gall Bladder Channel and the Yin Linking Vessel.- Foot Jue Yin Channel with the Foot Shao Yang Channel and Yin Wei Mai

Pos: Position of patient: supine.

Loc: a) On the anterior aspect of the torso.
b) On the mid-abdomen (the middle jiao).
c) Directly inferior to the nipple.
d) On the inferior edge of the thoracic cage.
e) Just medial to the inferior border of the ninth rib, where the costal cartilage meets the tenth rib.
f) At the level half way between Ren (CV) 11 and Ren (CV) 12

Tip: a) Locate Ren 12 by marking half way between the xiphisternal joint and the level of the centre of the umbilicus. This half way mark should be on the anterior median line (4 cun superior to the level of the umbilicus).

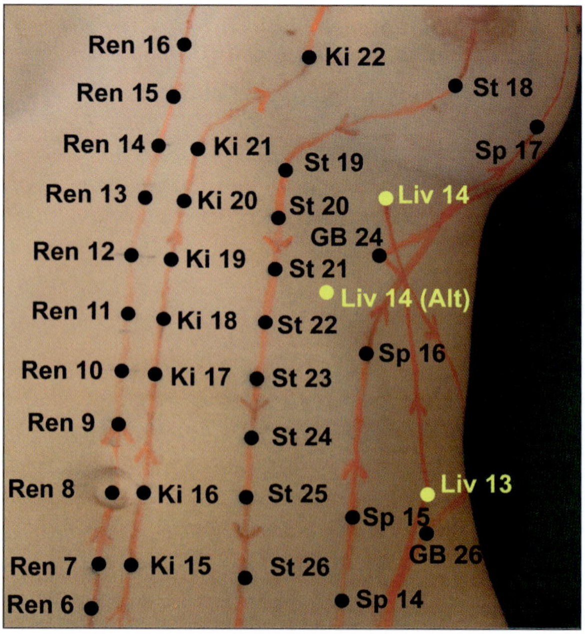

b) Divide in to 3 equal cun measurements from the level of the centre of the umbilicus to Ren 12.
c) Ren 11 is on the anterior median line, 3 cun superior to the level of the centre of the umbilicus (1 cun inferior to Ren 12).
d) Liv 14 is located on the inferior border of the thoracic cage, at the inferior border of the 9th rib which is halfway between Ren 11 and Ren 12. Draw a transverse line from the anterior median line to the rib cage.
e) The line should give an approximate level of the inferior edge of the thoracic cage which should be just medial to the inferior border of the 9th rib where the costal cartilage meets the 10th rib.
f) A notch can be palpated where the costal cartilage meets the 10th rib and Liv 14 can be palpated just medial to this notch.
g) The point should be directly inferior to the nipple. On women you may need to ask them to lift their breast (left breast, right hand; right breast, left hand) to allow you to visualise a "plumb" line inferior to the nipple which is at 4 cun.

Note: Soulié (1994) locates LR 14 on the anterolateral thorax: five FW (Finger Width) above the tip of the eleventh rib. Between the sixth and seventh ribs; two FW lateral to and below the nipple (men). In the angle between the lower edge of the sixth rib and the lateral edge of a vertical ligament (interosseous); in a hollow; four FW above and slightly lateral to LR 13; four FW lateral to ST 19; two FW below and lateral to SP 18; two FW anterior to GB 24.

Lawson-Wood (1973) locates VIII 14 below the nipple in the fifth intercostal space. Masayoshi (1975) locates LV 14 on the papillary line below the adhesive part of the costal cartilage. Huang (1993) locates Liv 14 at the tip of the angle of the second rib (this could be a printing error), one cun and five fen lateral to Not Contained (St 19), directly inferior to the breast. Located with the patient's arm raised. Voisin (1974) locates Liv 14 on the lower border of the eighth rib: 1 fb (finger breadth) lateral to the mammary line.

Worsley (1982) locates VIII 14 on the inferior edge of the thoracic cage, on the paramedian nipple line. The point lies at the level half-way between XIII 11 (Ren/CV 11) and XIII 12 (Ren/CV 12). Wu (1973) locates LI 14 upon a line vertical to the nipple at the lower edge of the thoracic cage . Lavier (1974) in an illustration locates LI 14 in the same location as Wu. Katsusuke (1983) locates LV 14 on the extremities of the ninth ribs. Or a place located at the boundary between the rib and the abdomen, directly below the nipple of the breast. The zone between the edge of the rib and the diaphragm.

Shanghai (1981) locate Li 14 at 6 units above the navel and 3 units lateral to Co 14 (Ren 14), in the sixth intercostal space. Lotan (2000) locates Liv 14 in the 6th intercostal 4 cun lateral to the front midline. Shandong (1982) locates Qimen directly below the nipple in the 6th intercostal space. Academy (1975) locate Liv 14 on the mamillary line, directly below the nipple, in the intercostal space of the 6th and 7th ribs. Eachou (1995) locates LIV 14 in the sixth intercostal space, and on the mid-clavicular line.

Deadman (1998) locate LIV 14 on the mamillary line, in the sixth intercostal space, 4 cun lateral to the midline. Li (1991) locates LIV 14 two ribs below the nipple, in the depression of the 6th intercostal space. So (1985) locates LV 14 up from the umbilicus six divisions and across from the midline four divisions; in between two ribs, between the sixth and seventh rib. bones.

REFERENCES FOR THE LIVER CHANNEL

Huang-fu Mi. Trans: Yang Shou-zhong and Charles Chace 1993 The Systematic Classic of Acupuncture & Moxibustion – Liv 1: 185; Liv 2: 186; Liv 3: 186; Liv 8: 187; Liv 14: 168

Ellis, Wiseman and Boss. 1991 Fundamentals of Chinese Acupuncture – LV 1: 334; LV 4: 336; LV 8: 338

Shanghai College of Traditional Chinese Medicine. 1993 Applied Anatomical Charts of Acupuncture and Moxibustion – LR 2: 154; LR 4: 156; LR 8: 158; LR 9: 158; LR 11

Shandong Medical College and Shandong College of Traditional Chinese Medicine 1982 Anatomical Atlas of Chinese Acupuncture Point – Xingjian (Liv 2): 56; Zhongfeng (Liv 4): 56; Xiguan (Liv 7): 56; Ququan (Liv 8): 56; Yinbao (Liv 9): 56; Femur-Wuli (Liv 10): 56; Yinlian (Liv 11): 56; Qimen (Liv 14): 56

Eachou Chen 1995 Cross-sectional Anatomy of Acupoints – LIV 2: 98; LIV 3: 94; LIV 4: 87; LIV 8: 62; LIV 9: 58; LIV 11: 52; LIV 12: 160; LIV 14: 159

Lotan, Alon 2000 Acupoint Location Guide – Liv 2: 151; Liv 5: 153; Liv 6: 153; Liv 7: 153; Liv 8: 153; Liv 9: 155; Liv 14: 155

So, James Tin Yau (Dr) 1985 The Book of Acupuncture Points – LV 2: 137; LV 3: 138; LV 4: 138; LV 5: 211; LV 8 : 139; LV 11: 69; LV 12: 212; LV 13: 48; LV 14: 46

Soulié De Morant, George. 1994 Chinese Acupuncture – LR 2: 501; LR 4: 502; LR 5: 503; LR 6: 503; LR 7: 504; LR 8: 504; LR 9: 505; LR 10: 505; LR 11: 506; LR 12: 506; LR 13: 506; LR 14: 507

Wu, Wei-P'ing 1973 Chinese Acupuncture – LI 2: 118; LI 4: 118; LI 5: 119; LI 6: 119; LI 7: 119; LI 8: 119; LI 9: 119; LI 10: 119; LI 11: 120; LI 12: 120; LI 14: 120

Voisin, Dr. H 1974 Essentials of Acupuncture – Liv 2: 76; Liv 4: 76; Liv 5: 76; Liv 6: 76; Liv 7: 76; Liv 8: 76; Liv 9: 76; Liv 10: 76; Liv 11: 76; Liv 12: 76; Liv 14: 76

Masayoshi Hyodo 1975 Ryodoraku Acupuncture – LV 2: 49; LV 7: 48; LV 8: 48; LV 9: 48; LV 10: 48; LV 11: 48; LV 14: 48

Shanghai College of Traditional Medicine 1981 Acupuncture – A Comprehensive Text – Li 3: 292; Li 4: 291; Li 8: 290; Li 12: 329; Li 13: 181; Li 14: 180

Jayasuriya, Anton 1982 Clinical Acupuncture – Liv 3: 405; Liv 4: 405; Liv 5: 405; Liv 6: 405; Liv 8: 405; Liv 12: 405

Legge, David 1999 Acupuncture Points and Meridians – Liv 4: 87; Liv 5: 87; Liv 6: 87; Liv 8: 87; Liv 13: 88

Academy of Traditional Chinese Medicine, The 1975 – Outline of Chinese Acupuncture, An. – Liv 3: 187; Liv 4: 187; Liv 5: 188; Liv 6: 188; Liv 8: 189; Liv 11: 190; Liv 12: 190; Liv 14: 191

Lawson-Wood 1973 Acupuncture Handbook – VIII 3 (Liv 3): 44; VIII 6 (Liv 5): 52; VIII 9 (Liv 8): 28; VIII 14 (Liv 14): 19

Cheng Xinnong (Editor) 1987 Chinese Acupuncture and Moxibustion – Liv 4: 212; Liv 8: 213/214

Li Ding (Prof.). 1991. Acupuncture, Meridian Theory and Acupuncture Points – LIV 4: 330; LIV 8: 331; LIV 9: 333; LIV 10: 333; LIV 11: 333; LIV 12: 333/334; LIV 13: 334; LIV 14: 334

Worsley, J R 1982 Traditional Chinese Acupuncture Volume 1 – Meridians and Points – VIII 4: 171; VIII 5: 171; VIII 6: 173; VIII 7: 173; VIII 8: 173; VIII 9: 173; VIII 10: 175; VIII 11: 175; VIII 12: 175; VIII 14: 175

Deadman, Peter; Al-Khafaji, Mazin; Baker, Kevin 1998 Manual of Acupuncture, An – LIV 4: 480; LIV 8: 485; LIV 12: 488; LIV 14: 490

Gray, H; Warwick, Roger; Williams, Peter L 1978 Gray's Anatomy 35th Edition. – (Liv 5) Tendocalcaneus: 575; (Liv 10) Adductor Longus Muscle: 565; (Liv 11) Adductor Longus Muscle: 565

Lavier, Dr. J 1974 Points of Chinese Acupuncture – LI 5: 39; LI 6: 39; LI 7: 39; LI 8: 39; LI 9: 31; LI 10: 25; LI 11: 53; LI 12: 53; LI 14: 55

Shudo Denmei. 1990 Japanese Classical Acupuncture (Introduction to Meridian Therapy) – Liv 8: Unknown Page Number.
Yang Jiasan (Prof) 1982 The Way to Locate Acu-Points – Liv 8: 62; Liv 9: 62
Qiu Mao-Liang 1996 – Chinese Acupuncture and Moxibustion – LIV 8: 149/150; LIV 9: 150; LIV 10: 150; LIV 11: 150
Katsusuke Serizawa 1983 Tsubo – Vital Points for Oriental Therapy – LV 8: 155; LV 14:241

THE CONCEPTION VESSEL (THE REN MAI)

Note: ***The Conception Vessel and the Governor Vessel are two of the 8 Extraordinary Vessels. They are different to the other Extraordinary Vessels in that they have their own points rather than using known points from other channels. Some texts and Schools include the Conception and Governor Vessels as primary channels along with the other twelve primary channels, and these are commonly called the Fourteen Channels.***

Primary channel

The Ren Mai starts at a deep level in the uterus in women, and in the lower abdomen (Ren 3) in men. It emerges in the centre of the perineum at Ren 1, and travels superficially up the anterior median line of the torso to Ren 24 in the middle of the chin, where bilateral deep branches travel round the angle of the mouth to the gums under the upper lip (Du 28), then ascend the cheeks to the optic foramen where they meet St 1.

A second branch is said to originate in the pelvic cavity, enter the spine, and ascend the back.

Note: Soulié (1994) – the two median lines are completely outside the double circle of the flow of energy. Together they constitute a distinct circle of energy. Indeed although their points have only one line, they are double, because each line is double, being composed of an ascending flow (right side of the body) and a descending flow (left side of the body).

Connecting Channel

This leaves the Conception vessel at the inferior border of the sternum at Ren 15, and spreads over the abdomen.

THE CONCEPTION VESSEL (THE REN MAI)

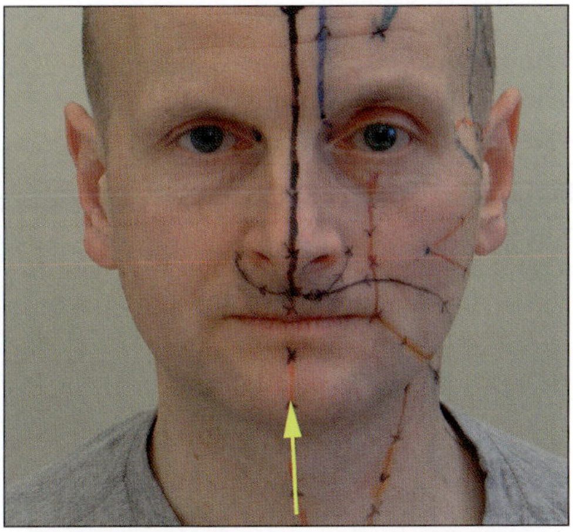

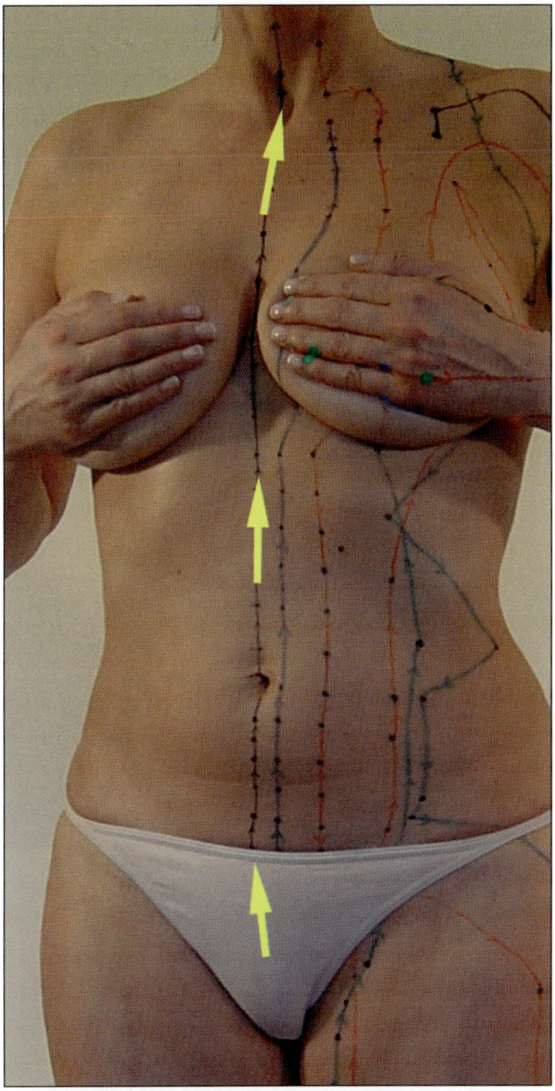

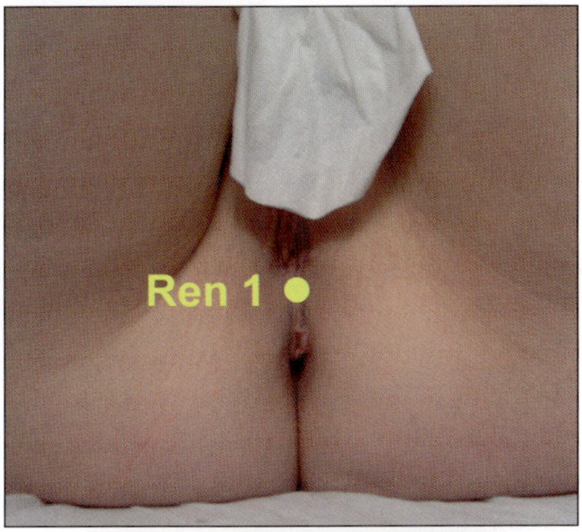

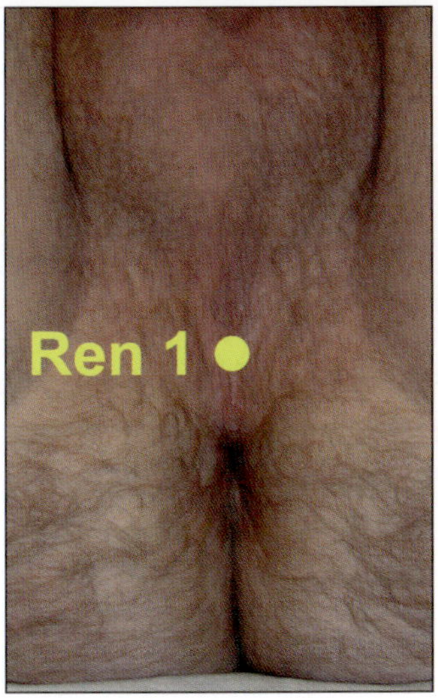

The Points of the Conception Vessel – Ren Mai
(Ren/REN/RN/CV/VC/Co/Conc/PIV/XIII)

All the points of the Ren Mai are found on the anterior median line of the torso/neck/face, and should be located with the patient in a supine position, with the legs relaxed. (The knees may be semi flexed for Ren 1.)

Ren 1 HUI YIN – MEETING OF YIN

⊥ *0.8 TO 1.2 CUN* △ *FORBIDDEN TO USE MOXA*

- ENTRY
- GENERAL JUNCTION/Luo/Connecting/Passage/Lo/Lê
- 8 EXTRAORDINARY VESSEL/Coalescent Point of Du Mai (Governor Vessel)
- 8 EXTRAORDINARY VESSEL/Coalescent Point of Penetrating Vessel (Chong Mai) – see note
- 8 EXTRAORDINARY VESSEL/Coalescent Point of the Yin Linking Vessel (Yin Wei Mai)
- RE-UNION/Crossing/Meeting Point of the Ren Mai with the Du Mai and the Penetrating Vessel – Conception/Directing Vessel with the Governor Vessel and the Chong Mai
- SUN SI-MIAO GHOST (Gui) – Ghost Point Name: Gui Cang – Ghost Store or Ghost's in the Hidden Place

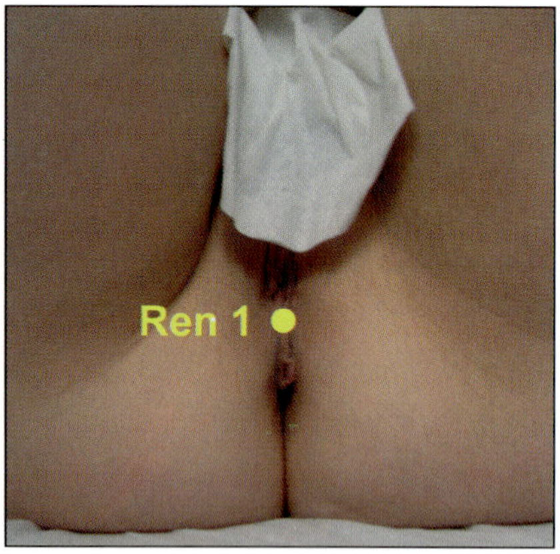

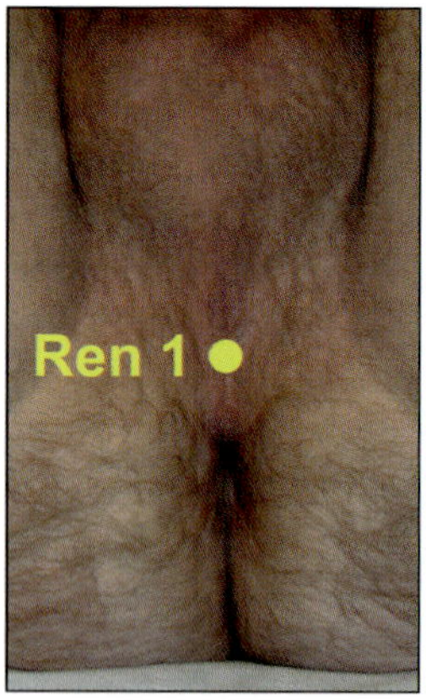

Pos: Position of patient: supine with both legs semi flexed. The legs should be approximately shoulder width apart from each other.

Loc: a) On the inferior pelvic aperture (pelvic outlet).
b) On the median line.
c) On the perineal body.
d) In the centre of the perineum.
e) Midway between the anus and the scrotum (in men).
f) Midway between the anus and the posterior commissure of the vagina (in women).

Tip:
a) ON WOMEN: You can often see a natural depression at the point location where the posterior commissure of the vagina and the anterior margin of the anus provide natural folds of skin. This forms a depression on the perineal body in the centre of the perineum. Palpate the point for confirmation of the point location.
b) ON WOMEN: If you cannot see a depression visualise midway between the anterior margin of the anus and the posterior commissure of the vagina, and palpate on the median line in the centre of the perineum.
c) ON MEN: Before palpating for the point, you can usually see the space between the scrotum and the anterior margin of the anus. The point is located midway between these two landmarks in the centre of the perineum on the median line .
d) The point may be difficult to locate on both men and women, therefore you may need to use palpation if visually you cannot identify where the point is.
e) The position of the patient is important when locating and needling the point as you need to have ease of access as well as making the patient as comfortable and the least exposed as possible. To ensure dignity is maintained you may like to give the patient a paper towel to cover their scrotum or vagina.

Note: In some texts Ren 1 is listed as an 8 EXTRAORDINARY VESSEL/Coalescent Point of Penetrating Vessel (Chong Mai), whereas in others it is omitted.

The longitudinal measurements of the anterior torso are:

9 cun from the xiphisternal joint to the suprasternal fossa (with the space between 2 ribs measuring approximately 1.6 cun in the lower chest, and 1 cun in the upper chest)

8 cun from the centre of the umbilicus to the xiphisternal joint
For the descriptions relating to the channels in the middle jiao, the longitudinal cun measurements are given from the centre of the umbilicus superiorly or from the xiphisternal joint inferiorly, depending on the direction of the flow of the channel.

5 cun from the centre of the umbilicus to the superior border of the symphysis pubis.
For the descriptions relating to the channels in the lower jiao, the longitudinal cun measurements are given from the centre of the umbilicus inferiorly or from the superior border of the symphysis pubis superiorly, depending on the direction of the flow of the channel.

Ren 2 QU GU – CROOKED BONE

⊥ ***0.5 TO 0.8 CUN*** Δ ***3 TO 7***

FORBIDDEN TO NEEDLE AND MOXA THIS POINT DURING PREGNANCY. ONLY NEEDLED IF THERE IS GREAT PUBIC PAIN

- RE-UNION/Crossing/Meeting Point of the Ren Mai with the Liver Channel – Conception/Directing Vessel with the Foot Jue Yin Channel

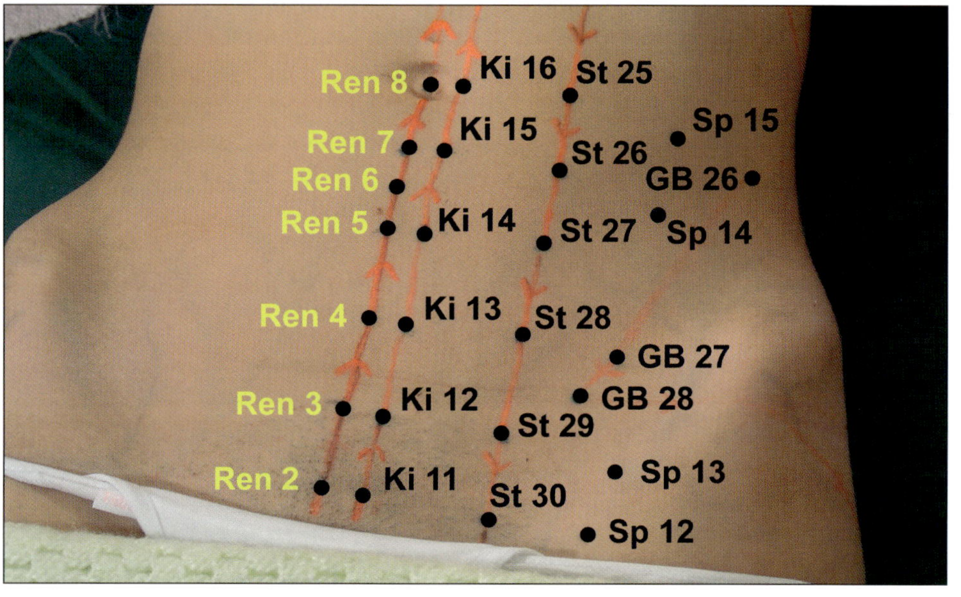

Pos: Position of patient: supine.

Loc:
a) On the anterior aspect of the torso.
b) On the lower abdomen (in the lower jiao).
c) On the anterior median line.
d) Just superior to the superior border of the symphysis pubis.
e) 5 cun inferior to the level of the centre of the umbilicus.

Cun:
a) The longitudinal measurement for the lower abdomen is 5 cun from the superior border of the symphysis pubis (Ren 2) to the centre of the umbilicus (Ren 8).

Tip:
a) First palpate for the superior border of the symphysis pubis by placing your finger on the lower abdomen just inferior to the umbilicus on the anterior median line.
b) Palpate gently but firmly towards the bottom of the lower abdomen until your finger meets resistance which is the superior border of the symphysis pubis.
c) If you find the patient's lower abdomen is rigid, ask them to bend their legs so the whole muscular region in this area is relaxed, then try palpating for the superior border of the symphysis pubis again.

d) Ren 2 is used as a reference for other points as they are described as being lateral to or in relation to the level at Ren 2. Other points can also be described as being located superior to the superior border of the symphysis pubis, on the anterior median line, and 5 cun inferior to the level of the centre of the umbilicus.
e) To ensure that you are on the anterior median line stand at the foot of the couch and visualise the anterior median line.

Ren 3 ZHONG JI – UTMOST MIDDLE

⊥ ***0.5 TO 0.8 CUN*** ***Δ 3 TO 15***
FORBIDDEN TO NEEDLE AND MOXA THIS POINT DURING PREGNANCY.

- ALARM/Front Collecting/Front Mu/Herald Point of Bladder
- RE-UNION/Crossing/Meeting Point of the Ren Mai with the Liver, Kidney and Spleen Channels – Conception/Directing Vessel with the Foot Jue Yin, Foot Shao Yin and Foot Tai Yin Channels

Pos: Position of patient: supine.

Loc: a) On the anterior aspect of the torso.
b) On the lower abdomen (in the lower jiao).
c) On the anterior median line.
d) 1 cun superior to the superior border of the symphysis pubis.
e) 4 cun inferior to the level of the centre of the umbilicus.

Cun: a) The longitudinal measurement for the lower abdomen is 5 cun from the superior border of the symphysis pubis (Ren 2) to the centre of the umbilicus (Ren 8).

Tip: a) First palpate for the superior border of the symphysis pubis by placing your finger on the lower abdomen just inferior to the umbilicus on the anterior median line.
b) Palpate gently but firmly towards the bottom of the lower abdomen until your finger meets resistance which is the superior border of the symphysis pubis.
c) If you find the patient's lower abdomen is rigid, ask them to bend their legs so the whole muscular region in this area is relaxed, then try palpating for the superior border of the symphysis pubis again.
d) Ren 2 is used as a reference for other points as they are described as being lateral to or in relation to the level at Ren 2. Other points can also be described as being located superior to the superior border of the symphysis pubis, on the anterior median line, and 5 cun inferior to the level of the centre of the umbilicus.
e) To ensure that you are on the anterior median line stand at the foot of the couch and visualise the anterior median line.
f) Once located Ren 2, divide 5 cun from Ren 2 to the level of the centre of the umbilicus into 5 equal measurements.
g) Ren 3 is on the anterior median line, 1 cun superior to Ren 2 (with the flow of the channel). Palpate for the point with the flow of the channel from Ren 2 and you should be able to feel a *men* (depression) 1 cun superior to Ren 2.

Note: Voisin (1974) locates Conc 3 on the midline of the body, at 1.5 fb (finger breadth) above the pubis. Lawson- Wood (1973) locates PIV 3 (Ren 3) on the median line, 4cm above the pubic symphysis.

Ren 4 GUAN YUAN – FIRST GATE

⊥ ***0.5 TO 1.0 CUN*** ***Δ 7 TO 15***
FORBIDDEN TO NEEDLE AND MOXA THIS POINT DURING PREGNANCY.

- ALARM/Front Collecting/Front Mu/Herald Point of Small Intestine
- RE-UNION/Crossing/Meeting Point of the Ren Mai with the Liver, Kidney and Spleen Channels – Conception/Directing Vessel with the Foot Jue Yin, Foot Shao Yin and Foot Tai Yin Channels

Pos: Position of patient: supine.

Loc: a) On the anterior aspect of the torso.
b) On the lower abdomen (in the lower jiao).
c) On the anterior median line.
d) 2 cun superior to the superior border of the symphysis pubis.
e) 3 cun inferior to the level of the centre of the umbilicus.

Cun: a) The longitudinal measurement for the lower abdomen is 5 cun from the superior border of the symphysis pubis (Ren 2) to the centre of the umbilicus (Ren 8).

Tip: a) First palpate for the superior border of the symphysis pubis by placing your finger on the lower abdomen just inferior to the umbilicus on the anterior median line.
b) Palpate gently but firmly towards the bottom of the lower abdomen until your finger meets resistance which is the superior border of the symphysis pubis.
c) If you find the patient's lower abdomen is rigid, ask them to bend their legs so the whole muscular region in this area is relaxed, then try palpating for the superior border of the symphysis pubis again.

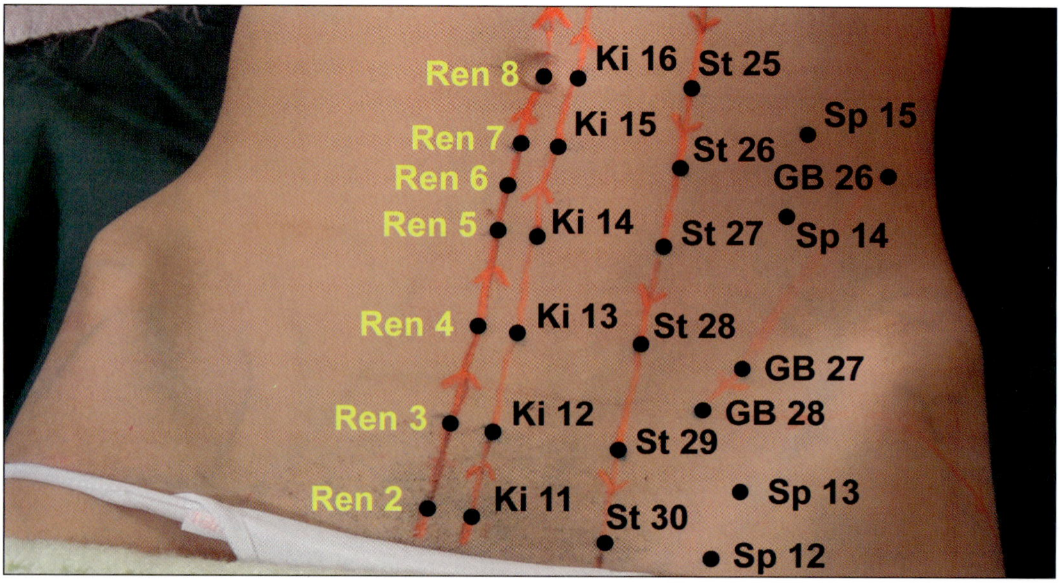

d) Ren 2 is used as a reference for other points as they are described as being lateral to or in relation to the level at Ren 2. Other points can also be described as being locatedsuperior to the superior border of the symphysis pubis, on the anterior median line, and 5 cun inferior to the level of the centre of the umbilicus.
e) To ensure that you are on the anterior median line stand at the foot of the couch and visualise the anterior median line.
f) Once located Ren 2, divide 5 cun from Ren 2 to the level of the centre of the umbilicus into 5 equal measurements.
g) Ren 4 is on the anterior median line, 2 cun superior to Ren 2 (with the flow of the channel). Palpate for the point with the flow of the channel from Ren 2 and you should be able to feel a *men* (depression) 2 cun superior to Ren 2.

Note: Voisin (1974) locates Conc 4 on the midline of the body, 3 fb (finger breadth) above the pubis. Lawson – Wood (1973) locates PIV 4 (Ren 4) on the median line, at the junction of the lower and middle third of a line drawn from the umbilicus to the upper border of the pubic symphysis.

Ren 5 SHI MEN – STONE GATE

⊥ ***0.5 TO 0.8 CUN*** Δ ***3 TO 15***
FORBIDDEN TO NEEDLE AND MOXA THIS POINT DURING PREGNANCY.

- ALARM/Front Collecting/Front Mu/Herald Point of Triple Heater (Main Alarm Point for the Upper, Middle and Lower Jiao of the Triple Heater)

Pos: Position of patient: supine.

Loc: a) On the anterior aspect of the torso.
b) On the lower abdomen (in the lower jiao).
c) On the anterior median line.
d) 3 cun superior to the superior border of the symphysis pubis.
e) 2 cun inferior to the level of the centre of the umbilicus.

Cun: a) The longitudinal measurement for the lower abdomen is 5 cun from the superior border of the symphysis pubis (Ren 2) to the centre of the umbilicus (Ren 8).

Tip: a) First palpate for the superior border of the symphysis pubis by placing your finger on the lower abdomen just inferior to the umbilicus on the anterior median line.
b) Palpate gently but firmly towards the bottom of the lower abdomen until your finger meets resistance which is the superior border of the symphysis pubis.
c) If you find the patient's lower abdomen is rigid, ask them to bend their legs so the whole muscular region in this area is relaxed, then try palpating for the superior border of the symphysis pubis again.

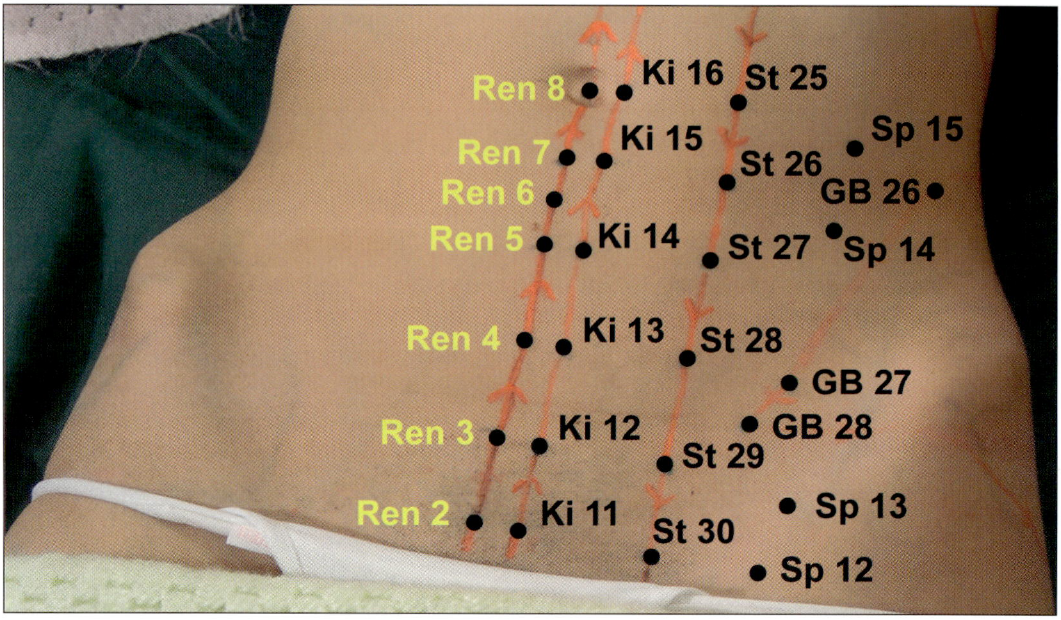

d) Ren 2 is used as a reference for other points as they are described as being lateral to or in relation to the level at Ren 2. Other points can also be described as being located superior to the superior border of the symphysis pubis, on the anterior median line, and 5 cun inferior to the level of the centre of the umbilicus.

e) To ensure that you are on the anterior median line stand at the foot of the couch and visualise the anterior median line.

f) Once located Ren 2, divide 5 cun from Ren 2 to the level of the centre of the umbilicus into 5 equal measurements.

g) Ren 5 is on the anterior median line, 3 cun superior to Ren 2 (with the flow of the channel). Palpate for the point with the flow of the channel from Ren 2 and you should be able to feel a *men* (depression) 3 cun superior to Ren 2.

Note: Voisin (1974) locates Conc 5 on the midline of the body, 3 fb (finger breadth) below the umbilicus. Lawson -Wood (1973) locates PIV 5 (Ren 5) on the median line, at the junction of the upper and middle quarter of a line drawn from the umbilicus to the lower border of the pubic symphysis.

Ren 6 QI HAI – SEA OF QI

⊥ ***0.5 TO 0.8 CUN*** **Δ** ***5 TO 15***
FORBIDDEN TO NEEDLE AND MOXA THIS POINT DURING PREGNANCY.

Pos: Position of patient: supine.

Loc: a) On the anterior aspect of the torso.
b) On the lower abdomen (in the lower jiao).
c) On the anterior median line.
d) 3.5 cun superior to the superior border of the symphysis pubis.
e) 1.5 cun inferior to the level of the centre of the umbilicus.

Cun: a) The longitudinal measurement for the lower abdomen is 5 cun from the superior border of the symphysis pubis (Ren 2) to the centre of the umbilicus (Ren 8).

Tip: a) First palpate for the superior border of the symphysis pubis by placing your finger on the lower abdomen just inferior to the umbilicus on the anterior median line.
b) Palpate gently but firmly towards the bottom of the lower abdomen until your finger meets resistance which is the superior border of the symphysis pubis.
c) If you find the patient's lower abdomen is rigid, ask them to bend their legs so the whole muscular region in this area is relaxed, then try palpating for the superior border of the symphysis pubis again.
d) Ren 2 is used as a reference for other points as they are described as being lateral to or in relation to the level at Ren 2. Other points can also be described as being located superior to the superior border of the symphysis pubis, on the anterior median line, and 5 cun inferior to the level of the centre of the umbilicus.
e) To ensure that you are on the anterior median line stand at the foot of the couch and visualise the anterior median line.
f) Once located Ren 2, divide 5 cun from Ren 2 to the level of the centre of the umbilicus into 5 equal measurements.
e) Ren 6 is on the anterior median line and is 3.5 cun superior to Ren 2 (with the flow of the channel). Palpate for the point with the flow of the channel from Ren 2 and you should be able to feel a *men* (depression) at midway between 3 cun and 4 cun (3.5 cun) superior to Ren 2.

Note: Voisin (1974) locates Conc 6 at 2 fb (finger breadth) below the umbilicus. Soulié (1994) locates CV 6 at 2 FW (Finger Width) below the umbilicus. About one quarter the distance to the pubic bone. In a hollow of the groove between the two rectus abdominus muscles; on the upper edge of a transverse bulge; two points separated by a small rise of the linea alba. One FW above CV 5 and one small FW below CV 7; at either side, at the two FW, KI 15. Lawson-Wood (1973) locates PIV 6 (Ren 6) on the median line, 4cm below the umbilicus.

Ren 7 YIN JIAO – YIN CROSSING

⊥ *0.5 TO 0.8 CUN* Δ *5 TO 7*
FORBIDDEN TO NEEDLE AND MOXA THIS POINT DURING PREGNANCY.

- ALARM/Front Collecting/Front Mu/Herald Point of Triple Heater Lower Jiao
- 8 EXTRAORDINARY VESSEL/Coalescent Point of Penetrating Vessel (Chong Mai) – see note
- RE-UNION/Crossing/Meeting Point of the Ren Mai with the Kidney Channel and the Penetrating Vessel – Conception/Directing Vessel with the Foot Shao Yin Channel and the Chong Mai

Pos: Position of patient: supine.

Loc: a) On the anterior aspect of the torso.
b) On the lower abdomen (in the lower jiao).
c) On the anterior median line.
d) 4 cun superior to the superior border of the symphysis pubis.
e) 1 cun inferior to the level of the centre of the umbilicus.

Cun: a) The longitudinal measurement for the lower abdomen is 5 cun from the superior border of the symphysis pubis (Ren 2) to the centre of the umbilicus (Ren 8).

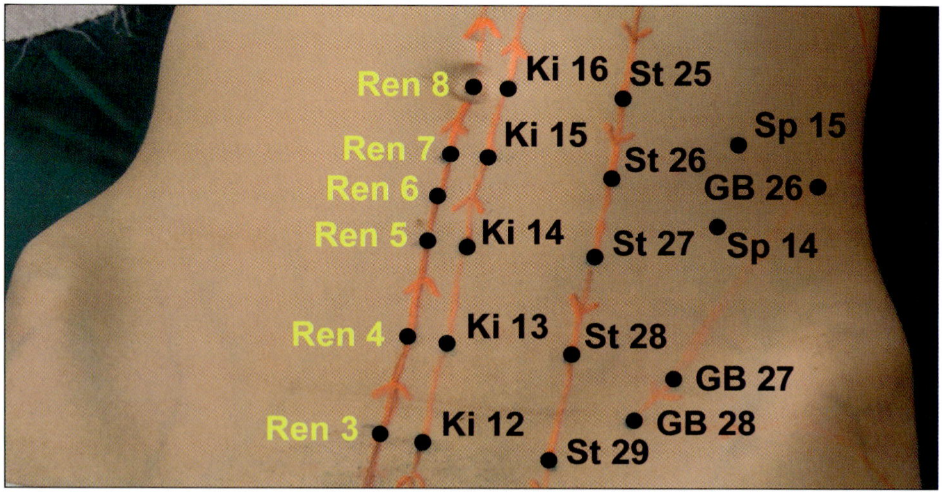

Tip: a) First palpate for the superior border of the symphysis pubis by placing your finger on the lower abdomen just inferior to the umbilicus on the anterior median line.
b) Palpate gently but firmly towards the bottom of the lower abdomen until your finger meets resistance which is the superior border of the symphysis pubis.
c) If you find the patient's lower abdomen is rigid, ask them to bend their legs so the whole muscular region in this area is relaxed, then try palpating for the superior border of the symphysis pubis again.

d) Ren 2 is used as a reference for other points as they are described as being lateral to or in relation to the level at Ren 2. Other points can also be described as being located superior to the superior border of the symphysis pubis, on the anterior median line, and 5 cun inferior to the level of the centre of the umbilicus.

e) To ensure that you are on the anterior median line stand at the foot of the couch and visualise the anterior median line.

f) Once located Ren 2, divide 5 cun from Ren 2 to the level of the centre of the umbilicus into 5 equal measurements.

e) Ren 7 is on the anterior median line and is 4 cun superior to Ren 2 (with the flow of the channel). Palpate for the point with the flow of the channel from Ren 2 and you should be able to feel a *men* (depression) 4 cun superior to Ren 2.

Note: In some texts Ren 7 is listed as an 8 EXTRAORDINARY VESSEL/Coalescent Point of Chong Mai (Penetrating Vessel), whereas in others it is omitted. Soulié (1994) locates CV 7 on the abdomen, medial line: just under the umbilicus at its (cartilaginous edge); in a hollow; between the two rectus abdominus muscles; two points separated by the rise of the linea alba; one small FW (Finger Width) above CV 6; one FW below CV 8, in the umbilicus. Lawson-Wood (1973) locates PIV 7 (Ren 7) on the median line, 2cm below the umbilicus. Vosin (1974) locates Conc 7 at 1 fb (finger breadth) below the umbilicus.

Ren 8 QI ZHONG – SPIRIT DEFICIENCY

⊥ ***FORBIDDEN TO NEEDLE*** Δ ***3 TO 30 (ON SALT)***
FORBIDDEN TO NEEDLE AND MOXA THIS POINT DURING PREGNANCY.

Pos: Position of patient: supine.

Loc:
a) On the anterior aspect of the torso.
b) In between the mid-abdomen and lower abdomen (in between the middle and lower jiao).
c) On the anterior median line.
d) In the centre of the umbilicus.
e) 5 cun superior to the superior border of the symphysis pubis (Ren 2)

Cun:
a) The longitudinal measurement of the mid abdomen is 8 cun from the centre of the umbilicus (Ren 8) to the xiphisternal joint (Ren 16).
b) The longitudinal measurement of the lower abdomen is 5 cun from the superior border of the symphysis pubis (Ren 2) to the centre of the umbilicus (Ren 8).

Tip:
a) Ren 8 is located in the centre of the umbilicus.
b) The level of the centre of the umbilicus is used as a reference for many point location descriptions of the upper and lower abdomen, therefore it is important that you locate the centre of the umbilicus correctly.
c) The point is located 5 cun superior to the upper border of the symphysis pubis.

Ren 9 SHUI FEN – WATER DIVISION

⊥ *0.5 TO 0.8 CUN* Δ *5 TO 15*
FORBIDDEN TO NEEDLE AND MOXA THIS POINT DURING PREGNANCY.

Pos: Position of patient: supine.

Loc: a) On the anterior aspect of the torso.
b) On the mid-abdomen (in the middle jiao).
c) On the anterior median line.
d) 1 cun superior to the level of the centre of the umbilicus.
e) 7 cun inferior to the level of the xiphisternal joint.

Cun: a) The longitudinal measurement for the mid-abdomen is 8 cun from the centre of the umbilicus to the level of the xiphisternal joint.

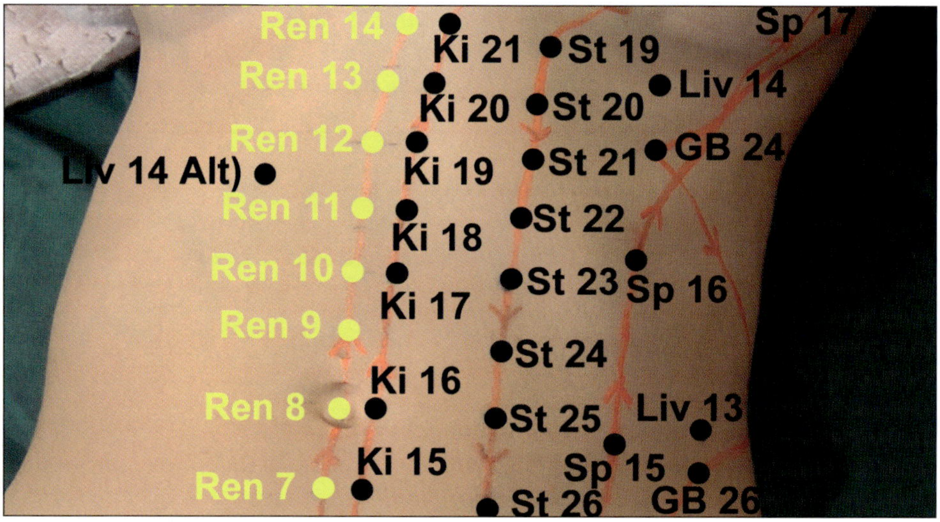

Tip: a) First palpate for the xiphisternal joint by placing a finger from both hands on both lower medial (inner) borders of the rib cage.
b) Palpate the edge of both rib cages superiorly until they meet on the chest. Note that some people have narrow rib cages. A frequent error is not palpating superiorly enough for the xiphisternal joint where Ren 16 is located.
c) If the patient's mid-abdomen is tense or rigid, there may be difficulty feeling for the anatomy. Ask the patient to bend their legs, which should help release some of the tension or rigidity.
d) Once you have located the xiphisternal joint, divide the distance from the level of the centre of the umbilicus to the xiphisternal joint in half to give 4 cun and Ren 12 location on the anterior median line.
e) Divide the lower half of the 4 cun measurement (from the level of the centre of the umbilicus to the level of Ren 12) in to 4 equal divisions.

f) Ren 9 is 1 cun superior to the level of the centre of the umbilicus. Palpate with the flow of the channel from the umbilicus to the 1 cun measurement and feel for a *men* (depression).
g) Make sure that you are on the anterior median line by standing at the foot of the couch and visualise where the anterior median line should be.

Note: Lavier (1974) measures 7 pouce between the tip of the xiphoid process and the umbilicus rather than 8 to the xiphisternal joint. Soulié (1994) locates CV 9 on the abdomen: medial line: just above the cartilaginous edge of the umbilicus. In a hollow; two points separated by the slight rise of the linea alba; on the lower edge of a transverse bulge; one FW (Finger Width) above CV 8, in the umbilicus; one FW below CV 10. Lawson-Wood (1973) locates PIV 9 (Ren 9) on the median line, 2cm above the umbilicus. Voisin (1974) locates Conc 9 at 1 fb (finger breadth) above the umbilicus.

Ren 10 XIA WAN – LOWER DUCT

⊥ ***0.5 TO 0.8 CUN*** **Δ *5 TO 15***
FORBIDDEN TO NEEDLE AND MOXA THIS POINT DURING PREGNANCY.

- RE-UNION/Crossing/Meeting Point of the Ren Mai with the Spleen Channel – Conception/Directing Vessel with the Foot Jue Yin and Foot Tai Yin Channels

Pos: Position of patient: supine.

Loc: a) On the anterior aspect of the torso.
b) On the mid-abdomen (in the middle jiao).
c) On the anterior median line.
d) 2 cun superior to the level of the centre of the umbilicus.
e) 6 cun inferior to the level of the xiphisternal joint.

Cun: a) The longitudinal measurement for the mid-abdomen is 8 cun from the centre of the umbilicus to the level of the xiphisternal joint.

Tip: a) First palpate for the xiphisternal joint by placing a finger from both hands on both lower medial (inner) borders of the rib cage.
b) Palpate the edge of both rib cages superiorly until they meet on the chest. Note that some people have narrow rib cages. A frequent error is not palpating superiorly enough for the xiphisternal joint where Ren 16 is located.
c) If the patient's mid-abdomen is tense or rigid, there may be difficulty feeling for the anatomy. Ask the patient to bend their legs, which should help release some of the tension or rigidity.
d) Once you have located the xiphisternal joint, divide the distance from the level of the centre of the umbilicus to the xiphisternal joint in half to give 4 cun and Ren 12 location on the anterior median line.

e) Divide the lower half of the 4 cun measurement (from the level of the centre of the umbilicus to the level of Ren 12) in half again.
f) Ren 10 is 2 cun superior to the level of the centre of the umbilicus. Palpate with the flow of the channel from the umbilicus to the 2 cun measurement and feel for a *men* (depression).
g) Make sure that you are on the anterior median line by standing at the foot of the couch and visualise where the anterior median line should be.

Note: Lavier (1974) measures 7 pouce between the tip of the xiphoid process and the umbilicus rather than 8 to the xiphisternal joint. Voisin (1974) locates Conc 10 on the midline of the body, 3 fb (finger breadth) above the umbilicus. Soulié (1994) locates CV 10 on the epigastrium, medial line: about one FW (Finger Width) above the umbilicus. About five FW below the sternum. In a hollow between two rectus abdominus muscles. Two points separated by a small rise of the linea alba; on the lower edge of a transverse bulge; one FW above CV 9; one FW below CV 11; about two FW on either side of KI 17. Lawson-Wood (1973) locates PIV 10 (Ren 10) on the median line, 5cm, above the umbilicus.

Ren 11 JIAN LI – ESTABLISHED MILE

⊥ ***0.5 TO 0.8 CUN*** **Δ** ***5 TO 15***
FORBIDDEN TO NEEDLE AND MOXA THIS POINT DURING PREGNANCY.

Pos: Position of patient: supine.

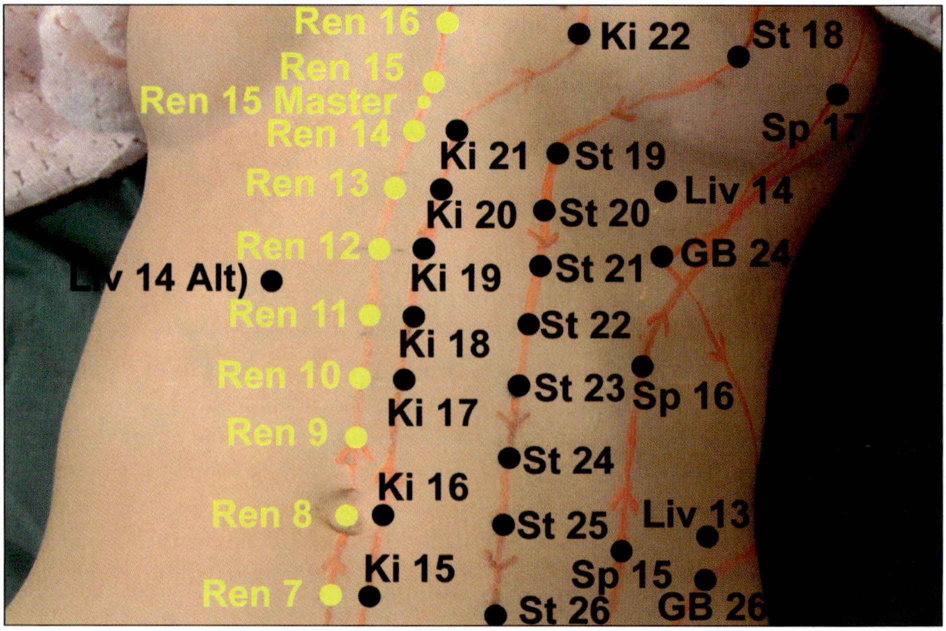

Loc: a) On the anterior aspect of the torso.
b) On the mid-abdomen (in the middle jiao).
c) On the anterior median line.
d) 3 cun superior to the level of the centre of the umbilicus.
e) 5 cun inferior to the level of the xiphisternal joint.

Cun: a) The longitudinal measurement for the mid-abdomen is 8 cun from the centre of the umbilicus to the level of the xiphisternal joint.

Tip: a) First palpate for the xiphisternal joint by placing a finger from both hands on both lower medial (inner) borders of the rib cage.
b) Palpate the edge of both rib cages superiorly until they meet on the chest. Note that some people have narrow rib cages. A frequent error is not palpating superiorly enough for the xiphisternal joint where Ren 16 is located.
c) If the patient's mid-abdomen is tense or rigid, there may be difficulty feeling for the anatomy. Ask the patient to bend their legs, which should help release some of the tension or rigidity.
d) Once you have located the xiphisternal joint, divide the distance from the level of the centre of the umbilicus to the xiphisternal joint in half to give 4 cun and Ren 12 location on the anterior median line.
e) Divide the lower half of the 4 cun measurement (from the level of the centre of the umbilcus to the level of Ren 12) in to 4 equal divisions.
f) Ren 11 is 3 cun superior to the level of the centre of the umbilicus. Palpate with the flow of the channel from the umbilicus to the 3 cun measurement and feel for a *men* (depression).
g) Make sure that you are on the anterior median line by standing at the foot of the couch and visualise where the anterior median line should be.

Note: Lavier (1974) measures 7 pouce between the tip of the xiphoid process and the umbilicus rather than 8 to the xiphisternal joint. Voisin (1974) locates Conc 11, 4 fb (finger Breadth) above the umbilicus; Soulié (1994) locates CV 11 on the epigastrium, medial line: two FW (Finger Width) above the umbilicus (about five FW below the sternum). In the groove between the rectus abdominus muscles. In a hollow; at the level of the union of the ninth rib with the tenth; two points separated by a rise on the line alba; one FW above CV 10; one FW below CV 12; Three FW medial to ST 23, two FW medial and above KI 17, two FW medial and below KI 18. Lawson-Wood (1973) has two location for this point.

The first location for PIV 11 (Ren 11) is on the median line, exactly halfway between the umbilicus and the superior part of the xiphoid process. The second location for PIV 11 is on the median line, 2cm, below the centre of a line drawn from the umbilicus to the superior part of the xiphoid process. Shandong (1982) locate Jianli at 1 cun below Pt. Zhongwan (Ren 12).

Ren 12 ZHONG WAN – MIDDLE DUCT

⊥ ***0.5 TO 0.8 CUN*** Δ ***7 TO 15***
FORBIDDEN TO NEEDLE AND MOXA THIS POINT DURING PREGNANCY.

- ALARM/Front Collecting/Front Mu/Herald Point of Stomach and Triple Heater Middle Jiao
- INFLUENTIAL/Hui – Meeting/Gathering/Assembling Point of the Yang or Fu (Hollow) Organs: Large Intestine, Stomach, Small Intestine, Bladder, Triple Heater and Gall Bladder – Hand Yang Ming, Foot Yang Ming, Hand Tai Yang, Foot Tai Yang, Hand Shao Yang and Foot Shao Yang
- RE-UNION/Crossing/Meeting Point of the Ren Mai with the Yang Channels: Large Intestine, Stomach, Small Intestine, Bladder, Triple Heater and Gall Bladder – Conception/Directing Vessel with theHand Yang Ming, Foot Yang Ming, Hand Tai Yang, Foot Tai Yang, Hand Shao Yang and Foot Shao Yang Channels

Pos: Position of patient: supine.

Loc: a) On the anterior aspect of the torso.
b) On the mid-abdomen (in the middle jiao).
c) On the anterior median line.
d) Midway between the level of the centre of the umbilicus and the xiphisternal joint.
e) 4 cun superior to the level of the centre of the umbilicus.
f) 4 cun inferior to the level of the xiphisternal joint.

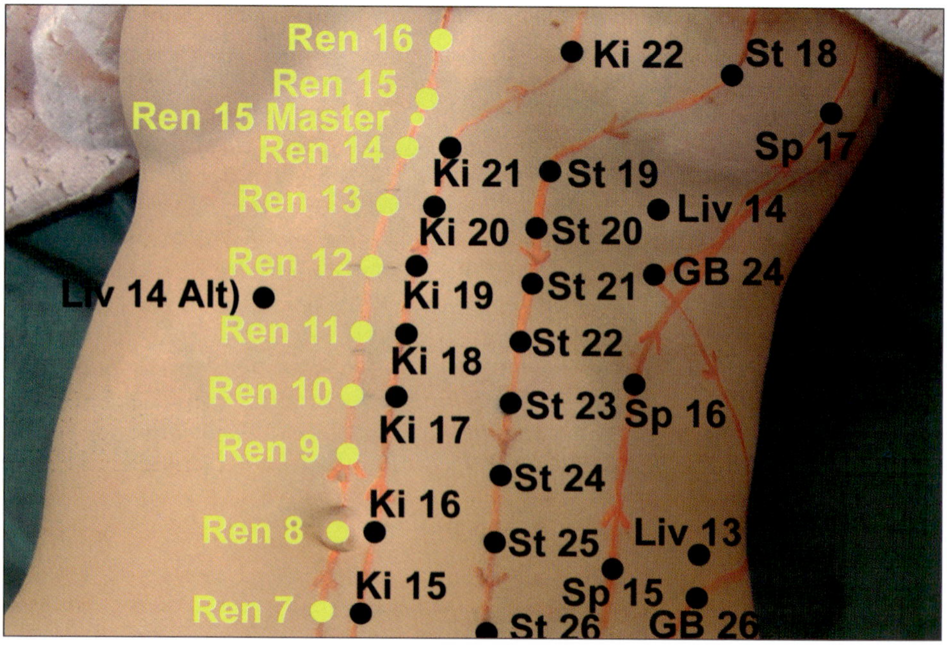

Cun: a) The longitudinal measurement for the mid-abdomen is 8 cun from the centre of the umbilicus to the level of the xiphisternal joint.

Tip: a) First palpate for the xiphisternal joint by placing a finger from both hands on both lower medial (inner) borders of the rib cage.

b) Palpate the edge of both rib cages superiorly until they meet on the chest. Note that some people have narrow rib cages. A frequent error is not palpating superiorly enough for the xiphisternal joint where Ren 16 is located.

c) If the patient's mid-abdomen is tense or rigid, there may be difficulty feeling for the anatomy. Ask the patient to bend their legs, which should help release some of the tension or rigidity.

d) Once you have located the xiphisternal joint, divide the distance from the level of the centre of the umbilicus to the xiphisternal joint in half to give 4 cun.

e) Ren 12 is 4 cun superior to the level of the centre of the umbilicus. Palpate with the flow of the channel from the umbilicus to the 4 cun measurement and feel for a *men* (depression).

f) Make sure that you are on the anterior median line by standing at the foot of the couch and visualise where the anterior median line should be.

g) Note that Ren 12 is always midway between the level of the centre of the umbilicus and the xiphisternal joint. The length of the xiphoid process makes no difference to the location of the point.

Note: Lavier (1974) measures 7 pouce between the tip of the xiphoid process and the umbilicus rather than 8 to the xiphisternal joint. Soulié (1994) locates CV 12 on the epigastrium, medial line: mid-distance from the umbilicus to the lower point of the xiphoid process (three FW (Finger Width) above the umbilicus, four large FW below the lower extremity of the sternum). In the groove between the two rectus abdominus muscles; two points separated by a slight rise of the linea alba. In a hollow; at the level of the mid-height of the medial edge of the ninth rib; one FW above CV 11; one large FW below CV 13; one and a half FW medial to KI 18; four FW medial and above ST 23; four FW medial and below ST 22. Voisin (1974) locates Conc 12 at 5 fb (finger breadth) above the umbilicus (midway between the umbilicus and the tip of the sternum). Lawson-Wood (1973) locates PIV 12 (Ren 12) on the median line, 2cm above the centre of the line drawn from the umbilicus to the superior part of the xiphoid process, at the level of the sterno-costal angles.

Ren 13 SHANG WAN – UPPER DUCT

⊥ ***0.5 TO 0.8 CUN*** Δ ***5 TO 15***
FORBIDDEN TO NEEDLE AND MOXA THIS POINT DURING PREGNANCY.

- RE-UNION/Crossing/Meeting Point of the Ren Mai with the Stomach and Small Intestine Channels – Conception/Directing Vessel with the Foot Yang Ming and Hand Tai Yang Channels

Pos: Position of patient: supine.

Loc:
a) On the anterior aspect of the torso.
b) On the mid-abdomen (in the middle jiao).
c) On the anterior median line.
d) 5 cun superior to the level of the centre of the umbilicus.
e) 3 cun inferior to the level of the xiphisternal joint.

Cun:
a) The longitudinal measurement for the mid-abdomen is 8 cun from the centre of the umbilicus to the level of the xiphisternal joint.

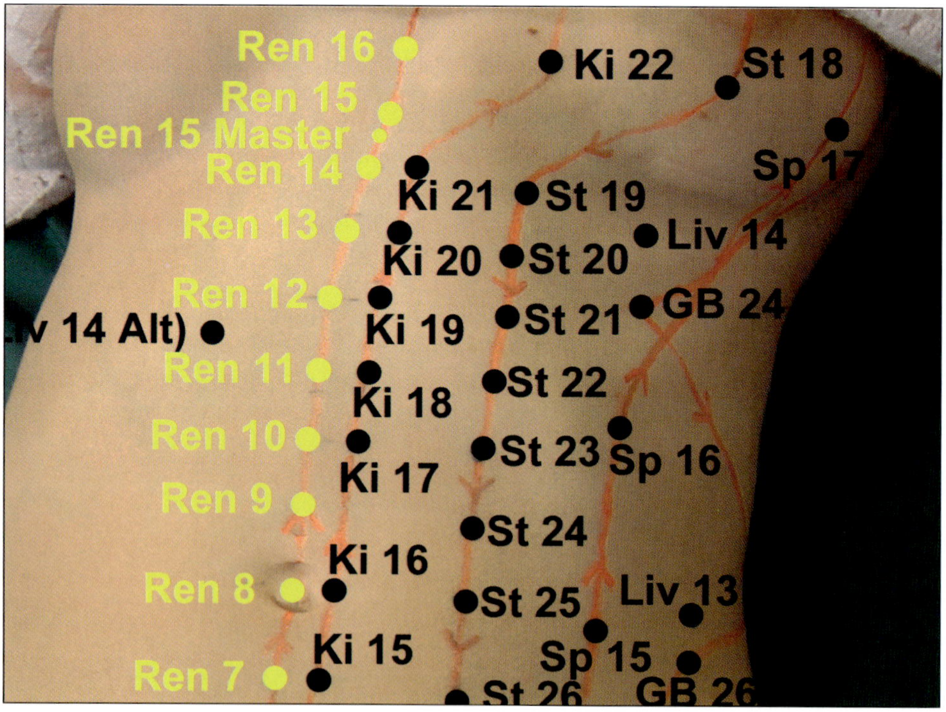

Tip:
a) First palpate for the xiphisternal joint by placing a finger from both hands on both lower medial (inner) borders of the rib cage.
b) Palpate the edge of both rib cages superiorly until they meet on the chest. Note that some people have narrow rib cages. A frequent error is not palpating superiorly enough for the xiphisternal joint where Ren 16 is located.

c) If the patient's mid-abdomen is tense or rigid, there may be difficulty feeling for the anatomy. Ask the patient to bend their legs, which should help release some of the tension or rigidity.
d) Once you have located the xiphisternal joint, divide the distance from the level of the centre of the umbilicus to the xiphisternal joint in half to give 4 cun.
e) Ren 12 is 4 cun superior to the level of the centre of the umbilicus. Palpate with the flow of the channel from the umbilicus to the 4 cun measurement and feel for a *men* (depression).
f) Make sure that you are on the anterior median line by standing at the foot of the couch and visualise where the anterior median line should be.
g) Note that Ren 12 is <u>always</u> midway between the level of the centre of the umbilicus and the xiphisternal joint. The length of the xiphoid process makes no difference to the location of the point.
h) The vast majority of people have a xiphoid process that is approximately 1 cun in length, if so then divide the distance between Ren 12 and the xiphisternal joint into 4. Palpate Ren 13 on the anterior median line, 5 cun superior to the level of the centre of the umbilicus. If the patient has a xiphoid process longer than 1 cun follow the tips below.
i) Locate the tip of the xiphoid process (location of Ren 15) by palpating superiorly from the superior edge of the umbilicus. Palpation should be gently inwards and upwards until you feel some resistance, which will be the tip of the xiphoid process.
j) Divide the distance between Ren 12 and the tip of the xiphoid process in to 3. This point is on the anterior median line approximately 5 cun superior to the level of the centre of the umbilicus. The cun measurements above Ren 12 may be smaller than those below Ren 12 depending on the size of the xiphoid process.
k) Palpation with the flow of the channel from the umbilicus will give you the accurate location for this point. You should be able to palpate a *men* (depression). The cun measurements are guides.
l) Make sure that you are on the anterior median line by standing at the base of the couch and visualise where this longitudinal line should be.
m) Note that the distance between the umbilicus and the xiphisternal joint is 8 cun. The Ki, St and Sp points on the middle abdomen are lateral to the cun measurements and not in relation to the length of the xiphoid process. Therefore the points will only be "crammed" together on the Ren channel if the xiphoid process is long.

Note: Lavier (1974) measures 7 pouce between the tip of the xiphoid process and the umbilicus rather than 8 to the xiphisternal joint. Voisin (1974) locates Conc 13 on the midline of the body, 7 fb (finger breadth) above the umbilicus. Soulié (1994) locates CV 13 on the epigastrium, medial line: two close FW (Finger Width) below the point of the xiphoid process (three FW below the lower extremity of the sternum), Four FW above the umbilicus; in the groove between the two rectus abdominus muscles; in a hollow, two points separated by the linea alba; one large FW above CV 12; one large FW below CV 14; about two FW on either side of ST 21, one large FW medial and below KI 19. Lawson-Wood (1973) locates PIV 13 (Ren 13) on the median line three eighths of the distance between the xiphoid process and umbilicus.

Ren 14 JU QUE – GREAT DEFICIENCY

⊥ ***0.3 TO 0.6 CUN*** ***Δ 5 TO 15***
FORBIDDEN TO NEEDLE AND MOXA THIS POINT DURING PREGNANCY.

- ALARM/Front Collecting/Front Mu/Herald Point of Heart

Pos: Position of patient: supine.

Loc: a) On the anterior aspect of the torso.
b) On the mid-abdomen (in the middle jiao).
c) On the anterior median line.
d) 6 cun superior to the level of the centre of the umbilicus.
e) 2 cun inferior to the level of the xiphisternal joint.

Cun: a) The longitudinal measurement for the mid-abdomen is 8 cun from the centre of the umbilicus to the level of the xiphisternal joint.

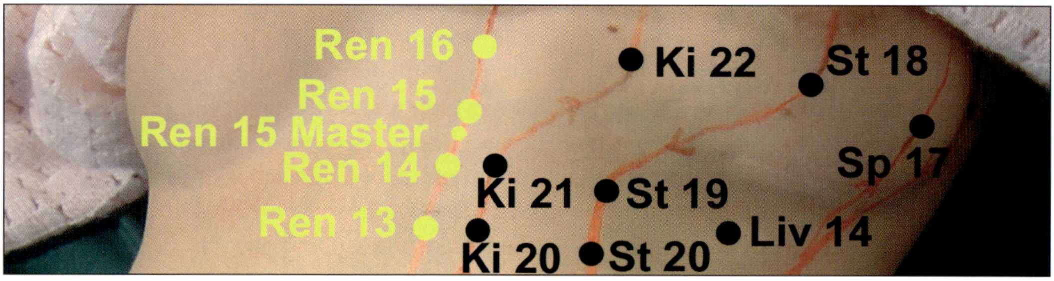

Tip: a) First palpate for the xiphisternal joint by placing a finger from both hands on both lower medial (inner) borders of the rib cage.
b) Palpate the edge of both rib cages superiorly until they meet on the chest. Note that some people have narrow rib cages. A frequent error is not palpating superiorly enough for the xiphisternal joint where Ren 16 is located.
c) If the patient's mid-abdomen is tense or rigid, there may be difficulty feeling for the anatomy. Ask the patient to bend their legs, which should help release some of the tension or rigidity.
d) Once you have located the xiphisternal joint, divide the distance from the level of the centre of the umbilicus to the xiphisternal joint in half to give 4 cun.
e) Ren 12 is 4 cun superior to the level of the centre of the umbilicus. Palpate with the flow of the channel from the umbilicus to the 4 cun measurement and feel for a *men* (depression).
f) Make sure that you are on the anterior median line by standing at the foot of the couch and visualise where the anterior median line should be.
g) Note that Ren 12 is <u>always</u> midway between the level of the centre of the umbilicus and the xiphisternal joint. The length of the xiphoid process makes no difference to the location of the point.

h) The vast majority of people have a xiphoid process that is approximately 1 cun in length, if so then divide the distance between Ren 12 and the xiphisternal joint into 4. Palpate Ren 14 on the anterior median line, 6 cun superior to the level of the centre of the umbilicus. If the patient has a xiphoid process longer than 1 cun follow the tips below.
i) Locate the tip of the xiphoid process (location of Ren 15) by palpating superiorly from the superior edge of the umbilicus. Palpation should be gently inwards and upwards until you feel some resistance, which will be the tip of the xiphoid process.
j) Divide the distance between Ren 12 and the tip of the xiphoid process in to 3. This point is on the anterior median line approximately 6 cun superior to the level of the centre of the umbilicus. The cun measurements above Ren 12 may be smaller than those below Ren 12 depending on the size of the xiphoid process.
k) Palpation with the flow of the channel from the umbilicus will give you the accurate location for this point. You should be able to palpate a *men* (depression). The cun measurements are guides.
l) Make sure that you are on the anterior median line by standing at the base of the couch and visualise where this longitudinal line should be.
m) Note that the distance between the umbilicus and the xiphisternal joint is 8 cun. The Ki, St and Sp points on the middle abdomen are lateral to the cun measurements and not in relation to the length of the xiphoid process. Therefore the points will only be "crammed" together on the Ren channel if the xiphoid process is long.

Note: Lavier (1974) measures 7 pouce between the tip of the xiphoid process and the umbilicus rather than 8 to the xiphisternal joint. Voisin (1974) locates Conc 14 on the midline of the body, 8 fb (finger breadth) above the umbilicus. Soulié (1994) locates CV 14 on the epigastrium, medial line: two close FW (Finger Width) under the lower extremity of the sternum (six FW above the umbilicus); just under the lower point (if there is one) of the xiphoid process. In a hollow of the groove between the two rectus abdominus muscles; two points separated by a small rise of the linea alba; at the level of the union of the eighth with the seventh rib; one large FW above CV 13; two tightened FW under CV 15. On either side, at the union of the eighth with the seventh rib (ST 21); one and a half FW medial and inferior to KI 20; one and a half FW superior and medial to KI 19.

Lawson-Wood (1973) has two locations for Ren 14: PIV 14 location one is on the median line, one eighth of the distance from the xiphoid process to the umbilicus, solar plexus. Location two is on the median line, just less than 2cm below the tip of the xiphoid process.

MASTER PT REN 15 (NO NAME)

⊥ ***0.3 TO 0.5 CUN*** ***Δ 3 TO 5***
FORBIDDEN TO NEEDLE AND MOXA THIS POINT DURING PREGNANCY.

- One of the 7 Internal Dragons (I.D's) Points (the other 6 points are St 25, St 32 and St 41 – bilateral)

Pos: Position of patient: supine.

Loc: a) On the anterior aspect of the torso.
b) On the mid-abdomen (in the middle jiao).
c) On the anterior median line.
d) Just inferior to the tip of the xiphoid process (Ren 15).
e) Approximately 0.1 to 0.3 cun inferior to Ren 15

Cun: a) The longitudinal measurement for the mid-abdomen is 8 cun from the centre of the umbilicus to the level of the xiphisternal joint.

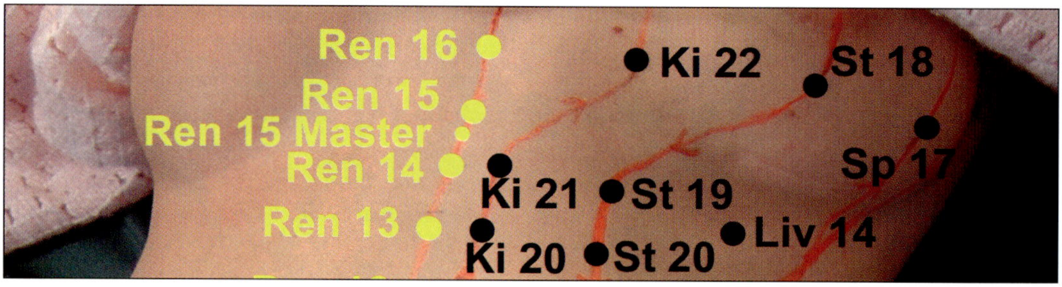

Tip: a) Locate the tip of the xiphoid process by palpating superiorly from the superior edge of the umbilicus. Palpation should be gently inwards and upwards. Eventually you should feel some resistance, this is the tip of the xiphoid process.
b) If the patient's mid-abdomen is tense or rigid, there may be difficulty feeling for the anatomy. Ask the patient to bend their legs, which should help release some of the tension or rigidity.
c) Ren 15 is located on the anterior median line, at the tip of the xiphoid process. Locate this before Ren 15 "Master" point.
d) Once you have located Ren 15, the "master" point is approximately 0.1 to 0.3 cun inferior to it. Palpation takes precedence over the cun measurement. Usually this point has a smaller *men* (depression) than Ren 15.
e) Make sure that you are on the anterior median line by standing at the base of the couch and visualise where this longitudinal line should be.

Note: This point is used by Five Element Practitioners as one of the seven points to release the Internal Dragons (I.D's). Even though it is used by Five Element practitioners, it is not of a Five Element patron.

There seems to be no other reference to this point except in Worsley (1982) – Traditional Chinese Acupuncture Volume 1 – Meridians and Points (Page 259 and 287).

Ren 15 JIU WEI – DOVE TAIL

⊥ ***0.3 TO 0.5 CUN*** Δ ***3 TO 5***
FORBIDDEN TO NEEDLE AND MOXA THIS POINT DURING PREGNANCY.

- JUNCTION/Luo/Connecting/Passage/Lo/Lê)
- ALARM/Front Collecting/Front Mu/Herald Point of Pericardium (Favoured by Five Element Practitioners)

Pos: Position of patient: supine.

Loc: a) On the anterior aspect of the torso.
b) On the mid-abdomen (in the middle jiao).
c) On the anterior median line.
d) At the tip of the xiphoidprocess.
e) 7 cun superior to the level of the centre of the umbilicus.
f) 1 cun inferior to the level of the xiphisternal joint.

Cun: a) The longitudinal measurement for the mid-abdomen is 8 cun from the centre of the umbilicus to the level of the xiphisternal joint.

Tip: a) First palpate for the xiphisternal joint by placing a finger from both hands on both lower medial (inner) borders of the rib cage.
b) Palpate the edge of both rib cages superiorly until they meet on the chest. Note that some people have narrow rib cages. A frequent error is not palpating superiorly enough for the xiphisternal joint where Ren 16 is located.
c) If the patient's mid-abdomen is tense or rigid, there may be difficulty feeling for the anatomy. Ask the patient to bend their legs, which should help release some of the tension or rigidity.
d) Once you have located the xiphisternal joint as a reference, on the vast majority of people the xiphoid process is approximately 1 cun in length. If so divide the distance between Ren 12 and the xiphisternal joint into 4. Palpate Ren 15 on the anterior median line, 7 cun superior to the level of the centre of the umbilicus. If the patient has a xiphoid process longer than 1 cun follow the tips below.
e) Locate the tip of the xiphoid process (location of Ren 15) by palpating superiorly from the superior edge of the umbilicus. Palpation should be gently inwards and upwards until you feel some resistance, which will be the tip of the xiphoid process.
f) Palpation with the flow of the channel from the umbilicus will give you the accurate location for this point. You should be able to palpate a *men* (depression). The cun measurements are guides.
g) Make sure that you are on the anterior median line by standing at the base of the couch and visualise where this longitudinal line should be.
h) Note that the distance between the umbilicus and the xiphisternal joint is 8 cun. The Ki, St and Sp points on the middle abdomen are lateral to the cun measurements and not in relation to the length of the xiphoid process. Therefore the points will only be "crammed" together on the Ren channel if the xiphoid process is long.

Note: Many Schools and texts use the Alarm Point of Pericardium as Ren (CV) 17 and not Ren (CV) 15. Many texts locate this point simply at 7 cun above the umbilicus , or at one cun below the xiphisternal joint, or inferior to the tip of the xiphoid process. Soulié (1994) locates CV 15 on the epigastrium, medial line: one FW (Finger Width) under the lower point of the sternum; mid-height and mid-width on the xiphoid process; in the hole of the xiphoid; two points separated by a slight rise; two tightened FW above CV 14; one large FW under CV 16; at one small FW on either side is KI 21.

Voisin (1974) locates Conc 15 just below the tip of the Xiphoid process. If process absent: 1.5 fb (finger breadth) below the tip of the sternum. Wu (1973) locates VC 15 upon the median line of the thorax, at one pouce below the sterno-xiphoid limit, upon the xiphoid process. So (1985) locates CV 15 one division below the xiphoid process, seven divisions above the umbilicus. He goes on to say that there are eight divisions from the umbilicus to the xiphoid process, not seven, as is shown on many charts.

Deadman (1998) locates REN 15 7 cun above the umbilicus and 1 cun below the sternocostal angle. In this case the cun takes precedemce, therefore if the patient has a long Xiphoid process it is possible that the point may lie on the xiphoid process itself. Lavier (1974) measures 7 pouce between the tip of the xiphoid process and the umbilicus rather than 8 to the xiphisternal joint.

Ren 16 ZHONG TING – MIDDLE HALL

⊥ ***0.3 CUN*** Δ **5**

Pos: Position of patient: supine.

Loc:
a) On the anterior aspect of the torso.
b) On the lower chest (in the upper jiao).
c) At the the inferior edge of the sternum.
d) At the xiphisternal joint.
e) On the anterior median line.
f) At the level of the fifth intercostal space.

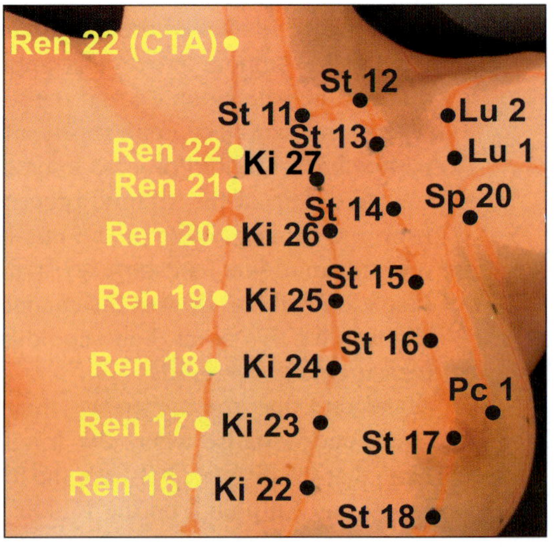

Cun: a) The longitudinal measurement for the mid-abdomen is 8 cun from the centre of the umbilicus to the level of the xiphisternal joint. The longitudinal measurement for the chest is 9 cun from the xiphisternal joint to the suprasternal fossa.

Tip:
a) First palpate for the xiphisternal joint by placing a finger from both hands on both lower medial (inner) borders of the rib cage.
b) Palpate the edge of both rib cages superiorly until they meet on the chest. Note that some people have narrow rib cages. A frequent error is not palpating superiorly enough for the xiphisternal joint where Ren 16 is located.
c) If the patient's mid-abdomen is tense or rigid, there may be difficulty feeling for the anatomy. Ask the patient to bend their legs, which should help release some of the tension or rigidity.
d) Ren 16 is located on the anterior median line, at the xiphisternal joint. Palpation with the flow of the channel towards the point from the umbilicus should give you the accurate location.
e) Make sure that you are on the anterior median line by standing at the base of the couch and visualise where this longitudinal line should be.
f) Ren 16 and the centre of the umbilcus (Ren 8) are used as a reference points for marking out the cun of the middle abdomen. The cun measurements are guides that will give you the area in which to palpate for points on the Ki, St and Sp channels.
g) Ren 16 may also be used as a reference point for marking out the cun of the chest, with the anatomy taking precedence over cun measurements. The longitudinal measurement for the chest is 9 cun from the xiphisternal joint to the suprasternal fossa with the space between the ribs measuring approximately 1.6 cun in the lower chest, and 1 cun in the upper chest.
h) Ren 16 can sometimes be located at the level of the 5th intercostal space, but is not always accurate. Palpating for the intercostal spaces can be challenging as the intercostal spaces can be hidden by muscle or excess tissue.
i) Note that the distance between the umbilicus and the xiphisternal joint is 8 cun. The Ki, St and Sp points on the middle abdomen are lateral to the cun measurements and not in relation to the length of the xiphoid process. Therefore the points will only be "crammed" together on the Ren channel if the xiphoid process is long.
j) An easy way to remember which Ren point lies level with each intercostal space is to remember the formula: 21 minus Ren point X equals intercostal space X.
For example, 21 – Ren 16 = 5th intercostal space; 21 – Ren 20 = 1st intercostal space; etc.

Note: Lavier (1974) measures 7 pouce between the tip of the xiphoid process and the umbilicus rather than 8 to the xiphisternal joint. Some texts simply locate this point at 1.6 cun below Ren (CV) 17. So (1985) locates CV 16 one rib bone below CV 17, at the fifth intercostal space, directly across from ST 18 on the midline. Academy (1975) locates Ren 16 in the midline of the sternum, at the level of the 5th intercostal space, 1.6 cun below Ren 17.

Lawson-Wood (1973) has two locations for Ren 16 – The first location is on the median line, on the superior base of the xiphoid. The second location is on the median line, on the sternum at the level of the fifth intercostal space. Soulié (1994) locates CV 16 on the sternum, midline: one FW above the lower extremity; just under the transverse rise connecting the two fifth ribs (upper part of the supra-xyphoidian fossa). In a narrow vertical groove; two points, one on either side of the groove; one large FW above CV 15; one FW under CV 17. On either side, in the angle between the sternum and the lower edge of the fifth rib, is KI 22.

Ren 17 SHAN ZHONG – WITHIN THE BREAST

⊥ ***0.3 CUN*** ***(EXTREME CAUTION!! WHEN NEEDLING THIS POINT)*** **Δ *3 TO 5***

- ALARM/Front Collecting/Front Mu/Herald Point of Pericardium and Triple Heater Upper Jiao
- A POINT OF THE SEA OF QI (There are two other Sea of Qi Points: Bl 10 and St 9)
- INFLUENTIAL/Hui – Meeting/Gathering/Assembling Point of Qi
- RE-UNION/Crossing/Meeting Point of the Ren Mai with the Spleen, Heart, Small Intestine, Kidney, Pericardium and Triple Heater Channels – Conception/Directing Vessel with the Foot Tai Yin, Hand Shao Yin, Hand Tai Yang, Foot Shao Yin, Hand Jue Yin and Hand Shao Yang Channels

Pos: Position of patient: supine.

Loc: a) On the anterior aspect of the torso.
b) On the chest (in the upper jiao).
c) On the body of the sternum.
d) On the anterior median line.
e) At the level of the fourth intercostal space.
f) Midway between the nipples.
g) Level with Ki 23.

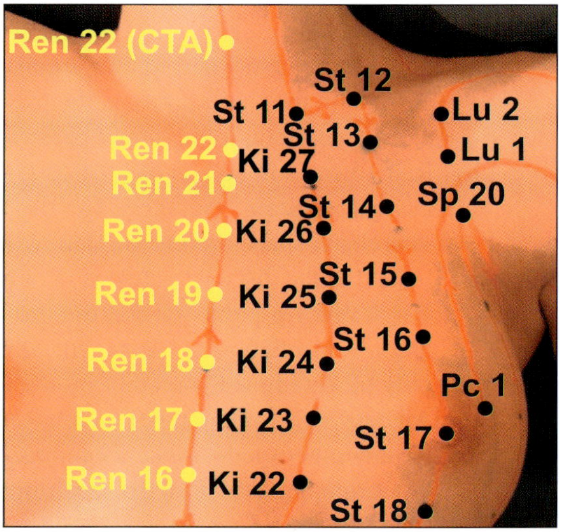

Cun: a) The longitudinal measurement for the chest is 9 cun from the xiphisternal joint to the suprasternal fossa. As the individual cun measurements can be inacurrate, they have not been included in the main location description.

Tip: a) There are two methods of locating Ren 17. The first is to locate Ren 16. Palpate for the xiphisternal joint by placing a finger from both hands on both lower medial (inner) borders of the rib cage.
b) Palpate the edge of both rib cages superiorly until they meet on the chest. Note that some people have narrow rib cages. A frequent error is not palpating superiorly enough for the xiphisternal joint where Ren 16 is located.
c) If the patient's mid-abdomen is tense or rigid, there may be difficulty feeling for the anatomy. Ask the patient to bend their legs, which should help release some of the tension or rigidity.
d) Ren 16 is located on the anterior median line, at the xiphisternal joint. Palpation with the flow of the channel towards the point from the umbilicus should give you accurate location.

e) Make sure that you are on the anterior median line by standing at the foot of the couch and visualise the anterior median line.
f) From Ren 16 palpate superiorly on to the body of the sternum.You should eventually be able to feel a slight contour on the bone of the sternum. As this contour changes you should be able to palpate for a *men* (depression) which is Ren 17.
g) The second method of locating Ren 17 is to count down the intercostal spaces until your finger is in the 4th intercostal space. When you have done this the point lies at the level with the 4th intercostal space, on the anterior median line.
h) To enable accurate point location, palpate with the flow of the Ren channel from the xiphisternal joint on the chest to the level of the 4th intercostal space. You should be able to feel a *men* (depression) on the body of the sternum.
i) You may have problems feeling for the intercostal spaces from the third intercostal space downwards, because of the pectoralis major muscle covering the surface of the ribs. To help you with this you can usually feel the first and second intercostal spaces quite easily from the sternal end of the ribs by placing two of your fingers in the first and second intercostal spaces.
j) Your fingers are now a "rib space" apart, so if you place one finger in the second intercostal space, your other finger should then give you a good approximation of the position of the third intercostal space as the intercostal spaces are of approximately equal width.
k) You can continue with this procedure of working your way down the intercostal spaces, but as you go down past the fourth intercostal space you will need to feel for the spaces more laterally. This is because at this level the costal cartilages of the lower ribs can merge together to attach to the sternum rather than having individual articulations with thesternum. The intercostal spaces are therefore only easily palpable more laterally, and will curve upwards as you palpate laterally from the sternum.
h) Note that the nipples on men or 'flat chested' women are generally located at the fourth intercostal space.
i) An easy way to remember which Ren point lies level with each intercostal space is to remember the formula: 21 minus Ren point X equals intercostal space X.
For example, 21 – Ren 17 = 4th intercostal space; 21 – Ren 20 = 1st intercostal space; etc.

Note: EXTREME CAUTION should be taken when needling this point, make sure that you do not exceed the maximum needle depth. Gray's (1978) The body of the sternum is made up of sternal plates. As we reach adulthood these sternal plates should all eventually fuse together, sometimes they don't. Incomplete fusion can result in a sternal foramen which is a hole between two plates. Therefore needling too deeply can be exceedingly dangerous as the heart lies in this region.

Note: Worsley (1982), the Alarm Point of Pericardium is CV (Ren) 15 and the Triple Heater Upper Jiao is the Alarm Point at CV (Ren) 17. The Ling Shu (Spiritual Pivot) Chapter 33 describes areas to needle rather than point numbers, therefore the middle of the chest is in the region of Ren 17. Ren 17 and St 9 locations seem to have universal agreement as Seas of Qi, but the other Sea of Qi point(s) in the region of the neck, Bl 10 or Du 14/Du 15 seem to have differences of opinion. The College of Traditional Acupuncture favours using Bl 10 in the region of the neck.

Worsley (1982) locates XIII 17 on the anterior median line, 1.6 ACI (Anatomical Chinese Inch) superior to XIII 16, at the level of the fourth intercostal space, and level with IV 23 (Ki 23).

Wu (1973) locates VC 17 upon the median line, at one pouce six fen above the sterno-xiphoid limit, at the height of the nipples.

Shanghai (1981) locate Co 17 on the sternum, level with the niples of the breasts; or just between and above the articulations of the right and left rib with the sternum. Soulié (1994) locates CV 17 on the chest, medial line. Men: mid-distance between the two nipples; two FW (Finger Width) above the lower edge of the lower extremity of the sternum; on the lower edge of the rise betweenthe fourth ribs. At the top of a triangular hollow; in a narrow vertical groove; two points, each one on the edge of the rise of the groove; one FW (Finger Width) above CV 16; one FW under CV 18; on either side, in the angle between the fourth rib and the sternum, is KI 23.

Ren 18 YU TANG – JADE COURT

⊥ ***0.3 CUN*** Δ **5**

Pos: Position of patient: supine.

Loc:
a) On the anterior aspect of the torso.
b) On the chest (in the upper jiao).
c) On the body of the sternum.
d) On the anterior median line.
e) At the level of the third intercostal space.
f) Level with Ki 24.

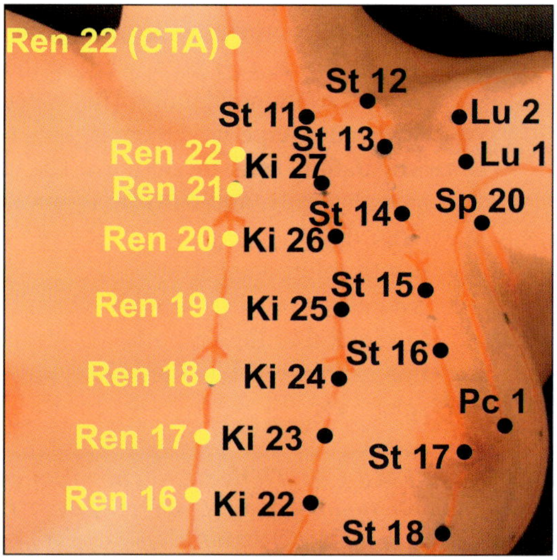

Cun: a) The longitudinal measurement for the chest is 9 cun from the xiphisternal joint to the suprasternal fossa. As the individual cun measurements can be inacurrate, they have not been included in the main location description.

Tip:
a) There are two methods of locating Ren 18. The first is to locate Ren 16. Palpate for the xiphisternal joint by placing a finger from both hands on both lower medial (inner) borders of the rib cage.
b) Palpate the edge of both rib cages superiorly until they meet on the chest. Note that some people have narrow rib cages. A frequent error is not palpating superiorly enough for the xiphisternal joint where Ren 16 is located.
c) If the patient's mid-abdomen is tense or rigid, there may be difficulty feeling for the anatomy. Ask the patient to bend their legs, which should help release some of the tension or rigidity.

d) Ren 16 is located on the anterior median line, at the xiphisternal joint. Palpation with the flow of the channel towards the point from the umbilicus should give you accurate location.
e) Make sure that you are on the anterior median line by standing at the foot of the couch and visualise the anterior median line.
f) From Ren 16 palpate superiorly on to the body of the sternum.You should eventually be able to feel a slight contour on the bone of the sternum. As this contour changes you should be able to palpate for a *men* (depression) which is Ren 17.
g) From Ren 17 palpate superiorly until you feel another contour change. You should be able to palpate for a *men* (depression) which is Ren 18.
h) The second method of locating Ren 18 is to count down the intercostal spaces until your finger is in the 3rd intercostal space. When you have done this the point lies at the level with the 3rd intercostal space, on the anterior median line.
i) To enable accurate point location, palpate with the flow of the Ren channel from the xiphisternal joint on the chest to the level of the 3rd intercostal space. You should be able to feel a *men* (depression) on the body of the sternum.
j) You may have problems feeling for the intercostal spaces from the third intercostal space downwards, because of the pectoralis major muscle covering the surface of the ribs. To help you with this you can usually feel the first and second intercostal spaces quite easily from the sternal end of the ribs by placing two of your fingers in the first and second intercostal spaces.
k) Your fingers are now a "rib space" apart, so if you place one finger in the second intercostal space, your other finger should then give you a good approximation of the position of the third intercostal space as the intercostal spaces are of approximately equal width.
l) You can continue with this procedure of working your way down the intercostal spaces, but as you go down past the third intercostal space you will need to feel for the spaces more laterally. This is because at this level the costal cartilages of the lower ribs can merge together to attach to the sternum rather than having individual articulations with the sternum. The intercostal spaces are therefore only easily palpable more laterally, and will curve upwards as you palpate laterally from the sternum.
m) Note that the nipples on men or 'flat chested' women are generally located at the fourth intercostal space.
n) An easy way to remember which Ren point lies level with each intercostal space is to remember the formula: 21 minus Ren point X equals intercostal space X. For example, 21 – Ren 18 = 3rd intercostal space; 21 – Ren 20 = 1st intercostal space; etc.

Note: Wu (1973) locates VC 18 upon the median line, at three pouce and two fen above the sterno-xiphoid limit, at the level of KI 24 and ST 16. So (1985) locates CV 18 on the median line, one intercostal space above CV 17, traditionally one and three eighth divisions above CV 17, between the 3rd and 4th rib bones.

Worsley (1982) locates XIII 18 on the anterior median line, 1.6 ACI (Anatomical Chinese Inch) superior to XIII 17, at the level of the third intercostal space, and level with IV 24 (Ki 24). Shanghai (1981) locate Co 18 at 1.6 units above Co 17, level with the 3rd intercostal space.

Soulié (1994) locates CV 18 on the chest, medial line: three FW (Finger Width) above the lower extremity of the sternum; on the lower edge of the rise connecting the third ribs; in the hollow of a vertical groove; one FW above CV 17; one FW under CV 19. On either side, in the angle between the third rib and the sternum, is KI 24. Academy (1975) locates Ren 18 on the midline of the abdomen, 1.6 cun above Ren 17, at the level of the 3rd intercostal space.

Ren 19 ZI GONG – PURPLE PALACE

⊥ ***0.3 CUN*** **Δ 5**

Pos: Position of patient: supine.

Loc:
a) On the anterior aspect of the torso.
b) On the chest (in the upper jiao).
c) On the body of the sternum.
d) On the anterior median line.
e) At the level of the second intercostal space.
f) Level with Ki 25.

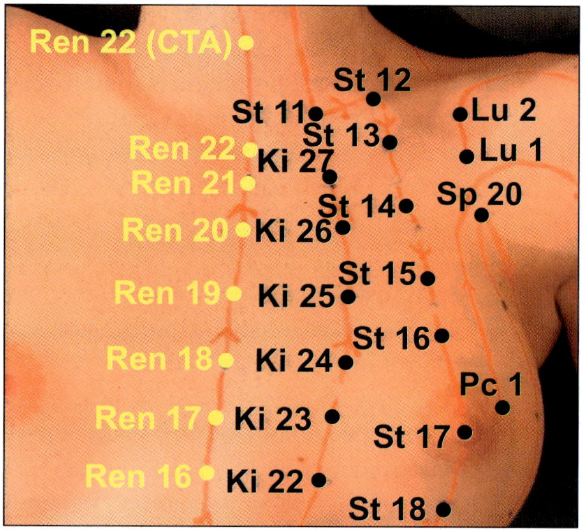

Cun: a) The longitudinal measurement for the chest is 9 cun from the xiphisternal joint to the suprasternal fossa. As the individual cun measurements can be inacurrate, they have not been included in the main location description.

Tip:
a) There are two methods of locating Ren 19. The first is to locate Ren 16. Palpate for the xiphisternal joint by placing a finger from both hands on both lower medial (inner) borders of the rib cage.
b) Palpate the edge of both rib cages superiorly until they meet on the chest. Note that some people have narrow rib cages. A frequent error is not palpating superiorly enough for the xiphisternal joint where Ren 16 is located.
c) If the patient's mid-abdomen is tense or rigid, there may be difficulty feeling for the anatomy. Ask the patient to bend their legs, which should help release some of the tension or rigidity.
d) Ren 16 is located on the anterior median line, at the xiphisternal joint. Palpation with the flow of the channel towards the point from the umbilicus should give you accurate location.
e) Make sure that you are on the anterior median line by standing at the foot of the couch and visualise the anterior median line.

f) From Ren 16 palpate superiorly on to the body of the sternum. You should eventually be able to feel a slight contour on the bone of the sternum. As this contour changes you should be able to palpate for a *men* (depression) which is Ren 17.

g) From Ren 17 palpate superiorly until you feel another contour change. You should be able to palpate for a *men* (depression) which is Ren 18.

h) From Ren 18 palpate superiorly until you feel another contour change. You should be able to palpate for a *men* (depression) which is Ren 19.

i) The second method of locating Ren 19 is to count down the intercostal spaces until your finger is in the 2nd intercostal space. When you have done this the point lies at the level with the 2nd intercostal space, on the anterior median line.

j) To enable accurate point location, palpate with the flow of the Ren channel from the xiphisternal joint on the chest to the level of the 2nd intercostal space. You should be able to feel a *men* (depression) on the body of the sternum.

k) Note that the nipples on men or 'flat chested' women are generally located at the fourth intercostal space.

l) An easy way to remember which Ren point lies level with each intercostal space is to remember the formula: 21 minus Ren point X equals intercostal space X.
For example, 21 – Ren 19 = 2nd intercostal space; 21 – Ren 20 = 1st intercostal space; etc.

Note: Wu (1973) locates VC 19 upon the median line of the sternum at three pouce and two fen below the upper edge of the manubrium at the level of KI 25 and ST 15. So (1985) locates CV 19 on the median line, one intercostal space (1 and 3/8 divisions) above CV 18, that is, at the second intercostal space.

Worsley (1982) locates XIII 19 on the anterior median line, 1.6 ACI (Anatomical Chinese Inch) superior to XIII 18, at the level of the second intercostal space, and level with IV 25 (Ki 25). Shanghai (1981) locate Co 19 at 1.6 units above Co 18, level with the 2nd intercostal space.

Soulié (1994) locates CV 19 on the chest, medial line of the sternum: at the lower edge of the rise connecting the second ribs. In the hollow of a vertcal groove; two points, each on the edge of the groove; one FW (Finger Width) above CV 18; one FW under CV 20; on either side, in the angle between the second rib and the sternum, is KI 25. Academy (1975) locates Ren 19 on the midline of the sternum, 3.3 cun above Ren 17, at the level of the 2nd intercostal space.

Ren 20 HUA GAI – FLOWER COVERING

⊥ *0.3 CUN* Δ *3 TO 5*

Pos: Position of patient: supine.

Loc:
a) On the anterior aspect of the torso.
b) On the chest (in the upper jiao).
c) On the anterior median line.
d) At the superior edge of the crest of the sternal angle.
e) At the level of the first intercostal space.
f) Level with Ki 26.

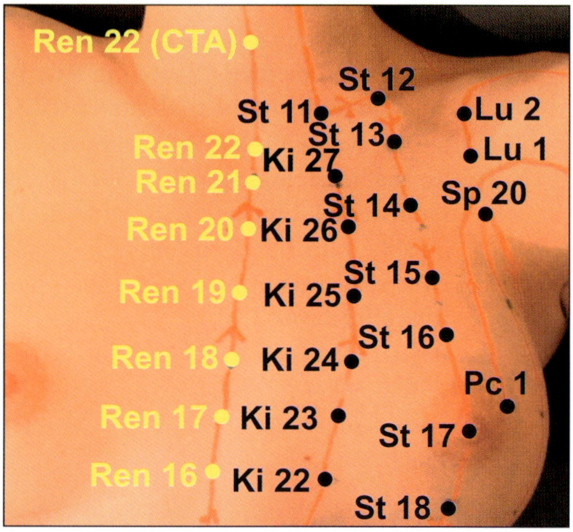

Cun: a) The longitudinal measurement for the chest is 9 cun from the xiphisternal joint to the suprasternal fossa. As the individual cun measurements can be inacurrate, they have not been included in the main location description.

Tip:
a) To locate Ren 20, place your finger in the 1st intercostal space. As the 1st rib can sometimes be hidden by the clavicle, your finger may be between the clavicle and the 2nd rib. This is still acceptable as long as you are able to palpate the space superior to the 2nd rib.When you have located the 1st intercostal space, draw a mark just lateral to the body of the manubrium, the point lies at the level of the 1st intercostal space, on the anterior median line.
b) To accurately locate this point, palpate with the flow of the Ren channel from the xiphisternal joint on the chest at the level of the 1st intercostal space. You should be able to feel a *men* (depression) on the manubrium of the sternum.
c) Note that the nipples on men or 'flat chested' women are generally located at the fourth intercostal space.
d) Another method of locating Ren 20 is to palpate for the sternal angle of the sternum. This can be done by palpating inferiorly from the suprasternal notch on the superior border of the manubrium until you feel a protruberance or crest. The height of the sternal angle is located at the middle of this crest where the superior part of the body of the sternum articulates with the manubrium. Ren 20 is located at the superior edge of the crest of the sternal angle, on the anterior median line.
e) The longitudinal measurement for the chest is 9 cun from the xiphisternal joint to the suprasternal fossa with the space between the ribs measuring approximately 1.6 cun in the lower chest, and 1 cun in the upper chest. Quite often these cun measurements are not accurate, so palpation of the anatomical region and palpation of the point itself will ensure accurate point location.

f) An easy way to remember which Ren point lies level with each intercostal space is to remember the formula: 21 minus Ren point X equals intercostal space X.
For example, 21 – Ren 20 = 1st intercostal space; 21 – Ren 17 = 4th intercostal space; etc.

Note: Wu (1973) locates VC 20 upon the median line, at one pouce and six fen below the upper edge of the manubrium at the level of KI 26 and ST 14. So (1985) locates CV 20 one intercostal space above CV 19 (1 and 3/8 divisions); at the first intercostal space, that is. Worsley (1982) locates XIII 20 on the anterior median line, 1.6 ACI (Anatomical Chinese Inch) superior to XIII 19, at the level of the first intercostal space, and level with IV 26 (Ki 26). Shanghai (1981) locate Co 20 at 1 unit below Co 21, level with the 1st intercostal space. Soulié (1994) locates CV 20 on the upper chest, midline: two FW (Finger Width) under the upper edge of the sternum. At the lower edge of the rise connecting the two first ribs. In the hollow of a vertcal groove; two points, each on the edge of the groove; one FW above CV 19; one FW under CV 21; on either side, in the angle between the first rib and the sternum, is KI 26. Qiu (1996) locates REN 20 on the anterior midline, at the midpoint of the sternal angle. Cheng (1987) locates Ren 20 on the anterior midline, at the midpoint of the sternal angle, at the level with the first intercostal space. Academy (1975) locates Ren 20 on the midline of the sternum, at the junction of the sternal manubrium and the body of the sternum.

Ren 21 XUAN JI – PEARL JADE

⊥ ***0.3 CUN*** **Δ *5***

Pos: Position of patient: supine.

Loc:
a) On the anterior aspect of the torso.
b) On the upper chest (in the upper jiao).
c) On the anterior median line.
d) On the manubrium of the sternum.
e) At the centre of the sternal manubrium.
f) Level with the articulation of the first rib.
g) 1 cun inferior to Ren 22.

Cun:
a) The longitudinal measurement for the chest is 9 cun from the xiphisternal joint to the suprasternal fossa. As the individual cun measurements can be inacurrate, they have not been included in the main location description.

Tip:
a) Palpate for the centre of the suprasternal fossa, which is a large hollow superior to the superior border of the manubrium. Place a mark in the centre of this hollow on the anterior median line (Ren 22).
b) Palpate for the sternal angle. If you palpate from the superior border of the manubrium down its length, you will eventually feel the contour begin elevate slightly like a crest. The height of the sternal angle is at the middle of this crest and is where the superior part of the body of the sternum articulates with the manubrium. Draw a mark at this level.

c) Measure midway between the two marks and palpate for the point. With the flow of the channel palpate for the point superiorly from the height of the sternal angle. The point should be at the centre of the sternal manubrium and level with the articulation of the 1st rib, where it meets the body of the sternal manubrium.

d) If you cannot feel a *men* (depression), locate Ren 20 and Ren 22, then halve the distance and draw a mark. The point can often be located on or in between your original mark (tip b) on the manubrium and your new mark halfway between Ren 20 and Ren 22 (this is why palpation is so important).

e) The longitudinal measurement for the chest is 9 cun from the xiphisternal joint to the suprasternal fossa with the space between the ribs measuring approximately 1.6 cun in the lower chest, and 1 cun in the upper chest. Quite often these cun measurements are not accurate, so palpation of the anatomical region and palpation of the point itself will give you accurate point location.

Note: Worsley (1982) locates XIII 21 on the anterior median line, in the suprasternal notch. Deadman (1998) locates REN 21 on the midline of the manubrium of the sternum, midway between REN 20 and REN 22. So (1985) locates CV 21 one intercostal space above CV 20 (1 and 3/8 divisions), between the clavicle and first rib bones.

Legge (1999) locates Ren 21 on the midline of the sternum, midway between Ren 22 and Ren 20. Lavier (1974) in an illustration locates VC 21 above the suprasternal notch. Soulié (1994) locates CV 21 on the upper sternum, midline: on the lower edge of the ligamentous rise connecting the two clavicle bones. In the hollow of a vertical groove; two points, each on the edge of the groove; one FW (Finger Width) above CV 20; one FW under CV 22. On either side, in the angle between the clavicle and the sternum, is KI 27.

Voisin (1974) locates Conc 21 in the suprasternal fossa: on the superior border of the sternum. Jayasuriya (1982) locates Ren 21 on the midline of the sternum, midway between Ren 22 and Ren 20. Ellis (1991) locates CV 21 on the anterior midline, midway between CV 22 and CV 20. At the centre of the manubrium. Wu (1973) locates VC 21 upon the median line, above the superior edge of the suprasternal notch. Shandong (1982) locate Xuanji on the midsternal line at the level of the superior margin of the first rib.

Ren 22 TIAN TU – HEAVEN RUSHING OUT

⊥ ***0.3 CUN*** **Δ** ***3 TO 7***

- WINDOW OF THE SKY/Window of Heaven
- 8 EXTRAORDINARY VESSEL/Coalescent Point of Yin Linking Vessel (Yin Wei Mai)
- RE-UNION/Crossing/Meeting Point of the Ren Mai with the Yin Linking Vessel – Conception/Directing Vessel with the Yin Wei Mai

Pos: Position of patient: supine.

Loc: **Traditional/Bronze Man/TCM location:**

a) On the anterior aspect of the torso.
b) On the upper chest (in the upper jiao).
c) On the anterior median line.
d) In the centre of the suprasternal fossa.
e) 0.5 cun superior to the suprasternal notch (jugular notch).

Cun: a) The longitudinal measurement for the chest is 9 cun from the xiphisternal joint to the suprasternal fossa. As the individual cun measurements can be inacurrate, they have not been included in the main location description.

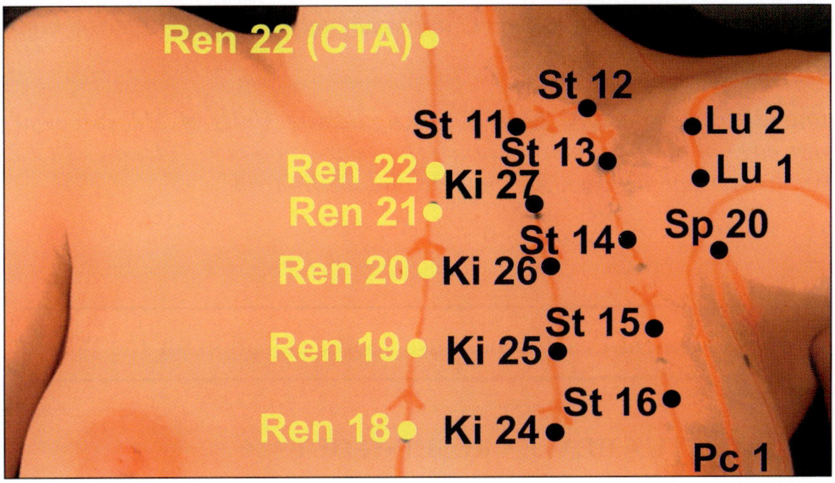

Tip: a) Locate the centre of the suprasternal fossa by palpating the body of the manubrium from the sternal angle (see Ren 21 tips for guidance) superiorly until you feel a notch towards the superior border of the manubrium. This is the suprasternal notch. Place a mark on the notch.

b) From the suprasternal notch palpate superiorly again until you are completely off the manubrium. You will feel a large hollow surrounded on three sides, one by the superior border of the manubrium and the other two by the sternal ends of the clavicles.

c) The point is in the deepest part of the hollow, therefore palpation is important.

d) Ren 22 is also 0.5 cun superior to the suprasternal notch. The cun measurement of the space between the 1st rib and 2nd rib, just lateral to the border of the manubrium is 1 cun. You can halve this measurement and transfer it to the suprasternal notch on the anterior median line and then palpate for the point superior to the notch.

e) The longitudinal measurement for the chest is 9 cun from the xiphisternal joint to the suprasternal fossa with the space between the ribs measuring approximately 1.6 cun in the lower chest, and 1 cun in the upper chest. Quite often these cun measurements are not accurate, so palpation of the anatomical region and palpation of the point itself will give you accurate point location.

Note: Voisin (1974) locates Conc 22 in the suprasternal notch: 1 fb (finger breadth) above the sternum. Worsley (1982) locates XIII 22 on the anterior median line, 1.6 ACI (Anatomical Chinese Inch) superior to XIII 21 (Ren 21), inferior to the cricoid cartilage – see the alternate Ren 21 location. Soulié (1994) locates CV 22 at the front of the neck, bottom, midline: on the posterior edge of the upper edge of the sternum; two points, each in the angle between the sternum and the posterior edge of the head of the clavicle. One FW (Finger Width) above CV 21; three FW under CV 23; one large FW medial and inferior to ST 11.

Wu (1973) locates VC 22 upon the anterior median line of the neck, at one pouce and six fen above the superior edge of the suprasternal notch. Ellis (1991) locates CV 22 on the anterior midline in the centre of the suprasternal notch. So (1985) locates CV 22 on the anterior median line of the neck, at the top of the sternum bone, in the hollow behind the bone. Lavier (1974) in an illustration locates VC 22 approximately halfway between VC 21 and VC 23, on the anterior median line of the neck, approximately where the inferior border of the cricoid cartilage would be located.

Chaitow (1976) locates CV 22 at 1.5 Acupuncture Units of Measurement proximal to the superior edge of the suprasternal notch. Lawson-Wood (1973) locates PIV 21 on the median line, on the sternum between the clavicle and the first rib.

Five Element Practitioners use another location for the Window point

---

Ren 22 TIAN TU – HEAVEN RUSHING OUT

⊥ ***0.3 CUN*** **Δ** ***3 TO 7***

- WINDOW OF THE SKY/Window of Heaven
- 8 EXTRAORDINARY VESSEL/Coalescent Point of Yin Linking Vessel (Yin Wei Mai)
- RE-UNION/Crossing/Meeting Point of the Ren Mai with the Yin Linking Vessel – Conception /Directing Vessel with the Yin Wei Mai

Pos: Position of patient: supine.

Loc: **Five Elements Location** (for use as the Window of the Sky of the Conception Vessel):

a) On the anterior aspect of the neck.

b) On the pharynx.

c) Directly inferior to the cricoid cartilage.

d) On the anterior median line.

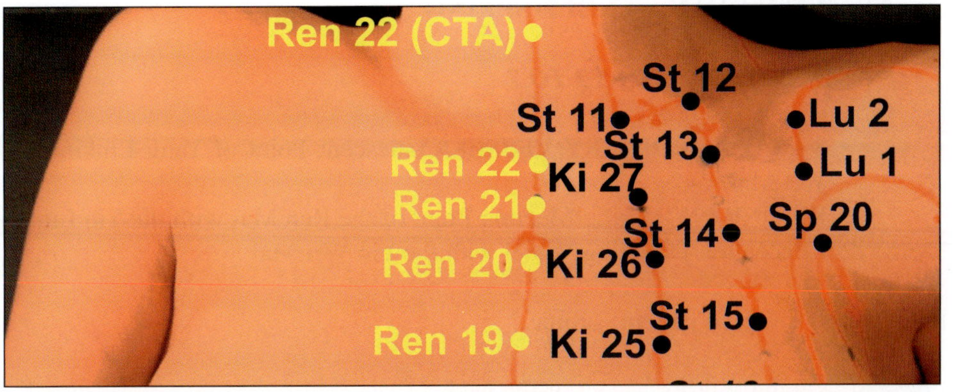

Tip: a) Gently palpate superiorly from the suprasternal fossa on to the neck along the anterior median line. On the neck you should be able to feel a smooth layer of tissue on the surface of the pharynx.

b) As you continue to palpate superiorly with the flow of the Ren channel, you should begin to feel the contour of the pharynx change from this smooth formation to where it feels more "bumpy", this is the inferior border of the cricoid cartilage. Make a mark where the contour changes at the inferior border of the cartilage.

c) Palpate again from the suprasternal fossa until just inferior to the mark. As you palpate towards the mark on the pharynx, you should feel a *men* (depression) which is Ren 22.

d) Lightly palpate for the point otherwise you could make the patient feel a little nauseous.

Note: Shanghai (1984) locates a point that may possibly be the same point as above. It calls the point N-HN-53 Zhiou (Stop Vomiting) which means it is a new point of the head and neck, number 53. The location of the point is midway between Co 23 and Co 22 (the Traditional/Bronze Man/TCM location). Low (1988) gives a 'non-meridial' point midway between CV 22 and CV 23 (OHN4).

Voisin (1974) locates Conc 22 in the suprasternal notch: 1 fb (finger breadth) above the sternum. Worsley (1982) locates XIII 22 on the anterior median line, 1.6 ACI (Anatomical Chinese Inch) superior to XIII 21 (Ren 21), inferior to the cricoid cartilage. Soulié (1994) locates CV 22 at the front of the neck, bottom, midline: on the posterior edge of the upper edge of the sternum; two points, each in the angle between the sternum and the posterior edge of the head of the clavicle.; one FW (Finger Width) above CV 21; three FW under CV 23; one large FW medial and inferior to ST 11.

Wu (1973) locates VC 22 upon the anterior median line of the neck, at one pouce and six fen above the superior edge of the suprasternal notch. Ellis (1991) locates CV 22 on the anterior midline in the centre of the suprasternal notch. So (1985) locates CV 22 on the anterior median line of the neck, at the top of the sternum bone, in the hollow behind the bone. Lavier (1974) in an illustration locates VC 22 approximately halfway between VC 21 and VC 23, on the anterior median line of the neck, approximately where the inferior border of the cricoid cartilage would be located.

Chaitow (1976) locates CV 22 at 1.5 Acupuncture Units of Measurement proximal to the superior edge of the suprasternal notch. Lawson-Wood (1973) locates PIV 22 on the median line 2cm above the superior border of the manubrium

Ren 23 LIAN QUAN – ANGLE SPRING

⊥ ***0.3 TO 0.5 CUN*** **Δ *3 TO 7***

- 8 EXTRAORDINARY VESSEL/Coalescent Point of Yang Linking Vessel (Yang Wei Mai)
- RE-UNION/Crossing/Meeting Point of the Ren Mai with the Yin Linking Vessel – Conception/Directing Vessel with the Yin Wei Mai

Pos: Position of patient: supine.

Loc: a) On the anterior aspect of the neck.
b) At the superior border of the hyoid bone.
c) On the anterior median line.

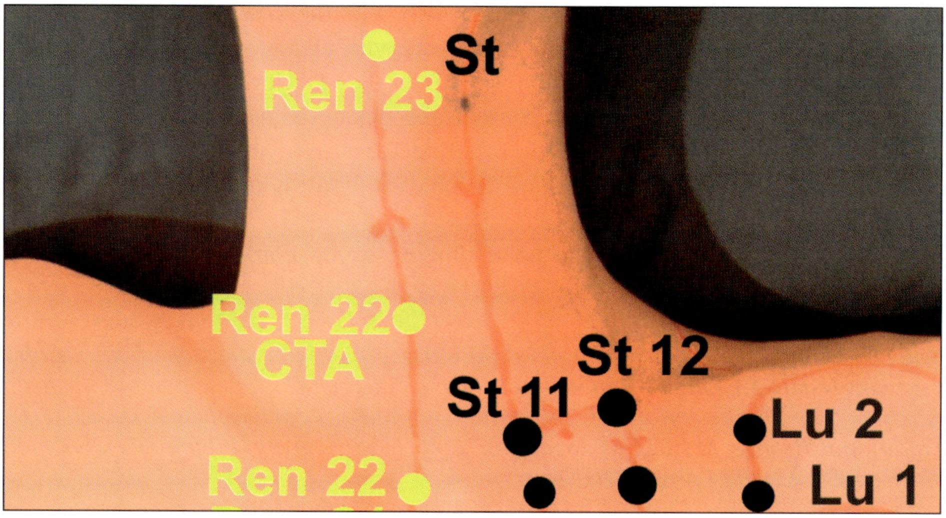

Tip: a) Gently palpate superiorly from the laryngeal prominence of the thyroid cartilage along the anterior median line of the neck. The laryngeal prominence or "Adam's Apple" is often located higher on women than on men.
b) As you palpate towards the jaw, the skin plane will change This is the approximate area of the hyoid bone location. The hyoid bone is a narrow U shaped bone that can be moved from side to side, although this is not advised as the patient may feel choked and vulnerable.
c) You should be able to feel the inferior and superior borders of the hyoid bone by light palpation. If you can't, place a rolled towel behind the neck so the head drops back a little more and the hyoid bone should be more palpable.
d) Palpate for Ren 23 at the superior border of the hyoid bone on the anterior median line.
e) Lightly palpate for the point otherwise you could make the patient feel a little nauseous.

Note: Some texts locate Ren 23 at the inferor border of the hyoid bone, at the superior border of the hyoid bone, or at the level of the hyoid bone.

Note: Lawson-Wood (1973) locates PIV 23 (Ren 23) on the median line, in the angle between the throat and underneath part of the chin. Legge (1999) locates Ren 23 superior to the upper border of the hyoid bone. This is about 1 cun superior to the thyroid cartilage (Adam's apple). Wu (1973) locates VC 23 at the level of the hyoid bone. Lavier (1974) in an illustration, locates VC 23 at the level of the hyoid bone. Voisin (1974) locates Conc 23 on the neck: upper border of the larynx. Shanghai (1981) locates Co 23 in the depression between the pharyngeal prominence and the lower margin of the hyoid bone.

Qiu (1996) locates REN 23 at the midpoint of the upper border of the hyoid bone. Masayoshi (1975) in an illustration locates CV 23 on the upper border of the laryngeal prominence. Academy (1975) locate Ren 23 in the midline of the neck, midway between the tip of the cricoid cartilage and the border of the mandible. Soulié (1994) locates CV 23 on the front of the neck, midline: mid-height above the prominence and the two horns of the thyroid cartilage, larynx, Adam's apple. At mid-height of the transverse cartilage (hyoid bone); in the hollow of a vertical groove between the insertions of the sternocleidohyoidian muscles; two points, on the edge of each insertion; three FW (Finger Width) above CV 22; two FW on either side and lower down is ST 9; three FW on either side and above is LI 18.

Yang (1982) locates Ren 23 between the Adam's apple and the mandible. Worsley (1982) locates XIII 23 on the anterior median line, directly inferior to the hyoid bone. Lotan (2000) locates CV (Ren) 23 in the centre of the hyoid superior border. Jayasuriya (1982) locates Ren 23 on the midline of the neck, midway between the upper border of the cricoid cartilage and the lower border of the mandible. So (1985) locates CV 23 upon the Adam's apple in the hollow of the "V." On females this bone is a little high and small.

Cheng (1987) locates Ren 23 above the Adam's apple, in the depression of the upper border of the hyoid bone. Shanghai (1993) locates RN 23 on the neck, on the anterior midline, on the upper border of the laryngeal protruberance, in the depression superior to the hyoid bone.

Eachou (1995) locates CV 23 in the fossa superior to the thyroid cartilage between the hyoid and mandibular bones. Li (1991) locates REN 23 in the depression above the Adam's apple. Put the transverse crease of the thumb upon the middle of the chin. The place where the tip of the thumb touches is Ren 23.

Deadman (1998) locates REN 23 on the anterior midline of the neck, in the depression above the hyoid bone. Ellis (1991) locates CV 23 on the anterior midline of the throat, above the Adam's apple, in the depression at the upper border of the hyoid bone.

Ren 24 CHENG JIANG – RECEIVING FLUID

⊥ ***0.2 TO 0.3 CUN*** ***Δ 3 TO 7***

- EXIT
- RE-UNION/Crossing/ Meeting Point of the Ren Mai with the Stomach Channel and Du Mai – Conception/Directing Vessel with the Foot Yang Ming Channel and the Governor Vessel
- SUN SI-MIAO GHOST (Gui) – Ghost Point Name: Gui Shi – Ghost Market

Pos: Position of patient: supine or seated.

Loc: a) On the face.
b On the mandible bone (lower jaw).
c) In the middle of the mentolabial groove.
d) Directly superior to the mental shelf.
e) At the inferior border of the orbicularis oris muscle.
f) On the anterior median line.

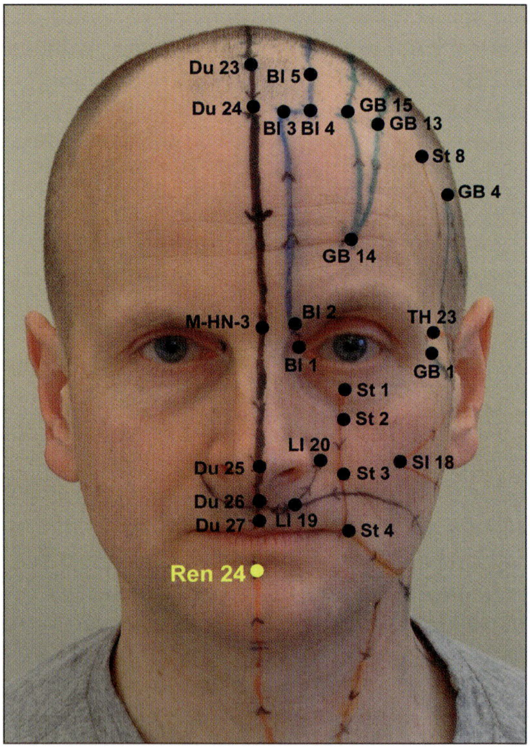

Tip: a) The location description may look complicated, but it is quite simple to locate. First of all draw a vertical mark on the chin showing the anterior median line.
c) Draw the mentolabial groove which is formed by the inferior border of the orbicularis oris muscle. The groove is inferior to the lower lip and it can be seen on may people as an inverted U shape or a horizontal line. If you cannot see the groove, ask your patient to lower their bottom lip (sulky expression).
d) You now have the vertical axis of the anterior medianline and the horizontal/curved axis of the groove. Palpate for the point where these two lines intersect.

Note: Another common location description is simply between the point of the chin and lower lip or just under the lower lip. Shandong (1982) locate Chengjiang on the mid-mandibular line, in the depression below the mental labial groove.

REFERENCES FOR THE REN MAI CONCEPTION VESSEL CHANNEL

Gray, H; Warwick, Roger; Williams, Peter L 1978 Gray's Anatomy 35th Edition. Ren 1: Inferior pelvic aperture (pelvic outlet) – 529; Ren 17: Sternum Ossification: 251

Voisin, Dr. H 1974 Essentials of Acupuncture – Conc 3: 58; Conc 4: 58; Conc 5: 58; Conc 6: 58; Conc 7: 58; Conc 9: 58; Conc 10: 58; Conc 11: 58; Conc 12: 58; Conc 13: 58; Conc 14: 58; Conc 15: 58; Conc 21: 58; Conc 22: 58; Conc 23: 58

Lawson-Wood 1973 Acupuncture Handbook – PIV 3 (Ren 3): 71; PIV 4 (Ren 4): 71; PIV 5 (Ren 5): 72; PIV 6 (Ren 6): 72; PIV 7 (Ren 7): 72; PIV 9 (Ren 9): 73; PIV 10 (Ren 10): 73; PIV 11 (Ren 11): 73; PIV 12 (Ren 12): 74; PIV 13 (Ren 13): 74; PIV 14 (Ren 14): 74; PIV 16 (Ren 16): 75; PIV 21 (Ren 21): 76; PIV 22 (Ren 22): 76; PIV 23 (Ren 23): 76

Soulié De Morant, George. 1994 Chinese Acupuncture – Conception Vessel Energy Description: 511; CV 6: 515; CV 7: 516; CV 9: 517; CV 10: 517; CV 11: 517; CV 12: 518; CV 13: 519; CV 14: 519; CV 15: 520; CV 16: 521; CV 17: 521; CV 18: 522; CV 19: 522/523; CV 20: 523; CV 21: 523; CV 22: 524; CV 23: 524/525

Lavier, Dr. J 1974 Points of Chinese Acupuncture – VC 8 to VC 15 (Ren 8 to Ren 15) Mid Abdomen(Epigastrium) Longitudinal Measurement: 50/51; VC 21: 49; VC 22: 63; VC 23: 63

Shandong Medical College and Shandong College of Traditional Chinese Medicine 1982 Anatomical Atlas of Chinese Acupuncture Point – Jianli (Ren 11): 63; Xuanji (Ren 21): 63; Chengjiang (Ren 24): 63

Wu, Wei-P'ing 1973 Chinese Acupuncture – VC 15: 123; VC 17: 123; VC 18: 123; VC 19: 124; VC 20: 124; VC 21: 125; VC 22: 125; VC 23: 125

So, James Tin Yau (Dr) 1985 The Book of Acupuncture Points – CV 15: 51; CV 16: 43; CV 18: 169; CV 19: 169; CV 20: 170; CV 21: 170; CV 22: 42

Deadman, Peter; Al-Khafaji, Mazin; Baker, Kevin 1998 Manual of Acupuncture, An – REN 15: 515/516; REN 21: 521; REN 23: 523

Worsley, J R 1982 Traditional Chinese Acupuncture Volume 1 – Meridians and Points – XIII 15 V Alarm Point: 259; XIII 17 VI (upper) Alarm Point: 259; XIII 17: 259; XIII 18: 259; XIII 19: 259; XIII 20 261; XIII 21: 261; XIII 22: 261; XIII 23: 261

Academy of Traditional Chinese Medicine, The. 1975 – Outline of Chinese Acupuncture, An. – Ren 16: 202; Ren 18: 202; Ren 19: 203; Ren 23: 203

Shanghai College of Traditional Medicine 1981 Acupuncture – A Comprehensive Text – Co 17: 177; Co 18: 332; Co 19: 332; Co 20: 332; N-HN-53: 340; Co 23: 332

Qiu Mao-Liang 1996 – Chinese Acupuncture and Moxibustion – REN 20: 164; REN 23: 165

Cheng Xinnong (Editor) 1987 Chinese Acupuncture and Moxibustion – Ren 20: 230; Ren 23: 230

Legge, David 1999 Acupuncture Points and Meridians – Ren 21: 93; Ren 23: 93

Jayasuriya, Anton 1982 Clinical Acupuncture – Ren 21: 408; Ren 23: 408

Ellis, Wiseman and Boss. 1991 Fundamentals of Chinese Acupuncture – CV 21: 362; CV 22: 363; CV 23: 364

Chaitow, Leon 1976 The Acupuncture Treatment of Pain – CV 22: Not Known

Low, Royston. 1988 The Non-Meridial Points of Acupuncture – OHN 4 (CTA Ren 22): Not Known

Masayoshi Hyodo 1975 Ryodoraku Acupuncture – CV 23: 68

Yang Jiasan (Prof) 1982 The Way to Locate Acu-Points – Ren 23: 69

Lotan, Alon 2000 Acupoint Location Guide – CV (Ren) 23: 163

Eachou Chen 1995 Cross-sectional Anatomy of Acupoints – CV 23: 131

Shanghai College of Traditional Chinese Medicine. 1993 Applied Anatomical Charts of Acupuncture and Moxibustion – RN 23: 72

Li Ding (Prof.). 1991. Acupuncture, Meridian Theory and Acupuncture Points – REN 23: 379

THE GOVERNOR VESSEL (THE DU MAI)

***Note:* The Governor Vessel and the Conception Vessel are two of the 8 Extraordinary Vessels. They are different to the other Extraordinary Vessels in that they have their own points rather than using known points from other channels. Some texts and Schools include the Conception and Governor Vessels as primary channels along with the other twelve primary channels, and these are commonly called the Fourteen Channels.**

Primary Channel

The Du Mai originates in the uterus/lower abdomen, descends as a deep channel to the genitals and perineum to meet Ren 1, then goes to the tip of the coccyx.

The Du Mai surfaces at the tip of the coccyx (Du 1), and travels up the spine and over the head to Du 28 on the upper gum. At Du 16, at the nape of the neck, a branch enters the brain, then emerges at the vertex (Du 20) to rejoin the main channel.

From Du 12 deep bilateral branches go to Bl 12, then turn medially to rejoin the main channel at Du 13.

Some texts attribute other channels to the Du Mai:

- *A branch from the coccyx to the gluteal region, meeting the Bladder and Kidney channels before returning to the spine and the kidneys.*

- *Two bilateral branches from the medial canthus of the eye (Bl 1), ascending the forehead to meet at the vertex, then descending through the brain and the neck to run parallel with the spine down to the kidneys.*

- *A branch from the lower abdomen ascending through the umbilicus, heart and trachea, then crossing the cheek, encircling the mouth, and ending just inferior to the centre of the eye.*

Note: Soulié (1994) – the Governor Vessel (Du Mai): Each of its points is double. On the spine, they are on the inferior, lateral edges of the vertebrae, in the angle of the lateral edge of the median tendon; on the skull they are on either side of a slight rise. They form two currents, a rising flow on the right side, and a descending flow on the left side. At their extremities they pass into the conception vessel (Ren Mai), changing side and direction of flow.

Connecting Channel

This leaves the main channel at Du 1 and travels bilaterally parallel to the spine to the nape of the neck, where it spreads over the top of the head. At the level of the scapula it joins the Bladder channel to diffuse through the spine.

THE GOVERNOR VESSEL

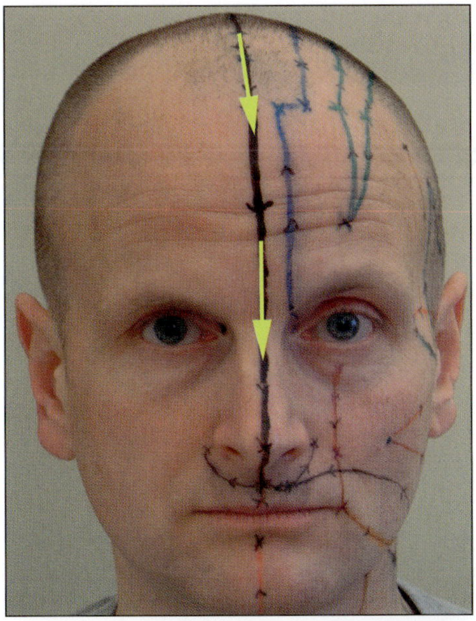

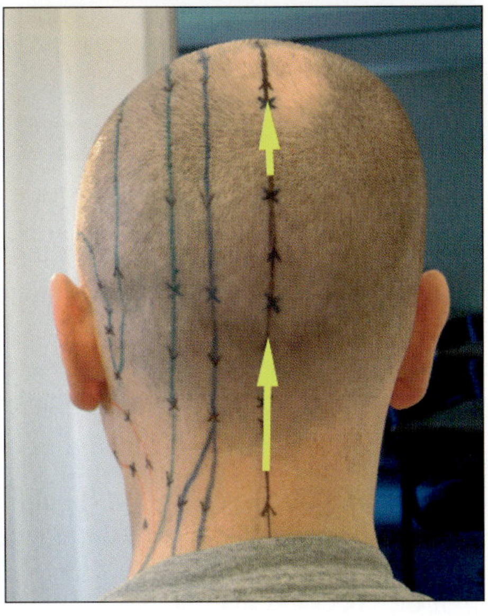

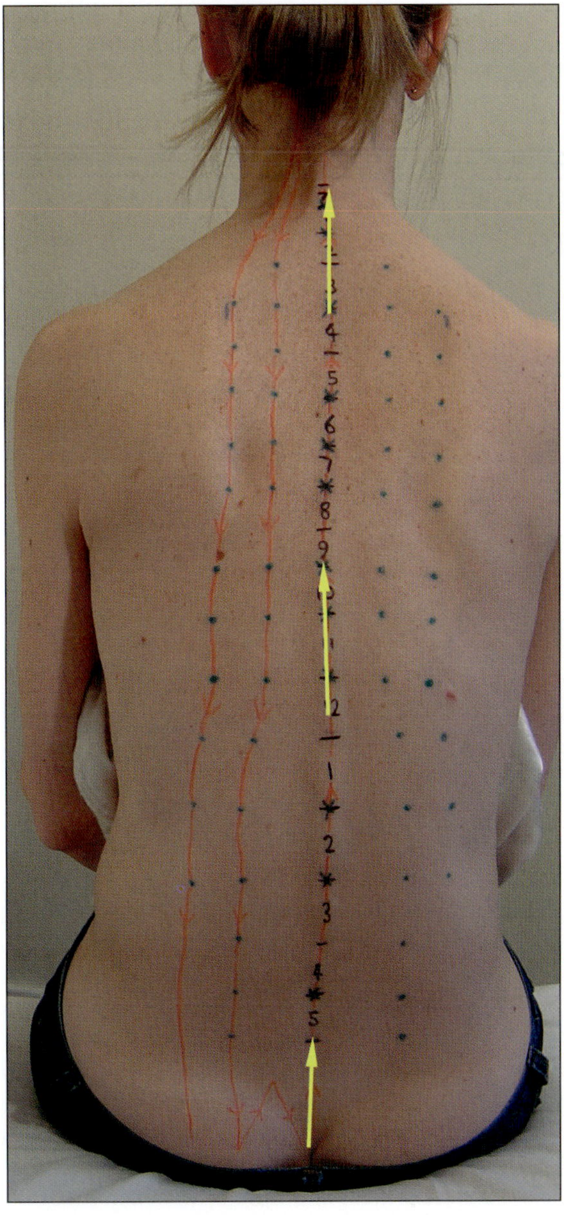

Points of the Governor Vessel – Du Mai (Du/DU/GV/Gov/VG/PIII/XIV)

All points lie on the median line, ascending the posterior median line of the torso, neck and head, and crossing over the vertex to the anterior median line of the forehead, nose and upper lip.

To locate Du 1, have the patient in a lateral recumbant position, with the knees flexed and pulled up towards the chin.

Du 1 CHANG QIANG – LONG STRENGTH

⊥ *0.3 TO 0.5 CUN* Δ *3 TO 15*

- ENTRY
- GENERAL JUNCTION/Luo/Connecting/Passage/Lo/Lê
- RE-UNION/Crossing/Meeting Point of the Du Mai with the Ren Mai, Kidney and Gall Bladder Channels – Governor Vessel with the Conception/Directing Vessel, Foot Shao Yin and Foot Shao Yang Channels

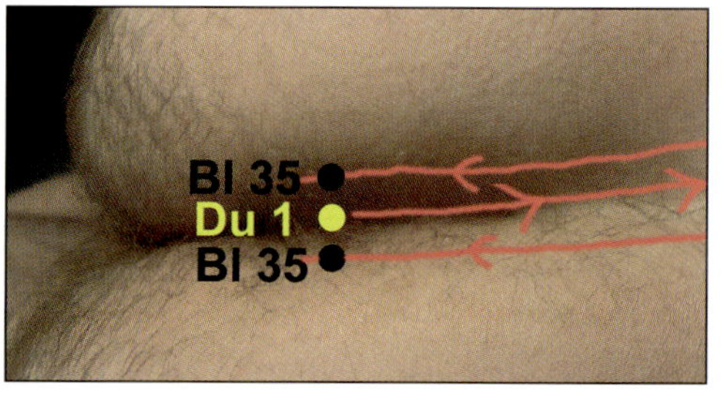

Pos: Position of patient: recumbent on their side with the knees flexed (pulled up towards the chin).

Loc: a) On the inferior pelvic aperture (pelvic outlet).
b) At the tip of the coccyx.
c) On the median line.

Tip: a) Recumbent with the knees flexed means that the patient should be lying down and on their side with their knees bent. The knees need to be bent and pulled up towards the chin to access the point.
b) Practitioners commonly needle this point too near to the tip of the coccyx, consequentially they hit the bone.
c) You may need to use both hands to locate and needle this point if the patient has an excess of flesh, (one to allow you access to the area and the other to palpate and locate the point).
d) When you have located the tip of the coccyx, visualise where the posterior aspect of the anus is, then palpate for Du 1 at the tip of the coccyx. Needle insertion should be midway from the tip of the coccyx to the anus angling the needle with the flow of the channel towards the spine.
e) The most common error when locating the tip of the coccyx is that the practitioner does not palpate sufficiently inferior, thus feeling a boney ridge that falls away in to flesh. This is often one of the spaces between the four fused vertebrae that make up the coccygeal body. The tip of the coccyx should be curved further round under the posterior torso so that you can feel a definate ending of the coccygeal body.
f) Palpate inferiorly from the sacrum or from the sacro-coccygeal articulation (the semi moveable joint of the sacrum and the coccyx) towards the anus. Palpate firmly but gently especially when you get towards the tip of the coccyx as this can sensitive area.

Note: Worsley (1982) locates XIV 1 on the posterior median line at the tip of the coccyx. Voisin (1974) locates Gov 1 on the midline of the body, at the coccyx: just below its tip. Lawson-Wood (1973) locates PIII 1 (Du 1) on the median line: on the point of the coccyx.

So (1985) locates GV 1 at a half inch behind the anus on the centre line. Qiu (1996) locates DU 1 at 0.5 cun below the tip of the coccyx, midway between the tip of the coccyx and the anus.

To locate Du 2-21, have the patient in a seated upright position.

Du 2 YAO SHU – LOINS CORRESPONDENCE

⊥ ***0.3 TO 0.5 CUN*** ∆ ***5 TO 15***

Pos: Position of patient: seated upright, or recumbent on their side with the knees flexed (pulled up towards the chin).

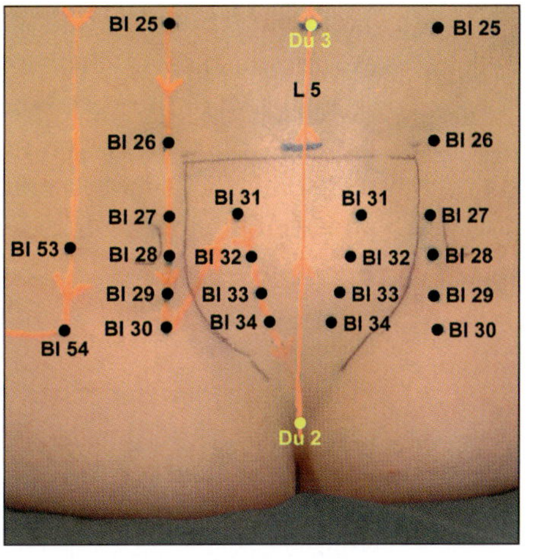

Loc: a) On the posterior torso.
b) In the sacro-coccygeal articulation.
c) At the sacral hiatus.
d) On the posterior median line.

Tip: a) Recumbent with the knees flexed means that the patient should be lying down and on their side with their knees bent. If in this position the knees need to be bent and pulled up towards the chin otherwise the patient can be seated upright to access the point.
b) Palpate inferiorly from the body of the sacrum on the posterior median line until you have reached the inferior border of the sacral bone. The contour of the sacrum can often be seen on people which will guide you to the inferior border of the sacrum.
c) The inferior border of the sacral bone and the superor border of the coccygeal body can be palpated as a small gap. This is is a semi moveable joint called the sacro-coccygeal articulation.
d) The sacral hiatus is located at the base of the sacrum. The superior border of the coccyx is inferior to the sacral hiatus. Du 2 is located at the sacral hiatus on the posterior median line in the sacro-coccygeal articulation.

Note: So (1985) locates GV 2 below the 21st vertebra, and above the top of the coccyx. Shandong (1982) locate Yaoshu below the 4th vertebra sacralis in the hiatuc sacralis.

HOW TO MARK OUT AND CHECK THE VERTEBRAE.

It is important to follow both the musculature of the torso, and any curvature/tilt of bony structures (scapula, spine, pelvis). You need to recognise any congenital or acquired conditions that can affect the alignment of the vertebrae such as scoliosis, lordosis, spinabifida and ankalosing spondilitis.

The distance between the medial border of the scapula and the posterior median line is measured as 3 cun at the level of the 3rd thoracic vertebra. There are 7 cevical, 12 thoracic and 5 lumbar vertebrae. The Du points lie in relation to the intervertebral spaces between two vertebrae, eg. T3/4.

Tip: Using the following landmarks to locate the intervertebral spaces of the upper thoracic vertebrae:

a) First mark out the intervertebral spaces of the thoracic vertebrae.
b) To locate the intervertebral space between C7 and T1, place your index finger on the prominence of the vertebra that may be T1 and your middle finger on the prominence of the vertebra which may be C7.
c) Now ask the patient to turn their head to the left and then to the right. You should feel some slight movement under your middle finger which is C7. You should feel no rotation under your index finger as T1 is attached to a rib whereas C7 is not.
d) A common error is to visualise C7 as being more prominent than T1. Gray's (1978) states it very often can be, but T1 is usually just as prominent and sometimes more so.
e) Place your four fingers from each hand vertically on the each side of the neck so that the radial borders of your fingers are uppermost and the pads are resting lightly against the lateral surface of the neck. Make sure that the ulnar border of the little fingers (5th digit) are resting on the top of the shoulder with the pads of your 5th digits resting on the lateral surface of the neck.
f) Then keeping your left and right 5th digits at this level, bring them together so their tips meet on the posterior median line. They should meet at the level of C7/T1 space or at the spinous process of C7.
g) The illustration below shows how you should have your fingers on the neck and shoulder before the 5th digits meet at the posterior median line:

o (2)	o (2)
o (3)	o (3)
o (4)	o (4)
<u>o</u> (5th digit)	<u>o</u> (5th digit)
(5th digit on top of left shoulder)	(5th digit on top of right shoulder)

h) When you have marked out the intervertebral spaces of the spine, step back and visualise the first place that you would be able to attach the first rib to T1. The first rib curves anteriorly and inferiorly to the inferior border of the clavicle, so T1 can seem more superior than you may realise. T1 should also be the first vertebra at the base of the neck.

i) Another method is to place your finger in the angle formed at the superior aspect of the shoulder by the acromial extremity of the clavicle and the scapular spine. From this angle, with the patient relaxed, run your finger across in a straight line until you meet an intervertebral space – this is the intervertebral space between T2/T3. A straight line means following the 3D curvature of the body, not as if you were drawing on a flat piece of paper – 2D image.

j) To locate the intervertebral space between T3/T4 run your finger from the acromial end of the scapular spine along its superior border towards the spine. You should meet the intervertebral space of T3/T4, however this is not always as accurate as tip i) as some scapula spines are almost horizontal. Therefore they may not slope downwards as you run your finger to the medial edge of the scapular spine.

k) To locate the intervertebral space between L2/L3 place your little finger (5th digit) on top of the iliac crest with your 1st, 2nd and 3rd fingers vertically on top of your little finger. Move your thumb horizontal (at a right angle) to the fingerswhich should bring the thumb in to alignment line with the intervertebral space of L2/L3 as illustrated below:

o (2) o – thumb L2/L3 thumb – o o (2)
o (3) o (3)
o (4) o (4)
o (5th digit) o (5th digit)
(left iliac crest) (right iliac crest)

l) To locate the intervertebral space between L3/L4 place your left and right index fingers on the top of the left and right iliac crests with your 1st, 3rd, 4th, and 5th digits at the same level (horizontal). Your thumbs should be at the level of L3/L4 intervertebral space, as illustrated below:

o o o o o – thumb L3/L4 thumb – o o o o o
5 4 3 2 1st digit 1st digit 2 3 4 5
l l
index fingers on top of the iliac crest

m) To locate the intervertebral space between L4/L5 place your left and right index (2nd) fingers on the top of the left and right iliac crests as above, but this time allowing your thumb to fall away naturally instead of keeping it horizontal with the other digits. The thumb then will be aligned with the intervertebral space of L4/L5, as illustrated below:

5 4 3 2 (digits) 2 3 4 5 (digits)
o o o o o o o o
o L4/L5 o
thumbs
index (2nd) fingers on top of the iliac crest

On tips g), k), l) and m) "=" is the top of the iliac crest.

n) From the base of L5 the vertebrae are fused and form the sacrum. The size of the sacrum longitudinally is approximately the size of the patient's fist from the knuckle (metacarpo-phalangeal joint) of the thumb to the knuckle (metacarpo-phalangeal joint) of the little finger. If the base of L5 vertebra to the bottom of the sacrum/superior border of the coccyx (sacral body) is longer than the person's fist then you need to re-check the intervertebral spaces again. The sacro-coccygeal articulation may be located at the level of the superior border of the gluteal fold.

Points on the posterior torso should be located with the patient in a seated position, with an upright posture.

Du 3 YAO YANG GUAN – LOINS YANG BORDER

⊥ ***0.3 TO 0.5 CUN*** **Δ** ***5 TO 15***

Pos: Position of patient: seated and upright.

Loc:
a) On the posterior torso.
b) On the posterior median line.
c) Between the 4th and 5th lumbar vertebrae (below the spinous process of the 4th lumbar vertebra).
d) Just below the level of the upper border of the iliac crest.

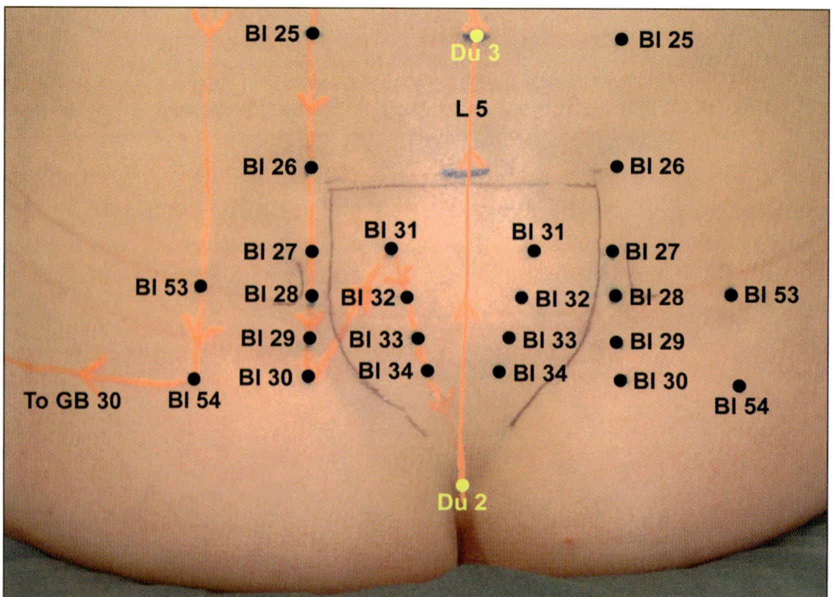

Tip: a) Please read **"HOW TO MARK OUT AND CHECK THE VERTEBRAE"**.

b) To help you to remember which Du point lies between which vertebrae, try remembering this numerical formula: 2•1•3•3•2•1. If you add up all the numbers and all of the '•', they should add up to 17 (12 thoracic + 5 lumbar spaces).

c) The numbers correspond to the points, and '•' corresponds to an intervertebral space where no point is located.

d) As a starting point for your formula, count down from C7/T1 (Du 14 location).

e) The last number in the formula '1' corresponds to Du 3 which is between L4/L5 vertebrae.

f) The first number in the formula '2'corresponds to two points, Du 14 and Du 13 (C7/T1 and T1/T2) followed by '•', a gap in the vertebrae with no point (T2/T3).

g) The next number '1' is Du 12 (T3/T4) followed by '•', another gap between the vertebrae with no point (T4/T5).

h) The next number in the formula is '3' which corresponds to three points in a row Du 11, Du 10 and Du 9 (T5/T6, T6/T7 and T7/T8) followed by '•' a gap between the vertebrae with no point (T8/T9).

i) The next number in the formula is '3' which corresponds to three points in a row Du 8, Du 7 and Du 6 (T9/T10, T10/T11 and T11/T12), followed by '•' a gap between the vertebrae with no point (T12/L1),

j) The next number in the formula is '2' which corresponds to three points in a row Du 5 and Du 4 (L1/L2 and L2/L3), followed by '•' a gap between the vertebrae with no point (L3/L4).

k) The last number in the formula is '1' which corresponds to one point Du 3 (L4/L5).

l) Once you have remembered the formula and have marked out the gaps or spaces in between the vertebrae, the rest should become easier.

m) When you palpate for the point make sure you are on the posterior median line.

n) For patient's with a structural problem you need to follow the 'V' (formed by the contour of the spinous erector muscles, each side of the vertebrae) of the back which is usually along the posteror median line. You may find that the 'V' has followed the curvature of the spine (where the spine is now), this usually means that the person has a long standing structural problem. With short term structural problems the spine may have a curvature, but the 'V' is still visible in the middle of the back. In most cases the 'V' determines where you locate the point. In some cases you may have to not only locate the point in the 'V' but also in between the vertebrae as you may not be getting the desired effect when needling.

o) In some cases you may have to needle the point in two locations in the 'V' and the intervertebral space.

p) Du 3 is located between L4/L5.

Note: Soulié (1994) locates GV 3 on the lower back, midline: between the fifth (last) lumbar and the upper edge of the sacrum. Two points separated by the median tendon; in the angle between the tendon and the sacrum; in a hollow; two FW (Finger Width) medial to BL 26. Lawson-Wood (1973) locates PIII 3 (Du 3) on the median line, on the point of the spinous process of the fifth lumbar.

Du 4 **MING MEN – GATE OF LIFE**

⊥ *0.3 TO 0.5 CUN* Δ *3 TO 15*

Pos: Position of patient: seated and upright.

Loc: a) On the posterior torso.
b) On the posterior median line.
c) Between the 2nd and 3rd lumbar vertebrae (below the spinous process of the 2nd lumbar vertebra).

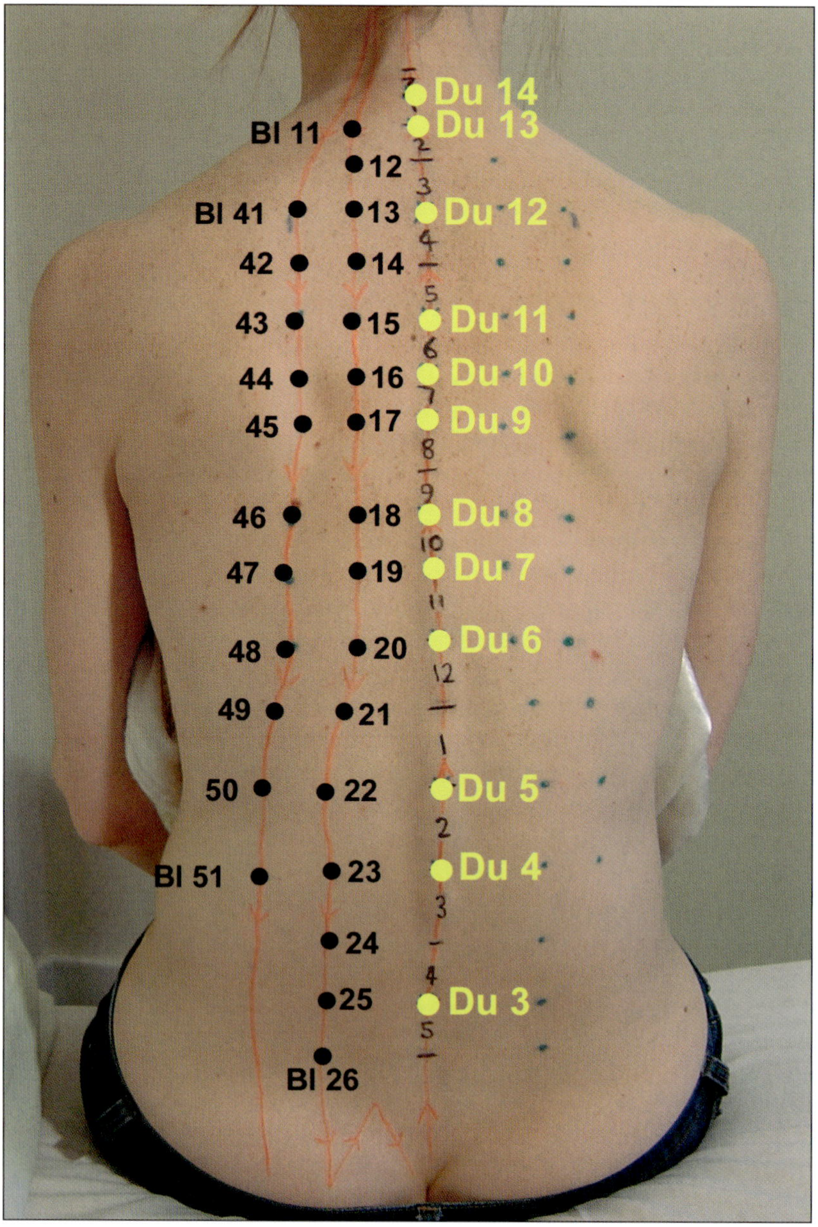

Tip:
a) Please read **"HOW TO MARK OUT AND CHECK THE VERTEBRAE"**.
b) To help you to remember which Du point lies between which vertebrae, try remembering this numerical formula: 2•1•3•3•2•1. If you add up all the numbers and all of the '•', they should add up to 17 (12 thoracic + 5 lumbar spaces).
c) The numbers correspond to the points, and '•' corresponds to an intervertebral space where no point is located.
d) As a starting point for your formula, count down from C7/T1 (Du 14 location).
e) The last number in the formula '1' corresponds to Du 3 which is between L4/L5 vertebrae.
f) The first number in the formula '2'corresponds to two points, Du 14 and Du 13 (C7/T1 and T1/T2) followed by '•', a gap in the vertebrae with no point (T2/T3).
g) The next number '1' is Du 12 (T3/T4) followed by '•', another gap between the vertebrae with no point (T4/T5).
h) The next number in the formula is '3' which corresponds to three points in a row Du 11, Du 10 and Du 9 (T5/T6, T6/T7 and T7/T8) followed by '•' a gap between the vertebrae with no point (T8/T9).
i) The next number in the formula is '3' which corresponds to three points in a row Du 8, Du 7 and Du 6 (T9/T10, T10/T11 and T11/T12), followed by '•' a gap between the vertebrae with no point (T12/L1),
j) The next number in the formula is '2' which corresponds to three points in a row Du 5 and Du 4 (L1/L2 and L2/L3), followed by '•' a gap between the vertebrae with no point (L3/L4).
k) The last number in the formula is '1' which corresponds to one point Du 3 (L4/L5).
l) Once you have remembered the formula and have marked out the gaps or spaces in between the vertebrae, the rest should become easier.
m) When you palpate for the point make sure you are on the posterior median line.
n) For patient's with a structural problem you need to follow the 'V' (formed by the contour of the spinous erector muscles, each side of the vertebrae) of the back which is usually along the posteror median line. You may find that the 'V' has followed the curvature of the spine (where the spine is now), this usually means that the person has a long standing structural problem. With short term structural problems the spine may have a curvature, but the 'V' is still visible in the middle of the back. In most cases the 'V' determines where you locate the point. In some cases you may have to not only locate the point in the 'V' but also in between the vertebrae as you may not be getting the desired effect when needling.
o) In some cases you may have to needle the point in two locations in the 'V' and the intervertebral space.
p) Du 4 is located between L2/L3.

Note: Worsley (1982) lists this point as a point of Chong Mo (Chong Mai – Penetrating Vessel). Lawson-Wood (1973) locates PIII 4 (Du 4) on the median line, on the spinous process of the third lumbar vertebra.

Du 5 XUAN SHU – SUSPENDED PIVOT

⊥ *0.3 TO 0.5 CUN* Δ *3 TO 15*

Pos: Position of patient: seated and upright.

Loc:
a) On the posterior torso.
b) On the posterior median line.
c) Between the 1st and 2nd lumbar vertebrae (below the spinous process of the 1st lumbar vertebra).

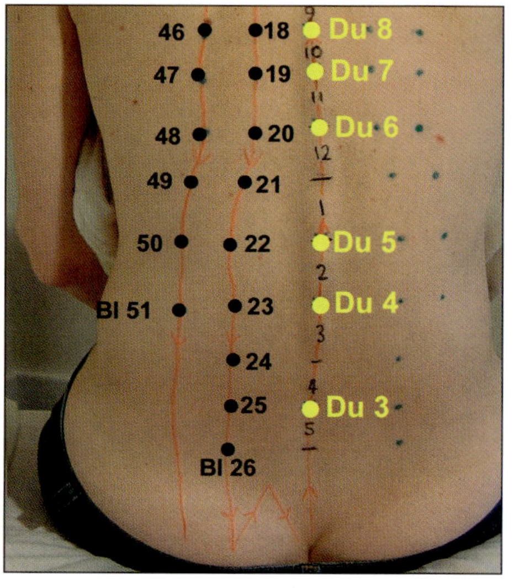

Tip:
a) Please read **"HOW TO MARK OUT AND CHECK THE VERTEBRAE"**.
b) To help you to remember which Du point lies between which vertebrae, try remembering this numerical formula: 2•1•3•3•2•1. If you add up all the numbers and all of the '•', they should add up to 17 (12 thoracic + 5 lumbar spaces).
c) The numbers correspond to the points, and '•' corresponds to an intervertebral space where no point is located.
d) As a starting point for your formula, count down from C7/T1 (Du 14 location).
e) The last number in the formula '1' corresponds to Du 3 which is between L4/L5 vertebrae.
f) The first number in the formula '2'corresponds to two points, Du 14 and Du 13 (C7/T1 and T1/T2) followed by '•', a gap in the vertebrae with no point (T2/T3).
g) The next number '1' is Du 12 (T3/T4) followed by '•', another gap between the vertebrae with no point (T4/T5).
h) The next number in the formula is '3' which corresponds to three points in a row Du 11, Du 10 and Du 9 (T5/T6, T6/T7 and T7/T8) followed by '•' a gap between the vertebrae with no point (T8/T9).
i) The next number in the formula is '3' which corresponds to three points in a row Du 8, Du 7 and Du 6 (T9/T10, T10/T11 and T11/T12), followed by '•' a gap between the vertebrae with no point (T12/L1),
j) The next number in the formula is '2' which corresponds to three points in a row Du 5 and Du 4 (L1/L2 and L2/L3), followed by '•' a gap between the vertebrae with no point (L3/L4).
k) The last number in the formula is '1' which corresponds to one point Du 3 (L4/L5).
l) Once you have remembered the formula and have marked out the gaps or spaces in between the vertebrae, the rest should become easier.

m) When you palpate for the point make sure you are on the posterior median line.
n) For patient's with a structural problem you need to follow the 'V' (formed by the contour of the spinous erector muscles, each side of the vertebrae) of the back which is usually along the posteror median line. You may find that the 'V' has followed the curvature of the spine (where the spine is now), this usually means that the person has a long standing structural problem. With short term structural problems the spine may have a curvature, but the 'V' is still visible in the middle of the back. In most cases the 'V' determines where you locate the point. In some cases you may have to not only locate the point in the 'V' but also in between the vertebrae as you may not be getting the desired effect when needling.
o) In some cases you may have to needle the point in two locations in the 'V' and the intervertebral space.
p) Du 5 is located between L1/L2.

Note: Lawson-Wood (1973) locates PIII 5 (Du 5) on the median line; on the spinous process of the second lumbar vertebra.

Du 6 JI ZHONG – MIDDLE OF THE SPINE

⊥ ***0.3 TO 0.5 CUN*** ***∆ FORBIDDEN TO USE MOXA***

Pos: Position of patient: seated and upright.

Loc: a) On the posterior torso.
b) On the posterior median line.
c) Between the 11th and 12th thoracic vertebrae (below the spinous process of the 11th thoracic vertebra).

Tip: a) Please read **"HOW TO MARK OUT AND CHECK THE VERTEBRAE"**.
b) To help you to remember which Du point lies between which vertebrae, try remembering this numerical formula: 2•1•3•3•2•1. If you add up all the numbers and all of the '•', they should add up to 17 (12 thoracic + 5 lumbar spaces).
c) The numbers correspond to the points, and '•' corresponds to an intervertebral space where no point is located.
d) As a starting point for your formula, count down from C7/T1 (Du 14 location).
e) The last number in the formula '1' corresponds to Du 3 which is between L4/L5 vertebrae.
f) The first number in the formula '2'corresponds to two points, Du 14 and Du 13 (C7/T1 and T1/T2) followed by '•', a gap in the vertebrae with no point (T2/T3).
g) The next number '1' is Du 12 (T3/T4) followed by '•', another gap between the vertebrae with no point (T4/T5).
h) The next number in the formula is '3' which corresponds to three points in a row Du 11, Du 10 and Du 9 (T5/T6, T6/T7 and T7/T8) followed by '•' a gap between the vertebrae with no point (T8/T9).
i) The next number in the formula is '3' which corresponds to three points in a row Du 8, Du 7 and Du 6 (T9/T10, T10/T11 and T11/T12), followed by '•' a gap between the vertebrae with no point (T12/L1),

j) The next number in the formula is '2' which corresponds to three points in a row Du 5 and Du 4 (L1/L2 and L2/L3), followed by '•' a gap between the vertebrae with no point (L3/L4).

k) The last number in the formula is '1' which corresponds to one point Du 3 (L4/L5).

l) Once you have remembered the formula and have marked out the gaps or spaces in between the vertebrae, the rest should become easier.

m) When you palpate for the point make sure you are on the posterior median line.

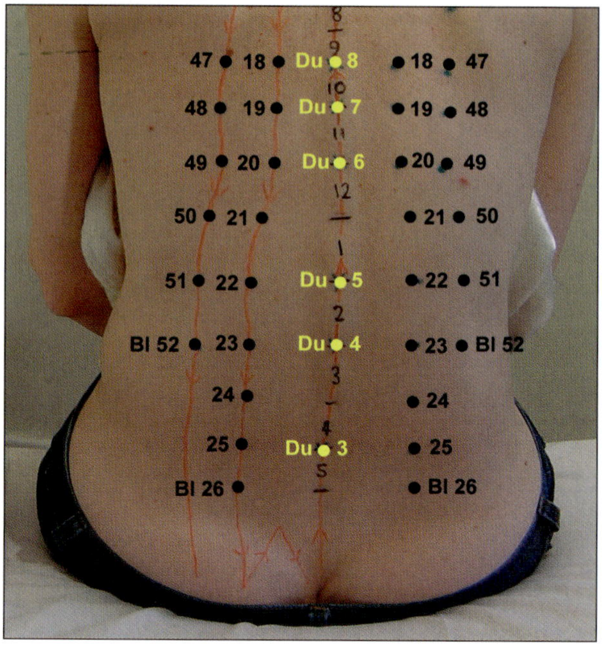

n) For patient's with a structural problem you need to follow the 'V' (formed by the contour of the spinous erector muscles, each side of the vertebrae) of the back which is usually along the posteror median line. You may find that the 'V' has followed the curvature of the spine (where the spine is now), this usually means that the person has a long standing structural problem. With short term structural problems the spine may have a curvature, but the 'V' is still visible in the middle of the back. In most cases the 'V' determines where you locate the point. In some cases you may have to not only locate the point in the 'V' but also in between the vertebrae as you may not be getting the desired effect when needling.

o) In some cases you may have to needle the point in two locations in the 'V' and the intervertebral space.

p) Du 6 is located between T11/T12.

Note: Lawson-Wood (1973) locates PIII 6 (Du 6) on the median line; on the spinous process of the twelfth dorsal vertebra. Voisin (1974) locates Gov 6 on the midline of the back, just below the spinous process of D 10 which is at the location of our Du 7. He locates Gov 5 at D 10 spinous process, just below it. This is lower than our Du 6. Soulié (1994) as well as locating GV 6 in a similar location, he also locates another point, GV 6a on the lower edge of the thoracic vertebra (spinous process), between the eleventh and twelfth thoracic vertebrae. There seems to be a discrepancy with the numbering of the vertebrae (it should say between the tenth and eleventh vertebrae) as he goes on to say that GV 6a is two FW (Finger Width) above GV 6 and two FW under his location for GV 7 (which is our Du 8), which would make the location where we locate Du 7. The name of the point for Souliés GV 6a is the same as our Du 7 location.

Du 7 ZHONG SHU – MIDDLE PIVOT

⊥ *FORBIDDEN TO NEEDLE* Δ *FORBIDDEN TO USE MOXA*

Pos: Position of patient: seated and upright.

Loc:
a) On the posterior torso.
b) On the posterior median line.
c) Between the 10th and 11th thoracic vertebrae (below the spinous process of the 10th thoracic vertebra).

Tip:
a) Please read **"HOW TO MARK OUT AND CHECK THE VERTEBRAE"**.
b) To help you to remember which Du point lies between which vertebrae, try remembering this numerical formula: 2•1•3•3•2•1. If you add up all the numbers and all of the '•', they should add up to 17 (12 thoracic + 5 lumbar spaces).
c) The numbers correspond to the points, and '•' corresponds to an intervertebral space where no point is located.
d) As a starting point for your formula, count down from C7/T1 (Du 14 location).
e) The last number in the formula '1' corresponds to Du 3 which is between L4/L5 vertebrae.
f) The first number in the formula '2'corresponds to two points, Du 14 and Du 13 (C7/T1 and T1/T2) followed by '•', a gap in the vertebrae with no point (T2/T3).
g) The next number '1' is Du 12 (T3/T4) followed by '•', another gap between the vertebrae with no point (T4/T5).
h) The next number in the formula is '3' which corresponds to three points in a row Du 11, Du 10 and Du 9 (T5/T6, T6/T7 and T7/T8) followed by '•' a gap between the vertebrae with no point (T8/T9).
i) The next number in the formula is '3' which corresponds to three points in a row Du 8, Du 7 and Du 6 (T9/T10, T10/T11 and T11/T12), followed by '•' a gap between the vertebrae with no point (T12/L1),
j) The next number in the formula is '2' which corresponds to three points in a row Du 5 and Du 4 (L1/L2 and L2/L3), followed by '•' a gap between the vertebrae with no point (L3/L4).
k) The last number in the formula is '1' which corresponds to one point Du 3 (L4/L5).
l) Once you have remembered the formula and have marked out the gaps or spaces in between the vertebrae, the rest should become easier.
m) When you palpate for the point make sure you are on the posterior median line.
n) For patient's with a structural problem you need to follow the 'V' (formed by the contour of the spinous erector muscles, each side of the vertebrae) of the back which is usually along the posteror median line. You may find that the 'V' has followed the curvature of the spine (where the spine is now), this usually means that the person has a long standing structural problem. With short term structural problems the spine may have a curvature, but the 'V' is still visible in the middle of the back. In most cases the 'V' determines where you locate the point. In some cases you may have to not only locate the point in the 'V' but also in between the vertebrae as you may not be getting the desired effect when needling.
o) In some cases you may have to needle the point in two locations in the 'V' and the intervertebral space.
p) Du 7 is located between T10/T11.

Note: Lawson-Wood (1973) locates PIII 7 (Du 7) on the median line, on the spinous process of the 9th dorsal vertebra. Voisin (1974) locates Gov 6 at D 10 spinous process: just below it. This is our Du 7. His Gov 7 is on the midline of the back, just below the spinous process of D 9 which is at the location of our Du 8. Soulié (1994) locates GV 6a (our Du 7) as a "new point, discovered in Japan", on the back, midline: lower edge of the thoracic vertebra (spinous process), between the eleventh and twelfth thoracic vertebrae; in the angle between the lower edge of the vertebra and the lateral edge of the median tendon: two points separated by the median tendon; two FW (Finger Width) above GV 6; two FW under GV 8; two FW medial to BL 19.

Du 8 JIN SUO – CONTRACTED MUSCLE

⊥ ***0.3 TO 0.5 CUN*** Δ **3**

Pos: Position of patient: seated and upright.

Loc: a) On the posterior torso.
b) On the posterior median line.
c) Between the 9th and 10th thoracic vertebrae (below the spinous process of the 9th thoracic vertebra).

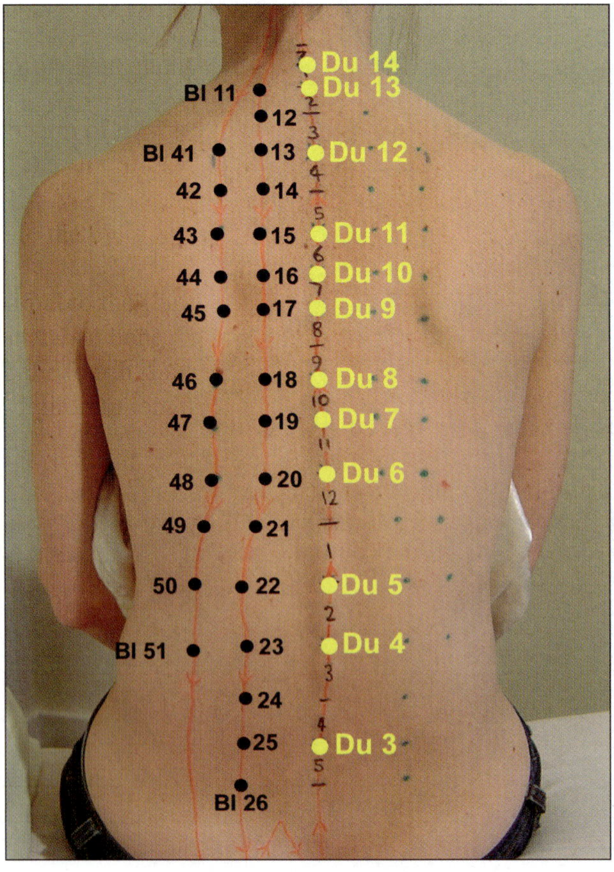

Tip: a) Please read **"HOW TO MARK OUT AND CHECK THE VERTEBRAE"**.

b) To help you to remember which Du point lies between which vertebrae, try remembering this numerical formula: 2•1•3•3•2•1. If you add up all the numbers and all of the '•', they should add up to 17 (12 thoracic + 5 lumbar spaces).

c) The numbers correspond to the points, and '•' corresponds to an intervertebral space where no point is located.

d) As a starting point for your formula, count down from C7/T1 (Du 14 location).

e) The last number in the formula '1' corresponds to Du 3 which is between L4/L5 vertebrae.

f) The first number in the formula '2'corresponds to two points, Du 14 and Du 13 (C7/T1 and T1/T2) followed by '•', a gap in the vertebrae with no point (T2/T3).

g) The next number '1' is Du 12 (T3/T4) followed by '•', another gap between the vertebrae with no point (T4/T5).

h) The next number in the formula is '3' which corresponds to three points in a row Du 11, Du 10 and Du 9 (T5/T6, T6/T7 and T7/T8) followed by '•' a gap between the vertebrae with no point (T8/T9).

i) The next number in the formula is '3' which corresponds to three points in a row Du 8, Du 7 and Du 6 (T9/T10, T10/T11 and T11/T12), followed by '•' a gap between the vertebrae with no point (T12/L1),

j) The next number in the formula is '2' which corresponds to three points in a row Du 5 and Du 4 (L1/L2 and L2/L3), followed by '•' a gap between the vertebrae with no point (L3/L4).

k) The last number in the formula is '1' which corresponds to one point Du 3 (L4/L5).

l) Once you have remembered the formula and have marked out the gaps or spaces in between the vertebrae, the rest should become easier.

m) When you palpate for the point make sure you are on the posterior median line.

n) For patient's with a structural problem you need to follow the 'V' (formed by the contour of the spinous erector muscles, each side of the vertebrae) of the back which is usually along the posteror median line. You may find that the 'V' has followed the curvature of the spine (where the spine is now), this usually means that the person has a long standing structural problem. With short term structural problems the spine may have a curvature, but the 'V' is still visible in the middle of the back. In most cases the 'V' determines where you locate the point. In some cases you may have to not only locate the point in the 'V' but also in between the vertebrae as you may not be getting the desired effect when needling.

o) In some cases you may have to needle the point in two locations in the 'V' and the intervertebral space.

p) Du 8 is located between T9/T10.

Note: Lawson-Wood (1973) locates PIII 8 (Du 8) on the median line; on the spinous process of the 8th dorsal vertebra. Voisin (1974) locates Gov 7 at D 9 spinous process: just below it. This is our Du 8. His Gov 8 is located on the midline of the back; just below the spinous process of D 7 which is the location of our Du 9. Soulié (1994) locates GV 7 (our Du 8) on the back, midline: on the lower edge of the ninth thoracic vertebra (spinous process); between the tenth and ninth vertebrae; in the angle between the lower edge of the vertebra and the lateral edge of the median tendon; two points separated by the median tendon; two FW above GV 6a (Du 7); four FW beneath GV 8; BL 18 is found at two FW on either side.

Du 9 ZHI YANG – UTMOST YANG

⊥ *0.3 TO 0.5 CUN* Δ *7*

Pos: Position of patient: seated and upright.

Loc:
a) On the posterior torso.
b) On the posterior median line.
c) Between the 7th and 8th thoracic vertebrae (below the spinous process of the 7th thoracic vertebra).
d) Approximately level with the inferior angle of the scapula.

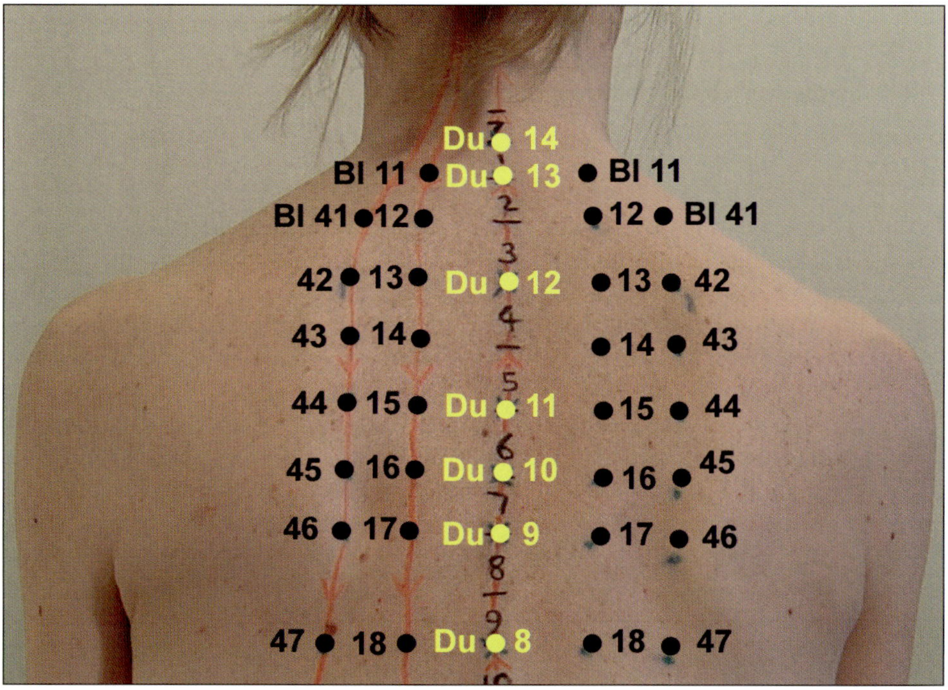

Tip:
a) Please read **"HOW TO MARK OUT AND CHECK THE VERTEBRAE"**.
b) To help you to remember which Du point lies between which vertebrae, try remembering this numerical formula: 2•1•3•3•2•1. If you add up all the numbers and all of the '•', they should add up to 17 (12 thoracic + 5 lumbar spaces).
c) The numbers correspond to the points, and '•' corresponds to an intervertebral space where no point is located.
d) As a starting point for your formula, count down from C7/T1 (Du 14 location).
e) The last number in the formula '1' corresponds to Du 3 which is between L4/L5 vertebrae.
f) The first number in the formula '2' corresponds to two points, Du 14 and Du 13 (C7/T1 and T1/T2) followed by '•', a gap in the vertebrae with no point (T2/T3).

g) The next number '1' is Du 12 (T3/T4) followed by '•', another gap between the vertebrae with no point (T4/T5).
h) The next number in the formula is '3' which corresponds to three points in a row Du 11, Du 10 and Du 9 (T5/T6, T6/T7 and T7/T8) followed by '•' a gap between the vertebrae with no point (T8/T9).
i) The next number in the formula is '3' which corresponds to three points in a row Du 8, Du 7 and Du 6 (T9/T10, T10/T11 and T11/T12), followed by '•' a gap between the vertebrae with no point (T12/L1),
j) The next number in the formula is '2' which corresponds to three points in a row Du 5 and Du 4 (L1/L2 and L2/L3), followed by '•' a gap between the vertebrae with no point (L3/L4).
k) The last number in the formula is '1' which corresponds to one point Du 3 (L4/L5).
l) Once you have remembered the formula and have marked out the gaps or spaces in between the vertebrae, the rest should become easier.
m) When you palpate for the point make sure you are on the posterior median line.
n) For patient's with a structural problem you need to follow the 'V' (formed by the contour of the spinous erector muscles, each side of the vertebrae) of the back which is usually along the posteror median line. You may find that the 'V' has followed the curvature of the spine (where the spine is now), this usually means that the person has a long standing structural problem. With short term structural problems the spine may have a curvature, but the 'V' is still visible in the middle of the back. In most cases the 'V' determines where you locate the point. In some cases you may have to not only locate the point in the 'V' but also in between the vertebrae as you may not be getting the desired effect when needling.
o) In some cases you may have to needle the point in two locations in the 'V' and the intervertebral space.
p) Du 9 is located between T7/T8.

Note: Soulié (1994) locates GV 8 (our Du 9) on the back, median line. On the inferior border of the seventh thoracic vertebra. Between T7 and T8. In the angle of the inferior border of the vertebrae and the lateral border of the median tendon. Two points separated by the median tendon; four FW (Finger Width) above GV 8; two FW under GV 10; at two FW on either side is BL 17. Voisin (1974) locates Gov 8 at D 7 spinous process: just below it. This is our Du 9 location. He locates Gov 9 on the midline of the back; just below the spinous process of D 6 which is the location of our Du 10.

Du 10 LING TAI – SUPERNATURAL TOWER

⊥ *FORBIDDEN TO NEEDLE* Δ *3 TO 7*

Pos: Position of patient: seated and upright.

Loc: a) On the posterior torso.
b) On the posterior median line.
c) Between the 6th and 7th thoracic vertebrae (below the spinous process of the 6th thoracic vertebra).

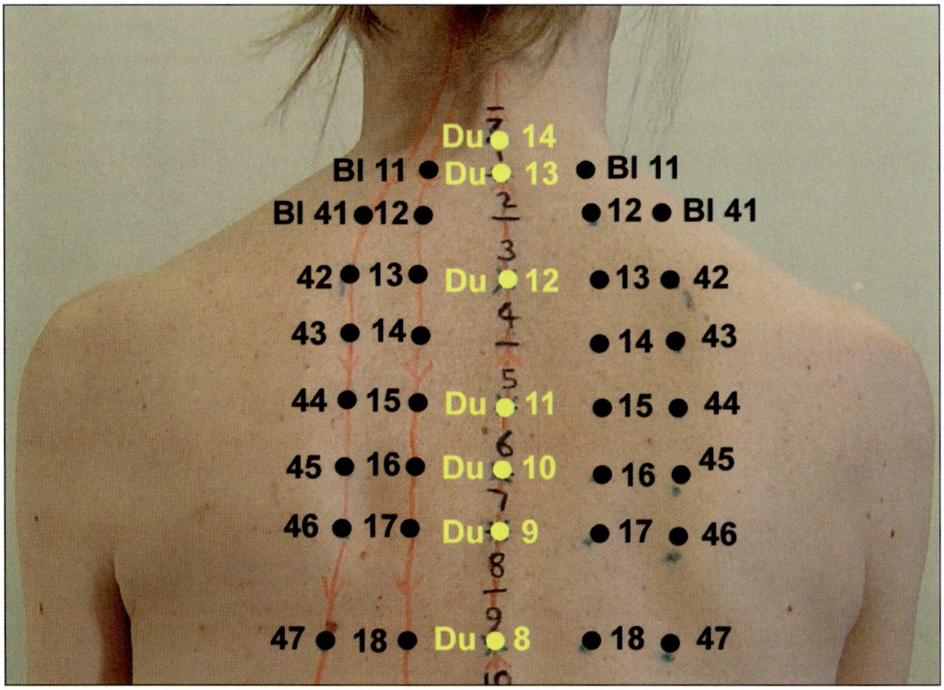

Tip: a) Please read **"HOW TO MARK OUT AND CHECK THE VERTEBRAE"**.
b) To help you to remember which Du point lies between which vertebrae, try remembering this numerical formula: 2•1•3•3•2•1. If you add up all the numbers and all of the '•', they should add up to 17 (12 thoracic + 5 lumbar spaces).
c) The numbers correspond to the points, and '•' corresponds to an intervertebral space where no point is located.
d) As a starting point for your formula, count down from C7/T1 (Du 14 location).
e) The last number in the formula '1' corresponds to Du 3 which is between L4/L5 vertebrae.
f) The first number in the formula '2' corresponds to two points, Du 14 and Du 13 (C7/T1 and T1/T2) followed by '•', a gap in the vertebrae with no point (T2/T3).
g) The next number '1' is Du 12 (T3/T4) followed by '•', another gap between the vertebrae with no point (T4/T5).

h) The next number in the formula is '3' which corresponds to three points in a row Du 11, Du 10 and Du 9 (T5/T6, T6/T7 and T7/T8) followed by '•' a gap between the vertebrae with no point (T8/T9).
i) The next number in the formula is '3' which corresponds to three points in a row Du 8, Du 7 and Du 6 (T9/T10, T10/T11 and T11/T12), followed by '•' a gap between the vertebrae with no point (T12/L1),
j) The next number in the formula is '2' which corresponds to three points in a row Du 5 and Du 4 (L1/L2 and L2/L3), followed by '•' a gap between the vertebrae with no point (L3/L4).
k) The last number in the formula is '1' which corresponds to one point Du 3 (L4/L5).
l) Once you have remembered the formula and have marked out the gaps or spaces in between the vertebrae, the rest should become easier.
m) When you palpate for the point make sure you are on the posterior median line.
n) For patient's with a structural problem you need to follow the 'V' (formed by the contour of the spinous erector muscles, each side of the vertebrae) of the back which is usually along the posteror median line. You may find that the 'V' has followed the curvature of the spine (where the spine is now), this usually means that the person has a long standing structural problem. With short term structural problems the spine may have a curvature, but the 'V' is still visible in the middle of the back. In most cases the 'V' determines where you locate the point. In some cases you may have to not only locate the point in the 'V' but also in between the vertebrae as you may not be getting the desired effect when needling.
o) In some cases you may have to needle the point in two locations in the 'V' and the intervertebral space.
p) Du 10 is located between T6/T7.

Note: Soulié (1994) locates GV 9 (our Du 10) on the back, median line: at the level of the mid-height between the spine of the scapula and its lower angle; on the lower edge of the sixth thoracic vertebra (spinous process). Between the seventh and sixth thoracic vertebrae. In the angle of the inferior border of the vertebrae and the lateral border of the median tendon; two points separated by the median tendon; Voisin (1974) locates Gov 9 at D 6 spinous process: just below it. This is our Du 10 location. He locates Gov 10 on the midline of the back; just below the spinous process of D 5 which is the location of our Du 11.

Du 11 SHEN DAO – SPIRIT PATH

⊥ 0.3 TO 0.5 CUN Δ 3 TO 5

Pos: Position of patient: seated and upright.

Loc:
a) On the posterior torso.
b) On the posterior median line.
c) Between the 5th and 6th thoracic vertebrae (below the spinous process of the 5th thoracic vertebra).

Tip:
a) Please read **"HOW TO MARK OUT AND CHECK THE VERTEBRAE"**.
b) To help you to remember which Du point lies between which vertebrae, try remembering this numerical formula: 2•1•3•3•2•1. If you add up all the numbers and all of the '•', they should add up to 17 (12 thoracic + 5 lumbar spaces).
c) The numbers correspond to the points, and '•' corresponds to an intervertebral space where no point is located.
d) As a starting point for your formula, count down from C7/T1 (Du 14 location).
e) The last number in the formula '1' corresponds to Du 3 which is between L4/L5 vertebrae.
f) The first number in the formula '2'corresponds to two points, Du 14 and Du 13 (C7/T1 and T1/T2) followed by '•', a gap in the vertebrae with no point (T2/T3).
g) The next number '1' is Du 12 (T3/T4) followed by '•', another gap between the vertebrae with no point (T4/T5).

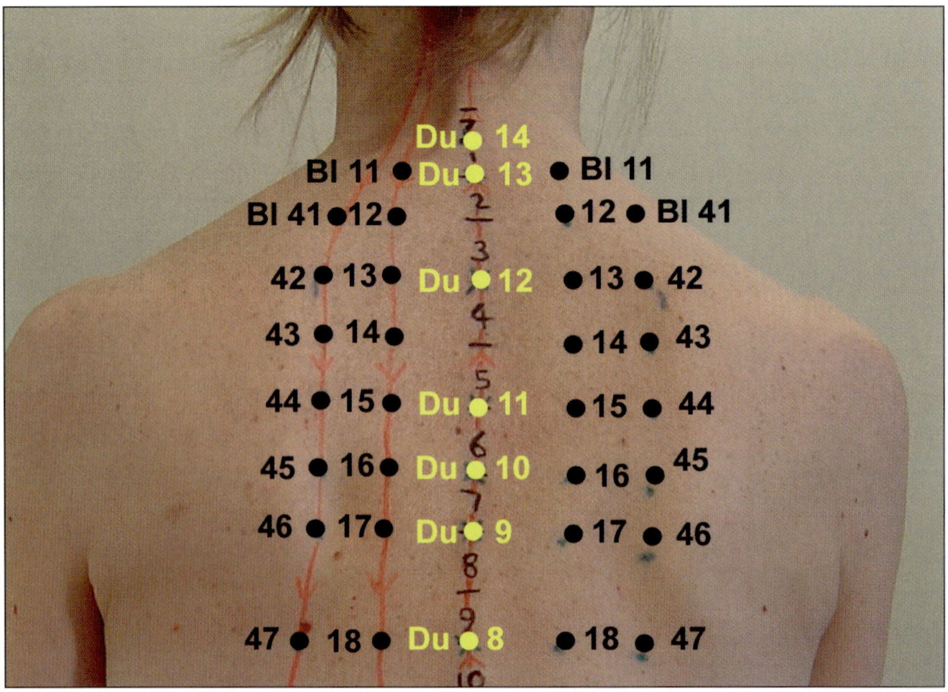

h) The next number in the formula is '3' which corresponds to three points in a row Du 11, Du 10 and Du 9 (T5/T6, T6/T7 and T7/T8) followed by '•' a gap between the vertebrae with no point (T8/T9).

i) The next number in the formula is '3' which corresponds to three points in a row Du 8, Du 7 and Du 6 (T9/T10, T10/T11 and T11/T12), followed by '•' a gap between the vertebrae with no point (T12/L1),

j) The next number in the formula is '2' which corresponds to three points in a row Du 5 and Du 4 (L1/L2 and L2/L3), followed by '•' a gap between the vertebrae with no point (L3/L4).

k) The last number in the formula is '1' which corresponds to one point Du 3 (L4/L5).

l) Once you have remembered the formula and have marked out the gaps or spaces in between the vertebrae, the rest should become easier.

m) When you palpate for the point make sure you are on the posterior median line.

n) For patient's with a structural problem you need to follow the 'V' (formed by the contour of the spinous erector muscles, each side of the vertebrae) of the back which is usually along the posteror median line. You may find that the 'V' has followed the curvature of the spine (where the spine is now), this usually means that the person has a long standing structural problem. With short term structural problems the spine may have a curvature, but the 'V' is still visible in the middle of the back. In most cases the 'V' determines where you locate the point. In some cases you may have to not only locate the point in the 'V' but also in between the vertebrae as you may not be getting the desired effect when needling.

o) In some cases you may have to needle the point in two locations in the 'V' and the intervertebral space.

p) Du 11 is located between T5/T6.

Note: Lawson-Wood (1973) locates PIII 11 (Du 11) on the median line, on the spinous process of the 4th dorsal vertebra. Soulié (1994) locates GV 10 (our Du 11) on the midline of the back: at the level of one third the distance from the spine of the scapula to its lower angle; on the lower edge of the fifth vertebra (spinous process). Between the sixth and fifth vertebrae; in the angle of the inferior border of the vertebrae and the lateral border of the median tendon; two points separated by the median tendon; two FW (Finger Width) above GV 10; four FW below GV 12; at two FW on either side is BL 15. Voisin (1974) locates Gov 10 at D 5 spinous process: just below it. This is our Du 11 location. He locates Gov 11 on the midline of the back; just below the spinous process of D 3 which is the location of our Du 12.

Du 12 SHEN ZHU – BODY PILLAR

⊥ *0.3 TO 0.5 CUN* Δ *5 TO 30*

Pos: Position of patient: seated and upright.

Loc: a) On the posterior torso.
b) On the posterior median line.
c) Between the 3rd and 4th thoracic vertebrae (below the spinous process of the 3rd thoracic vertebra).

Tip: a) Please read **"HOW TO MARK OUT AND CHECK THE VERTEBRAE"**.
b) To help you to remember which Du point lies between which vertebrae, try remembering this numerical formula: 2•1•3•3•2•1. If you add up all the numbers and all of the '•', they should add up to 17 (12 thoracic + 5 lumbar spaces).
c) The numbers correspond to the points, and '•' corresponds to an intervertebral space where no point is located.
d) As a starting point for your formula, count down from C7/T1 (Du 14 location).
e) The last number in the formula '1' corresponds to Du 3 which is between L4/L5 vertebrae.
f) The first number in the formula '2' corresponds to two points, Du 14 and Du 13 (C7/T1 and T1/T2) followed by '•', a gap in the vertebrae with no point (T2/T3).

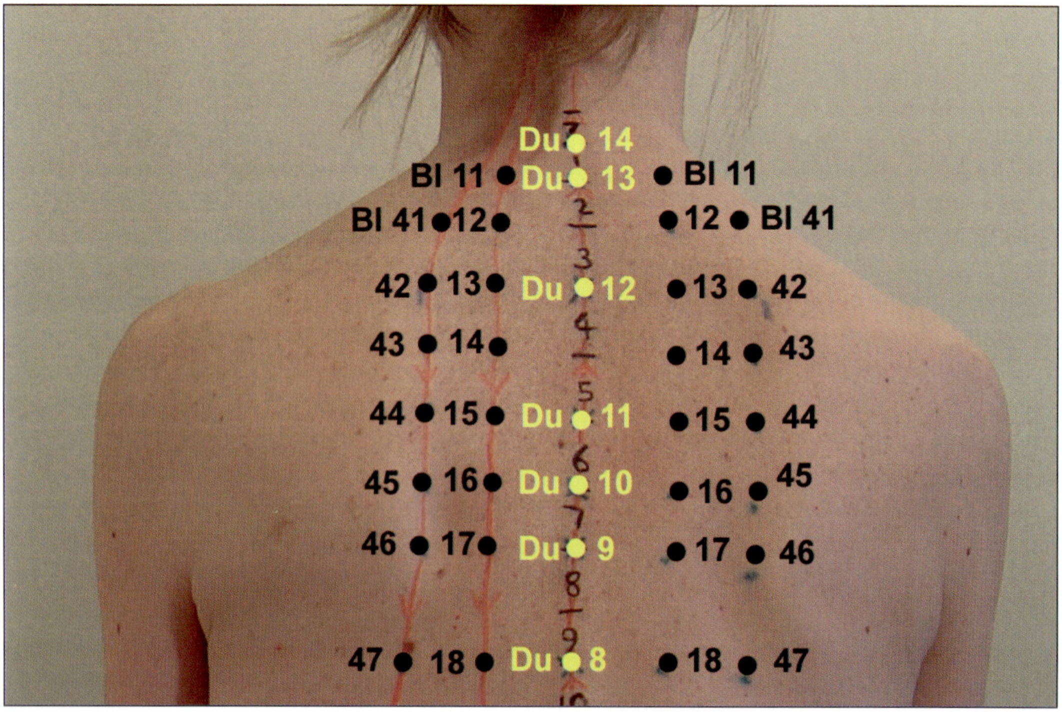

g) The next number '1' is Du 12 (T3/T4) followed by '•', another gap between the vertebrae with no point (T4/T5).
h) The next number in the formula is '3' which corresponds to three points in a row Du 11, Du 10 and Du 9 (T5/T6, T6/T7 and T7/T8) followed by '•' a gap between the vertebrae with no point (T8/T9).
i) The next number in the formula is '3' which corresponds to three points in a row Du 8, Du 7 and Du 6 (T9/T10, T10/T11 and T11/T12), followed by '•' a gap between the vertebrae with no point (T12/L1),
j) The next number in the formula is '2' which corresponds to three points in a row Du 5 and Du 4 (L1/L2 and L2/L3), followed by '•' a gap between the vertebrae with no point (L3/L4).
k) The last number in the formula is '1' which corresponds to one point Du 3 (L4/L5).
l) Once you have remembered the formula and have marked out the gaps or spaces in between the vertebrae, the rest should become easier.
m) When you palpate for the point make sure you are on the posterior median line.
n) For patient's with a structural problem you need to follow the 'V' (formed by the contour of the spinous erector muscles, each side of the vertebrae) of the back which is usually along the posteror median line. You may find that the 'V' has followed the curvature of the spine (where the spine is now), this usually means that the person has a long standing structural problem. With short term structural problems the spine may have a curvature, but the 'V' is still visible in the middle of the back. In most cases the 'V' determines where you locate the point. In some cases you may have to not only locate the point in the 'V' but also in between the vertebrae as you may not be getting the desired effect when needling.
o) In some cases you may have to needle the point in two locations in the 'V' and the intervertebral space.
p) Du 12 is located between T3/T4.

Note: Lawson-Wood (1973) locates PIII 12 (Du 12) on the median line, on the spinous process of the 2nd dorsal vertebra. Soulié (1994) locates GV 11 (our Du 12) is on the back, median line: at the level of the superior inferior angle of the scapula. Lower edge of the third dorsal vertebra (spinous process). Between the fourth and third vertebrae. In the angle between the lower edge of the vertebra and the lateral edge of the median tendon; four FW (Finger Width) above GV 11; four FW under GV 13, BL 13 is two FW on either side. He locates his GV 12 (Du 13 name only) on the upper back, midline: on the lower edge of the second thoracic vertebra (spinous process). Between the second and third vertebrae and the lateral edge of the median tendon; four FW above GV 12; two FW below GV 14; at two FW on either side is BL 12. Voisin (1974) locates Gov 11 at D 3 spinous process: just below it. This is our Du 12 location. He locates Gov 12 on the midline of the back; just below the spinous process of D 1 which is the location of our Du 13.

Du 13 TAO DAO – KILN PATH

⊥ ***0.3 TO 0.5 CUN*** Δ ***5 TO 10***

- RE-UNION/Crossing/Meeting Point of the Du Mai with the Bladder Channel – Governor Vessel with the Foot Tai Yang Channel

Pos: Position of patient: seated and upright.

Loc: a) On the posterior torso.
b) On the posterior median line.
c) Between the 1st and 2nd thoracic vertebrae (below the spinous process of the 1st thoracic vertebra).

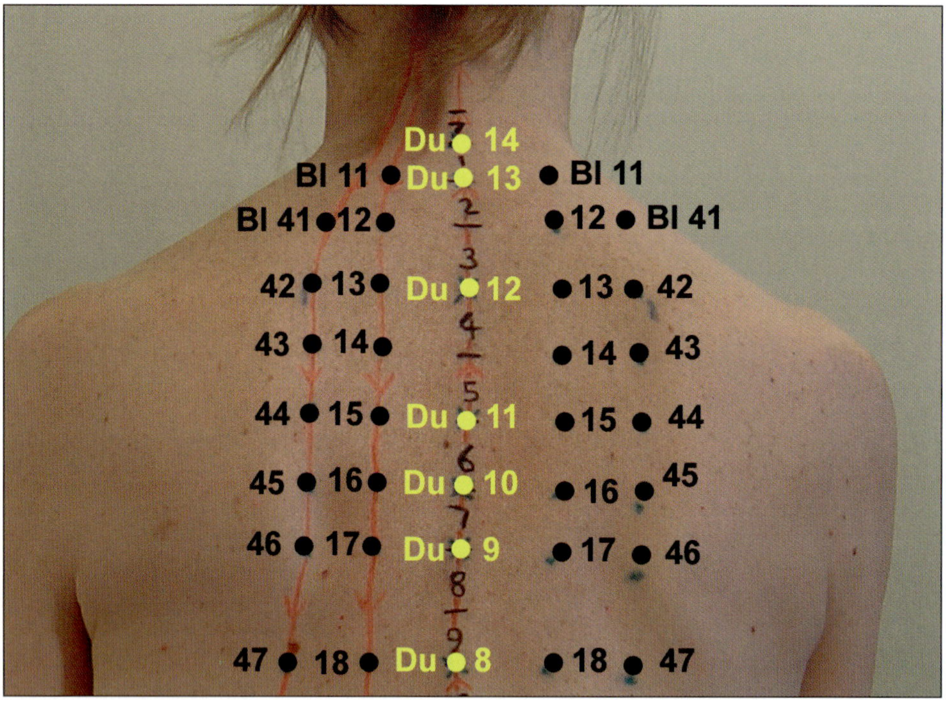

Tip: a) Please read **"HOW TO MARK OUT AND CHECK THE VERTEBRAE"**.
b) To help you to remember which Du point lies between which vertebrae, try remembering this numerical formula: 2•1•3•3•2•1. If you add up all the numbers and all of the '•', they should add up to 17 (12 thoracic + 5 lumbar spaces).
c) The numbers correspond to the points, and '•' corresponds to an intervertebral space where no point is located.
d) As a starting point for your formula, count down from C7/T1 (Du 14 location).
e) The last number in the formula '1' corresponds to Du 3 which is between L4/L5 vertebrae.

f) The first number in the formula '2'corresponds to two points, Du 14 and Du 13 (C7/T1 and T1/T2) followed by '•', a gap in the vertebrae with no point (T2/T3).
g) The next number '1' is Du 12 (T3/T4) followed by '•', another gap between the vertebrae with no point (T4/T5).
h) The next number in the formula is '3' which corresponds to three points in a row Du 11, Du 10 and Du 9 (T5/T6, T6/T7 and T7/T8) followed by '•' a gap between the vertebrae with no point (T8/T9).
i) The next number in the formula is '3' which corresponds to three points in a row Du 8, Du 7 and Du 6 (T9/T10, T10/T11 and T11/T12), followed by '•' a gap between the vertebrae with no point (T12/L1),
j) The next number in the formula is '2' which corresponds to three points in a row Du 5 and Du 4 (L1/L2 and L2/L3), followed by '•' a gap between the vertebrae with no point (L3/L4).
k) The last number in the formula is '1' which corresponds to one point Du 3 (L4/L5).
l) Once you have remembered the formula and have marked out the gaps or spaces in between the vertebrae, the rest should become easier.
m) When you palpate for the point make sure you are on the posterior median line.
n) For patient's with a structural problem you need to follow the 'V' (formed by the contour of the spinous erector muscles, each side of the vertebrae) of the back which is usually along the posteror median line. You may find that the 'V' has followed the curvature of the spine (where the spine is now), this usually means that the person has a long standing structural problem. With short term structural problems the spine may have a curvature, but the 'V' is still visible in the middle of the back. In most cases the 'V' determines where you locate the point. In some cases you may have to not only locate the point in the 'V' but also in between the vertebrae as you may not be getting the desired effect when needling.
o) In some cases you may have to needle the point in two locations in the 'V' and the intervertebral space.
p) Du 13 is located between T1/T2.

Note: Lawson-Wood (1973) locates PIII 13 (Du 13) on the median line, on the spinous process of the 7th cervical vertebra. Soulié (1994) locates GV 13 on the top of the back, midline: between the second and first thoracic vertebrae. Soulié's numbering is slightly different to the International Standard. His GV 13 location is the same but the name of the point is "Bailao" "Hundred Fatigues". Soulié also numbers a point as GV 13a but locates this between C7 and T1 (where we locate Du 14).

Voisin (1974) locates Gov 12 at D 1 spinous process: just below it. This is our Du 13 location. He locates Gov 13 on the midline of the back; just below the spinous process of C 7 which is the location of our Du 14.

Du 14 DA ZHUI – GREAT HAMMER

⊥ *0.3 TO 0.5 CUN (SEATED) 0.5 CUN (SUPINE)* Δ *3 TO 7*

- A POINT OF THE SEA OF QI (and Du 15 or Bl 10- see note) There are two other Sea of Qi Points: Ren 17 and St 9)
- RE-UNION/Crossing/Meeting Point of the Du Mai with the Six Yang Channels: Large Intestine, Stomach, Small Intestine, Bladder, Triple Heater and Gall Bladder Channels – Governor Vessel with the Hand Yang Ming, Foot Yang Ming, Hand Tai Yang, Foot Tai Yang, Hand Shao Yang and Foot Shao Yang Channels

Pos: Position of patient: seated and upright.

Loc: a) On the posterior torso.
b) On the posterior median line.
c) Between the 7th cervical and 1st thoracic vertebrae (below the spinous process of the 7th cervical vertebra).

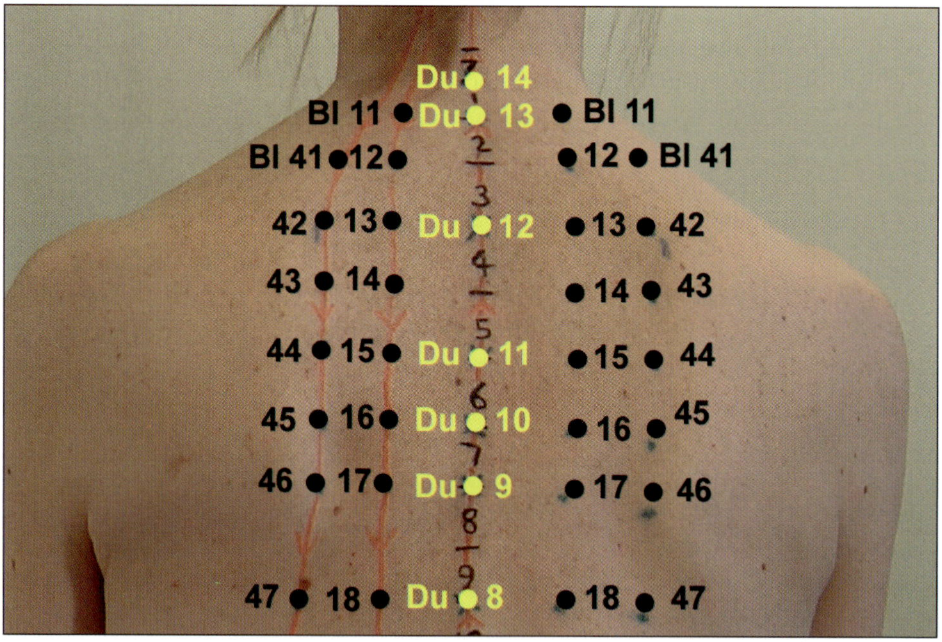

Tip: a) Please read **"HOW TO MARK OUT AND CHECK THE VERTEBRAE"**.
b) To help you to remember which Du point lies between which vertebrae, try remembering this numerical formula: 2•1•3•3•2•1. If you add up all the numbers and all of the '•', they should add up to 17 (12 thoracic + 5 lumbar spaces).
c) The numbers correspond to the points, and '•' corresponds to an intervertebral space where no point is located.
d) As a starting point for your formula, count down from C7/T1 (Du 14 location).
e) The last number in the formula '1' corresponds to Du 3 which is between L4/L5 vertebrae.

f) The first number in the formula '2'corresponds to two points, Du 14 and Du 13 (C7/T1 and T1/T2) followed by '•', a gap in the vertebrae with no point (T2/T3).
g) The next number '1' is Du 12 (T3/T4) followed by '•', another gap between the vertebrae with no point (T4/T5).
h) The next number in the formula is '3' which corresponds to three points in a row Du 11, Du 10 and Du 9 (T5/T6, T6/T7 and T7/T8) followed by '•' a gap between the vertebrae with no point (T8/T9).
i) The next number in the formula is '3' which corresponds to three points in a row Du 8, Du 7 and Du 6 (T9/T10, T10/T11 and T11/T12), followed by '•' a gap between the vertebrae with no point (T12/L1),
j) The next number in the formula is '2' which corresponds to three points in a row Du 5 and Du 4 (L1/L2 and L2/L3), followed by '•' a gap between the vertebrae with no point (L3/L4).
k) The last number in the formula is '1' which corresponds to one point Du 3 (L4/L5).
l) Once you have remembered the formula and have marked out the gaps or spaces in between the vertebrae, the rest should become easier.
m) When you palpate for the point make sure you are on the posterior median line.
n) For patient's with a structural problem you need to follow the 'V' (formed by the contour of the spinous erector muscles, each side of the vertebrae) of the back which is usually along the posteror median line. You may find that the 'V' has followed the curvature of the spine (where the spine is now), this usually means that the person has a long standing structural problem. With short term structural problems the spine may have a curvature, but the 'V' is still visible in the middle of the back. In most cases the 'V' determines where you locate the point. In some cases you may have to not only locate the point in the 'V' but also in between the vertebrae as you may not be getting the desired effect when needling.
p) Du 14 is located between C7/T1.

Note: The Ling Shu (Spiritual Pivot) Chapter 33 describes areas to needle rather than point numbers, eg. the middle of the chest is in the region of Ren 17. Ren 17 and St 9 locations seem to have universal agreement as Seas of Qi, but the other Sea of Qi point(s) in the region of the neck, Bl 10 or Du 14/Du 15 seem to have differences of opinion.

Note: Lawson-Wood (1973) locates PIII 14 (Du 14) on the median line, on the spinous process of the 3rd cervical vertebra. Soulié (1994) numbers a point as GV 13a (our Du 14 location only) and locates this on the lower nape, midline: between C7 and T1; in the angle between the lower edge of C7 (the seventh cervical vertebra is the first very prominent vertebra) and either edge of the median tendon. Two points; in a hollow; one large FW above GV 13; one large FW under GV 13b; one FW medial to SI 14. The Chinese name is the same as our Du 14 but the English translation he uses is "C7-pituitary".

Soulié also has extra points located between our Du 14 and Du 15. They are numbered as GV 13b, GV 13c, GV 14 and GV 15. GV 13b is called "C6-parathyroid", there is no Chinese name for this point, It is located on the lower nape, midline: between C6 and C7; lower edge of C6. GV 13c is called "C5-thyroid", again there is no Chinese name for this point. He locates the point on the nape, midline: between C5 and C6, on the lower edge of C5. GV 14 is called

"Yamen", "Door of Muteness", which is the name for our Du 15 "Gate of Dumbness". Soulié locates GV 14 (our Du 15 name only) on the nape, midline: between the fourth and third cervical vertebrae, on the lower edge of the third vertebra; in the angle of the median tendon; two points separated by the tendon; one FW (Finger Width) above C5-thyroid (CV 13c); one FW under GV 16. GV 15 is named as "Fengfu" "Workshop of the Wind" which is the name for our Du 16, "Wind Palace".

Soulié's GV 15 location is on the nape, midline: between the third and second vertebrae; on the lower edge of the second vertebra. Voisin (1974) locates Gov 13 at C 7 spinous process. This is our Du 14 location. He locates Gov 14 on the midline of the nape; just below the spinous process of C 2.

Longitudinal bone proportional measurements of the head:

- **3 cun from between the two eyebrows (Du 24.5/M-HN-3/Yin Tang) to the natural anterior hairline on the anterior median line.**
- **12 cun from the natural anterior hairline to the posterior hairline on the median line.**
- **3 cun from the posterior hairline to the space between the 7th cervical and 1st thoracic vertebrae (Du 14) on the posterior median line.**
- **15 cun (anterior natural hairline to the space between C7/T1);**
- **18 cun (between the two eyebrows at Du 24.5 or Yin Tang to the space between C7/T1).**

Transverse bone proportional measurements of the head:

- **(Anterior) 9 cun between the two corners of the forehead (St 8).**
- **(Posterior) 9 cun between the bilateral mastoid processes.**

It may be easier to use a strip of paper so that you can draw on the cun measurements as opposed to drawing the measurements on the scalp itself.

Note: The measurements of the head medical literature prior to the Song Dynasty, tend to place Du 15 on the posterior hairline. All subsequent texts measure 12 cun from the posterior hairline to the anterior hairline, but locate Du 15 in the depression 0.5 cun superior to the posterior hairline, and Du 16 1 cun superior to the hairline.

Du 15 YA MEN – GATE OF DUMBNESS

⊥ *0.3 CUN* *Δ FORBIDDEN TO USE MOXA*

- A POINT OF THE SEA OF MARROW (see note) There are three other Sea of Marrow Points: Du 16, Du 19 and Du 20
- 8 EXTRAORDINARY VESSEL/Coalescent Point of Yang Linking Vessel (Yang Wei Mai)
- RE-UNION/Crossing/Meeting Point of the Du Mai with the Yang Linking Vessel – Governor Vessel with the Yang Wei Mai

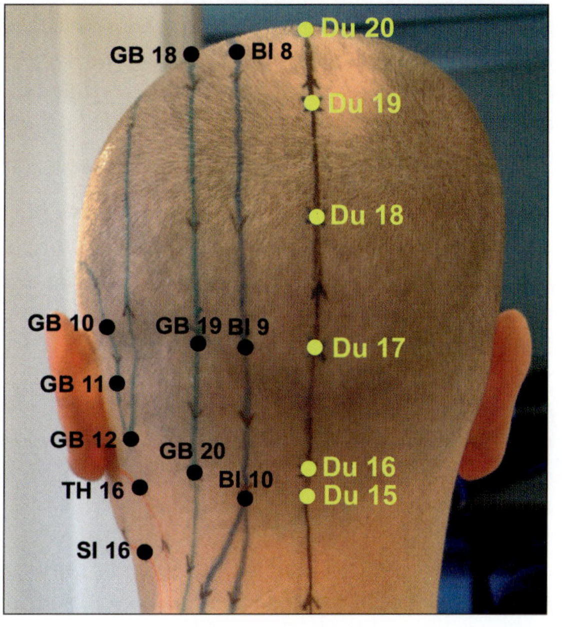

Pos: Position of patient: seated and upright.

Loc:
a) On the posterior torso.
b) On the nape of the neck.
c) On the posterior median line.
d) Between the first and second cervical vertebrae (below the spinous process of the 1st cervical vertebra) (the atlas and the axis).
e) 0.5 cun superior to the natural posterior hairline (11.5 cun posterior to the natural anterior hairline).
f) 0.5 cun inferior to Du 16.
g) Level with Bl 10.

Tip:
a) To locate Du 15 first mark the median line on the anterior and posterior aspects of the head at the natural anterior and posterior hairline. Many head points are in relation to the natural hairline. The natural hairline may not be apparent due to the hairline receding. Sometimes you can see a definite change in skin texture from the forehead to the scalp, which is usually where the natural hairline was previously.
b) Measure 12 cun from the natural anterior hairline to the natural posterior hairline on the median line.
c) Place a mark at 0.5 cun superior to the natural posterior hairline.
d) Du 15 is located between C1 and C2 vertebrae which should be either on or very close to your mark.
e) Palpation with the flow of the channel from shoulder level on the posterior median line to the area of your mark will assist you in accurate point location.
f) Another method of locating Du 15 is to ask the patient to bend their head forward slightly and then place your finger on the posterior median line, just inferior to the external occipital protuberance of the occipital bone (base of the skull). Your finger will not go any more superior due to the bone forming a resistance.

g) With your finger still just inferior to the external occipital protuberance of the occipital bone, ask the patient to bring their head backwards so they are just past the upright position (looking upwards). Your finger should automatically move inferiorly as the base of the skull pushes it downwards.
h) Ask the patient to straighten their head again, your finger should be placed at the 'hinge' of the head and neck where Du 16 is located (just inferior to the external occipital protuberance of the occipital bone).
i) Palpation at 0.5 cun inferior to Du 16 should help you to locate Du 15, between C1 (atlas) and C2 (axis) vertebrae.

Note: The Ling Shu (Spiritual Pivot) Chapter 33 describes areas where the Seas are located rather than point numbers, eg. the middle of the chest is in the region of Ren 17. There are regions where the Sea of Marrow can be located and in many cases just two points are used as the Sea of Marrow, these are Du 16 and Du 20,. The College of Traditional Acupuncture uses these two points as well as using Du 15 and Du 19. Du 15 is classified in some texts as a Sea of Qi point.

Note: Lawson-Wood (1973) locates PIII 15 (Du 15) on the median line, on the spinous process of the 2nd cervical vertebra. Soulié (1994) numbers a point as GV 13a but locates this between C7 and T1 (where we locate Du 14), it has the same Chinese name as our Du 14 but the translation is C7 – pituitary. Soulié also has extra points located between our Du 14 and Du 15. They are numbered as GV 13b, GV 13c, GV 14 and GV 15. GV 13b is called "C6-parathyroid", there is no Chinese name for this point, It is located on the lower nape, midline: between C6 and C7; lower edge of C6. GV 13c is called "C5-thyroid", again there is no Chinese name for this point. He locates the point on the nape, midline: between C5 and C6, on the lower edge of C5. Soulié's GV 14 is called "Yamen", "Door of Muteness", which is the name for our Du 15 "Gate of Dumbness".

Soulié locates GV 14 (our Du 15 name only) on the nape, midline: between the fourth and third cervical vertebrae, on the lower edge of the third vertebra; in the angle of the median tendon; two points, separated by the tendon; one FW above C5-thyroid (GV 13c); one FW under GV 16. GV 15 is named as "Fengfu" "Workshop of the Wind" which is the name for our Du 16, "Wind Palace". Soulié's GV 15 location (our Du 16 name only) is on the nape, midline: between the third and second vertebrae; on the lower edge of the second vertebra; two points; in the angle on the lateral edge of the medial tendon; one FW (Finger Width) above GV 15 by name; one FW under GV 17 by name, GV 15 by location; one small FW medial to BL 10. Souliés name for GV 16 is our Du 17 name, and the location for his GV 16 is our Du 15 location which is on the nape, midline: one large FW (Finger Width) under the skull; between the first and second vertebrae; two points; in the angle between the lateral edge of the medial tendon and the lower edge of the first vertebra (hardly perceptible); in a hollow.

Voisin (1974) locates Gov 15 on the midline of the nape; just below the spinous process of C 1 which is the same location as our Du 15. Here you can see that the numbering and location match up again with ours. Wu (1973) locates VG 15 upon the posteio-median line of the neck, at three pouce above VG 14. Jayasuriya (1982) locates Du 15 as in the main location. He also locates it at 3.5 cun above the spinous process of the 7th cervical vertebra when the head is held erect. Shandong (1982) locate Yamen at 0.5 cun above the mid-point of the posterior hairline, directly below the protruberantia occipitalis externa.

Du 16 FENG FU – WIND PALACE

⊥ *0.3 TO 0.5 CUN* Δ *FORBIDDEN TO USE MOXA*

- WINDOW OF THE SKY/Window of Heaven
- A POINT OF THE SEA OF MARROW (see note) There are three other Sea of Marrow Points: Du 15, Du 19 and Du 20
- 8 EXTRAORDINARY VESSEL/Coalescent Point of Yang Linking Vessel (Yang Wei Mai)
- RE-UNION/Crossing/Meeting Point of the Du Mai with the Yang Linking Vessel – Governor Vessel with the Yang Wei Mai
- SUN SI-MIAO GHOST (Gui) – Ghost Point Name: Gui Zhen – Ghost Pillow, Ghost Hole or Ghost Forest

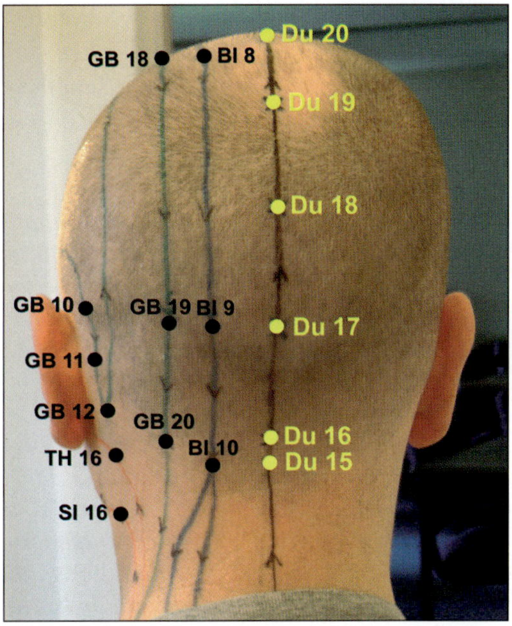

Pos: Position of patient: seated and upright.

Loc: a) On the posterior torso.
b) At the junction of the head and neck (nape of the neck).
c) Between the attachments of the trapezius muscle (left and right bands).
d) On the posterior median line.
e) Just inferior to the base of the external occipital protuberance of the occipital bone.
f) 1 cun superior to the natural posterior hairline (11 cun posterior to the natural anterior hairline).
g) 0.5 cun superior to Du 15.

Tip: a) The simplest method of locating Du 16 is to place your finger just inferior to the external occipital protuberance of the occipital bone and ask the patient to bring their head backwards so they are just past the upright position (looking upwards). Your finger should automatically move inferiorly as the base of the skull pushes it downwards.
b) Ask the patient to straighten their head again, your finger should be placed at the 'hinge' of the head and neck where Du 16 is located (just inferior to the external occipital protuberance of the occipital bone).
c) Palpating for a *men* (depression) between the left and right bands of the trapezius muscle on the posterior median line should assist point location.
d) Another method to locate Du 16 is to use the longitudinal measurement of the head.
e) First mark the median line on the anterior and posterior aspects of the head at the natural anterior and posterior hairline. Many head points are in relation to the

natural hairline. The natural hairline may not be apparent due to the hairline receding. Sometimes you can see a definite change in skin texture from the forehead to the scalp, which is usually where the natural hairline was previously.

f) Measure 12 cun from the natural anterior hairline to the natural posterior hairline on the median line.
g) Place a mark at 1 cun superior to the natural posterior hairline. Du 16 should be located on or near to your mark. Palpation with the flow of the channel from shoulder level on the posterior median line to the area of your mark will assist in accurate point location, as well as palpation of the external occipital protruberence of the occipital bone.
h) There are other combinations of longitudinal measurements you can use other than 12 cun eg.:
15 cun (anterior natural hairline to the space between C7/T1);
18 cun (between the two eyebrows at Du 24.5, M-HN-3 or Yin Tang to the space between C7/T1).
i) It may be easier to use a length of string or strip of paper so that you can draw on the cun measurements as opposed to drawing the measurements on the scalp itself.

Note: The Ling Shu (Spiritual Pivot) Chapter 33 describes areas where the Seas are located rather than point numbers, eg. the middle of the chest is in the region of Ren 17. There are regions where the Sea of Marrow can be located and in many cases just two points are used as the Sea of Marrow, these are Du 16 and Du 20,. The College of Traditional Acupuncture uses these two points as well as using Du 15 and Du 19. Du 15 in some texts is classified as a Sea of Qi point.

Note: Soulié (1994), the location for GV 17 (is our Du 16 location only) is on the nape, midline: in the angle between the lower edge of the cranium and the lateral edge of the medial tendon; one large FW below and medial to BL 9. Soulié's GV 15 is named as "Fengfu" "Workshop of the Wind", this is the name for our Du 16, "Wind Palace". His GV 15 location (our Du 16 name only) is on the nape, midline: between the third and second vertebrae; on the lower edge of the second vertebra; two points; in the angle on the lateral edge of the medial tendon; one small FW medial to BL 10. Souliés name for GV 16 – "Naohu" is our Du 17 (name only), and the location for his GV 16 is our Du 15 (location only) which is on the nape, midline: one large FW (Finger Width) under the skull; between the first and second vertebrae; two points; in the angle between the lateral edge of the medial tendon and the lower edge of the first vertebra (hardly perceptable); in a hollow. Souliés name for GV 17 is "Qiangjian" "Stiff Interval" which is the name of our Du 18 "Strength Divider".

Jayasuriya (1982) locates Du 16 as in the main location, but also adds that the point is at 4 cun above the vertebra prominens. Voisin (1974) locates Gov 16 on the atlanto-occipital joint. Wu (1973) locates VG 16 upon the posterio-median line of the neck, just below the occipital basis. Worsley (1982) locates XIV 16 on the median line of the head, just inferior to the base of the occipital bone, 0.5 ACI (Anatomical Chinese Inch) superior to XIV 15 (Du/GV 15).

Du 17 NAO HU – BRAIN DOOR

⊥ *0.3 CUN* ∆ *FORBIDDEN TO USE MOXA*

- RE-UNION/Crossing/Meeting Point of the Du Mai with the Bladder Channel – Governor Vesse with the Foot Tai Yang

Pos: Position of patient: seated.

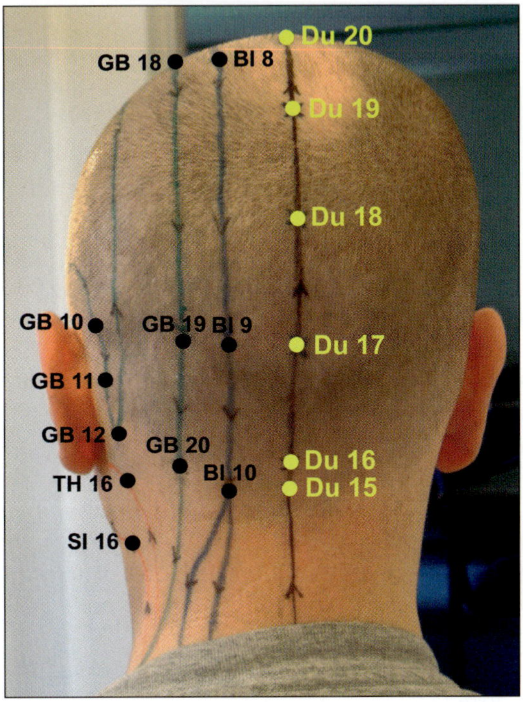

Loc:
a) On the posterior aspect of the head.
b) On the occipital bone.
c) On the level of the superior border of the external occipital protruberance of the occipital bone and Bl 9.
d) On the posterior median line of the head.
e) 1.5 cun superior to Du 16.
f) 2.5 cun superior to the natural posterior hairline (9.5 cun posterior to the natural anterior hairline).

Tip:
a) To locate Du 17 mark the posterior median line which is the Du (GV) line at the natural posterior hairline. Many head points are in relation to the natural hairline.
b) With your finger on the posterior median line at the natural posterior hairline run your finger superiorly on to the skull, the bone you are on is the occipital bone. If you carry on superiorly you will eventually come to a bump where the smooth contour has given way to a roughened area, this is the external occipital protruberance.
c) At the superior border of the external occipital protruberance on the posterior median line is Du 17 which can be palpated relatively easily.
d) Another method to locate Du 17 which is at 2.5 cun superior to the natural posterior hairline or 1.5 cun superior to Du 16 is to use the longitudinal measurement of the head.
e) First mark the median line on the anterior and posterior aspects of the head at the natural anterior and posterior hairline. Many head points are in relation to the natural hairline. The natural hairline may not be apparent due to the hairline receding. Sometimes you can see a definite change in skin texture from the forehead to the scalp, which is usually where the natural hairline was previously.
f) Measure 12 cun from the natural anterior hairline to the natural posterior hairline on the median line.

g) Place a mark at 2.5 cun superior to the natural posterior hairline (or 1.5 cun superior to Du 16), Du 17 should located on or near the mark. Palpation with the flow of the channel from shoulder level on the posterior median line to the area of your mark will assist in accurate point location, as well as palpation of the external occipital protruberence of the occipital bone.
h) Bl 9 has the same location description as Du 17, but is1.3 cun lateral to it.
i) There are other combinations of longitudinal measurements you can use other than 12 cun eg.:
   15 cun (anterior natural hairline to the space between C7/T1);
   18 cun (between the two eyebrows at Du 24.5, M-HN-3 or Yin Tang to the space between C7/T1).
j) It may be easier to use a length of string or strip of paper so that you can draw on the cun measurements as opposed to drawing the measurements on the scalp itself.

Note: Soulié (1994), his name for GV 17 "Qiangjian" "Stiff Interval" is the name of our Du 18 "Strength Divider". The location for GV 17 (our Du 16 location only) is on the nape, midline: in the angle between the lower edge of the cranium and the lateral edge of the medial tendon; two FW (Finger Width) above GV 17 by name and GV 16 by location; four FW below GV 19; one large FW below and medial to BL 9. The location of Soulié's GV 18 is on the posterior top of the skull, midline: two FW posterior to the occipitoparietal suture; at the upper edge of a large protruberance; two points on either side of a vertical groove.

Note that some other texts and schools may locate this point as Du 19, but this point is near to the location of our Du 18. Wu (1973) locates VG 17 upon the median line of the occiput, at five pouce and a half above VG 14. Worsley (1982) locates XIV 17 on the median line of the head, 2.5 ACI (Anatomical Chinese Inch) superior to XIV 15 (Du/GV 15).

So (1985) locates GV 17 at 4.5 divisions down from GV 20 on the median line of the head. Voisin (1974) locates Gov 17 on the occiput: just above the protruberance.

Du 18 QIANG JIAN – STRENGTH DIVIDER

⊥ ***0.3 CUN*** ***∆ FORBIDDEN TO USE MOXA***

Pos: Position of patient: seated.

Loc: a) On the posterior aspect of the head.
b) At the junction of the sagittal and lambdoid sutures (lambda suture).
c) On the posterior median line of the head.
d) 1.5 cun superior to Du 17.
e) 4 cun superior to the natural posterior hairline (8 cun posterior to the natural anterior hairline).
f) Approximately midway between Du 16 and Du 20.

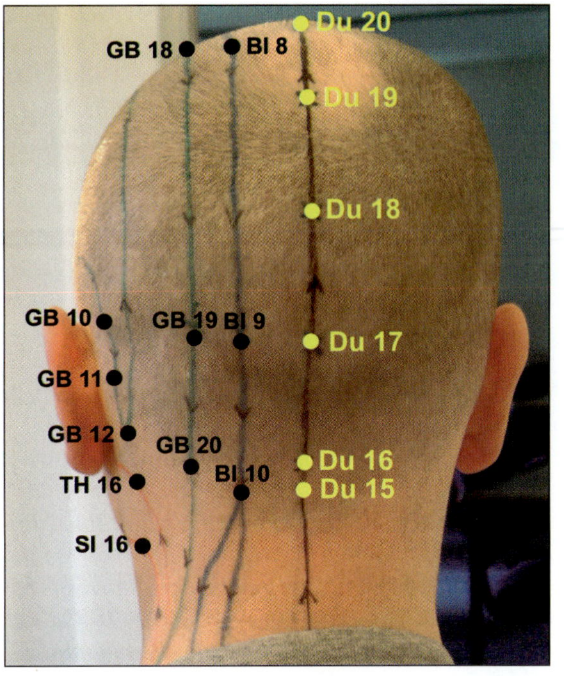

Tip:

a) The lamdoid suture joins the posterior borders of the parietal bones to the superior border of the occipital bone, whereas the saggital suture interlocks the most medial aspect of the two parietal bones together.

b) The point is located at the junction formed by the medial aspect of the lambdoid suture and the posterior aspect of the saggital suture is where the formation of the lambda suture is. The lambda suture is the shape of the Greek letter lambda 'Λ'

c) On the posterior median line palpate the lambda suture at the junction of the sagittal and lambdoid sutures, if so palpate for Du 18. To feel the anatomy, try palpating superiorly from the external occipital protruberence of the occipital bone until you can feel a *men* (depression).

d) Often the cun measurements can guide you to the area to the proximity of the point, but anatomy takes precedence.

e) Du 18 is 4 cun superior to the natural posterior hairline or 1.5 cun superior to Du 17. For the longitudinal measurement of the head see below.

f) First mark the median line on the anterior and posterior aspects of the head at the natural anterior and posterior hairline. Many head points are in relation to the natural hairline. The natural hairline may not be apparent due to the hairline receding. Sometimes you can see a definite change in skin texture from the forehead to the scalp, which is usually where the natural hairline was previously.

g) Measure 12 cun from the natural anterior hairline to the natural posterior hairline on the median line.

h) Place a mark at 4 cun superior to the natural posterior hairline (or 1.5 cun superior to Du 17), Du 18 should located on or near to the mark. Palpation with the flow of the channel from shoulder level on the posterior median line to the area of your mark will assist in accurate point location, as well as palpation of the external occipital protruberence of the occipital bone.

i) There are other combinations of longitudinal measurements you can use other than 12 cun eg.:
15 cun (anterior natural hairline to the space between C7/T1);
18 cun (between the two eyebrows at Du 24.5, M-HN-3 or Yin Tang to the space between C7/T1).

j) It may be easier to use a length of string or strip of paper so that you can draw on the cun measurements as opposed to drawing the measurements on the scalp itself.

Note: Lawson-Wood (1973) locates PIII 18 (Du 18) on the median line, on the external occipital protruberance. Soulié (1994), the name of his GV 18 is the name of our Du 19, "Houding" "Posterior Summit of the Head", His location for GV 18 is on the posterior top of the skull, midline: two FW (Finger Width) posterior to the occipitoparietal suture; at the upper edge of a large protruberance. The location of his GV 19 is our Du 18 location only. His location for GV 19 (our Du 18 location only) is on the head, posterior top: posterior fontanelle; midline; suture of the occiput and parietal bones. At the level of the posterior edge of two small rises; in a hollow; two points on either side of the groove. Note that some other texts and schools may locate this point as being Du 19, but this point is near to the location of our Du 18. The name of Soulié's GV 19 is the name of our Du 20 only. , "Baihui" – "Hundred Meetings".

Soulié's location for GV 20 is in a similar location to our Du 21, on the head, top, midline: mid-distance between the frontal and occipital bones; in a transverse fissure (sagittal plane); on the anterior edge of the posterior relief; two points on either side of the groove between the parietal bones. The name of his GV 20 is the same name as our Du 21 ("Qianding"). Wu (1973) locates VG 18 upon the median line of the cranium, at 7 pouce above VG 14.

Worsley locates XIV 18 on the median line of the head, 4 ACI (Anatomical Chinese Inch) superior to XIV 15 (Du/GV 15). So (1985) locates GV 18 at three divisions below GV 20. Voisin (1974) locates Gov 18 on the occiput: 2 fb (finger breadth) above the preceding point which is just over the protruberance of the occiput.

Du 19 HOU DING – POSTERIOR SUMMIT

⊥ 0.3 TO 0.5 CUN Δ 5 TO 7

- A POINT OF THE SEA OF MARROW (see note) There are three other Sea of Marrow Points: Du 15, Du 16 and Du 20

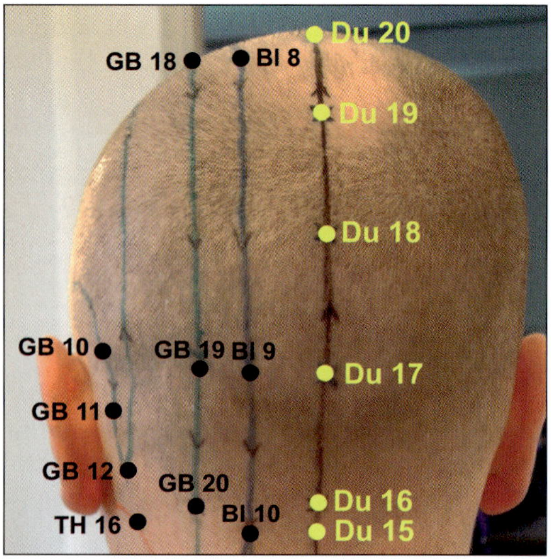

Pos: Position of patient: seated.

Loc:
a) On the posterior aspect of the head.
b) On the parietal bone.
c) On the posterior median line of the head.
d) 1.5 cun superior to Du 18.
e) 5.5 cun superior to the natural posterior hairline (6.5 cun posterior to the natural anterior hairline).

Tip:
a) Du 19 is often located on the most superior part of the posterior aspect of the head, in other words at the top of the back of the head.

b) Stand back and view the shape of the skull. Quite often you can see the contour of the shape of the skull change. If so palpate for the point where you can see this change on the posterior median line.
c) As there are left and right parietal bones, their most medial aspects join together either on or near to the median line. The joining of the parietal bones are referred as the sagittal suture, and the point may or may not be located on this suture as the line may "wiggle" from side to side (like a river meandering).
d) Often the cun measurements canindicate the area where to palpate for the point.
e) Du 19 is 5.5 cun superior to the natural posterior hairline or 1.5 cun superior to Du 18. For the longitudinal measurement of the head see below.
f) First mark the median line on the anterior and posterior aspects of the head at the natural anterior and posterior hairline. Many head points are in relation to the natural hairline. The natural hairline may not be apparent due to the hairline receding. Sometimes you can see a definite change in skin texture from the forehead to the scalp, which is usually where the natural hairline was previously.
g) Measure 12 cun from the natural anterior hairline to the natural posterior hairline on the median line.
h) Place a mark at 5.5 cun superior to the natural posterior hairline (or 1.5 cun superior to Du 18), Du 19 should located on or near to your mark. Palpation with the flow of the channel from shoulder level on the posterior median line to the area of your mark will assist in accurate point location, as well as palpation of the external occipital protruberence of the occipital bone.
i) There are other combinations of longitudinal measurements you can use other than 12 cun eg.:
   15 cun (anterior natural hairline to the space between C7/T1);
   18 cun (between the two eyebrows at Du 24.5, M-HN-3 or Yin Tang to the space between C7/T1).
j) It may be easier to use a length of string or strip of paper so that you can draw on the cun measurements as opposed to drawing the measurements on the scalp itself.

Note: The Ling Shu (Spiritual Pivot) Chapter 33 describes areas where the Seas are located rather than point numbers, eg. the middle of the chest is in the region of Ren 17. There are regions where the Sea of Marrow can be located and in many cases just two points are used as the Sea of Marrow, these are Du 16 and Du 20. The College of Traditional Acupuncture uses these two points as well as using Du 15 and Du 19. Du 15 in some texts is classified as a Sea of Qi point.

Note: Lawson-Wood (1973) locates PIII 19 (Du 19) on the median line, at the parieto-occipital suture (lambda). This is where we locate our Du 18. Soulié (1994), the name of his GV 18 is our Du 19, "Houding" "Posterior Summit of the Head". The name of his GV 19 "Baihui", "Hundred Meetings" is the name of our Du 20. The location of Soulié's GV 19 is similar to the location of our Du 18, on the head, posterior top: posterior fontanelle; midline; suture of the occiput and parietal bones. At the level of the posterior edge of two small rises; in a hollow; two points on either side of the groove.. Note that some other texts and schools may locate Du 18 as Du 19, but this point is near to the location of our Du 18.

Soulié's location for GV 20 is in a similar location to our Du 21, on the head, top, midline: mid-distance between the frontal and occipital bones; in a transverse fissure (sagittal plane); on the anterior edge of the posterior relief; two points on either side of the groove between the parietal bones. The name of his GV 20 is the same name as our Du 21 ("Qianding").

Voisin (1974) locates Gov 19 on the midline of the cranium, on the Calvarium: 1 fb (finger breadth) behind the highest point (Gov 20), in a hollow. Wu (1973) locates VG 19 upon the median line of the cranium, at eight and one-half pouce above VG 14. Worsley (1982) locates XIV 19 on the median line of the head, 5.5 ACI (Anatomical Chinese Inch) superior to XIV 15.

Du 20 BAI HUI – ONE HUNDRED MEETINGS

⊥ ***0.3 CUN*** Δ ***5 TO 7***

- A Seven External Dragons (E.D's) Point (the other points are Bl 11, Bl 23 and Bl 61)
- A POINT OF THE SEA OF MARROW (see note) There are three other Sea of Marrow Points: Du 15, Du 16 and Du 19
- RE-UNION/Crossing/Meeting Point of the Du Mai with the Large Intestine, Stomach, Small Intestine, Bladder, Triple Heater, Gall Bladder and Liver Channels – Governor Vessel with the Hand Yang Ming, Foot Yang Ming, Hand Tai Yang, Foot Tai Yang, Hand Shao Yang, Foot Shao Yang and Foot Jue Yin Channels

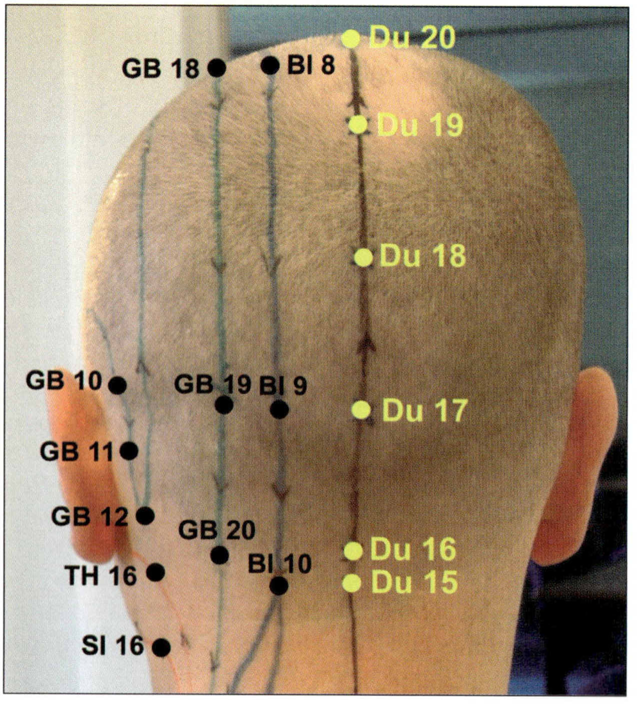

Pos: Position of patient: seated.

Loc:
a) On top of the head.
b) On the parietal bone.
c) On the median line of the head.
d) 1.5 cun superior and anterior to Du 19.
e) 7 cun superior to the natural posterior hairline.
f) 5 cun posterior to the natural anterior hairline.

Tip: a) Du 20 is located on the parietal bone, halfway between Du 19 and Du 21. Du 19 is on the most superior part of the posterior aspect of the head, in other words at the top of the back of the head, and Du 21 is on the most posterior aspect of the top of the head (back of the top of the head).

b) Locate Du 19 and Du 21 first (see separate descriptions), then palpate for the point on the median line, halfway between these two points.

c) As there are left and right parietal bones, their most medial aspects join together either on or near to the median line. The joining of the parietal bones are referred to as the sagittal suture, and the point may or may not be located on this suture as the line may "wiggle" from side to side (like a river meandering).

d) There are other useful methods of locating Du 20: Run your finger directly superior from the highest part of the helix of the ear to the median line, this is the approximate location of Du 21. Locate Du 19 using the top of the back of the head method where you should be able to palpate for the point. Then halfway between Du 21 and Du 19 is the location of Du 20.

e) The line from the ear lobe, through the highest part of the helix of the ear goes slightly diagonally towards the median line. Place the flat part of a pen on the ear lobe, then pass the length of the pen through the highest part of the helix of the ear, carrying on to the median line. This will be in the area of Du 20. Palpate for accurate point location.

f) Another common method is to think of the skull as a box where the superior and posterior aspects meet. This is done by placing the palm of one hand on the superior aspect of the head, and the other palm of the hand on the posterior part of the head. By keeping your fingers straight on both hands, they should meet together so it looks like you have the corner of a box. The corner of the box should place you in the area of Du 20. Again palpation will accurately locate this point.

g) Often the cun measurements can indicate the area where to palpate for the point.

h) Du 20 is at 7 cun superior to the natural posterior hairline (5 cun posterior to the natural anterior hairline) or 1.5 cun superior to Du 19. For the longitudinal measurement of the head see below.

i) First mark the median line on the anterior and posterior aspects of the head at the natural anterior and posterior hairline. Many head points are in relation to the natural hairline. The natural hairline may not be apparent due to the hairline receding. Sometimes you can see a definite change in skin texture from the forehead to the scalp, which is usually where the natural hairline was previously.

j) Measure 12 cun from the natural anterior hairline to the natural posterior hairline on the median line.

k) Place a mark at 7 cun superior to the natural posterior hairline (5 cun posterior to the natural anterior hairline) or 1.5 cun superior to Du 19, Du 20 should be located on or near to your mark. Palpation with the flow of the channel on the posterior median line from the external occipital protruberence of the occipital bone to the area of your mark will assist with the point location.

l) There are other combinations of longitudinal measurements you can use other than 12 cun: 15 cun (anterior natural hairline to the space between C7/T1); 18 cun (between the two eyebrows at Du 24.5, M-HN-3 or Yin Tang to the space between C7/T1).

m) It may be easier to use a length of string or strip of paper so that you can draw on the cun measurements as opposed to drawing the measurements on the scalp itself.

Note: The Ling Shu (Spiritual Pivot) Chapter 33 describes areas where the Seas are located rather than point numbers, eg. the middle of the chest is in the region of Ren 17. There are regions where the Sea of Marrow can be located and in many cases just two points are used as the Sea of Marrow, these are Du 16 and Du 20,. The College of Traditional Acupuncture uses these two points as well as using Du 15 and Du 19. Du 15 in some texts is classified as a Sea of Qi point.

Note: There are texts that locate Du 20 on the median line of the head on a line connecting the apexes of the ears. These texts also locate the point at the same measurements as above. In practice the apexes may seem to be on a line nearer to Du 21 than Du 20, it depends on the shape of the persons helix.

Note: Lawson-Wood (1973) locates PIII 20 (Du 20) on the median line, half-way between lambda and bregma; about 6cm above the parieto-occipital suture. This is approximately midway between our Du 18 and Du 22, which is the same location as our Du 20. Soulié (1994), the name of his GV 18 is our Du 19, "Houding" "Posterior Summit of the Head". The name of his GV 19 "Baihui" "Hundred Meetings" is the name of our Du 20. The location of Soulié's GV 19 (our Du 18) is on the head, posterior top: posterior fontanelle; midline; suture of the occiput and parietal bones. At the level of the posterior edge of two small rises; in a hollow; two points on either side of the groove.

Soulié's location for GV 20 is the approximate location of our Du 21, on the head, top, midline: mid-distance between the frontal and occipital bones; in a transverse fissure (sagittal plane); on the anterior edge of the posterior relief; two points on either side of the groove between the parietal bones. The name of GV 20 is the same as our Du 21 ("Qianding"). Soulié's GV 21 (our Du 22) is located on the head, anterior top, midline: posterior edge of the frontal bone between the two parietal bones (fontanelles).

The name of his GV 21 is similar to the name of our Du 22. His name for GV 21 is "Chuanghui " (Wade -Giles spelling) , "Xinhui" (Pin Yin spelling) which translated means "Meeting of the Brain" or "Skull Meeting". Voisin (1974) locates Gov 20 on the midline of the cranium, on the Calvarium: the highest point.

Wu (1973) locates VG 20 upon the median line of the head, at the parietal eminence in the sagittal suture, at 10 pouce above VG 14. Deadman (1998) also states that you can measure this point as 8 cun posterior to the glabella and 6 cun superior to the external occipital protruberance. Lavier (1974) locates VG 20 where there is a separation of the upper cranial region from the occipital region. Worsley (1982) locates XIV 20 on the median line of the head, 7 ACI (Anatomical Chinese Inch) superior to XIV 15.

Li (1991) locates DU 20 at five cun within the frontal hairline on the midsagittal line, or midway between the posterior hairline and the landmark one finger's width superior to Yintang (Du 24.5/M-HN-3). Lotan (2000) locates GV 20 at 7 cun superior to the neck hairline, midpoint, 5 cun posterior to the forehead hairline, on the straight line that connects the two ear auricles (helix) posterior borders. Jayasuriya (1982) locates Du 20 as in the main location, he also adds that it can be located at the vertex of the skull, 8 cun above and behind the glabella, and at 10 cun above the vertebra prominens.

Shandong (1982) locate Baihui at the junction between the line connecting the apexes of both ears and the top point of the sutura sagittalis.

Du 21 QIAN DING – ANTERIOR SUMMIT

⊥ *0.3 CUN (Not on infants as their fontanelle may not yet be closed)* Δ *3 TO 7*

Pos: Position of patient: seated.

Loc: a) On top of the head.
b) On the parietal bone.
c) On the median line of the head.
d) 1.5 cun anterior to Du 20.
e) 3.5 cun posterior to the natural anterior hairline.
f) 8.5 cun anterior to the natural posterior hairline.

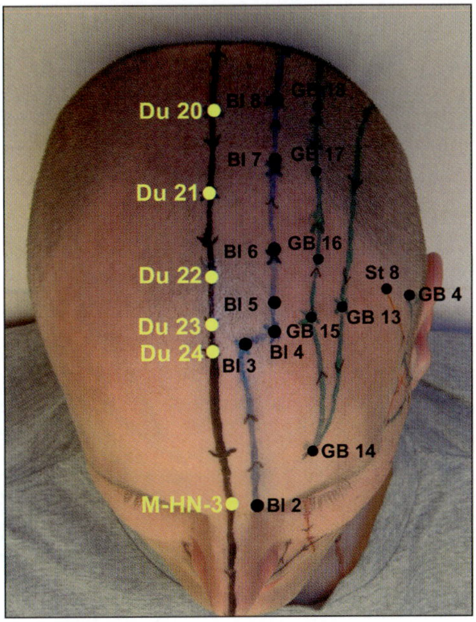

Tip: a) Du 21 is located on the parietal bone, and is on the back of the top of the head.
b) As there are left and right parietal bones, their most medial aspects join together either on or near to the median line. The joining of the parietal bones are referred to as the sagittal suture, and the point may or may not be located on this suture as the line may "wiggle" from side to side (like a river meandering).
d) Run your finger directly superior from the highest part of the helix of the ear on to the median line of the head.
e) Palpate with the the flow of the channel from the back of the head to the area of the point until you are able to locate Du 21.
f) Often the cun measurements can assist you to the area where you can palpate for the point.
g) Du 21 is 8.5 cun anterior to the natural posterior hairline (3.5 cun posterior to the natural anterior hairline) or 1.5 cun anterior to Du 20. For the longitudinal measurement of the head, see below.
h) First mark the median line on the anterior and posterior aspects of the head at the natural anterior and posterior hairline. Many head points are in relation to the natural hairline. The natural hairline may not be apparent due to the hairline receding. Sometimes you can see a definite change in skin texture from the forehead to the scalp, which is usually where the natural hairline was previously.
i) Measure 12 cun from the natural anterior hairline to the natural posterior hairline on the median line.
j) Place a mark at 7 cun anterior to the natural posterior hairline (5 cun posterior to the natural anterior hairline) or 1.5 cun anterior to Du 20, Du 21 should be located

on or near to your mark. Palpation with the flow of the channel on the posterior median line from the external occipital protruberence of the occipital bone to the area of your mark will assist with the point location.

k) There are other combinations of longitudinal measurements you can use other than 12 cun:
15 cun (anterior natural hairline to the space between C7/T1);
18 cun (between the two eyebrows at Du 24.5, M-HN-3 or Yin Tang to the space between C7/T1).

l) It may be easier to use a length of string or strip of paper so that you can draw on the cun measurements as opposed to drawing the measurements on the scalp itself.

Note: Lawson-Wood (1973) locates PIII 21 (Du 21) on the median line, at the meeting of the sagittal suture and the frontal bone, (the bregma), our Du 22. Soulié (1994), the name and location of his GV 20 is the name and approximate location of our Du 21. Soulié's location of GV 20 (near to our Du 21) is on the head, top, midline: mid-distance between the frontal and occipital bones; in a transverse fissure (sagittal plane) on the anterior edge of the posterior relief, between the parietal bones. The name of Soulié's GV 21 is similar to the name of our Du 22. His name for GV 21 is "Chuanghui " (Wade -Giles spelling), "Xinhui" (Pin Yin spelling) which translated means "Meeting of the Brain" or "Skull Meeting". He locates GV 21 (our Du 22) on the head, anterior top, midline: posterior edge of the frontal bone between the two parietal bones (fontanelles). Two points on either side of the groove between the parietal bones (acts on the opposite half of the brain).

Voisin (1974) locates Gov 21 on the midline of the cranium, on the coronal suture. This is where we locate Du 22. Wu (1973) locates VG 21 upon the median line of the cranium, at one and a half pouce in front of VG 20. Worsley (1982) locates XIV 21 on the median line of the head, 8.5 ACI superior to XIV 15. Shandong (1982) locate Qianding on the midline of the vertex, 1.5 cun anterior to Pt. Baihui.

Du 22 XIN HUI – SKULL MEETING

⊥ ***0.1 TO 0.3 CUN*** ***(Not on infants as their fontanelle may not yet be closed)***
Δ ***3 TO 5***

Pos: Position of patient: seated or supine.

Loc:
a) On top of the head.
b) At the junction of the coronal and sagittal suture (bregma).
c) On the median line of the head.
d) 2 cun posterior to the natural anterior hairline.
e) 10 cun anterior to the natural posterior hairline.
f) 1.5 cun anterior to Du 21.
g) 3 cun anterior to Du 20.

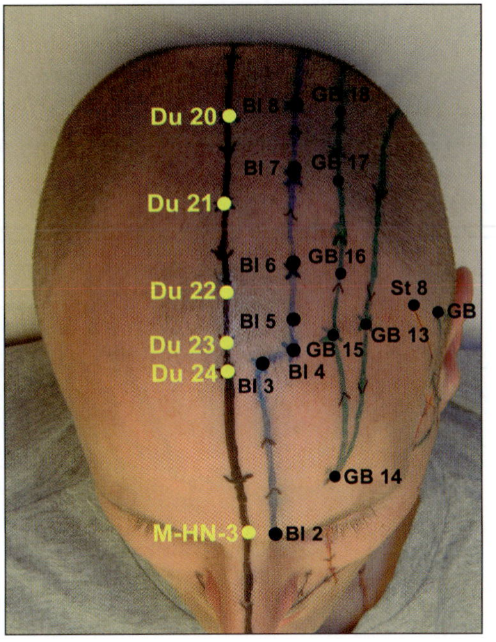

Tip:
a) Du 22 is located at the junction of the coronal and sagittal suture (bregma). The coronal suture is formed by the joint between the posterior edge of the frontal bone and the anterior borders of the parietal bones. The sagittal suture is formed by the meeting of the medial borders of the left and right parietal bones On the median line these two sutures meet at a junction called the "bregma". The point is located on the bregma.
b) The cun measurements can assist you to the area where you can palpate for the point.
c) Du 22 is 10 cun anterior to the natural posterior hairline (2 cun posterior to the natural anterior hairline) or 1.5 cun anterior to Du 21. For the longitudinal measurement of the head (see tip i).
d) First mark the median line on the anterior and posterior aspects of the head at the natural anterior and posterior hairline. Many head points are in relation to the natural hairline. The natural hairline may not be apparent due to the hairline receding. Sometimes you can see a definite change in skin texture from the forehead to the scalp, which is usually where the natural hairline was previously.
e) Measure 12 cun from the natural anterior hairline to the natural posterior hairline on the median line.
f) Place a mark at 10 cun anterior to the natural posterior hairline or 2 cun posterior to the natural anterior hairline or 1.5 cun anterior to Du 21, Du 22 should be located on or near to your mark. Palpation with the flow of the channel on the posterior median line from the external occipital protruberence of the occipital bone to the area of your mark will assist with the point location.
g) There are other combinations of longitudinal measurements you can use other than 12 cun:
15 cun (anterior natural hairline to the space between C7/T1);
18 cun (between the two eyebrows at Du 24.5, M-HN-3 or Yin Tang to the space between C7/T1).
h) It may be easier to use a length of string or strip of paper so that you can draw on the cun measurements as opposed to drawing the measurements on the scalp itself.

Note: Lawson-Wood (1973) locates PIII 22 (Du 22) on the median line, on the frontal bone, 3cm from PIII 21. This is at the approximate location of our Du 23, The location of PIII 21 is at the location of our Du 22. Soulié (1994), The name of his GV 21 is similar to the name of our Du 22. His name for GV 21 is "Chuanghui " (Wade -Giles spelling) , "Xinhui" (Pin Yin spelling) which means "Meeting of the Brain" or "Skull Meeting".

Soulié's location of GV 21 is similar to the location of our Du 22. He locates GV 21 (our Du 22) on the head, anterior top, midline: posterior edge of the frontal bone between the two parietal bones (fontanelles). Two points on either side of the groove between the parietal bones (acts on the opposite half of the brain). The name and location of his GV 22 is the same name and location as our Du 23 ("Shangxing"), on the head, anterior top, onthe frontal bone; at about two FW (Finger Width) in front of its suture with the two parietal bones (fontanelle); posterior (upper) edge of a slight rise on a plateau in a little hollow; two points on either side of the hollow. Voisin (1974) locates Gov 22 on the midline of the cranium, on the frontal bone: 1 fb (finger breadth) in front of the coronal suture.

Wu (1973) locates VG 22 upon the median line of the cranium, at three pouce in front of VG 20. Worsley (1982) locates XIV 22 on the median line of the head, 10 ACI (Anatomical Chinese Inch) superior to XIV 15.

Du 23 SHANG XING – UPPER STAR

⊥ ***0.2 TO 0.3 CUN*** **∆ 5**

- SUN SI-MIAO GHOST (Gui) – Ghost Point Name: Gui Tang – Ghost Hall

Pos: Position of patient: seated or supine.

Loc:
a) On top of the head.
b) On the frontal bone.
c) On the anterior median line.
d) 1 cun posterior to the natural anterior hairline.
e) 11 cun anterior to the natural posterior hairline.
f) 0.5 cun posterior to Du 24
g) 4 cun anterior to Du 20.
h) 1 cun anterior to Du 22.

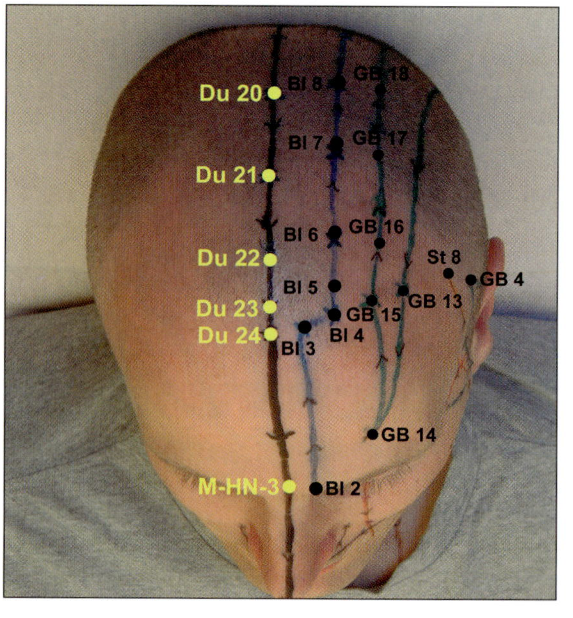

Tip: a) On the median line palpate posteriorly from the natural anterior hairline. You should be able to palpate a *men* (depression) just posterior to the natural anterior hairline which is Du 24 (at 0.5 cun), from here palpate posteriorly the same distance again, this should be Du 23, at 1 cun posterior to the natural anterior hairline (or 0.5 cun posterior to Du 24).

b) If you cannot feel a depression, use the cun measurements as a guide as these may assist you to the area to palpate for the point on the frontal bone.
c) Du 23 is 11 cun anterior to the natural posterior hairline or 1 cun posterior to the natural anterior hairline or 1 cun anterior to Du 22. For the longitudinal measurement of the head, see below.
d) First mark the median line on the anterior and posterior aspects of the head at the natural anterior and posterior hairline. Many head points are in relation to the natural hairline. The natural hairline may not be apparent due to the hairline receding. Sometimes you can see a definite change in skin texture from the forehead to the scalp, which is usually where the natural hairline was previously.
e) Measure 12 cun from the natural anterior hairline to the natural posterior hairline on the median line.
f) Place a mark at 11 cun anterior to the natural posterior hairline or 1 cun posterior to the natural anterior hairline or 1 cun anterior to Du 22, Du 23 should be located on or near to your mark. Palpation with the flow of the channel on the posterior median line from the external occipital protruberence of the occipital bone to the area of your mark will assist with the point location.
g) There are other combinations of longitudinal measurements you can use other than 12 cun:
   15 cun (anterior natural hairline to the space between C7/T1);
   18 cun (between the two eyebrows at Du 24.5, M-HN-3 or Yin Tang to the space between C7/T1).
h) It may be easier to use a length of string or strip of paper so that you can draw on the cun measurements as opposed to drawing the measurements on the scalp itself.

Note: Lawson-Wood (1973) locates PIII 23 (Du 23) on the median line, on the frontal bone, halfway between the bregma and glabella. This is the approximate location of our Du 24. The location of PIII 22 is at the approximate location of our Du 23. Soulié (1994), the name and location of his GV 22 is the same name and location as our Du 23 ("Shangxing"), on the head, anterior top, onthe frontal bone; at about two FW (Finger Width) in front of its suture with the two parietal bones (fontanelle); posterior (upper) edge of a slight rise on a plateau in a little hollow; two points on either side of the hollow. Even though there is a slight difference in the location description, the result of the location of the point seems to be in a same place as Du 23.

Soulié's location of GV 23 has a different description to the location of our Du 24 but it seems to be in a similar location. He locates GV 23 on the top of the forehead, midline: on the upper edge of the vertical medial relief; about mid-distance from the line of the eyebrow to the posterior (upper) edge of the frontal bone. The name of his GV 23 is the name of our Du 24, "Shenting". The English name is a little different, he calls it "Palace of the Evolved Man", whereas we call it "Spirit Hall".

Voisin (1974) locates Gov 23 on the midline of the cranium, on the frontal bone: normal hairline. This is the location of our Du 24. (His Gov 22 is located on the midline of the cranium, on the frontal bone: 1 fb (finger breadth) in front of the coronal suture.) Wu (1973) locates VG 23 upon the median line of the cranium, at four pouce in front of VG 20. Eachou (1995) there is a possibility that the locations for GV 23 and GV 24 should be swapped around, if so then the locations are more or less the same. Worsley (1982) locates XIV 23 on the median line of the head, 11 ACI (Anatomical Chinese Inch) superior to XIV 15.

Du 24 SHEN TING – SPIRIT HALL

⊥ *FORBIDDEN TO NEEDLE* Δ *3 TO 5*

- RE-UNION/Crossing/Meeting Point of the Du Mai with the Stomach and Bladder Channels – Governor Vessel with the Foot Yang Ming and Foot Tai Yang Channels

Pos: Position of patient: seated or supine.

Loc:
a) On top of the head.
b) On the frontal bone.
c) On the anterior median line.
d) 0.5 cun posterior to the natural anterior hairline.
e) 11.5 cun anterior to the natural posterior hairline.
f) 0.5 cun anterior to Du 23.

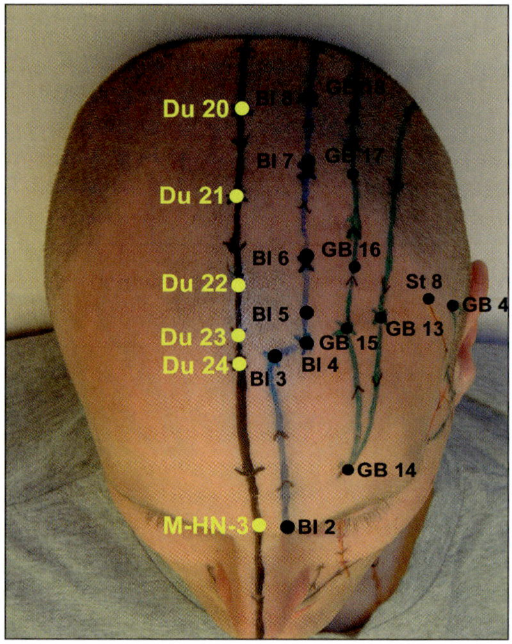

Tip:
a) On the median line palpate posteriorly from the natural anterior hairline. You should be able to palpate a *men* (depression) just posterior to the natural anterior hairline which is Du 24 at 0.5 cun.
b) If you cannot feel a depression, use the cun measurements as a guide as these may assist you to the area to palpate for the point on the frontal bone.
c) Du 24 is 0.5 cun posterior to the natural anterior hairline or 11.5 cun anterior to the natural posterior hairline or 1 cun anterior to Du 22. For the longitudinal measurement of the head, see below.
d) First mark the median line on the anterior and posterior aspects of the head at the natural anterior and posterior hairline. Many head points are in relation to the natural hairline. The natural hairline may not be apparent due to the hairline receding. Sometimes you can see a definite change in skin texture from the forehead to the scalp, which is usually where the natural hairline was previously.
e) Measure 12 cun from the natural anterior hairline to the natural posterior hairline on the median line.
f) Place a mark at 0.5 cun posterior to the natural anterior, or 11.5 cun anterior to the natural posterior hairline or hairline or 0.5 cun anterior to Du 23, Du 24 should be located on or near to your mark. Palpation with the flow of the channel on the posterior median line from the external occipital protruberence of the occipital bone to the area of your mark will assist with the point location.

g) There are other combinations of longitudinal measurements you can use other than 12 cun:
   15 cun (anterior natural hairline to the space between C7/T1);
   18 cun (between the two eyebrows at Du 24.5, M-HN-3 or Yin Tang to the space between C7/T1).
h) It may be easier to use a length of string or strip of paper so that you can draw on the cun measurements as opposed to drawing the measurements on the scalp itself.

Note: Lawson-Wood (1973) locates PIII 24 (Du 24) on the median line, on the tip of the nose. This is at our Du 25 location. The location of PIII 23 is at the location of our Du 24. Soulié (1994), the name of his GV 23 is the same Chinese name ("Shenting") as our Du 24, but the English name is a little different. He calls it, "Palace of the Evolved Man", whereas we call it "Spirit Hall". Soulié's location of GV 23 has a different description to the location of our Du 24 but seems to be in a similar location to our Du 24. He locates GV 23 on the top of the forehead, midline: on the upper edge of the vertical medial relief; about mid-distance from the line of the eyebrow to the posterior (upper) edge of the frontal bone.

Soulié numbers his next point to GV 23 as GV 23a, called "Yintang", this is more commonly known as an extra point on this GV/Du vessel and is numbered M-HN-3 or Du 24.5/GV 24.5. He locates GV 23a between the eyebows, midline: in the suture of the frontal and vomer bonesVoisin (1974) locates Gov 23 on the midline of the cranium, on the frontal bone: normal hairline. This is the location of our Du 24. Soulié's GV 24 is our Du 25, located at the tip of the nose, midline: just above the small ball formung the tip of the nose; two points acting on the opposite sides. The name of GV 24 is"Suliao" , this is the name of our Du 25.

Voisin (1974) locates Gov 24 at the location of our Du 24.5/M-HN-3/Yin Tang on the midline of the cranium, on the frontal bone: between the eyebrows. Wu (1973) locates VG 24 upon the median line of the cranium, at four and a half pouce in front of VG 20. Eachou (1995) there is a possibility that the locations for GV 23 and GV 24 should be swapped around, if so then the locations are more or less the same, except on GV 24 (on both possible locations) the point is located 1 inch posterior to the anterior hairline. Worsley (1982) locates XIV 24 on the median line of the head, 11.5 ACI superior to XIV 15.

(M-HN-3 / Du 24.5 / GV 24.5 / GV 23a / XIV 24.5 / XF-3 / Gov 24)

M-HN-3 YIN TANG – SEAL HALL

⊥ ***0.3 TO 0.5 CUN (SEATED) 0.5 CUN (SUPINE)*** **Δ** ***3 TO 5***

Pos: Position of patient: seated or supine.

Loc:
a) On the anterior aspect of the head.
b) On the frontal bone.
c) On the anterior median line.
d) At the midpoint between the medial borders of the two eyebrows.
e) On the glabella.

Tip:
a) Measure midway between the medial borders of the eyebrows and palpate for the point on the anterior median line. The point is located on the glabella.
b The eyebrows are situated on two superciliary arches, and these arches give the shape of the eyebrows. Between the medial ends of the superciliary arches there is a smooth elevation, called the glabella. The point is located on this elevation on the anterior median line, transversely level with the medial ends of the eyebrows.

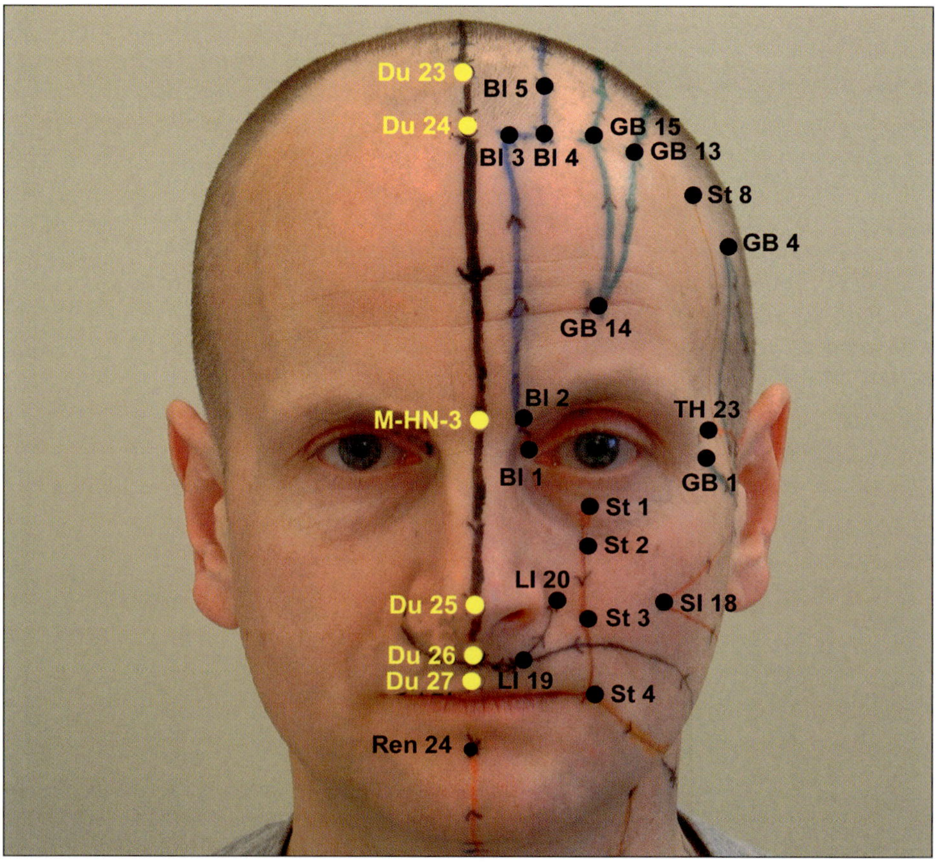

c) A common error is to locate this point just inferior to the glabella. There is a suture formed by the nasal bone and the glabella of the frontal bone called the nasion, the point lies superior to this.

d) This point can be used as a reference for marking the cun measurements of the head.
Longitudinal bone proportional measurements of the head:
3 cun from between the two eyebrows (Du 24.5, M-HN-3 or Yin Tang) to the natural anterior hairline on the anterior median line.
12 cun from the natural anterior hairline to the posterior hairline on the median line.
3 cun from the posterior hairline to the space between the 7th cervical and 1st thoracic vertebrae (Du 14) on the posterior median line.

Note: Worsley (1982) refers to this point as XIV (GV) 24.5; Soulié (1994), refers to this point as GV 23a and locates it between the eyebrows, midline; in the suture of the frontal and vomer bones; two points each in the angle of the upper edge between the extremity of the brow ridge and a vertical relief; acts on the opposite side; four FW (Finger Width) below GV 24; one FW on either side of BL 2. He locates GV 24 at our Du 25 location, at the tip of the nose. Voisin (1974) calls this point Gov 24. Gov 23 is at our Du 24 location.

Du 25 SU LIAO – PLAIN BONE

⊥ ***0.2 TO 0.3 CUN*** ***∆ FORBIDDEN TO USE MOXA***

Pos: Position of patient: seated or supine.

Loc:
a) On the anterior aspect of the face.
b) At the tip of the nose.
c) On the anterior median line.
d) At the apex of the cartilage of the major alar nasi.
e) At the apex of the septal cartilage of the septum of the nose.

Tip:
a) Palpate for the point on the anterior median line. You should be able to palpate a *men* (depression) at the tip of the nose where the two lateral parts of the major alar nasi unite. The cartilage should part when you press the tip of the nose.
b) The major alar nasi, minor alar nasi and the septal cartilages lie on the anterior aspect of the nose. On a skeleton these cartilages disappear to leave a hole surrounded by the bones of the face.
c) To help you to palpate for the *men* (depression) run the tip of your finger from the natural anterior hairline on the anterior median line (Du channel) to the tip of the nose where the point is located.
d) Occasionally the point may be located just superior to the tip of the nose, so palpating for the *men* is of utmost importance.

Note: Lawson-Wood (1973) locates PIII 25 (Du 25) on the median line, on the orbicularis oris, just under the anterior nasal spine. This is the approximate location of our Du 26. The location of PIII 24 is at the location of our Du 25. Soulié (1994), The name of Soulié's GV 24 is the name of our Du 25 ("Suliao"), located at the tip of the nose, midline: just above the small ball forming the tip of the nose; two points acting on the opposite sides. He locates GV 25 at our Du 26, on the face, a little below the nose, midline: on the upper edge of a flat muscle (orbicular muscle of the lips); in a vertical groove of the upper lip; two points on either side of this groove; one FW (Finger Width) on either side is LI 19. The name of GV 25 is "Shuigou", this is different to our Du 26 name,"Renzhong".

Worsley (1982) locates XIV 25 on the median line of the nose, at the inferior edge of the alar cartilage, just superior to the tip of the nose. Wu (1973) locates VG 25 upon the median line of the nose, at the extreme edge of the cartilage above the tip.

Du 26 REN ZHONG – MIDDLE OF THE MAN

⊥ ***0.3 CUN*** Δ ***3***

- RE-UNION/Crossing/Meeting Point of the Du Mai with the Large Intestine and Stomach Channels – Governor Vessel with the Hand Yang Ming and Foot Yang Ming Channels
- SUN SI-MIAO GHOST (Gui) – Ghost Point Name: Gui Gong – Ghost Palace or Ghost Reception Room

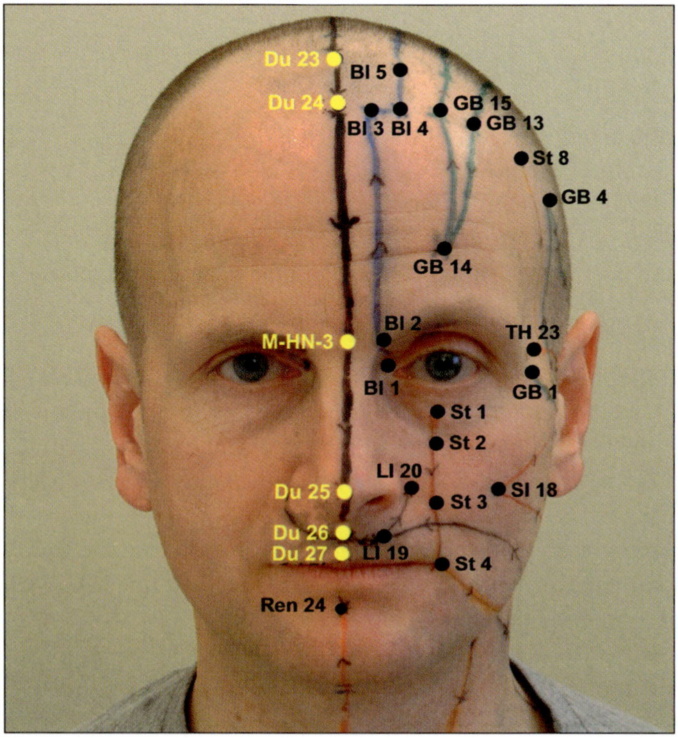

Pos: Position of patient: seated or supine.

Loc: a) On the anterior aspect of the face.
b) On the philtrum.
c) On the anterior median line.
d) One third of the distance from the root of the nasal spine to the vermillion border of the upper lip.

Tip: a) On the anterior median line between the base of the nose and the upper part of the lip is a vertical groove called the philtrum. The point is located on the philtrum.
b) The point is located one third of the distance from the root of the nasal spine of the nose and the vermillion border of the upper lip on the philtrum.
c) The root of the nasal spine is on the anterior median line and can be palpated for by feeling for the contour of the maxilla bone. Draw a mark where the contour of the bone flattens just inferior to base of the nose.
d) The vermillion border of the upper lip is the most superior part of the upper lip where the skin texture changes from the face to the lip.
e) Measure one third of the distance from the root of the nasal spine to the vermillion border of the upper lip and then palpate for the point on the philtrum (which is also on the anterior median line).

Note: Lawson-Wood (1973) locates PIII 26 (Du 26) on the median line, on the upper lip, below the lower extremity of the naso-labial fold. This is the location of our Du 27. The location of his PIII 25 is at the approximate location of our Du 26, Soulié (1994) locates his GV 25 at the same location as our Du 26 but calls this point "Shuigou" – "Drainage Ditch", this makes sense in a way when we think of what the philtrum does with waste from our nose. This name is different to our Du 26 name,"Renzhong", which means "Middle of Man". He locates GV 25 (our Du 26), on the face, a little below the nose, midline: on the upper edge of a flat muscle (orbicular muscle of the lips); in a vertical groove of the upper lip; two points on either side of this groove; one FW (Finger Width) on either side is LI 19. The location of his GV 26 is our Du 27 , located on the upper lip (fold), midline: just at the upper edge of the red mucosal tissue. The name of his GV 26 is the same name as our Du 27, "Duiduan".

Wu (1973) locates VG 26 upon the median line of the face, below the nose, in the centre of the philtrum. Cheng (1987) and Shanghai (1993) states that this point is known as "Shuigou" with "Renzhong" as an alternative name. Worsley (1982) locates this point on the anterior median line, inferior to the nose, in the centre of the philtrum. So (1985) locates GV 26 in the centre of the philtrum.

Du 27 DUI DUAN – CORRECT EXCHANGE

⊥ ***0.2 CUN*** Δ ***1 TO 3***

Pos: Position of patient: seated or supine.

Loc: a) On the anterior aspect of the face.
b) On the tubercle of the philtrum.
c) On the anterior median line.
d) At the junction of the philtrum and the vermillion border of the upper lip.

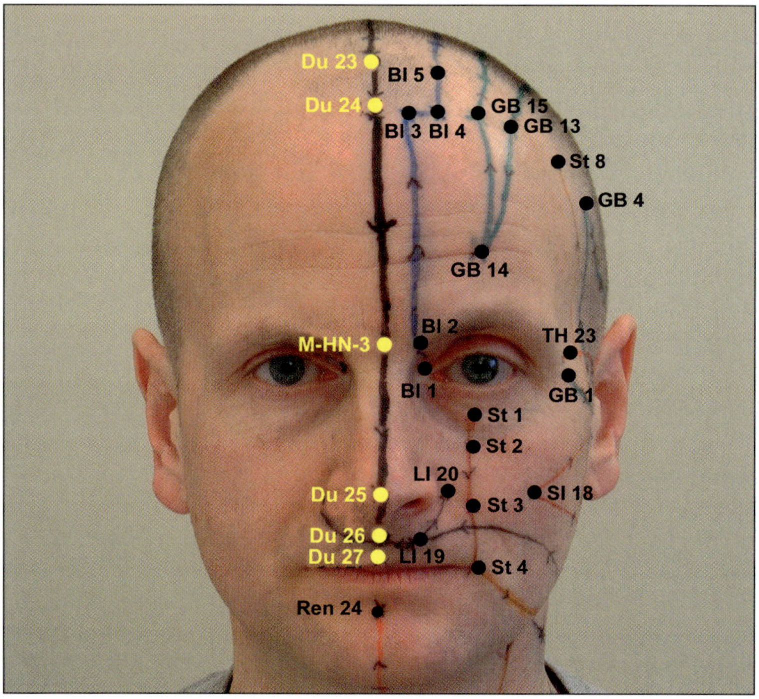

Tip: a) On the anterior median line between the base of the nose and the upper part of the lip is a vertical groove called the philtrum.
b) The vermillion border of the upper lip is the most superior part of the upper lip where the skin texture changes from the face to the lip.
e) The point is located on the anterior median line, on the inferior border of the philtrum where it tends to slightly prominate. This is at the junction where the philtrum and the vermillion border of the the upper lip meet.

Note: Lawson-Wood (1973) locates PIII 27 (Du 27) on the median line, inside the mouth, on the front of the gum just above the first incisors of the upper jaw. This is at the location of our Du 28, Lawson-Wood has no PIII 28 as his PIII 27 ends at our Du 28, Soulié (1994) locates his GV 26 at our Du 27. He calls GV 26 "Duiduan" – "Prominent Extremity". The location of his GV 26 (our Du 27) is on the upper lip (fold), midline: just at the upper edge of the red mucosal tissue. He locates and names GV 27 at our Du 28, called "Yinjiao", located on the upper gum, midline: lower edge of the septum; between the two large incisors; two points.

Du 28 YIN JIAO – MOUTH CROSSING

⊥ ***0.1 TO 0.2 CUN*** Δ ***FORBIDDEN TO USE MOXA***

- EXIT
- 8 EXTRAORDINARY VESSEL/Coalescent Point of Ren Mai (Conception/Directing Vessel)
- RE-UNION/Crossing/Meeting Point of the Du Mai with the Stomach Channel and the Ren Mai – Governor Vessel with Foot Yang Ming Channel and the Conception/Directing Vessel

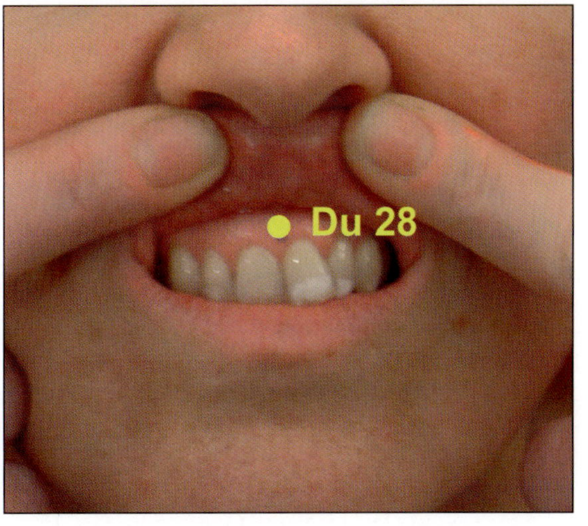

Pos: Position of patient: seated or supine.

Loc: a) On the anterior aspect of the face.
b) At the junction of the frenulum of the upper lip and the upper gum
c) On the anterior median line.

Tip: a) To have access to the point you will need to ask the patient to hold up their upper lip for you to see their upper gum.
b) If the patient has false teeth, they will need to drop them down enough so you can locate and needle the point where the frenulum of the upper lip attaches to the upper gum.
c) There are two frenulum, one upper and one lower. They are part of the inner surface of the upper and lower lips and they attach to the upper and lower gums, The frenulum of the upper lip is the one we use for locating Du 28.
d) The point is located on the anterior median line, at the junction of the frenulum and the upper gum. Some frenulum vary in length, the shorter the frenulum the easier it is to locate Du 28.
e) If your patient has a long frenulum that seems to run down to the inferior border of the upper gum, you still will need to needle the point on the anterior gum. The point will be on the anterior median line, therefore you will need to angle the needle towards the anterior median line and hence the frenulum, and also with or against the flow of the channel.

Note: Lawson-Wood (1973) has no PIII 28 (Du 28) as his PIII 27 is located at our Du 28, Soulié (1994) locates GV 27 at our Du 28. He names this point"Yinjiao" – "Crossing of the gums". He locates and names his GV 27 as our Du 28, located on the upper gum, midline: lower edge of the septum; between the two large incisors; two points. Shandong (1982) locate Yinjiao by taking up the upper lip, at the labial end of the frenulum labii superiors, it is slightly above the cleft between the incisors.

REFERENCES FOR THE DUMAI GOVERNOR CHANNEL

Worsley, J R 1982 Traditional Chinese Acupuncture Volume 1 – Meridians and Points – XIV 1: 271; XIV 4 – Chong Mo Point: 294; XIV 16: 277; XIV 17: 277; XIV 18: 279; XIV 19: 279; XIV 20: 279; XIV 21: 279; XIV 22: 281; XIV 23: 281; XIV 24: 281; XIV 24.5: 281; XIV 25: 283; XIV 26: 283

Voisin, Dr. H 1974 Essentials of Acupuncture – Gov 1: 66; Gov 5: 66; Gov 6 (Du 7): 66; Gov 7 (Du 8): 66; Gov 8 (Du 9): 66; Gov 9 (Du 10): 66; Gov 10 (Du 11) : 66; Gov 11 (Du 12): 66; Gov 12 (Du 13): 66; Gov 13 (Du 14): 66 Gov 14: 66; Gov 15; 66; Gov 16: 66; Gov 17: 66; Gov 18: 66; Gov 19: 66; Gov 20: 66; Gov 21 (Du 22): 66; Gov 22: 66; Gov 23 (Du 24): 66; Gov 24 (Du 24.5/M-HN-3/Yin Tang): 66

Lawson-Wood 1973 Acupuncture Handbook – PIII 1 (Du 1): 62; PIII 3 (Du 3): 62; PIII 4 (Du 4): 64; PIII 5 (Du 5): 64; PIII 6 (Du 6): 64; PIII 7 (Du 7): 65; PIII 8 (Du 8): 65; PIII 9 (Du 9): 65; PIII 10 (Du 10): 65; PIII 11 (Du 11): 66; PIII 12 (Du 12): 66; PIII 13 (Du 13): 66; PIII 14: 67; PIII 15: 67; PIII 18: 69; PIII 19 (Du 18): 69; PIII 20: 69; PIII 21 (Du 22): 70; PIII 22 (Du 23): 70; PIII 23 (Du 24): 70; PIII 24 (Du 25): 70; PIII 25 (Du 26): 70; PIII 26 (Du 27): 70; PIII 27 (Du 28): 70

So, James Tin Yau (Dr) 1985 The Book of Acupuncture Points – GV 1: 80; GV 2: 79; GV 17: 172; GV 18: 172; GV 26: 31

Qiu Mao-Liang 1996 – Chinese Acupuncture and Moxibustion – DU 1: 151

Gray, H; Warwick, Roger; Williams, Peter L 1978 Gray's Anatomy 35th Edition – (Du 1) Inferior Pelvic Aperture (Pelvic Outlet): 529; (Du 18) – Lamboid, Sagittal and Lambda Sutures (Norma Verticalis): 261; (Du 24.5/M-HN-3/Yin Tang): Superciliary Arches/ Glabella – 298, Nasion Illustration – 257;

Shandong Medical College and Shandong College of Traditional Chinese Medicine 1982 Anatomical Atlas of Chinese Acupuncture Point – Yaoshu (Du 2): 58; Yamen (Du 15): 59; Baihui (Du 20): 59; Qianding (Du 21): 59; Yinjiao (Du 28) 60

Soulié De Morant, George. 1994 Chinese Acupuncture – GV 3: 528; GV 6a (Du 7): 530; GV 7 (Du 8): 530; GV 8 (Du 9): 530; GV 9 (Du 10): 531; GV 10 (Du 11): 531; GV 11 (Du 12): 532; GV 12 (Du 13 Name Only): 532; GV 13 (Du 13): 533; GV 13a (Du 14 Location): 533; GV 13b: 534; GV 13c: 535; GV 14 (Du 15 Name Only): 536; GV 15 (Du 16 Name Only): 537; GV 16 (Du 15 Location, Du 17 Name): 538; GV 17 (Du 16 Location, Du 18 Name): 539; GV 18 (Du 17 Location, Du 19 Name Only): 539; GV 19 (Du 18 Location, Du 20 Name): 540; GV 20 (Du 21); GV 21 (Du 22): 541; GV 22 (Du 23): 541; GV 23 (Du 24): 541; GV 23a (Du 24.5 or M-HN-3): 542; GV 24 (Du 25): 542; GV 25 (Du 26): 542/543; GV 26 (Du 27): 543; GV 27 (Du 28): 543

Wu, Wei-P'ing 1973 Chinese Acupuncture – VG 15: 128; VG 16: 128; VG 17: 129; VG 18: 129; VG 19: 129; VG 20: 129; VG 21: 129; VG 22: 129; VG 23: 130; VG 24: 130; VG 25: 130; VG 26: 130

Jayasuriya, Anton 1982 Clinical Acupuncture – Du 15: 406; Du 16: 406; Du 20: 406/407

Deadman, Peter; Al-Khafaji, Mazin; Baker, Kevin 1998 Manual of Acupuncture, An – DU 20: 552

Lavier, Dr. J 1974 Points of Chinese Acupuncture – VG 20: 76/77

Li Ding (Prof.). 1991. Acupuncture, Meridian Theory and Acupuncture Points – DU 20: 357

Lotan, Alon 2000 Acupoint Location Guide – GV (Du) 20: 171

Eachou Chen 1995 Cross-sectional Anatomy of Acupoints – GV 23: 105; GV 24: 104

Cheng Xinnong (Editor) 1987 Chinese Acupuncture and Moxibustion – Du 26: 224

Shanghai College of Traditional Chinese Medicine. 1993 Applied Anatomical Charts of Acupuncture and Moxibustion – DU 26: 186

THE EXTRAORDINARY VESSELS

<u>Note:</u> The Governor Vessel and the Conception Vessel are two of the 8 Extraordinary Vessels. They are different to the other Extraordinary Vessels in that they have their own points rather than using known points from other channels. Some texts and Schools include the Conception and Governor Vessels as primary channels along with the other twelve primary channels, and these are commonly called the Fourteen Channels.

Note: Points given in brackets appear in certain, but not all, Acupuncture texts.

If you require tips for any of these points, please refer to their main channels eg. Pc or St etc.

THE CHONG MAI (Penetrating Vessel)

The Chong Mai starts inside the lower abdomen and emerges at the perineum. Rising, it runs inside the spinal column where its superficial branch crosses the region of St 30 and communicates with the Kidney channel. Passing along both sides of the abdomen it reaches the middle of the thorax and diffuses there. From there, a branch rises up to the throat and curves around the lips.

The coalescent points of the Chong Mai are: (Ren 1), (Ren 7), (St 30), Ki 11, Ki 12, Ki 13, Ki 14, Ki 15, Ki 16, Ki 17, Ki 18, Ki 19, Ki 20, Ki 21.

Note: Some texts talk of the "five routes" of the Chong Mai, including two channels which descend the medial and lateral borders of the tibia to the foot.

(Ren 1) HUI YIN – MEETING OF YIN

⊥ ***0.8 TO 1.2 CUN*** ***∆ FORBIDDEN TO USE MOXA***

- ENTRY
- GENERAL JUNCTION/Luo/Connecting/Passage/Lo/Lê
- 8 EXTRAORDINARY VESSEL/Coalescent Point of Du Mai (Governor Vessel)
- 8 EXTRAORDINARY VESSEL/Coalescent Point of Penetrating Vessel (Chong Mai) – see note
- 8 EXTRAORDINARY VESSEL/Coalescent Point of the Yin Linking Vessel (Yin Wei Mai)
- RE-UNION/Crossing/Meeting Point of the Ren Mai with the Du Mai and the Penetrating Vessel.- Conception/Directing Vessel with the Governor Vessel and the Chong Mai

Pos: Position of patient: supine with both legs semi flexed. The legs should also be at the approximate shoulder width apart from each other.

Loc: a) On the inferior pelvic aperture (pelvic outlet) – (Grays 1978-p.529).
b) On the perineal body.
c) In the centre of the perineum.
d) On the median line.
e) Midway between the anus and the scrotum (in men).
f) Midway between the anus and the posterior commissure of the vagina (in women).

Note: In some texts Ren 1 is listed as an 8 EXTRAORDINARY VESSEL/Coalescent Point of Chong Mai (Penetrating Vessel), whereas in others it is omitted.

(Ren 7) YIN JIAO – YIN CROSSING

⊥ ***0.5 TO 0.8 CUN*** Δ ***5 TO 7***
FORBIDDEN TO NEEDLE AND MOXA THIS POINT DURING PREGNANCY

- ALARM/Front Collecting/Front Mu/Herald Point of Triple Heater Lower Jiao
- 8 EXTRAORDINARY VESSEL/Coalescent Point of Penetrating Vessel (Chong Mai) – see note
- RE-UNION/Crossing/Meeting Point of the Ren Mai with the Kidney Channel and the Penetrating Vessel – Conception/Directing Vessel with the Foot Shao Yin Channel and the Chong Mai

Pos: Position of patient: supine.

Loc: a) On the anterior aspect of the torso.
b) On the lower abdomen (in the lower jiao).
c) On the anterior median line.
d) 4 cun superior to the superior border of the symphysis pubis.
e) 1 cun inferior to the level of the centre of the umbilicus.

Note: In some texts Ren 7 is listed as an 8 EXTRAORDINARY VESSEL/Coalescent Point of Chong Mai (Penetrating Vessel), whereas in others it is omitted.

(St 30) QI CHONG – QI RUSHING

⊥ ***0.3 TO 0.5 CUN*** **Δ** ***3 TO 7***
FORBIDDEN TO NEEDLE AND MOXA THIS POINT DURING PREGNANCY

- 8 EXTRAORDINARY VESSEL/Coalescent Point of Penetrating Vessel (Chong Mai) – see note
- RE-UNION/Crossing/Meeting Point of the Stomach Channel with the Penetrating Vessel – Foot Yang Ming with the Chong Mai
- A POINT OF THE SEA OF NOURISHMENT (Waters and Grains) (There is one other Sea of Nourishment Point: St 36)

Pos: Position of patient: supine.

Loc:
a) On the anterior aspect of the torso.
b) On the lower abdomen (in the lower jiao).
c) On the lateral border of the rectus abdominis muscle.
d) Level with the superior border of the symphysis pubis bone.
e) 2 cun lateral to the anterior median line.
f) 5 cun inferior to the level of the centre of the umbilicus.
g) Level with Ren 2 (which is on the anterior median line, at 5 cun inferior to the level of thecentre of the umbilicus.

Note: In some texts St 30 is listed as an 8 EXTRAORDINARY VESSEL/Coalescent Point of Chong Mai (Penetrating Vessel), whereas in others it is omitted.

Ki 11 HENG GU – TRANSVERSE BONE

⊥ ***0.3 TO 0.5 CUN*** **Δ** ***5 TO 15***
FORBIDDEN TO NEEDLE AND MOXA THIS POINT DURING PREGNANCY.

- 8 EXTRAORDINARY VESSEL/Coalescent Point of Chong Mai (Penetrating Vessel)
- RE-UNION/Crossing/Meeting Point of the Kidney Channel with the Penetrating Vessel – Foot Shao Yin Channel with the Chong Mai.

Pos: Position of patient: supine.

Loc:
a) On the anterior aspect of the torso.
b) On the lower abdomen (in the lower jiao).
c) On the superior border of the symphysis pubis bone.
d) 0.5 cun lateral to the anterior median line.
e) 5 cun inferior to the level of the centre of the umbilicus.
f) Level with Ren 2 (which is on the anterior median line, at 5 cun inferior to the level of centre of the umbilicus and is on the superior border of the symphysis pubis bone.

Ki 12 DA HE – GREAT BRIGHTNESS

⊥ ***0.5 TO 1.0 CUN*** Δ ***5 TO 10***
FORBIDDEN TO NEEDLE AND MOXA THIS POINT DURING PREGNANCY.

- 8 EXTRAORDINARY VESSEL/Coalescent Point of Penetrating Vessel (Chong Mai)
- RE-UNION/Crossing/Meeting Point of the Kidney Channel with the Penetrating Vessel – Foot Shao Yin Channel with the Chong Mai

Pos: Position of patient: supine.

Loc: a) On the anterior aspect of the torso.
b) On the lower abdomen (in the lower jiao).
c) 0.5 cun lateral to the anterior median line.
d) 1 cun superior to the superior border of the symphysis pubis bone.
e) 1 cun superior to Ki 11.
f) 4 cun inferior to the level of the centre of the umbilicus.
g) Level with Ren 3 (see separate location).

Ki 13 QI XUE – DOOR OF INFANTS

⊥ ***0.5 TO 1.0 CUN*** Δ ***5 TO 10***
FORBIDDEN TO NEEDLE AND MOXA THIS POINT DURING PREGNANCY.

- 8 EXTRAORDINARY VESSEL/Coalescent Point of Penetrating Vessel (Chong Mai)
- RE-UNION/Crossing/Meeting Point of the Kidney Channel with the Penetrating Vessel – Foot Shao Yin Channel with the Chong Mai

Pos: Position of patient: supine.

Loc: a) On the anterior aspect of the torso.
b) On the lower abdomen (in the lower jiao).
c) 0.5 cun lateral to the anterior median line.
d) 2 cun superior to the superior border of the symphysis pubis bone.
e) 2 cun superior to Ki 11.
f) 3 cun inferior to the level of the centre of the umbilicus.
g) Level with Ren 4 (see separate location).

Ki 14 SI MAN – FOUR FULL

⊥ ***0.5 TO 1.0 CUN*** ***Δ 5 TO 30***
FORBIDDEN TO NEEDLE AND MOXA THIS POINT DURING PREGNANCY.

- 8 EXTRAORDINARY VESSEL/Coalescent Point of Penetrating Vessel (Chong Mai)
- RE-UNION/Crossing/Meeting Point of the Kidney Channel with the Penetrating Vessel – Foot Shao Yin Channel with the Chong Mai

Pos: Position of patient: supine.

Loc: a) On the anterior aspect of the torso.
b) On the lower abdomen (in the lower jiao).
c) 0.5 cun lateral to the anterior median line.
d) 3 cun superior to the superior border of the symphysis pubis bone.
e) 3 cun superior to Ki 11.
f) 2 cun inferior to the level of the centre of the umbilicus.
g) Level with Ren 5 (see separate location).

Ki 15 ZHONG ZHU – MIDDLE FLOWING OUT

⊥ ***0.5 TO 1.0 CUN*** ***Δ 5 TO 15***
FORBIDDEN TO NEEDLE AND MOXA THIS POINT DURING PREGNANCY.

- 8 EXTRAORDINARY VESSEL/Coalescent Point of Penetrating Vessel (Chong Mai)
- RE-UNION/Crossing/Meeting Point of the Kidney Channel with the Penetrating Vessel – Foot Shao Yin Channel with the Chong Mai

Pos: Position of patient: supine.

Loc: a) On the anterior aspect of the torso.
b) On the lower abdomen (in the lower jiao).
c) 0.5 cun lateral to the anterior median line.
d) 4 cun superior to the superior border of the symphysis pubis bone.
e) 4 cun superior to Ki 11.
f) 1 cun inferior to the level of the centre of the umbilicus.
g) Level with Ren 7 (see separate location).

Ki 16 HUANG SHU – VITALS CORRESPONDENCE

⊥ ***0.5 TO 1.0 CUN*** **Δ *5 TO 7***
FORBIDDEN TO NEEDLE AND MOXA THIS POINT DURING PREGNANCY.

- 8 EXTRAORDINARY VESSEL/Coalescent Point of Penetrating Vessel (Chong Mai)
- RE-UNION/Crossing/Meeting Point of the Kidney Channel with the Penetrating Vessel – Foot Shao Yin Channel with the Chong Mai

Pos: Position of patient: supine.

Loc: a) On the anterior aspect of the torso.
b) In between the mid-abdomen and lower abdomen (in between the middle and lower jiao).
c) 0.5 cun lateral to the anterior median line.
d) Level with the centre of the umbilicus.
e) Level with Ren 8 (which is in the centre of the umbilicus).

Ki 17 SHANG QU – MERCHANT CROOKED

⊥ ***0.5 TO 1.0 CUN*** **Δ *5 TO 7***
FORBIDDEN TO NEEDLE AND MOXA THIS POINT DURING PREGNANCY.

- 8 EXTRAORDINARY VESSEL/Coalescent Point of Penetrating Vessel (Chong Mai)
- RE-UNION/Crossing/Meeting Point of the Kidney Channel with the Penetrating Vessel – Foot Shao Yin Channel with the Chong Mai

Pos: Position of patient: supine.

Loc: a) On the anterior aspect of the torso.
b) On the mid-abdomen (in the middle jiao).
c) 0.5 cun lateral to the anterior median line.
d) 2 cun superior to the level of the centre of the umbilicus.
e) Level with Ren 10 (which is on the anterior median line, at 2 cun superior to the level of the centre of the umbilicus).

Ki 18 SHI GUAN – STONE BORDER

⊥ ***0.5 TO 1.0 CUN*** ***Δ 5 TO 7***
FORBIDDEN TO NEEDLE AND MOXA THIS POINT DURING PREGNANCY.

- 8 EXTRAORDINARY VESSEL/Coalescent Point of Penetrating Vessel (Chong Mai)
- RE-UNION/Crossing/Meeting Point of the Kidney Channel with the Penetrating Vessel – Foot Shao Yin Channel with the Chong Mai

Pos: Position of patient: supine.

Loc: a) On the anterior aspect of the torso.
b) On the mid-abdomen (in the middle jiao).
c) 0.5 cun lateral to the anterior median line.
d) 3 cun superior to the level of the centre of the umbilicus.
e) Level with Ren 11 (which is on the anterior median line, at 3 cun superior to the level of the centre of the umbilicus).

Ki 19 YIN DU – YIN CAPITAL

⊥ ***0.5 TO 1.0 CUN*** ***Δ 5 TO 10***
FORBIDDEN TO NEEDLE AND MOXA THIS POINT DURING PREGNANCY.

- 8 EXTRAORDINARY VESSEL/Coalescent Point of Penetrating Vessel (Chong Mai)
- RE-UNION/Crossing/Meeting Point of the Kidney Channel with the Penetrating Vessel – Foot Shao Yin Channel with the Chong Mai

Pos: Position of patient: supine.

Loc: a) On the anterior aspect of the torso.
b) On the mid-abdomen (in the middle jiao).
c) 0.5 cun lateral to the anterior median line.
d) 2 cun superior to the level of the centre of the umbilicus.
e) Level with Ren 12 (which is on the anterior median line, at 4 cun superior to the level of the centre of the umbilicus).

Ki 20 FU TONG GU – THROUGH THE VALLEY

⊥ ***0.5 TO 0.7 CUN*** **Δ *7 TO 10***
FORBIDDEN TO NEEDLE AND MOXA THIS POINT DURING PREGNANCY.

- 8 EXTRAORDINARY VESSEL/Coalescent Point of Penetrating Vessel (Chong Mai)
- RE-UNION/Crossing/Meeting Point of the Kidney Channel with the Penetrating Vessel – Foot Shao Yin Channel with the Chong Mai

Pos: Position of patient: supine.

Loc: a) On the anterior aspect of the torso.
b) On the mid-abdomen (in the middle jiao).
c) 0.5 cun lateral to the anterior median line.
d) 5 cun superior to the level of the centre of the umbilicus.
e) Level with Ren 13 (which is on the anterior median line, at 5 cun superior to the level of the centre of the umbilicus).

Ki 21 YOU MEN – DARK GATE

⊥ ***0.3 TO 0.5 CUN*** **Δ *5 TO 10***
FORBIDDEN TO NEEDLE AND MOXA THIS POINT DURING PREGNANCY.

- 8 EXTRAORDINARY VESSEL/Coalescent Point of Penetrating Vessel (Chong Mai)
- RE-UNION/Crossing/Meeting Point of the Kidney Channel with the Penetrating Vessel – Foot Shao Yin Channel with the Chong Mai

Pos: Position of patient: supine.

Loc: a) On the anterior aspect of the torso.
b) On the mid-abdomen (in the middle jiao).
c) 0.5 cun lateral to the anterior median line.
d) 6 cun superior to the level of the centre of the umbilicus.
e) Level with Ren 14 (which is on the anterior median line, at 5 cun superior to the level of the centre of the umbilicus).

THE DAI MAI (Girdle Vessel)

The Dai Mai arises below the hypochondriacal region in the area of the 11th and 12th ribs, and runs obliquely downward through GB 26, GB 27 and GB 28; it traverses the waist like a belt.

The coalescent points of the Dai Mai are: GB 26, GB 27 and GB 28.

GB 26 DAI MAI – GIRDLE VESSEL

⊥ ***0.5 TO 0.8 CUN Δ 5 TO 15***
FORBIDDEN TO NEEDLE AND MOXA THIS POINT DURING PREGNANCY

- 8 EXTRAORDINARY VESSEL/Coalescent Point of the Girdle Vessel (Dai Mai)
- RE-UNION/Crossing/Meeting Point of the Gall Bladder Channel with the Girdle Vessel.- Foot Shao Yang Channel with the Dai Mai

Pos: Position of patient: supine.

Loc: a) On the anterior aspect of the torso.
b) In between the mid-abdomen and lower abdomen (in between the middle and lower jiao).
c) At the level of the umbilicus.
d) Inferior to the tip of the eleventh rib (where Liv 13 is located).
e) On a line from GB 25 to GB 27.

GB 27 WU SHU – FIVE PIVOTS

⊥ ***0.5 TO 0.7 CUN Δ 3 TO 10***
FORBIDDEN TO NEEDLE AND MOXA THIS POINT DURING PREGNANCY

- 8 EXTRAORDINARY VESSEL/Coalescent Point of the Girdle Vessel (Dai Mai)
- RE-UNION/Crossing/Meeting Point of the Gall Bladder Channel with the Girdle Vessel.- Foot Shao Yang Channel with the Dai Mai

Pos: Position of patient: supine.

Loc: a) On the anterior aspect of the torso.
b) On the lower abdomen (lower jiao).
c) Just anterior to the border of the anterior superior iliac spine of the ilium.
d) 3 cun inferior to the level of the umbilicus.
e) Transversely level with Ren 4.

GB 28 WEI DAO – BINDING PATH

⊥ ***0.5 TO 0.7 CUN*** **Δ** ***3 TO 7***
FORBIDDEN TO NEEDLE AND MOXA THIS POINT DURING PREGNANCY

- 8 EXTRAORDINARY VESSEL/Coalescent Point of the Girdle Vessel (Dai Mai)
- RE-UNION/Crossing/Meeting Point of the Gall Bladder Channel with the Girdle Vessel.- Foot Shao Yang Channel with the Dai Mai

Pos: Position of patient: supine.

Loc: a) On the anterior aspect of the torso.
b) On the lower abdomen (lower jiao).
c) Anterior to the border of the anterior superior iliac spine of the ilium.
d) Inferior to GB 27.
e) Approximately 0.5 cun medial to GB 27.

THE YIN QIAO MAI (Yin Heel/Yin Motility Vessel)

The Yin Qiao Mai starts in the middle of the heel and rises to the proximal aspect of the navicular bone. Travelling superior to the medial malleolus it goes straight upwards, along the posterior border of the medial aspect of the thigh to the external genitalia and from there through the chest to the supraclavicular fossa (St 12). It ascends and passes anterior to St 9, then goes along the zygoma to reach the inner canthus and communicate with the Bladder channel and the Yang Qiao Mai.

The coalescent points of the Yin Qiao Mai are: Ki 6, Ki 8 and Bl 1.

Ki 6Z HAO HAI – ILLUMINATED SEA

⊥ ***0.3 TO 0.5 CUN*** **Δ** ***3 TO 5***

- 8 EXTRAORDINARY VESSEL/Coalescent Point of Yin Qiao Mai (Yin Heel/Yin Motility Vessel)
- 8 EXTRAORDINARY CHANNELS CONFLUENT/8 Extraordinary Meridians Confluent/8 Extraordinary Vessels Opening/Master Point of the Yin Heel/Yin Motility Vessel (Yin Qiao Mai)
- 8 EXTRAORDINARY VESSEL/Coupled Point of the Ren Mai (Conception/ Directing Vessel)

Pos: Position of patient: supine or seated.

Loc: a) On the foot.
b) On the medial aspect of the foot.
c) On the superior border of the sustentaculum tali of the calcaneus bone.
d) Immediately inferior to the talus bone.
e) 1 cun inferior to the prominence of the medial malleolus.

Ki 8J IAO XIN – EXCHANGE PLEDGES

⊥ ***0.3 TO 0.5 CUN*** **Δ *3 TO 5***

- ACCUMULATION/Xi Cleft/Gueki Point of the Yin Heel/Yin Motility Vessel (Yin Qiao Mai)
- 8 EXTRAORDINARY VESSEL/Coalescent Point of thc Yin IIeel/Yin Motility Vessel (Yin Qiao Mai)

Pos: Position of patient: supine (at 15 cun), or in a seated position with the leg bent at 90 degrees (at 13 cun).

Loc: a) On the lower leg.
b) On the medial aspect of the lower leg.
c) Posterior to the medial border of the tibia.
d) 2 cun superior to the prominence of the medial malleolus.
e) 2 cun superior to Ki 3.
f) 0.5 cun anterior to Ki 7.

Bl 1 JING MING – EYES BRIGHT

⊥ ***0.3 CUN*** **Δ *FORBIDDEN TO USE MOXA***

- ENTRY
- 8 EXTRAORDINARY VESSEL/Coalescent Point of Yin Heel/Yin Motility Vessel (Yin Qiao Mai)
- 8 EXTRAORDINARY VESSEL/Coalescent Point of the Yang Heel/Yang Motility Vessel (Yang Qiao Mai)
- RE-UNION/Crossing/Meeting Point of the Bladder Channel with the Small Intestine, Triple Heater, Gall Bladder and Stomach Channels, the Du Mai, Yang Motility/Yang Heel Vessel and the Yin Motility/Yin Heel Vessel – Foot Tai Yang Channel with the Hand Tai Yang, Hand Shao Yang, Foot Shao Yang and Foot Yang Ming Channels, the Governor Vessel, Yang Qiao Mai and the Yin Qiao Mai

Pos: Position of patient: supine.

Loc: a) On the face.
b) 0.1 cun superior and medial to the medial canthus of the eye.

THE YANG QIAO MAI (Yang Heel/Yang Motility Vessel)

The Yang Qiao Mai starts at the middle of the heel and rises to the lateral side of the heel. It runs upward along the lateral malleolus, passing the posterior border of the fibula, then it continues along the lateral side of the thigh and the posterior side of the hypochondrium to the shoulder and the posterior axillary crease. From there it ascends the neck to the corner of the mouth, and enters the inner canthus to communicate with the Yin Qiao Mai. It runs onward and upward along the Bladder channel to the forehead, and meets the Gallbladder channel at GB 20. Some texts say it enters the brain at Du 16.

The coalescent points of the Yang Qiao Mai are: Bl 62, Bl 61, (Bl 55), Bl 59, GB 29, SI 10, LI 15, LI 16, (TH 15), St 4, St 3, St 1, Bl 1 and GB 20.

Bl 62 SHEN MAI – EXTENDED MERIDIAN

⊥ ***0.3 CUN*** ***Δ FORBIDDEN TO USE MOXA***

- 8 EXTRAORDINARY VESSEL/Coalescent Point of Yang Heel/Yang Motility Vessel (Yang Qiao Mai)
- 8 EXTRAORDINARY CHANNELS CONFLUENT/8 Extraordinary Meridians Confluent/8 Extraordinary Vessels Opening/Master Point of the Yang Heel/Yang Motility Vessel (Yang Qiao Mai)
- 8 EXTRAORDINARY VESSEL/Coupled Point of the Du Mai (Governor Vessel)

Pos: Position of patient: supine.

Loc: a) On the lateral aspect of the foot.
b) Directly inferior to the prominence of the lateral malleolus.
c) Approximately 0.5 cun inferior to the inferior border of the lateral malleolus.

Bl 61 PU SHEN – SERVANT'S AIDE

⊥ ***0.3 CUN*** ***Δ 3 TO 7***

- A Seven External Dragons (E.D's) Point (the other points are Du 20, Bl 11 and Bl 23)
- 8 EXTRAORDINARY VESSEL/Coalescent Point of Yang Heel/Yang Motility Vessel (Yang Qiao Mai)
- RE-UNION/Crossing/Meeting Point of the Bladder Channel with the Yang Motility/Yang Heel Vessel – Foot Tai Yang Channel with the Yang Qiao Mai.

Pos: Position of patient: supine or prone with the feet hanging over the end of the couch.

Loc: a) On the lateral aspect of the foot.
b) On the calcaneus.
c) Approximately 1.5 cun directly inferior to Bl 60 (at the level of the prominence of the lateral malleolus)
d) At the junction of the change in skin colour.

(Bl 55) HE YANG – UNITING YANG

⊥ ***0.5 TO 0.7 CUN*** Δ ***3 TO 7***

- 8 EXTRAORDINARY VESSEL/Coalescent Point of Yang Heel/Yang Motility Vessel (Yang Qiao Mai) – see note

Pos: Position of patient: prone with the feet hanging over the end of the couch.

Loc: a) On the posterior aspect of the lower leg.
b) On the posterior median line of leg
c) On the line connecting Bl 40 and Bl 57.
d) Between the medial and lateral heads of the gastrocnemius muscle.
e) 2 cun inferior to Bl 40 (with the flow of the channel).
f) 14 cun proximal to the prominence of the lateral malleolus bone.

Note: In some texts Bl 55 is listed as an 8 EXTRAORDINARY VESSEL/Coalescent Point of Yang Qiao Mai (Yang Heel/Yang Motility Vessel), whereas in others it is omitted.

Bl 59 FU YANG – FOOT BONE YANG

⊥ ***0.5 TO 0.7 CUN*** Δ ***3 TO 7***

- ACCUMULATION/Xi Cleft/Gueki Point of the Yang Linking/Yang Heel Vessel (Yang Qiao Mai)
- 8 EXTRAORDINARY VESSEL/Coalescent Point of the Yang Linking/Yang Heel Vessel (Yang Qiao Mai)

Pos: Position of patient: prone with the feet hanging over the end of the couch.

Loc: a) On the lateral aspect of the lower leg.
b) In a seam between the tendo calcaneus (achilles tendon) and the posterior border of the fibula bone.
c) Directly superior to Bl 60.
d) Approximately 13 cun inferior to Bl 40 (with the flow of the channel).
e) Approximately 3 cun proximal to the prominence of the lateral malleolus bone.

GB 29 JU LIAO – DWELLING IN THE BONE

⊥ ***0.5 TO 0.8 CUN*** **Δ** ***3 TO 7***

- 8 EXTRAORDINARY VESSEL/Coalescent Point of Yang Heel/Yang Motility Vessel (Yang Qiao Mai)
- RE-UNION/Crossing/Meeting Point of the Gall Bladder Channel with the Yang Heel/Yang Motility Vessel.- Foot Shao Yang Channel with the Yang Qiao Mai

Pos: Position of patient: supine.

Loc: a) On the lateral aspect of the torso.
b) On the lateral aspect of the hip.
c) Midway between the anterior superior iliac spine of the ilium and the prominence of the greater trochanter of the femur.
d) Approximately 3 cun posterior to GB 28.
e) Traditionally described in the anterior fossa of the greater trochanter of the femur.

SI 10 NAO SHU – SHOULDER BLADE

⊥ ***0.5 TO 0.7 CUN*** **Δ** ***3 TO 7***

- 8 EXTRAORDINARY VESSEL/Coalescent Point of the Yang Heel/Yang Motility Vessel (Yang Qiao Mai)
- 8 EXTRAORDINARY VESSEL/Coalescent Point of Yang Linking Vessel (Yang Wei Mai)
- RE-UNION/Crossing/Meeting Point of the Small Intestine Channel with the Bladder Channel, Yang Linking Vessel and Yang Heel/Yang Motility Vessel – Hand Tai Yang Channel with the, Foot Tai Yang Channel, Yang Wei Mai and Yang Qiao Mai

Pos: Position of patient: seated with the forearm adducted against the torso.

Loc: a) On the posterior torso.
b) On the posterior aspect of the shoulder.
c) Superior to the posterior axillary crease.
d) In a depression that is just inferior to the neck of the acromion.
e) Approximately 1 cun medial to TH 14 (which is at the inferolateral corner of the acromion process at the acromial angle).

LI 15 JIAN YU – SHOULDER JOINT

⊥ ***0.5 TO 1.0 CUN*** ***Δ 7***

- 8 EXTRAORDINARY VESSEL/Coalescent Point of the Yang Heel/Yang Motility Vessel (Yang Qiao Mai)
- RE-UNION/Crossing/Meeting Point of the Large Intestine Channel with the Yang Heel/Yang Motility Vessel – Hand Yang Ming Channel with the Yang Qiao Mai

Pos: Position of patient: supine or seated with the forearm positioned so that the medial surface of the upper arm is against the torso with the elbow flexed at an angle of 90 degrees. Alternatively, with the patient supine, the forearm can be extended and partially pronated so that the radial border of the radius is uppermost.

Loc: a) On the lateral aspect of the shoulder.
b) Inferior to the acromion.
c) Between the acromion process of the scapula bone and the greater tuberosity of the humerus.
d) At the centre of the upper portion of the deltoid muscle.

LI 16 JU GU – GREAT BONE

⊥ ***0.5 TO 0.7 CUN*** ***Δ 3 TO 7***

- 8 EXTRAORDINARY VESSEL/Coalescent Point of the Yang Heel/Yang Motility Vessel (Yang Qiao Mai)
- RE-UNION/Crossing/Meeting Point of the Large Intestine Channel with the Yang Heel/Yang Motility Vessel – Hand Yang Ming Channel with the Yang Qiao Mai

Pos: Position of patient: supine or seated with the arms at their side.

Loc: a) On the superior aspect of the shoulder.
b) In the depression between the acromial extremity of the clavicle and the scapular spine.

(TH 15) TIAN LIAO – HEAVENLY BONE

⊥ ***0.3 TO 0.5 CUN*** Δ ***3 TO 7***

- 8 EXTRAORDINARY VESSEL/Coalescent Point of the Yang Linking Vessel (Yang Wei Mai)
- 8 EXTRAORDINARY VESSEL/Coalescent Point of the Yang Heel/Yang Motility Vessel (Yang Qiao Mai) – see note
- RE-UNION/Crossing/Meeting Point of the Triple Heater Channel with the Gall Bladder Channel and the Yang Linking Vessel – Hand Shao Yang Channel with the Foot Shao Yang Channel and Yang Wei Mai

Pos: Position of patient: seated with the shoulders in a relaxed position.

Loc: a) On the shoulder.
b) On the trapezius muscle.
c) At the transverse mid-point between Du 14 (at the posterior median line) and the lateral tip of the acromion of the scapula.
d) Also midway between SI 13 (at the medial end of the supraspinous fossa) and GB 21 (at the highest point of the shoulder).
e) On a vertical line from SI 13 to TH 15, ending at GB 21.

Note: In some texts TH 15 is listed as an 8 EXTRAORDINARY VESSEL/Coalescent Point of Yang Qiao Mai (Yang Heel/Yang Motility Vessel), whereas in others it is omitted.

St 4 DI CANG – EARTH GRANARY

⊥ ***0.1 TO 0.4 CUN*** Δ ***5***

- 8 EXTRAORDINARY VESSEL/Coalescent Point of the Yang Heel/Yang Motility Vessel (Yang Qiao Mai)
- RE-UNION/Crossing/Meeting Point of the Stomach Channel with the Large Intestine Channel, the Ren Mai andYang Heel/Yang Motility Vessels – Foot Yang Ming Channel with the Hand Yang Ming Channel, Conception/Directing Vessel and Yang Qiao Mai

Pos: Position of patient: supine.

Loc: a) On the face.
b) Inferior to the centre of the pupil of the eye when the person is looking directly ahead.
c) Inferior to St 1, St 2 and St 3.
d) Level with the corner of the mouth.
e) Traditionally 0.4 cun lateral to the corner of the mouth.

St 3 JU LIAO – GREAT CHEEKBONE

⊥ ***0.1 TO 0.5 CUN*** **Δ *5***

- 8 EXTRAORDINARY VESSEL/Coalescent Point of the Yang Heel/Yang Motility Vessel (Yang Qiao Mai)
- RE-UNION/Crossing/Meeting Point of the Stomach Channel with the Yang Heel/Yang Motility Vessel – Foot Yang Ming Channel with the Yang Qiao Mai

Pos: Position of patient: supine.

Loc: a) On the face.
b) On the maxilla bone.
c) Directly inferior to the centre of the pupil of the eyes when the person is looking directly ahead.
d) Inferior to St 1, and St 2,
e) Level with the inferior border of the nostrils.

St 1 CHENG QI – RECEIVE TEARS

⊥ ***0.1 TO 0.3 CUN*** ***Δ FORBIDDEN TO USE MOXA***

- ENTRY
- 8 EXTRAORDINARY VESSEL/Coalescent Point of Yang Heel/Yang Motility Vessel (Yang Qiao Mai)
- 8 EXTRAORDINARY VESSEL/Coalescent Point of Ren Mai (Conception/ Directing Vessel)
- RE-UNION/Crossing/Meeting Point of the Stomach Channel with the Ren Mai andYang Heel/Yang Motility Vessels – Foot Yang Ming Channel with the Conception/Directing Vessel and Yang Qiao Mai

Pos: Position of patient: supine.

Loc: a) On the face.
b) Inferior to the centre of the pupil with the eyes looking straight forward.
c) Between the eyeball and the infraorbital margin formed by the zygomatic bone and maxilla bone (these two bones form the inferior border of the orbit).
d) Traditionally 0.7 cun below the pupil.

Bl 1 JING MING – EYES BRIGHT

⊥ ***0.3 CUN*** ***Δ FORBIDDEN TO USE MOXA***

- ENTRY
- 8 EXTRAORDINARY VESSEL/Coalescent Point of Yin Heel/Yin Motility Vessel (Yin Qiao Mai)
- 8 EXTRAORDINARY VESSEL/Coalescent Point of the Yang Heel/Yang Motility Vessel (Yang Qiao Mai)
- RE-UNION/Crossing/Meeting Point of the Bladder Channel with the Small Intestine, Triple Heater, Gall Bladder and Stomach Channels, the Du Mai, Yang Motility/Yang Heel Vessel and the Yin Motility/Yin Heel Vessel – Foot Tai Yang Channel with the Hand Tai Yang, Hand Shao Yang, Foot Shao Yang and Foot Yang Ming Channels, the Governor Vessel, Yang Qiao Mai and the Yin Qiao Mai

Pos: Position of patient: supine.

Loc: a) On the face.
b) 0.1 cun superior and medial to the medial canthus of the eye.

GB 20 FENG CHI – WIND POND

⊥ ***0.3 TO 0.5 CUN Δ 3 TO 10***

- 8 EXTRAORDINARY VESSEL/Coalescent Point of Yang Heel/Yang Motility Vessel (Yang Qiao Mai)
- 8 EXTRAORDINARY VESSEL/Coalescent Point of Yang Linking Vessel (Yang Wei Mai)
- RE-UNION/Crossing/Meeting Point of the Gall Bladder Channel with the Yang Linking and Yang Heel/Motility Vessels.- Foot Shao Yang Channel with the Yang Wei Mai and Yang Qiao Mai

Pos: Position of patient: seated.

Loc: a) On the posterior aspect of the head.
b) Inferior to the occipital bone.
c) Between the trapezius and sternocleidomastoid muscles.
d) Level with Du 16.
e) 2.25 cun lateral to the posterior median line.
f) 1 cun superior to the natural posterior hairline.

THE YIN WEI MAI (Yin Linking Vessel)

The Yin Wei Mai starts from the medial aspect of the leg, ascending the medial aspect of the thigh to the abdomen to communicate with the Spleen channel. It then goes along the chest and communicates with the Ren Mai at the neck.

The coalescent points of the Yin Wei Mai are: Ki 9, (Sp 12), Sp 13, Sp 15, Sp 16, Liv 14, Ren 22 and Ren 23.

Ki 9 ZHU BIN – BUILDING GUEST

⊥ ***0.3 TO 0.7 CUN*** ***Δ 3 TO 7***

- ACCUMULATION/Xi Cleft/Gueki Point of the Yin Linking Vessel (Yin Wei Mai)

Pos: Position of patient: supine (at 15 cun), or in a seated position with the leg bent at 90 degrees (at 13 cun).

Loc:
a) On the lower leg.
b) On the medial aspect of the lower leg.
c) On a line from Ki 3 to Ki 10.
d) In a seam on the medial border of the gastrocnemius (calf) and the soleus muscles, or on some people the medial border of the tendocalcaneus (achilles tendon) and the soleus muscle.
e) 5 cun superior to the prominence of the medial malleolus.
f) 5 cun superior to Ki 3.
g) Level with Liv 5 (see separate location).

(Sp 12) CHONG MEN – RUSHING GATE

⊥ ***0.5 TO 0.7 CUN*** ***Δ 5***
FORBIDDEN TO NEEDLE AND MOXA THIS POINT DURING PREGNANCY

- 8 EXTRAORDINARY VESSEL/Coalescent Point of Yin Linking Vessel (Yin Wei Mai) – see note
- RE-UNION/Crossing/Meeting Point of the Spleen Channel with the Liver Channel and the Yin Linking Vessel – Foot Tai Yin Channel with the Foot Jue Yin Channel and the Yin Wei Mai

Pos: Position of patient: supine.

Loc: a) On the anterior torso.
b) On the lower abdomen (lower jiao)
c) Level with the superior border of the symphysis pubis bone (at Ren 2).
d) On the lateral edge of the femoral artery.
e) Superior to the lateral end of the inguinal groove.
f) 3.5 cun lateral to the anterior median line.

Note: In some texts Sp 12 is listed as an 8 EXTRAORDINARY VESSEL/Coalescent Point of Yin Wei Mai (Yin Linking Vessel), whereas in others it is omitted.

Sp 13 FU SHE – OFFICIAL RESIDENCE

⊥ ***0.5 TO 0.7 CUN*** Δ ***5 TO 10***
FORBIDDEN TO NEEDLE AND MOXA THIS POINT DURING PREGNANCY

- 8 EXTRAORDINARY VESSEL/Coalescent Point of Yin Linking Vessel (Yin Wei Mai)
- RE-UNION/Crossing/Meeting Point of the Spleen Channel with the Liver Channel and the Yin Linking Vessel – Foot Tai Yin Channel with the Foot Jue Yin Channel and the Yin Wei Mai

Pos: Position of patient: supine.

Loc: a) On the anterior aspect of the torso.
b) On the lower abdomen (in the lower jiao).
c) On the lateral edge of the rectus abdominis muscle.
d) 4 cun lateral to the anterior median line.
e) 0.5 cun lateral to and 0.7 cun superior to Sp 12 (separate description).
f) 0.7 cun superior to the superior border of the symphysis pubis bone (at Ren 2)
g) 4.3 cun inferior to the level of the centre of the umbilicus or Sp 15 (separate description).
h) 3 cun inferior to Sp 14 (separate location).

Sp 15 DA HENG – GREAT HORIZONTAL

⊥ ***0.7 TO 1.0 CUN*** **Δ** ***5 TO 10***
FORBIDDEN TO NEEDLE AND MOXA THIS POINT DURING PREGNANCY

- 8 EXTRAORDINARY VESSEL/Coalescent Point of Yin Linking Vessel (Yin Wei Mai)
- RE-UNION/Crossing/Meeting Point of the Spleen Channel with the Yin Linking Vessel – Foot Tai Yin Channel with the Yin Wei Mai

Pos: Position of patient: supine.

Loc: a) On the anterior aspect of the torso.
b) In between the mid-abdomen and lower abdomen (in between the middle and lower jiao).
c) On the lateral edge of the rectus abdominis muscle.
d) 4 cun lateral to the anterior median line or 4 cun lateral to the level of the centre of the umbilicus and Ren 8.

Sp 16 FU AI – ABDOMEN SORROW

⊥ ***0.5 TO 0.7 CUN*** **Δ** ***5 TO 10***
FORBIDDEN TO NEEDLE AND MOXA THIS POINT DURING PREGNANCY

- 8 EXTRAORDINARY VESSEL/Coalescent Point of Yin Linking Vessel (Yin Wei Mai)
- RE-UNION/Crossing/Meeting Point of the Spleen Channel with the Yin Linking Vessel – Foot Tai Yin Channel with the Yin Wei Mai

Pos: Position of patient: supine.

Loc: a) On the anterior aspect of the torso.
b) On the mid-abdomen (in the middle jiao).
c) On the lateral edge of the rectus abdominis muscle.
d) 4 cun lateral to the anterior median line.
e) 3 cun superior to Sp 15.
f) Level with Ren 11 (which is 3 cun superior to the level of the centre of the umbilicus).

Liv 14 QI MEN – GATE OF HOPE

⊥ ***0.3 TO 0.5 CUN*** Δ ***5 TO 7***

- EXIT
- ALARM/Front Collecting/Front Mu/Herald Point of Liver
- 8 EXTRAORDINARY VESSEL/Coalescent Point of the Yin Linking Vessel (Yin Wei Mai)
- RE-UNION/Crossing/Meeting Point of the Liver Channel with the Gall Bladder Channel and the Yin Linking Vessel.- Foot Jue Yin Channel with the Foot Shao Yang Channel and Yin Wei Mai

Pos: Position of patient: supine.

Loc: a) On the anterior aspect of the torso.
b) On the mid-abdomen (in the middle jiao).
c) Directly inferior to the nipple.
d) In the sixth intercostal space.
e) 4 cun lateral to the anterior median line.
f) Directly superior to GB 24 (which is in the seventh intercostal space).

Ren 22 TIAN TU – HEAVEN RUSHING OUT

⊥ ***0.3 CUN*** Δ ***3 TO 7***

- WINDOW OF THE SKY/Window of Heaven
- 8 EXTRAORDINARY VESSEL/Coalescent Point of Yin Linking Vessel (Yin Wei Mai)
- RE-UNION/Crossing/Meeting Point of the Ren Mai with the Yin Linking Vessel – Conception/Directing Vessel with the Yin Wei Mai

Pos: Position of patient: supine.

Loc: a) On the anterior aspect of the torso.
b) On the upper chest (in the upper jiao).
c) On the anterior median line.
d) In the centre of the suprasternal fossa.
e) 0.5 cun superior to the suprasternal notch (jugular notch).

Ren 23 LIAN QUAN – ANGLE SPRING

⊥ ***0.3 TO 0.5 CUN*** ***Δ 3 TO 7***

- 8 EXTRAORDINARY VESSEL/Coalescent Point of Yang Linking Vessel (Yang Wei Mai)
- RE UNION/Crossing/Meeting Point of the Ren Mai with the Yin Linking Vessel – Conception/Directing Vessel with the Yin Wei Mai

Pos: Position of patient: supine.

Loc: a) On the anterior aspect of the neck.
b) On the pharynx.
c) At the superior border of the hyoid bone.
d) On the anterior median line.

THE YANG WEI MAI (Yang Linking Vessel)

The Yang Wei Mai starts at the lateral aspect of the heel. Emerging from the lateral malleolus it ascends along the Gallbladder channel, passes through the hip region, then goes further upward along the posterior aspect of the hypochondriacal and costal regions. It crosses the posterior aspect of the axilla to the shoulder and to the forehead, then turns backward to the posterior aspect of the neck where it communicates with the Du Mai.

The coalescent points of the Yang Wei Mai are: Bl 63, GB 35, SI 10, TH 15, GB 21, (St 8), GB 13, GB 14, GB 15, GB 16, GB 17, GB 18, GB 19, GB 20, Du 16 and Du 15.

Bl 63 JIN MEN – GOLDEN GATE

⊥ ***0.3 CUN*** ***Δ 3 TO 5***

- ACCUMULATION/Xi Cleft/Gueki
- 8 EXTRAORDINARY VESSEL/Coalescent Point of Yang Linking Vessel (Yang Wei Mai)
- RE-UNION/Crossing/Meeting Point of the Bladder Channel with the Yang Linking Vessel – Foot Tai Yang Channel with the Yang Wei Mai.

Pos: Position of patient: supine.

Loc: a) On the lateral aspect of the foot.
b) Proximal to the tuberosity of the fifth metatarsal bone.
c) Just inferior to the inferior border of the cuboid bone.
d) Anterior and inferior to Bl 62 (see separate description).

GB 35 YANG JIAO – YANG CROSSING

⊥ ***0.5 TO 0.7 CUN*** Δ ***3 TO 7***

- ACCUMULATION/Xi Cleft/Gueki Point of the Yang Linking Vessel (Yang Wei Mai)
- 8 EXTRAORDINARY VESSEL/Coalescent Point of Yang Linking Vessel (Yang Wei Mai)

Pos: Position of patient: supine with the leg semi flexed.

Loc: a) On the lateral aspect of the lower leg.
b) Posterior to the posterior border of the fibula.
c) Posterior to and on a level with GB 36.
d) 7 cun proximal to the prominence of the lateral malleolus.

SI 10 NAO SHU – SHOULDER BLADE

⊥ ***0.5 TO 0.7 CUN*** Δ ***3 TO 7***

- 8 EXTRAORDINARY VESSEL/Coalescent Point of the Yang Heel/Yang Motility Vessel (Yang Qiao Mai)
- 8 EXTRAORDINARY VESSEL/Coalescent Point of Yang Linking Vessel (Yang Wei Mai)
- RE-UNION/Crossing/Meeting Point of the Small Intestine Channel with the Bladder Channel, Yang Linking Vessel and Yang Heel/Yang Motility Vessel – Hand Tai Yang Channel with the, Foot Tai Yang Channel, Yang Wei Mai and Yang Qiao Mai

Pos: Position of patient: seated with the forearm adducted against the torso.

Loc: a) On the posterior torso.
b) On the posterior aspect of the shoulder.
c) Superior to the posterior axillary crease.
d) In a depression that is just inferior to the neck of the acromion.
e) Approximately 1 cun medial to TH 14 (which is at the inferolateral corner of the acromion process at the acromial angle).

TH 15 TIAN LIAO – HEAVENLY BONE

⊥ ***0.3 TO 0.5 CUN*** Δ ***3 TO 7***

- 8 EXTRAORDINARY VESSEL/Coalescent Point of the Yang Linking Vessel (Yang Wei Mai)
- 8 EXTRAORDINARY VESSEL/Coalescent Point of the Yang Heel/Yang Motility Vessel (Yang Qiao Mai) – see note
- RE-UNION/Crossing/Meeting Point of the Triple Heater Channel with the Gall Bladder Channel and the Yang Linking Vessel – Hand Shao Yang Channel with the Foot Shao Yang Channel and Yang Wei Mai

Pos: Position of patient: seated with the shoulders in a relaxed position.

Loc: a) On the shoulder.
b) On the trapezius muscle.
c) At the transverse mid-point between Du 14 (at the posterior median line) and the lateral tip of the acromion of the scapula.
d) Also midway between SI 13 (at the medial end of the supraspinous fossa) and GB 21 (at the highest point of the shoulder).
e) On a vertical line from SI 13 to TH 15, ending at GB 21.

Note: In some texts TH 15 is listed as an 8 EXTRAORDINARY VESSEL/Coalescent Point of Yang Qiao Mai (Yang Heel/Yang Motility Vessel), whereas in others it is omitted.

GB 21 JIAN JING – SHOULDER WELL

⊥ ***0.3 TO 0.5 CUN*** Δ ***5 TO 15***

- 8 EXTRAORDINARY VESSEL/Coalescent Point of Yang Linking Vessel (Yang Wei Mai)
- RE-UNION/Crossing/Meeting Point of the Gall Bladder Channel with the Triple Heater Channel and the Yang Linking Vessel.- Foot Shao Yang Channel with the Hand Shao Yang Channel and Yang Wei Mai

Pos: Position of patient: seated.

Loc: a) On the shoulder.
b) At the highest point of the shoulder.
c) On the trapezius muscle.
d) Midway between Du 14 and the lateral extremity of the acromion of the scapula.
e) On a line with SI 13 and TH 15.

(St 8) TOU WEI – HEAD TIED

⊥ ***0.3 TO 0.5 CUN*** ***Δ FORBIDDEN TO USE MOXA***

- 8 EXTRAORDINARY VESSEL/Coalescent Point of Yang Linking Vessel (Yang Wei Mai) – see note
- RE-UNION/Crossing/Meeting Point of the Stomach Channel with the Gall Bladder Channel and the Yang Linking Vessel – Foot Yang Ming Channel with the Foot Shao Yang Channel and the Yang Wei Mai

Pos: Position of patient: supine.

Loc: a) On the head.
b) At the corner of the forehead.
c) In a groove formed by the frontal bone of the skull and the medial border of the temporalis muscle.
d) 4.5 cun lateral to the anterior median line.
e) 0.5 cun posterior to the natural anterior hairline.
e) At the level of Du 24.

Note: In some texts St 8 is listed as an 8 EXTRAORDINARY VESSEL/Coalescent Point of Yang Wei Mai (Yang Linking Vessel), whereas in others it is omitted.

GB 13 BEN SHEN – ROOT SPIRIT

⊥ ***0.3 CUN*** ***Δ 3 TO 7***

- 8 EXTRAORDINARY VESSEL/Coalescent Point of Yang Linking Vessel (Yang Wei Mai)
- RE-UNION/Crossing/Meeting Point of the Gall Bladder Channel with the Yang Linking Vessel.- Foot Shao Yang Channel with the Yang Wei Mai

Pos: Position of patient: supine or seated.

Loc: a) On the anterior aspect of the head.
b) On the frontal bone.
c) Two thirds of the distance from Du24 to St 8.
d) 3 cun lateral to Du 24 (anterior median line).
e) 0.5 cun posterior to the natural anterior hairline.

GB 14 YANG BAI – YANG WHITE

⊥ ***0.3 CUN*** **Δ *3***

- 8 EXTRAORDINARY VESSEL/Coalescent Point of Yang Linking Vessel (Yang Wei Mai)
- RE-UNION/Crossing/Meeting Point of the Gall Bladder Channel with the Triple Heater Channel and the Yang Linking Vessel.- Foot Shao Yang Channel with the Hand Shao Yang Channel and Yang Wei Mai

Pos: Position of patient: supine or seated.

Loc: a) On the anterior aspect of the head.
b) On the frontal bone.
c) Directly superior to the centre of the pupil of the eye when the person is looking straight ahead.
d) Approximately1 cun superior to the eyebrow.

GB 15 TOU LIN QI – HEAD ABOVE TEARS

⊥ ***0.3 CUN*** **Δ *3***

- 8 EXTRAORDINARY VESSEL/Coalescent Point of Yang Linking Vessel (Yang Wei Mai)
- RE-UNION/Crossing/Meeting Point of the Gall Bladder Channel with the Bladder Channel and the Yang Linking Vessel. Foot Shao Yang Channel with the Foot Tai Yang Channel and the Yang Wei Mai

Pos: Position of patient: supine or seated.

Loc: a) On the anterior aspect of the head.
b) On the frontal bone.
c) At the mid-point of the distance from Du24 to St 8.
d) Directly superior to GB 14.
e) 0.5 cun posterior to the natural anterior hairline.
f) 2.25 cun lateral to Du 24 or the anterior median line.

GB 16 MU CHUANG – EYE WINDOW

⊥ ***0.3 CUN*** **Δ *5***

- 8 EXTRAORDINARY VESSEL/Coalescent Point of Yang Linking Vessel (Yang Wei Mai)
- RE-UNION/Crossing/Meeting Point of the Gall Bladder Channel with the Yang Linking Vessel.- Foot Shao Yang Channel with the Yang Wei Mai

Pos: Position of patient: supine or seated.

Loc: a) On the anterior aspect of the head.
b) On the coronal suture.
c) 1.5 cun posterior to the natural anterior hairline.
d) 1 cun posterior to GB 15.
e) 2.25 cun lateral to the anterior median line.

GB 17 ZHEN YING – UPRIGHT LIVING

⊥ ***0.3 CUN*** **Δ *5***

- 8 EXTRAORDINARY VESSEL/Coalescent Point of Yang Linking Vessel (Yang Wei Mai)
- RE-UNION/Crossing/Meeting Point of the Gall Bladder Channel with the Yang Linking Vessel.- Foot Shao Yang Channel with the Yang Wei Mai

Pos: Position of patient: seated.

Loc: a) On the superior aspect of the head.
b) On the parietal bone.
c) 2.5 cun posterior to the natural anterior hairline.
d) 1 cun posterior to GB 16.
e) 2 cun posterior to GB 15.
f) 2.25 cun lateral to the superior median line.

GB 18 CHENG LING – RECEIVING SPIRIT

⊥ ***0.3 CUN*** Δ ***5***

- 8 EXTRAORDINARY VESSEL/Coalescent Point of Yang Linking Vessel (Yang Wei Mai)
- RE-UNION/Crossing/Meeting Point of the Gall Bladder Channel with the Yang Linking Vessel.- Foot Shao Yang Channel with the Yang Wei Mai

Pos: Position of patient: seated.

Loc: a) On the superior aspect of the head.
b) On the parietal bone.
c) 4 cun posterior to the natural anterior hairline.
d) 1.5 cun posterior to GB 17.
e) 3.5 cun posterior to GB 15.,
f) 2.25 cun lateral to the superior median line.

GB 19 NAO KONG – BRAIN HOLLOW

⊥ ***0.3 CUN*** Δ ***3***

- 8 EXTRAORDINARY VESSEL/Coalescent Point of Yang Linking Vessel (Yang Wei Mai)
- RE-UNION/Crossing/Meeting Point of the Gall Bladder Channel with the Yang Linking Vessel.- Foot Shao Yang Channel with the Yang Wei Mai

Pos: Position of patient: seated.

Loc: a) On the posterior aspect of the head.
b) On the level of the upper border of the external occipital protruberance of the occipital bone.
c) Level with Du 17.
d) 1.5 cun superior to GB 20.
e) 2.5 cun superior to the natural posterior hairline.
f) 2.25 cun lateral to the posterior median line.

GB 20 FENG CHI – WIND POND

⊥ ***0.3 TO 0.5 CUN*** **Δ** ***3 TO 10***

- 8 EXTRAORDINARY VESSEL/Coalescent Point of Yang Heel/Yang Motility Vessel (Yang Qiao Mai)
- 8 EXTRAORDINARY VESSEL/Coalescent Point of Yang Linking Vessel (Yang Wei Mai)
- RE-UNION/Crossing/Meeting Point of the Gall Bladder Channel with the Yang Linking and Yang Heel/Motility Vessels.- Foot Shao Yang Channel with the Yang Wei Mai and Yang Qiao Mai

Pos: Position of patient: seated.

Loc: a) On the posterior aspect of the head.
b) Inferior to the occipital bone.
c) Between the trapezius and sternocleidomastoid muscles.
d) Level with Du 16.
e) 2.25 cun lateral to the posterior median line.
f) 1 cun superior to the natural posterior hairline.

Du 16 FENG FU – WIND PALACE

⊥ ***0.3 CUN*** ***Δ FORBIDDEN TO USE MOXA***

- WINDOW OF THE SKY/Window of Heaven
- A POINT OF THE SEA OF MARROW (see note) There are three other Sea of Marrow Points: Du 15, Du 19 and Du 20
- 8 EXTRAORDINARY VESSEL/Coalescent Point of Yang Linking Vessel (Yang Wei Mai)
- RE-UNION/Crossing/Meeting Point of the Du Mai with the Yang Linking Vessel – Governor Vessel with the Yang Wei Mai

Pos: Position of patient: seated and upright.

Loc: a) On the posterior torso.
b) At the junction of the head and neck (nape of the neck).
c) On the posterior median line.
d) Just inferior to the external occipital protuberance of the occipital bone.
e) 1 cun superior to the natural posterior hairline (11 cun posterior to the natural anterior hairline).
f) 0.5 cun superior to Du 15.

Note: The Ling Shu (Spiritual Pivot) Chapter 33 describes areas where the Seas are located rather than point numbers, eg. the middle of the chest is in the region of Ren 17. There are regions where the Sea of Marrow can be located and in many cases just two points are used as the Sea of Marrow, these are Du 16 and Du 20,. The College of Traditional Acupuncture uses these two points as well as using Du 15 and Du 19. Du 15 in some texts is classified as a Sea of Qi point.

Du 15 YA MEN – GATE OF DUMBNESS

⊥ ***0.3 CUN*** **∆ *FORBIDDEN TO USE MOXA***

- A POINT OF THE SEA OF MARROW (see note) There are three other Sea of Marrow Points: Du 16, Du 19 and Du 20
- 8 EXTRAORDINARY VESSEL/Coalescent Point of Yang Linking Vessel (Yang Wei Mai)
- RE-UNION/Crossing/Meeting Point of the Du Mai with the Yang Linking Vessel – Governor Vessel with the Yang Wei Mai

Pos: Position of patient: seated and upright.

Loc: a) On the posterior torso.
b) On the neck.
c) On the posterior median line.
d) Between the first and second cervical vertebrae (the atlas and the axis).
e) 0.5 cun superior to the natural posterior hairline (11.5 cun posterior to the natural anterior hairline).
f) Level with Bl 10.

Note: The Ling Shu (Spiritual Pivot) Chapter 33 describes areas where the Seas are located rather than point numbers, eg. the middle of the chest is in the region of Ren 17. There are regions where the Sea of Marrow can be located and in many cases just two points are used as the Sea of Marrow, these are Du 16 and Du 20,. The College of Traditional Acupuncture uses these two points as well as using Du 15 and Du 19. Du 15 is classified in some texts as a Sea of Qi point.

THE DU MAI (Governing Vessel)

<u>Note:</u> The Governor Vessel and the Conception Vessel are two of the 8 Extraordinary Vessels. They are different to the other Extraordinary Vessels in that they have their own points rather than using known points from other channels. Some texts and Schools include the Conception and Governor Vessels as primary channels along with the other twelve primary channels, and these are commonly called the Fourteen Channels.

As this book includes the Du Mai as a primary channel, please see separate chapter for the main Du Mai points.

The coalescent points of the Du Mai are:
Bl 12 and Ren 1.

Bl 12 FENG MEN – WIND GATE

⊥ ***0.3 TO 0.5 CUN*** Δ ***5 TO 10***

- 8 EXTRAORDINARY VESSEL/Coalescent Point of Du Mai (Governor Vessel)
- RE-UNION/Crossing/Meeting Point of the Bladder Channel with the Du Mai – Foot Tai Yang Channel with the Governor Vessel.

Pos: Position of patient: seated and upright.

Loc: a) On the posterior torso.
b) On the inner line or the medial branch of the Bladder channel.
c) 1.5 cun lateral to the posterior median line.
d) Between the 2nd and 3rd thoracic vertebrae.

Ren 1 HUI YIN – MEETING OF YIN

⊥ ***0.8 TO 1.2 CUN*** Δ ***FORBIDDEN TO USE MOXA***

- ENTRY
- GENERAL JUNCTION/Luo/Connecting/Passage/Lo/Lê
- 8 EXTRAORDINARY VESSEL/Coalescent Point of Du Mai (Governor Vessel)
- 8 EXTRAORDINARY VESSEL/Coalescent Point of Penetrating Vessel (Chong Mai) – see note
- 8 EXTRAORDINARY VESSEL/Coalescent Point of the Yin Linking Vessel (Yin Wei Mai)
- RE-UNION/Crossing/Meeting Point of the Ren Mai with the Du Mai and the Penetrating Vessel.- Conception/Directing Vessel with the Governor Vessel and the Chong Mai

Pos: Position of patient: supine with both legs semi flexed. The legs should also be at the approximate shoulder width apart from each other.

Loc: a) On the inferior pelvic aperture (pelvic outlet) – (Grays 1978-p.529).
b) On the perineal body.
c) In the centre of the perineum.
d) On the median line.
d) Midway between the anus and the scrotum (in men).
e) Midway between the anus and the posterior commissure of the vagina (in women).

Note: In some texts Ren 1 is listed as an 8 EXTRAORDINARY VESSEL/Coalescent Point of Chong Mai (Penetrating Vessel), whereas in others it is omitted.

THE REN MAI (Conception Vessel)

***Note:* The Conception Vessel and the Governor Vessel are two of the 8 Extraordinary Vessels. They are different to the other Extraordinary Vessels in that they have their own points rather than using known points from other channels. Some texts and Schools include the Conception and Governor Vessels as primary channels along with the other twelve primary channels, and these are commonly called the Fourteen Channels.**

As this book includes the Ren Mai as a primary channel, please see separate chapter for the main Ren Mai points.

The coalescent points of the Ren Mai are:
St 1 and Du 28.

St 1 CHENG QI – RECEIVE TEARS

⊥ ***0.1 TO 0.3 CUN*** **∆ *FORBIDDEN TO USE MOXA***

- ENTRY
- 8 EXTRAORDINARY VESSEL/Coalescent Point of Yang Heel/Yang Motility Vessel (Yang Qiao Mai)
- 8 EXTRAORDINARY VESSEL/Coalescent Point of Ren Mai (Conception/ Directing Vessel)
- RE-UNION/Crossing/Meeting Point of the Stomach Channel with the Ren Mai andYang Heel/Yang Motility Vessels – Foot Yang Ming Channel with the Conception/Directing Vessel and Yang Qiao Mai

Pos: Position of patient: supine.

Loc: a) On the face.
b) Inferior to the centre of the pupil with the eyes looking straight forward.
c) Between the eyeball and the infraorbital margin formed by the zygomatic bone and maxilla bone (these two bones form the inferior border of the orbit).
d) Traditionally 0.7 cun below the pupil.

Du 28 YIN JIAO – MOUTH CROSSING

⊥ ***0.1 TO 0.2 CUN*** **Δ *FORBIDDEN TO USE MOXA***

- EXIT
- 8 EXTRAORDINARY VESSEL/Coalescent Point of Ren Mai (Conception/Directing Vessel)
- RE-UNION/Crossing/Meeting Point of the Du Mai with the Stomach Channel and the Ren Mai – Governor Vessel with Foot Yang Ming Channel and the Conception/Directing Vessel

Pos: Position of patient: seated or supine.

Loc: a) On the anterior aspect of the face.
b) At the junction of the frenulum of the upper lip and the upper gum.
c) On the anterior median line.

EXTRA POINTS

M = Miscellaneous point; BW = Back/Waist

M-BW-1 DING CHUAN – STOP WHEEZING

⊥ ***0.5 CUN – oblique towards the vertebral body***

Pos: Position of patient: seated and upright.

Loc: a) On the posterior torso.
b) Level with Du 14 (which is between the 7th cervical and 1st thoracic vertebrae).
c) 0.5 to 1 cun lateral to the posterior median line.

Note: Ellis (1991) lists this point as M-BW-1b. M-BW-1a is listed as "Chuan Xi – Gasping" and this is located on the back, 1" lateral to the inferior border of the spinous process of C7 vertebra. There is no M-BW-1 listed as a separate point.

No Number WAI DING CHUAN – OUTER STOP WHEEZING

⊥ ***0.5 CUN – slanted towards the spine***

Pos: Position of patient: seated with the forearm relaxed against the torso.

Loc: a) On the posterior torso.
b) Level with the intervertebral space between C7 and T1 vertebra.
c) 1.5 cun lateral to the posterior median line.
d) Level with Du 14 (which is on the posterior median line in the depression formed by the intervertebral space between C7 and T1 vertebra).
e) 0.5 cun medial to SI 15.
f) 0.5 to 1 cun lateral to DING CHUAN (M-BW-1)

M-BW-12 WEI GUAN XIA SHU – PANCREAS BACK SHU POINT

⊥ ***0.5 CUN***

Pos: Position of patient: seated and upright.

Loc: a) On the posterior torso.
b) 1.5 cun lateral to the posterior median line.
c) Between the 8th and 9th thoracic vertebrae (level with the base of the spinous process of the 8th thoracic vertebrae).

M-BW-25 SHI QI ZHUI – BELOW SEVENTEENTH VERTEBRA

⊥ ***0.5 CUN – vertically – can also use Δ or heated needle***

Pos: Position of patient: seated and upright.

Loc: a) On the posterior torso.
b) On the posterior median line.
c) Between the 8th and 9th thoracic vertebrae (level with the base of the spinous process of the 8th thoracic vertebrae).

M-BW-35 HUA TUO JIA JI – HUA TUO BACK-FILLING POINTS – LINING THE SPINE

⊥ ***0.3 TO 0.5 CUN – in cervical and thoracic areas***

⊥ ***0.5 TO 0.8 CUN – in lumbar and sacral areas***

Pos: Position of patient: seated and upright.

Loc: a) On the posterior torso.
b) On the neck, back and sacrum (running longitudinally parallel with the vertebrae).
c) 0.5 to 1 cun lateral to the posterior median line.
d) On a level between the spaces of each vertebrae (level with the base of the spinous process of each vertebrae, from the 1st cervical to the 4th sacral vertebrae) – C1 to S4.

Note: In some texts these points are limited in that they are located from the 1st thoracic to the 5th lumbar vertebrae. Hua Tuo, a famous Chinese physician from the Han dynasty period discovered these points, and used them to treat various regions of the body, not dissimilar to the Back Shu points.

N = New point; BW = Back/Waist

N-BW-2 XUE YA DIAN – BLOOD PRESSURE POINTS

⊥ ***0.5 CUN – vertically***

Pos: Position of patient: seated.

Loc: a) On the posterior torso.
b) 2 cun lateral to the posterior median line.
c) On a level between the 6th and 7th cervical vertebrae (level with the base of the spinous process of the 6th cervical vertebrae).

N-BW-2 1AN MIAN 3 – PEACEFUL SLEEP 3

⊥ ***0.5 CUN – slanted towards Bl 17***

Pos: Position of patient: seated.

Loc: a) On the posterior torso.
b) 0.5 cun lateral to the inner line or the medial branch of the Bladder channel.
c) 0.5 cun lateral to Bl 17
d) 2 cun lateral to the posterior median line.
e) Between the 7th and 8th thoracic vertebrae (level with the base of the spinous process of the 7th thoracic vertebrae).

No Number WU MING – FIVE BRIGHTNESSES

⊥ ***0.5 CUN – obliquely upwards***

Pos: Position of patient: seated.

Loc: a) On the back.
b) On the posterior median line.
c) Between the 2nd and 3rd thoracic vertebrae (level with the base of the spinous process of the 2nd thoracic vertebrae).
d) Located with the neck bent forward.

No Number JING GONG – PALACE OF ESSENCE

⊥ ***0.5 – 0.8 CUN – vertically***

Pos: Position of patient: seated and upright.

Loc: a) On the posterior torso.
b) On the outer line or the lateral branch of the Bladder channel.
c) Approximately 3.5 cun lateral to the posterior median line.
d) Approximately 0.5 cun lateral to Bl 52.
e) Between the 2nd and 3rd lumbar vertebrae (level with the base of the spinous process of the 2nd lumbar vertebra).

M = Miscellaneous point; HN = Head/Neck

M-HN-1 SI SHEN CONG – FOUR CLEVER SPIRITS

⊥ ***0.2 TO 0.3 CUN – towards Du 20***

Pos: Position of patient: seated.

Loc: There are 4 points:
a) On the superior aspect of the head.
b) Each at 1 cun anterior, posterior and lateral to Du 20.

M-HN-3 YIN TANG – SEAL HALL (Du 24.5)

⊥ ***0.3 CUN – downwards or towards Bl 2***

Pos: Position of patient: seated or supine.

Loc:
a) On the anterior aspect of the head.
b) On the frontal bone.
c) On the anterior median line.
d) At the midpoint between the medial borders of the two eyebrows.
e) On the glabella.

M-HN-6 YU YAO – FISH SPINE

⊥ ***0.2 CUN – towards either Bl 2 or TH 23***

Pos: Position of patient: seated or supine.

Loc:
a) On the anterior aspect of the head.
b) On the frontal bone.
c) On the eyebrow (on the superciliary arch).
d) Directly superior to the centre of the pupil when the person is looking directly ahead.
e) Directly inferior to GB 14.

M-HN-8 QIU HOU – BEHIND THE BALL

⊥ ***0.3 TO 0.3 CUN – vertical towards the orbit, slightly medially***

Pos: Position of patient: seated or supine.

Loc: a) On the face.
b) On the infraorbital margin of the zygomatic bone.
c) At the junction of the lateral 1/4 and medial 3/4 of the inferior border of the orbit.
d) Inferior and slightly medial to the level of the lateral canthus of the eye.
e) Lateral to St 1 and inferior to GB 1.

M-HN-9 TAI YANG – GREATER YANG or SUN

⊥ ***0.5 CUN – perpendicular or downwards towards St 6***

Pos: Position of patient: seated or supine.

Loc: a) On the temporal region of the head.
b) Posterior to the lateral orbital ridge of the zygomatic bone.
c) 1 cun posterior to the midpoint between the lateral canthus and the lateral extremity of the eyebrow.
d) Approximately midway between and posterior to TH 23 and GB 1.

M-HN-10 ER JIAN – EAR TIP

⊥ ***0.1 TO 0.2 CUN – vertically, or bleed for conjunctivitis***

Pos: Position of patient: seated or supine.

Loc: a) On the ear.
b) At the tip of the helix of the ear, when the ear is bent forward.
c) Immediately inferior to TH 20.

M-HN-13 YI MING – SHIELDING BRIGHTNESS

⊥ ***0.5 CUN – vertically***

Pos: Position of patient: supine.

Loc: a) On the neck.
b) Posterior to the ear lobe.
c) 1 cun posterior to TH 17.

M-HN-14 BI TONG – NOSE PASSAGE

⊥ ***0.3 CUN – slanting either upwards or downwards***

Pos: Position of patient: seated or supine.

Loc: a) On the face.
b) On the inferior border of the nasal bone.
c) At the superior end of the nasolabial sulcus or groove.
d) Superior to LI 20.

M-HN-37 HAI QUAN – SEA'S SPRING

⊥ ***0.2 CUN – needs to be slightly bled***

- SUN SI-MIAO GHOST (Gui) – Ghost Point Name: Gui Feng – Ghost Seal or Ghost's in the Enclosed Territory

Pos: Position of patient: seated or supine.

Loc: a) On the face.
b) In the mouth.
c) On the underside of the body of the tongue.
d) In the centre of the frenulum.

M-HN-41 JING BI – NECK AND ARM

⊥ ***0.5 TO O.8 CUN – vertically (caution: do <u>not</u> needle downwards towards the apex of the lung)***

Pos: Position of patient: seated or supine.

Loc: a) On the base of the neck.
b) At the posterior margin of the sternocleidomastoid muscle.
c) 1 cun superior tothe clavicle.
d) One third of the distance from the medial end of the clavicle to its lateral end.

N = New point; HN = Head/Neck

N-HN-8 TING XUE – HEARING ORIFICE

⊥ ***0.3 TO 0.5 CUN – vertical, with the mouth slightly open***

Pos: Position of patient: seated or supine with the mouth slightly open.

Loc: a) On the lateral aspect of the face.
b) Anterior to the ear.
c) On the posterior border of the condyle of the mandible bone.
d) Between the middle of the tragus and the intertragic incisure of the ear.
e) Midway between SI 19 and GB 2.

N-HN-9 TING LING – HEARING'S INSPIRATION

⊥ ***0.5 CUN – vertical, with the mouth slightly open***

Pos: Position of patient: seated or supine with the mouth slightly open.

Loc: a) On the lateral aspect of the face.
b) Anterior to the ear.
c) On the posterior border of the condyle of the mandible bone.
d) Between the middle of the tragus and the intertragic incisure of the ear.
e) Between SI 19 and GB 2.
f) 3/4 of the distance from SI 19 to GB 2 (therefore closer to GB 2).
g) Midway between N-HN-8 (Ting Xue) and GB 2.

N-HN-22 (a) AN MIAN 1 – PEACEFUL SLEEP 1

⊥ ***0.5 CUN – vertically***

Pos: Position of patient: supine.

Loc: a) On the neck.
b) Posterior to the ear lobe.
c) Midway between M-HN-13 – Yi Ming (1 cun posterior to TH 17) and TH 17.

N-HN-22 (b) AN MIAN 2 – PEACEFUL SLEEP 2

⊥ ***0.5 CUN – vertically***

Pos: Position of patient: supine.

Loc: a) On the neck.
b) Posterior to the ear lobe.
c) Midway between M-HN-13 – Yi Ming (1 cun posterior to TH 17) and GB 20.

N-HN-54 AN MIAN – PEACEFUL SLEEP

⊥ ***0.3 TO 0.5 CUN – vertically***

Pos: Position of patient: supine.

Loc: a) On the neck.
b) Posterior to the ear lobe.
c) On the prominence of the insertion of the tendon of the sternocleidomastoid muscle.
d) Midway between GB 20 and TH 17.

M = Miscellaneous point; CA = Chest/Abdomen

M-CA-18 ZI GONG – PALACE OF THE CHILD (UTERUS)

⊥ ***0.5 TO 0.8 CUN – vertical*** Δ ***highly recommended***

Pos: Position of patient: supine.

Loc: a) On the anterior aspect of the torso.
b) On the lower abdomen (in the lower jiao).
c) 3 cun lateral to the anterior median line.
d) Level with Ren 3.
e) 4 cun inferior to the level of the centre of the umbilicus.
f) 1 cun superior to the superior border of the symphysis pubis.

M-CA-23 SAN JIAO JIU – TRIANGLE MOXIBUSTION

Δ *ONLY*

Pos: Position of patient: supine.

Loc: a) On the anterior aspect of the torso.
b) On the lower-abdomen (in the lower jiao).
c) An equilateral triangle using the navel as the apex.
d) Each side of the equilateral triangle is approximately 3 cun in length.
e) These three points are located at each corner of the equilateral triangle.
f) The two points located at each end of the base line of the equilateral triangle are called "N-CA-12 – TI TUO XUE – LIFT AND SUPPORT ORIFICE". When you include Ren 8 as the third point these two points become M-CA-23.

N = New point; CA = Chest/Abdomen

N-CA-1 SHUI SHANG – ABOVE WATER

⊥ ***1.0 TO 1.5 CUN – straight insertion***

Pos: Position of patient: supine.

Loc: a) On the anterior aspect of the torso.
b) On the mid-abdomen (in the middle jiao).
c) On the anterior median line.
d) 1.5 cun superior to the level of the centre of the umbilicus.
e) 6.5 cun inferior to the level of the xiphisternal joint.
f) Midway between Ren 9 and Ren 10.

N-CA-3 ZHI XIE – STOP DIARRHOEA

⊥ ***1.0 TO 1.5 CUN – straight insertion***

Pos: Position of patient: supine.

Loc:
a) On the anterior aspect of the torso
b) On the lower abdomen (in the lower jiao).
c) On the anterior median line.
d) Midway between Ren 4 and Ren 5.
e) Approximately halfway between the superior border of the symphysis pubis and the level of the centre of the umbilicus.
f) 2.5 cun superior to the superior border of the symphysis pubis.
g) 2.5 cun inferior to the level of the centre of the umbilicus.

N-CA-4 TI TUO XUE – LIFT AND SUPPORT ORIFICE

⊥ ***0.5 TO 0.8 CUN – vertically***

Pos: Position of patient: supine.

Loc:
a) On the anterior aspect of the torso.
b) On the lower abdomen (in the lower jiao).
c) 4 cun lateral to the anterior median line.
d) Level with Ren 4.
e) 2 cun superior to the superior border of the symphysis pubis.
f) 3 cun inferior to the level of the centre of the umbilicus.

N-CA-5 CHONG JIAN – POUR BETWEEN

⊥ ***0.5 TO 1.0 CUN – vertically***

Pos: Position of patient: supine.

Loc:
a) On the anterior aspect of the torso.
b) On the lower abdomen (in the lower jiao).
c) 3 cun lateral to the anterior median line.
d) Level with Ren 2.
e) Level with the superior border of the symphysis pubis.
f) 5 cun inferior to the level of the centre of the umbilicus.

N-CA-6 SHU XI – MOUSE PATH

⊥ ***0.5 TO 0.8 CUN – vertically***

Pos: Position of patient: supine.

Loc:
a) On the anterior aspect of the torso.
b) On the lower abdomen (in the lower jiao).
c) Between 5 and 6 cun lateral to the anterior median line.
d) Level with Ren 3.
e) 1 cun superior to the superior border of the symphysis pubis.
f) 4 cun inferior to the level of the centre of the umbilicus.

N-CA-12 XING QI XUE – NEW QI ORIFICE

⊥ ***0.5 TO 0.8 CUN – vertically***

Pos: Position of patient: supine.

Loc:
a) On the anterior aspect of the torso.
b) On the lower abdomen (in the lower jiao).
c) An equilateral triangle using the navel as the apex.
d) Each side of the equilateral triangle is 3 cun in length.
e) The points are located at each end of the base line of the equilateral triangle.

M = Miscellaneous point; UE = Upper Extremity (Upper Limb)

M-UE-1 SHI XUAN – TEN SPREADINGS
very shallow or bleeding

Pos: Position of patient: supine, in the anatomical position (arms at the side and flat on the couch with the palms facing upwards).

Loc:
a) Ten points, five on each hand.
b) At the tip of each digit.
c) Approximately 0.1 cun distance from the nail.

M-UE-9 SI FENG – FOUR SEAMS

prick to draw a small amount of serum (yellow/white in colour)

Pos: Position of patient: supine, in the anatomical position (arms at the side and flat on the couch with the palms facing upwards) with the fingers in a relaxed position.

Loc:
a) Eight points, four on each hand.
b) On the palmar surface of the four fingers (not the thumb).
c) In the joint between the intermediate (middle) phalanges and the proximal phalanges of each finger.
d) At the centre of each proximal crease formed at the joint between the intermediate (middle) phalanges and the proximal phalanges.

M-UE-19 YAO TONG XUE -LOW BACK PAIN (also known as YAO TONG DIAN – LUMBAR PAIN POINT)

⊥ ***0.5 TO 1.0 CUN – perpendicular***

Pos: Position of patient: supine with the forearm fully pronated.

Loc:
a) Four points, two on each hand.
b) On the posterior surface of the hand.
c) Two points between and just distal to the flares of the bases of the second and third metacarpal bones.
d) Other two points between and just distal to the flares of the bases of the fourth and fifth metacarpal bones.

M-UE-22 BA XIE – EIGHT EVILS

⊥ ***0.5 TO 1.0 CUN – with the hand in a clenched fist insert between and along the heads of the metacarpals***

Pos: Position of patient: supine, in the anatomical position (arms at the side and flat on the couch with the palms facing upwards) with the hands in a clenched fist.

Loc:
a) On the posterior surface of the hand.
b) Four points on each hand, proximal to the web margin between the head of each metacarpal bone.
c) In the deepest part of the valley formed between each metacarpophalangeal joint.

M-UE-24 LUO ZHEN – STIFF NECK

⊥ ***0.5 TO 1.0 CUN – with the hand in a clenched fist insert between and along the heads of the metacarpals***

Pos: Position of patient: supine with the hands in a clenched fist.

Loc: a) On the posterior surface of the hand.
b) Between the heads of the second and third metacarpal bones.
c) Proximal to the flares of the heads of the second and third metacarpal bones.
d) Proximal to the second and third metacarpo-phalangeal joints.
e) Level with TH 3.

M-UE-29 ER BAI – TWO WHITES

⊥ ***0.5 CUN Δ recommended (especially combined with Δ on Du 1 and Du 20)***

Pos: Position of patient: supine.

Loc: a) On the anterior surface of the forearm.
b) Between the ulna and radius bones.
c) Two points, one just lateral and the other just medial to the tendon of the flexor carpi radialis muscle.
d) 4 cun proximal to the flexure of the wrist at Pc 7.

M-UE-33 ZHONG QUAN – MIDDLE SPRING

⊥ ***0.3 TO 0.5 CUN – vertically***

Pos: Position of patient: supine.

Loc: a) On the anterior surface of the forearm.
b) Between the ulna and radius bones.
c) Two points: one just lateral and the other just medial to the tendon of the flexor carpi radialis muscle.
d) 4 cun proximal to the flexure of the wrist at Pc 7.

M-UE-48 JIAN NEI LING – INNER SHOULDER MOUND (JIAN QIAN – FRONT OF THE SHOULDER)

⊥ ***0.5 TO 1.0 CUN – vertically towards the back of the shoulder***

Pos: Position of patient: supine or seated.

Loc:
a) On the anterior aspect of the shoulder.
b) On the anterior surface of the deltoid muscle.
c) Midway between LI 15 and the superior border of the anterior axillary crease (with the arm hanging at the side).

N = New point; UE = Upper Extremity (Upper Limb)

N-UE-1 YA TONG – TOOTHACHE

⊥ ***0.3 CUN – vertically***

Pos: Position of patient: supine, in the anatomical position (arms at the side and flat on the couch with the palms facing upwards).

Loc:
a) On the palmar surface of the hand.
b) Between the third and fourth metacarpal bones.
c) Approximately 1 cun proximal to the metacarpophalangeal crease.
d) Distal to the proximal transverse crease (or the "headline" of the hand)

N-UE-19 YAO TONG 1, 2, 3 -LOW BACK PAIN 1, 2, 3

⊥ ***UP TO 1.0 CUN – slanted towards the wrist***

Pos: Position of patient: supine with the forearm fully pronated.

Loc:
a) Six points, three on each hand.
b) On the posterior surface of the hand.
c) Three points between and just distal to the flares of the bases of the second and third (YAO TONG 1), third and fourth (YAO TONG 2) and fourth and fifth (YAO TONG 3) metacarpal bones.
d) YAO TONG 1 and 3 are known points – M-UE-19 YAO TONG XUE

M = Miscellaneous point; LE = Lower Extremity (Lower Limb)

M-LE-8 BA FENG – EIGHT WINDS

⊥ ***0.5 CUN – angled towards St 42***

Pos: Position of patient: supine.

Loc: a) Eight points, four on each foot.
b) On the dorsal aspect of the foot.
c) Between the toes.
d) Proximal to each web margin.
e) Three of the four points are known channel points: Liv 2, St 44 and GB 43.
f) The fourth point is between the third and fourth digits, distal to the metatarso-phalangeal joints and just distal to the flare of the base of the proximal phalanx of the third and fourth digits.
g) Liv 2 is between the first and second digits, distal to the metatarso-phalangeal joints and just distal to the flare of the base of the proximal phalanx of the first and second and digits. St 44 is between the second and third digits, distal to the metatarso-phalangeal joints and just distal to the flare of the base of the proximal phalanx of the second and third and digits. GB 43 is between the fourth and fifth digits, distal to the metatarso-phalangeal joints and just distal to the flare of the base of the proximal phalanx of the fourth and fifth digits.

M-LE-13 LAN WEI XUE – APPENDIX ORIFICE

⊥ ***0.8 TO 1.0 CUN – vertically***

Pos: Position of patient: supine.

Loc: a) On the RIGHT leg only.
b) On the anterolateral aspect of the lower leg.
c) Lateral to the anterior crest of the tibia bone.
d) On the medial border of the tibialis anterior muscle.
c) Approximately 2 cun inferior to St 36 (which is inferior to the inferior border of the tibial tuberosity of the tibia bone.
e) Approximately 11 cun proximal to the prominence of the lateral malleolus (St 36 is approximately 13 cun proximal to the prominence of the lateral malleolus).
f) Gently but firmly palpate for a tender spot.

M-LE-16 XI YAN – EYES OF THE KNEE

⊥ ***0.5 TO 1.0 CUN – with the knee semiflexed***

Pos: Position of patient: supine with the knee semiflexed.

Loc: a) Four points, two on each leg.
b) At the inferior corners of the patella (inferolateral and inferomedial corners).
c) In a depression (*men*) on the lateral and medial borders of the patellar ligament.
d) The lateral point is a known point, St 35 (DU BI – CALF NOSE).

M-LE-23 DAN NANG XUE – GALLBLADDER ORIFICE

⊥ ***0.8 TO 1.0 CUN – vertically***

Pos: Position of patient: supine with the leg semi flexed.

Loc: a) On the RIGHT leg only.
b) On the lateral aspect of the lower leg.
c) Inferior and anterior to the head of the fibula.
d) 13 to 14 cun proximal to the prominence of the lateral malleolus.
e) 1 to 2 cun distal to GB 34 (or 1 to 2 cun inferior and anterior to the head of the fibula).
f) Between the muscles of the peroneus longus and extensor digitorum longus.
g) Gently but firmly palpate for a tender spot.

M-LE-27 HE DING – CRANE'S TOP

⊥ ***0.5 CUN – vertically with the knee bent***

Pos: Position of patient: supine with the knee flexed.

Loc: a) On the leg.
c) On the anterior midline of the leg.
b) On the anterior aspect of the knee.
d) On the superior border of the patella.
e) Also known as the "top point of Bachman Knee Points".

N = New point; LE = Lower Extremity (Lower Limb)

N-LE-4 NAO QUING – BRAIN'S CLEARING

⊥ ***0.5 CUN – vertically***

Pos: Position of patient: supine.

Loc: a) On the anterior aspect of the lower limb.
b) On the lateral border of the tibia.
c) Approximately 1.5 cun (or 2 finger widths) proximal to St 41(which is at the anterior aspect of the flexure of the ankle and between the tendons of the extensor digitorum longus and extensor hallucis longus muscles).